HANDBOOK OF
Nutrition in the Aged
Third Edition

CRC SERIES IN MODERN NUTRITION
Edited by Ira Wolinsky and James F. Hickson, Jr.

Published Titles

Manganese in Health and Disease, Dorothy J. Klimis-Tavantzis

Nutrition and AIDS: Effects and Treatments, Ronald R. Watson

Nutrition Care for HIV-Positive Persons: A Manual for Individuals and Their Caregivers, Saroj M. Bahl and James F. Hickson, Jr.

Calcium and Phosphorus in Health and Disease, John J.B. Anderson and Sanford C. Garner

Edited by Ira Wolinsky

Published Titles

Handbook of Nutrition in the Aged, Ronald R. Watson

Practical Handbook of Nutrition in Clinical Practice, Donald F. Kirby and Stanley J. Dudrick

Handbook of Dairy Foods and Nutrition, Gregory D. Miller, Judith K. Jarvis, and Lois D. McBean

Advanced Nutrition: Macronutrients, Carolyn D. Berdanier

Childhood Nutrition, Fima Lifschitz

Nutrition and Health: Topics and Controversies, Felix Bronner

Nutrition and Cancer Prevention, Ronald R. Watson and Siraj I. Mufti

Nutritional Concerns of Women, Ira Wolinsky and Dorothy J. Klimis-Tavantzis

Nutrients and Gene Expression: Clinical Aspects, Carolyn D. Berdanier

Antioxidants and Disease Prevention, Harinda S. Garewal

Advanced Nutrition: Micronutrients, Carolyn D. Berdanier

Nutrition and Women's Cancers, Barbara Pence and Dale M. Dunn

Nutrients and Foods in AIDS, Ronald R. Watson

Nutrition: Chemistry and Biology, Second Edition, Julian E. Spallholz, L. Mallory Boylan, and Judy A. Driskell

Melatonin in the Promotion of Health, Ronald R. Watson

Nutritional and Environmental Influences on the Eye, Allen Taylor

Laboratory Tests for the Assessment of Nutritional Status, Second Edition, H.E. Sauberlich

Advanced Human Nutrition, Robert E.C. Wildman and Denis M. Medeiros

Handbook of Dairy Foods and Nutrition, Second Edition, Gregory D. Miller, Judith K. Jarvis, and Lois D. McBean

Nutrition in Space Flight and Weightlessness Models, Helen W. Lane and Dale A. Schoeller

Forthcoming Titles

Eating Disorders in Women and Children: Prevention, Stress Management, and Treatment, Jacalyn J. Robert

Childhood Obesity: Prevention and Treatment, Jana Parizkova and Andrew Hills

Alcohol and Substance Abuse in the Aging, Ronald R. Watson

Nutritional Anemias, Usha Ramakrishnan

Advances in Isotope Methods for the Analysis of Trace Elements in Man, Malcolm Jackson and Nicola Lowe

Handbook of Nutrition for Vegetarians, Joan Sabate and Rosemary A. Ratzin-Tuner

Tryptophan: Biochemicals and Health Implications, Herschel Sidransky

Handbook of Nutraceuticals and Functional Foods, Robert E. C. Wildman

The Mediterranean Diet, Antonia L. Matalas, Antonios Zampelas, Vasilis Stavrinos, and Ira Wolinsky

Handbook of Nutrition and the Aged, Third Edition, Ronald R. Watson

Handbook of Nutraceuticals and Nutritional Supplements and Pharmaceuticals, Robert E. C. Wildman

Inulin and Oligofructose: Functional Food Ingredients, Marcel B. Roberfroid

Micronutrients and HIV Infection, Henrik Friis

Vegetables, Fruits, and Herbs in Health Promotion, Ronald R. Watson

Nutrition and AIDS, 2nd Edition, Ronald R. Watson

Nutrition Gene Interactions in Health and Disease, Niama M. Moussa and Carolyn D. Berdanier

HANDBOOK OF
Nutrition in the Aged
Third Edition

Edited by
Ronald R. Watson

CRC Press
Boca Raton   London   New York   Washington, D.C.

Library of Congress Cataloging-in-Publication Data

Handbook of nutrition in the aged / edited by Ronald R. Watson. --3rd ed.
    p.   cm. (Modern Nutrition)
Includes bibliographical references and index.
ISBN 0-8493-2228-6 (alk. paper)
    1. Aging--Nutritional aspects--Handbooks, manuals, etc. 2.
Aged--Nutrition--Handbooks, manuals, etc. 3. Nutrition disorders in the aged--Handbooks,
manuals, etc. I. Watson, Ronald R. (Ronald Ross) II. Modern nutrition (Boca Raton, Fla.
QP86 .C7 2000
613.2′084′6—dc21   00-034233
                                                                                     CIP

© 2001 by CRC Press LLC

No claim to original U.S. Government works
International Standard Book Number 0-8493-2228-6
Library of Congress Card Number 00-034233
Printed in the United States of America 1 2 3 4 5 6 7 8 9 0
Printed on acid-free paper

Series Preface for Modern Nutrition

The CRC Series in Modern Nutrition is dedicated to providing the widest possible coverage of topics in nutrition. Nutrition is an interdisciplinary, interprofessional field par excellence. It is noted by its broad range and diversity. We trust the titles and authorship in this series will reflect that range and diversity.

Published for a scholarly audience, the volumes in the CRC Series in Modern Nutrition are designed to explain, review, and explore present knowledge and recent trends, developments, and advances in nutrition. As such, they will also appeal to the educated layman. The format for the series will vary with the needs of the author and the topic, including, but not limited to, edited volumes, monographs, handbooks, and texts.

Contributors from any bona fide area of nutrition, including the controversial, are welcome.

We welcome the contribution *Handbook of Nutrition in the Aged, Third Edition*, edited by my ever-productive colleague Ronald R. Watson. Scientific interest in aging, especially nutritional aspects, continues unabated. I am sure this volume will make a scholarly contribution to the field, as have the prior two very worthy editions.

Ira Wolinsky, Ph.D.
University of Houston
Series Editor

Preface

As we age, lower levels of physical activity and food consumption accentuate changes associated with aging. Lower levels of income and finances substantially reduce nutritional state and ability to maintain health via adequate nutrition. Therefore, the main focus of this book is understanding the role of nutrition, as well as supplementation and undernutrition, in health in the elderly. Intuitively and scientifically, adequate diet and thus nutrition, education, and nutritional supplementation should improve the amount and quality of life in seniors.

Undernutrition and very low food intake, leading sometimes to malnutrition and starvation, are significant problems of seniors, especially when institutionalized. Therefore, the needs of the elderly, which differ from those of young adults and growing children, are defined for key nutrients. In addition, support mechanisms and ways to provide improved dietary intake in the institutionalized are described and evaluated. Assessment of nutritional status in the elderly presents special problems.

The association of diet and hypertension in seniors is important to increasing longevity, as are other nutritional problems including undernutrition. The aging adult offers a number of nutritional challenges, such as determining which nutrients or combination will promote health and how they affect cell structure and function. Nutritional support for surgery patients or those with anorexia are special needs of seniors, not just healthy young adults. Cells in older people have altered nutritional needs and biochemical activities, including protein turnover. Key systems that protect the individual, such as immune defenses, decline with age even under adequate nutrition. Therefore, knowledge of the changing composition of the body, its needs for micro- and macronutrients, and its nutritional state facilitates care and survival of older people. The overall focus of this book is on the role of altered nutritional intake and needs in health promotion in older people.

About the Editor

Ronald R. Watson, Ph.D., has edited 50 books, including three books on aging. He worked for 20 years on research relating to nutrition and its role in moderating aging and immunosenescence.

Dr. Watson attended the University of Idaho but graduated from Brigham Young University in Provo, Utah with a degree in chemistry in 1966. He completed his Ph.D. degree in 1971 in biochemistry at Michigan State University. His postdoctoral schooling was completed at the Harvard School of Public Health in nutrition and microbiology, including a 2-year postdoctoral research experience in immunology. He was an assistant professor of immunology and did research at the University of Mississippi Medical Center in Jackson from 1973 to 1974. He was an assistant professor of microbiology and immunology at the Indiana University Medical School from 1974 to 1978 and an associate professor at Purdue University in the Department of Food and Nutrition from 1978 to 1982. In 1982, he joined the faculty at the University of Arizona in the Department of Family and Community Medicine. He is also a research professor in the University of Arizona's newly formed College of Public Health. He has published 450 research papers and review chapters. Dr. Watson initiated and directed the Specialized Alcohol Research Center at the University of Arizona College of Medicine for 6 years.

Dr. Watson is a member of several national and international nutrition, immunology, and cancer research societies. He has directed a program studying ways to slow aging, funded by Wallace Genetics Foundation, for 22 years. He is also currently studying the role of nutrition and antioxidants to moderate heart disease in a model of aging.

Contributors

Hemmi N. Bhagavan, Ph.D., FACN
Lancaster, PA
Hemmin@msn.com

Meredith C. Bogert, D.M.D.
Department of Restorative Dentistry
Temple University School of Dentistry
Philadelphia, PA

Wayne W. Campbell, Ph.D.
Assistant Professor
Department of Foods and Nutrition
Purdue University
West Lafayette, IN

Marvin Cohen, Ph.D.
Hoffmann-La Roche, Inc.
Nutley, NJ
Marvin.cohen@roche.com

Cyrus Cooper, Ph.D.
MRC Environmental
Epidemiology Unit
University of Southampton
Southampton General Hospital
Southampton, U.K.

Francisco Jose Hidalgo Correas, Ph.D.
Servicio de Farmacia
Hospital Severo Ochoa
Madrid, Spain
fhidalgo@hsvo.insalud.es

Debashish Kumar Dey, Ph.D.
Department of Geriatric Medicine
Vasa Hospital
Göteborg University
Gothenburg, Sweden
debashish.dey@geriatrik.gu.se

Adam Drewnowski Ph.D.
Nutritional Sciences program
Department of Epidemiology
School of Public Health and Community
  Medicine
University of Washington
Seattle, WA
adamdrew@u.washington.edu

P. Ghugre, Ph.D
Department of Food Science and Nutrition
S.N.D.T. Women's University
Mumbai, India

Mark Haub, Ph.D.
Nutrition, Metabolism, and Exercise Laboratory
Department of Geriatrics
University of Arkansas for
  Medical Sciences
Little Rock, AR
haubmarkd@exchange.uam.edu

Charles K. Herman, M.D.
Department of Plastic and Reconstructive
  Surgery
Montefiore Medical Center
Albert Einstein College of Medicine
Bronx, NY
charleshermanmd@hotmail.com

H. Hoskote, Ph.D
Department of Food Science and Nutrition
S.N.D.T. Women's University
Mumbai, India

Adele Huls, Ph.D., RD
Professional Nutrition & Health
  Care Services
Chadron, NE
ahuls@prairieweb.com

Katsumi Kano, Ph.D.
Department of Epidemiology
Graduate School of MedicineUniversity of
  Tsukuba
Ibaraki-ken, Japan
kano@md.tsukuba.ac.jp

M. Keelan, Ph.D.
Department of Medicine
Division of Gastroenterology
University of Alberta
Edmonton, Alberta
Canada
Alan.thomson@ualberta.ca

K. Kenjle, Ph.D.
Department of Food Science and Nutrition
S.N.D.T. Women's University
Mumbai, India

Evan W. Kligman, M.D.
Longevity Medicine
Tucson, AZ
Agewell100@aol.com
Cazadoro568@aol.com

U. Beate Krinke, Ph.D.
Public Health Nutrition
University of Minnesota
Div. of Epidemiology
Minneapolis MN
Krinke@epi.umn.edu

Bruno M. Lesourd, M.D., Ph.D.
Head of Geriatric Nutrition Unit
Hôpital Charles Foix
Ivry-sur-Seine, France
Bruno.lesourd@cfx.ap-hop-paris.fr

Roger B. McDonald, Ph.D.
Department of Nutrition
University of California, Davis
Davis, CA
Rbmcdonald@ucdavis.edu

Federico Mecchia, Ph.D.
Department of Internal Medicine and
  Gastroenterology
University of Bologna
S. Orsola Hospital
Bologna, Italy

Waithira Mirie, Ph.D.
University of Nairobi
Faculty of Medicine
Dept. of Nursing Science
Nairobi, Kenya
mirierw@hotmail.com

Marthe J. Moseley, Ph.D., RN, CCRN, CCNS
Clinical Nurse Specialist, Critical Care
South Texas Veterans
  Health Care System
Audie L. Murphy Memorial Division
San Antonio, TX
Marthe.Moseley@med.va.gov

Loris Pironi, M.D.
Department of Internal Medicine and
  Gastroenterology
University of Bologna
S. Orsola Hospital
Bologna, Italy
pironi@med.unibo.it

Arlan Richardson
Department of Physiology
University of Texas
  Health Science Center
San Antonio, TX
richardsona@uthscsa.edu

Enrico Ruggeri, Ph.D.
Department of Internal Medicine and
  Gastroenterology
University of Bologna
S. Orsola Hospital
Bologna, Italy

Rodney C. Ruhe, Ph.D.
Department of Nutrition
University of California, Davis
Davis, CA

Carlene Russell, MS, RD, FADA
Mason City, IA
carlene@netconx.net

Avan Aihie Sayer, Ph.D.
MRC Environmental
Epidemiology Unit
University of Southampton
Southampton General Hospital
Southampton, U.K.
Aas@mrc.soton.ac.uk

Bertil Steen, Ph.D.
Department of Geriatric Medicine
Vasa Hospital
Göteborg University
Gothenburg, Sweden
bertil.steen@geriatrik.gu.se

William A. Stini, Ph.D.
Department of Anthropology
University of Arizona
Tucson, AZ
stini@u.arizona.edu

Thomas M. Stulnig, M.D.
Department of Internal Medicine III
University of Vienna
Vienna, Austria
Thomas.stulnig@akh-wien.ac.at

A.B.R. Thomson, Ph.D.
Department of Medicine
Division of Gastroenterology
University of Alberta
Edmonton, Alberta
Canada

Satoshi Toyokawa, Ph.D.
Department of Epidemiology
Graduate School of Medicine
University of Tsukuba
Ibaraki-ken, Japan
toyokawa@hotmail.com

S.A. Udipi, Ph.D
Department of Food Science and Nutrition
S.N.D.T. Women's University
Mumbai, India

Teresa Bermejo Vicedo, Ph.D.
Servicio de Farmacia
Hospital Severo Ochoa
Madrid, Spain
Tbermejo@hsvo.insalud.es

Walter Ward
Department of Physiology
University of Texas Health
  Science Center
San Antonio, TX

Victoria Warren-Mears, Ph.D.
Department of Nutrition and Food Services
Harborview Medical Center
Seattle, WA
victoria_warren@email.msn.com

Sheldon Winkler, D.D.S.
Department of Restorative Dentistry
Temple University School of Dentistry
Philadelphia, PA
Swinkdent@aol.com

M. Anne Woodtli, Ph.D.
College of Nursing
University of Arizona
Tucson, AZ
Awoodtli@nursing.arizona.edu

Hunter Yost, M.D.
Functional Medicine
Tucson, AZ
Agewell100@aol.com
Cazadoro568@aol.com

Acknowledgments

Appreciation is expressed to Jessica Stant, editorial assistant, for multiple efforts in the preparation of this volume, which included working with contributors for a year and preparing its index. Dr. Watson's research on prevention of aging using nutrients has been graciously supported by the Wallace Genetics Foundation, Inc. for 22 years. The resulting research stimulated this series of books.

Contents

III Mechanistic Studies of Nutrition and Health in the Elderly

IV Nutritional Therapies and Promotion of Health

Section I

Nutritional Supplementation
and Health

1 Nutrition and Electrolytes in the Elderly

Marthe J. Moseley

CONTENTS

Nutrition plays a pivotal role in health promotion, disease prevention, and chronic disease management. The normal physiologic changes of aging place the elder at risk for potential complications regarding altered nutritional state and electrolyte imbalance. The most important principle in limiting the possibility of complications at any time throughout the age span is prevention.

I. INTRODUCTION

The population of older persons has risen dramatically and will continue to grow rapidly throughout the world. In 1990, more than 31 million Americans were over the age of 65; by 2040 this number will exceed 75 million (1). One of the major reasons for increased life expectancy and longevity includes increased emphasis on health promotion and disease prevention (2). Although longevity has increased, whether the added years of life are filled with health and vigor or chronic disease and limited functional status or disability is unknown (1).

There is a trend toward increased life expectancy in the aged, yet chronic conditions are prevalent and influence older people's ability to maintain their functional state (3). Good health is the key factor in maintaining an independent and productive life in the elderly. The expected outcome of good health reaches beyond longevity to the goal of an acceptable quality of life, without debilitating disabilities. For those with chronic illness, optimizing functional status is cornerstone in preventing a downward functional decline (4).

II. BACKGROUND

Dietary and nutritional factors underlie many elements that contribute to health disparities in elders (5). In the past, national health care expenditures have totaled more than $666 billion, for which

30% are associated with inappropriate diet (6). Those at risk for diminished quality of life and functional status due to the effects of an altered nutrition intake include individuals who have chronic disease conditions (6). Presence of nutrition risk factors may extend into chronic disability (7). Some data indicate that many of the continued health problems associated with the elderly are preventable through dietary intervention (8).

Inappropriate dietary intake is associated with 5 of the 10 leading causes of death in the U.S.: coronary artery disease, certain cancers, stroke, diabetes mellitus (noninsulin-dependent), and atherosclerosis (9,10). Many of the health problems associated with the elderly are preventable or controllable through dietary changes (9–11).

III. IMPORTANCE OF ADEQUATE NUTRITION

Adequate nutritional status has been recognized as an important factor in the prevention and treatment of chronic disease (12). The elderly are particularly prone to inadequate nutritional status because of age-related physiologic (13,14) and social changes, development of chronic diseases (15), use of medications (16–18), and decreased mobility (19,20). These factors may lead to subclinical malnutrition, which is not easy to recognize or separate from changes resulting from the aging process itself. If undetected, subclinical malnutrition among older people may result in more rapid deterioration of health and early death.

Factors affecting nutritional status are multidimensional and interrelated. For older adults, age-related changes in body function (gastrointestinal changes) (21,22), lifestyle, medication use (23,24), and the prevalence of chronic disease challenge maintenance of good nutrition. Psycho-social factors including income (25), social interactions, and access to transportation all can affect the client's nutritional state (26,27). Measures to promote good nutrition must specifically address the interrelated and multifactoral factors that affect nutritional status.

Nutrition plays a pivotal role in health promotion (28), disease prevention, chronic and disease management (29,30). Older Americans experience a variety of nutritional problems related to changes associated with aging. These changes are related to social, environmental, economic and physical alterations (17,31–33). Major physiologic changes that occur comprise a decrease in total body protein, a reduction in total body water, a loss in bone density, and an increase in the proportion of total body fat with a redistribution of fat stores (29). Cumulatively, these changes place a substantial number of elderly at high risk for poor nutrition status (28,34,35).

More specifically, many elderly patients requiring hospitalization show signs of malnutrition on admission or develop malnutrition during hospitalization (36–39). Malnutrition from any cause impacts on the recovery and rehabilitation after surgery and is not limited to protein-calorie deficiency but also low intakes of iron, vitamins, and minerals (29,38). Management of periop-erative care in geriatric patients is typically more complex than in younger patients, due to changes associated with advancing age (40). One in four elderly suffer from malnutrition, which is costly in the surgical patient because it leads to impaired immune system, poor wound healing, infections, complications, multi-system organ failure, prolonged hospitalizations, catastrophic costs, and death (29,40–44). Factors that are critical for obtaining the best outcomes from surgical treatment of elderly patients include avoidance of disturbances in nutritional and electrolyte status (40).

Immune response, typically a protective pattern, is impaired in old age, resulting in an augmented risk of infection (29,40,45). Nutrition is a significant determinant of immunocom-petence. Functional adaptations include decreased lymphocyte proliferation, reduced production of interleukin-2, impaired mixed lymphocyte reaction, and decreased natural killer cell activity (45–48).

IV. DETECTION OF NUTRITIONAL RISK

The DETERMINE your nutritional health checklist (Figure 1.1) completed during an assessment phase may detect high nutritional risk (36,49). The elderly can complete this form during an annual checkup in a primary care clinic, upon admission to the hospital or during the pre-admission work-up (50). The checklist depicts a series of warning signs of poor nutritional status for elder Americans. A foundation for further assessment and intervention is also provided. Elders with higher checklist scores are more likely to have the poorest levels of nutrient intake and increased threat of adverse health risks (35). The checklist, developed by the Nutrition Screening Initiative, can be used by a wide range of social service and health care professionals (18). Specifically, the Level II Screen helps to distinguish those individuals with nutritional problems that can have a profound impact upon nutritional health for the hospitalized elder. A thorough history and physical examination, including use of the Level II Screen alerts the health care provider of abnormal values, including anthropometric measurements and laboratory data; drug use, including use of over-the-counter medications; and clinical features including eating habits, living environment, functional status and mental/cognitive status issues affecting nutritional status in the elder (18,51).

THE DETERMINE YOUR NUTRITIONAL HEALTH CHECKLIST.

The warning signs of poor nutritional health are often overlooked. Use this checklist to find out if you or someone you know is at risk.

Read the statements below. Circle the number in the yes column for those that apply to you or someone you know. For each yes answer, score the number in the box. Total your nutritional score.

	YES
I have an illness or condition that made me change the kind and/or amount of food I eat.	2
I eat fewer than 2 meals per day.	3
I eat few fruits or vegetables, or milk products.	2
I have 3 or more drinks of beer, liquor, or wine almost every day.	2
I have tooth or mouth problems that make it hard for me to eat.	2
I don't always have enough money to buy the food I need.	4
I eat alone most of the time.	1
I take 3 or more different prescribed or over-the-counter drugs a day.	1
Without wanting to, I have lost or gained 10 pounds in the last 6 months.	2
I am not always physically able to shop, cook, and/or feed myself.	2
Total	

FIGURE 1.1 Determine Your Nutritional Health chart. (*Source*: Nutrition Screening Initiative, 1991. *Nutrition Screening Manual for Professionals Caring for Older Americans*. Washington, DC: Green Margolis, Mitchell, Burns and Associates. With permission.)

In those elders who are identified as having a poor nutritional status, screening identifies the need for additional support (28). An outcome of poor nutritional status may lead to functional impairment and disability, which, in turn, may reduce quality of life and increase morbidity and mortality (36,40,53,54).

V. OPTIMAL INTERVENTION

Interventions are taken to improve an elderly individual's nutritional status once a nutrition problem has been identified. Nutritional intervention planning begins with estimating the patient's nutrient balance, for example, nutrient intake vs. nutrient loss. Calorie and protein intake calculated through a diet history is essential in estimating the nutrient intake (49,55). Many times, nutrient loss is predicted as a total of all output excreted from the elder.

Harris and Benedict equation (HB) estimates basal energy expenditure (BEE) through parameters such as gender, age, height, and weight (56). A correction factor is added to the BEE to determine calorie needs conditional on the degree of metabolic stress the elder exhibits. The relationship between resting metabolic rate (RMR) and the HB was explored in a study that suggested that the World Health Organization (WHO) equations appear more precise than the HB equations (57). The FAO/WHO/UNU Expert Group recommendations determined weight to be the most useful and practical index for predicting BEE within a given gender and age range (Table 1.1) (58). The BEE is multiplied by factors that account for energy costs to determine total energy requirement (Table 1.2).

TABLE 1.1
Estimate of BEE (kcal) by Age and Gender

Age Range	Men	Women
18–30	15.3 W + 679	14.7 W + 496
30–60	11.6 W + 879	8.7 W + 829
60+	13.5 W + 487	10.5 W + 596

Note: W = body weight in kilograms

Source: FAO/WHO/UNU. 1985. *Energy and Protein Requirements*. Technical Report Series #724. Geneva, Switzerland: World Health Organization.

TABLE 1.2
Energy Costs of Physical Activity Expressed as Multiples of BEE

Level of Activity	Men	Women
Light work	1.7	1.7
Moderate work	2.7	2.2
Heavy work	3.8	2.8
Residual time (no activity, but awake)	1.4	1.4
Sleeping	1.0	1.0

Source: FAO/WHO/UNU. 1985. *Energy and Protein Requirements*. Technical Report Series #724. Geneva, Switzerland: World Health Organization.

Protein is the main nutrient used as a reference point for determination of the nutritional requirements in the elderly surgical patient (38). It is well known that amino acids are the building blocks of proteins and are essential in the metabolic response to stress (38). Nitrogen balance is used as an index of protein nutritional status (48). Nitrogen is released when amino acids are catabolized and excreted in the urine as urea. Nitrogen balance determination is indicated when an elder is anabolic (positive nitrogen balance) or catabolic (negative nitrogen balance), and is an indication of depletion of the lean body mass. Nitrogen balance is essential and the human body must maintain an adequate supply.

Prospects for achieving positive or even neutral nitrogen balance are unlikely when there is greater stress on an elder (31). The amount of replacement nitrogen to consider to be administered to an elder with a calculated loss is determined by measuring nitrogen lost in urine, feces, and through the skin. Protein requirements can be estimated without actual measurements of nitrogen lost through these body substances. The minimum requirement for the elderly for protein amount to 1 g/kg/day (59). When necessary, protein intake must be increased to fulfill the demand of disease or illness. The requirement for this increase is 1.5 to 2.0 g/kg/day (31,60).

VI. ROUTE SELECTION

If nutritional support is indicated in an elderly person, the most appropriate route must be determined. A nutrition support consultation may be indicated for older individuals who, because of anatomical, physiological or mental health problems, cannot meet their nutritional needs by eating a nutritionally balanced diet. Nutrition support consultation may provide for interventions that include altering usual food intake by modification of nutrient content or optimizing nutrient density or food consistency or form. The goal of nutritional support is to maintain adequate nutritional state, to determine and institute dietary modifications needed for prevention of energy and nutrient deficiencies, and for management of the elder with the most efficient method possible (35).

The enteral route is the preferred route and the optimal route for nutrition administration. The estimation of the nutrient balance accomplished when completing the calorie count might reveal at least 50% ingestion of nutritional needs; supplementation may be sufficient to increase intake to an optimal nutrient level. If, however, less than 50% of nutritional needs are ingested, tube feedings may become a necessity (38,61). Tube feedings can be instigated if gastric output is not more than 600 ml per day on gravity drainage (38). In the hospital or acute care setting the gastric residuals are obtained every 4 hours to determine that the residual does not exceed 50% of the volume infused. At the start of gastric feedings, rates are initially slow to determine tolerance. Increases by 20 to 25 ml/h are completed every day until the patient's nutrient requirements are met (38). Other options for feeding access include nasoenteric tubes or jejunostomies in the compromised elder. It is well known and documented that bowel rest causes intestinal mucosa atrophy with increased permeability to bacteria and endotoxins, thus the phenomenon of bacterial translocation and endotoxemia (31). As a result of this, one may need to consider, for example, that if all nutritional needs cannot be met intestinally, whenever possible, the intestine should be stimulated with some amount of enteral nutrition as a preventive measure (38). A balanced diet administered continuously over 24 hours in the elderly should include an optimally balanced polymeric formula of the three major nutrients — protein, carbohydrates, and lipids (38).

VII. WATER AND ELECTROLYTE BALANCE

Total body water accounts for 60% of body weight in young men and somewhat less in young women. Declining with age, water content reaches 50% and 45% of body weight in men and women over 60 years old, respectively (62). This reduction in body water is associated with the decrease in lean body mass, as water composes 72% of muscle tissue (13).

Age, body size, fluid intake, diet composition, solute load presented for renal excretion, metabolic and respiratory rates, body temperature, and presence and extent of abnormal fluid losses — for example, diarrhea, wound drainage, and fever — in part determine fluid and electrolyte balance (13). The body gains water via the gastrointestinal tract (GI) with additional water produced as a result of oxidation. Oral intake encompasses approximately two-thirds of the intake and usually is in the form of pure water or some other beverage, and the remainder is via ingested food (13). Water is mainly lost through the skin, lungs, GI tract, and kidneys. These fluid losses are coupled with varying losses of electrolytes, which must also be replaced.

The kidneys primarily regulate homeostasis, the maintenance of body fluids. There is a progressive decrease in kidney function, in particular the glomerular filtration rate (GFR), as a result of aging (63). The reduction in GFR is equivalent to the decline in muscle mass explanatory of the normal creatinine associated with aging (63).

Cardiac output (CO) in part determines renal blood flow and GFR. Thus, any alteration in CO, such as hypothermia, that results in a decrease in CO will result in a reduced renal blood flow and GFR (63). Acute renal failure (ARF) is one indicator for increased mortality in the elder patient. The characteristics of ARF are a rise in the blood urea nitrogen (BUN) and creatinine, with or without oliguria. In the elder patient, an immediate evaluation of the cause of increased BUN or creatinine to correct or remove reversible factors is required.

VIII. PREVENTIVE INTERVENTION

Prevention is the most practical approach to fluid and electrolyte balance in the elderly. Although the recommended amount of water ingested is not different for adults across the lifespan, the elder is prone to an inadequate water intake, with dehydration manifesting as the most common disturbance (60).

The elderly in general are less able to restore and maintain fluid, as the handling of water is less effective and the physiological response of aldosterone and vasopressin is altered (61). There is some justification for increased requirements for water in older patients as a result of increased loss through thinned skin and impairment of the concentrating ability of the kidneys (61).

An elder individual should be encouraged to consume 2 l of fluid per day or 1 ml of fluid per kilocalorie ingested to approximate at least 1500 ml/day. Adequate water intake is 30 ml/k of actual body weight and is essential for normal renal and bowel function (29).

The kidney plays a critical role in control of fluid balance regulating electrolyte homeostasis as well. The physiological capability of an elder to deal with extremes in sodium load has not been well studied. A wide variety of disease states commonly found in the elderly are linked to the incidence of altered sodium levels (64). Components of the excretion of sodium are affected by GFR. As the GFR decreases in the elderly, the ability of the kidneys to handle wide ranges in sodium load is diminished. This may be related to a decrease in the sensitivity to sodium or an altered response of the angiotensin–aldosterone system (63,64).

As in sodium regulation, the kidney is responsible for maintaining the potassium balance and metabolic acid levels in the body. Gastrointestinal losses of potassium and acids are at times common in the elderly especially those undergoing a surgical event. Serum concentrations of potassium and hydrogen ion may not reflect the severity of the deficit due to a simultaneous dehydration. Potassium depletion predisposes the elder to dysrhythmias. The risk of an alteration in rhythm status is compounded and particularly dangerous if the patient is also on digitalis medications (13). Hyperkalemia in itself is a serious dilemma for elderly persons on potassium-sparing diuretics.

Whether acute or chronic, many illnesses are accompanied by exaggerated additions in metabolic acid production. The aging kidney may not excrete the hydrogen ion load as effectively, thus increasing the severity of metabolic acidosis (63). The usually predictable compensatory response by the lungs to hyperventilate may be inadequate with the addition of pulmonary disease.

Severe imbalances of electrolyte concentrations are often accompanied by serious clinical manifestations (64). Particularly in the older patient, clinical improvement may lag behind correction of the electrolyte abnormality (63). Therefore, electrolyte imbalances should be recognized and corrected as soon as possible.

IX. CONCLUSION

Physiologic changes associated with the normal process of aging place the elder at risk for complications, particularly during illness. Prevention is the most important principle in limiting the possibility of complications. The goals for the elderly person include maintaining nitrogen balance, sustaining intravascular volume, and preserving electrolyte status. Scrupulous attention must be placed on screening and assessment to prevent untoward events from occurring. Awareness with the circumstances of the elderly plus routine and regular screening offers the best guarantee for timely identification of nutritional risk and electrolyte imbalance, which leads to prompt, appropriate intervention. Nutritional and electrolyte status maintenance in the elderly improves health status and quality of life.

REFERENCES

1. Abrams, W.B., Beers, M.H., and Berkow, R. 1995. *The Merck Manual of Geriatrics*, (2nd ed.). Whitehouse Station, NJ: Merck Research Laboratories.
2. Dellefield, M.E. 1996. Demographic trends: Issues and trends in gerontological nursing. In A.S. Luggen (Ed.). *Core Curriculum for Gerontological Nursing*. St. Louis: Mosby.
3. Matteson, M.A. 1997. Psychosocial aging changes. In M.A. Matteson, E.S. McConnell and A.D. Linton (Eds). *Gerontological Nursing: Concepts and Practice*, 2nd ed. Philadelphia: W.B. Saunders.
4. Bell, M.L. 1997. Nutritional Considerations. In M.A. Matteson, E.S. McConnell and A.D. Linton (Eds). *Gerontological Nursing: Concepts and Practice*, 2nd ed. Philadelphia: W.B. Saunders.
5. Kumanyika, S.K. 1993. Diet and nutrition as influences on the morbidity/mortality gap. *Ann. Epidem.*, 3, 154.
6. Bidlack, W.R. 1996. Interrelationships of food, nutrition, diet and health: The National Association of State Universities and Land Grant Colleges White Paper. *J. Am. Coll. Nutrit.*, 15, 422.
7. Frank, J.W., Brooker, A.S., DeMaio, S.E., et al. 1996. Disability resulting from occupational low back pain. Part II: What do we know about secondary prevention? A review of the scientific evidence on prevention after disability begins. *Spine,* 21, 2918.
8. Khaw, K.T. 1997. Epidemiological aspects of ageing. *Philosophical Transactions of the Royal Society of London — Series B: Biological Sciences,* 352, 1829.
9. U.S. Department of Health and Human Services Public Health Service. 1991a. *Healthy People 2000* (DHHS Publication No. 287-303/21332). Washington, DC: U.S. Government Printing Office.
10. U.S. Department of Health and Human Services, Public Health Service. 1991. *Healthy People 2000 — Summary Report* (DHHS Publication No. PHS 91-50213). Washington, DC: U.S. Government Printing Office.
11. Cope, K.A. 1994. Nutritional status: A basic "vital sign." *Home Healthcare Nurse, 12, 29.*
12. The Surgeon General's Workshop on Health Promotion and Aging. 1988. Washington, DC: U.S. Department of Health and Human Services.
13. Guyton, A.C. 1996. *The Textbook of Medical Physiology*, 9th ed. Philadelphia: W.B. Saunders.
14. Martin, W.E. 1995. The oral cavity and nutrition. In J.E. Morley, Z. Glick, and L.Z. Rubenstein, (Eds.). *Geri. Nut.,* 2nd ed. New York: Raven Press.
15. Boult, C., Kane, R.L., Louis, T.A., Boult, L. and McCaffrey, D. 1994 Chronic conditions that lead to functional limitation in the elderly. *J. Geront. Med. Sc.,* 49, M28.
16. Gilbride, J.A., Amella, E.J., Breines, E.B., Mariano, C. and Mezey, M. 1998. Nutrition and health status assessment of community-residing elderly in New York City: A pilot study. *J. Am. Diet. Assoc.,* 98, 554.
17. Nutrition Screening Initiative. 1991. Nutrition Screening Manual for Professionals Caring for Older Americans. Washington, DC: Green Margolis, Mitchell, Burns and Associates.
18. Nutrition Screening Initiative. 1992. Nutrition Screening Manual for Professionals Caring for Older Americans. Executive Summary. Washington, DC, Green Margolis, Mitchell, Burns and Associates.
19. Dwyer, J.T. 1991. *Screening Older Americans' Nutritional Health: Current Practices and Future Possibilities*. Washington, DC: Nutrition Screening Initiative.
20. Keller, H.H. 1993. Malnutrition in institutionalized elderly: How and why? *J. Am. Geri. Soc.*, 41, 1212.

21. Cashman, M.D. 1991. The aging gut. In R. Chernoff (Ed.). *Geriatric Nutrition: The Health Professional's Handbook*, Gaithersburg, MD: Aspen.

22. Martin, W.E. 1991. Oral health in the elderly. In R. Chernoff (Ed.). *Geriatric Nutrition: The Health Professional's Handbook*, Gaithersburg, MD: Aspen.

23. Ausman, L.M. and Russell, R.M. 1994. Nutrition in the elderly. In M.E. Shils, J.A. Olson and J. Shike, (Eds.). *Modern Nutrition in Health and Disease*, vol. 1, 8th ed. Philadelphia: Lea & Febiger.

24. Chernoff, R. 1991. *Geriatric Nutrition: The Health Professional's Handbook*, Gaithersburg, MD: Aspen.

25. White, J.V. 1991. Risk factors for poor nutritional status in older Americans. *Am. Fam. Phys.*, 44, 2087.

26. Horwath, C.C. 1991. Nutrition goals for older adults: A review. *Gerontologists*, 31, 811.

27. Walker, D. and Beauchene, R.E. 1991. The relationship of loneliness, social isolation, and physical health to dietary adequacy of independently living elderly. *J. Am. Diet. Assoc.*, 91, 300.

28. Posner, B.M., Jette, A., Smigelski, C., Miller, D., and Mitchell, P. 1994. Nutritional risk in New England elders. *J. Gerontology*, 49, M123.

29. Chernoff, R. 1995. Effects of age on nutrient requirements. *Clin. Geriatr. Med.*, 11, 641.

30. The Geriatric Research Education and Clinical Center, St. Louis VA Medical Center. 1991. Why do physicians fail to recognize and treat malnutrition in older persons? *JAGS* 39, 1139.

31. Opper, F.H. and Burakoff, R. 1994. Nutritional support of the elderly patient in an intensive care unit. *Clin. Geriatr. Med.*, 10:31.

32. Schlienger, J.L., Pradignac, A., and Grunenberger, F. 1995. Nutrition of the elderly: A challenge between facts and needs. *Hormone Res.*, 43:46.

33. Zylstra, R.C., Beerman, K., Hillers, V., and Mitchell, M. 1995. Who's at risk in Washington state? Demographic characteristics affect nutritional risk behaviors in elderly meal participants. *J. Am. Diet. Assoc.*, 95, 358.

34. Fleming, K.C., Evans, J.M., Weber, D.C., and Chutka, D.S. 1995. Practical functional assessment of elderly persons: a primary-care approach. *Mayo Clinic Proc.*, 70:890.

35. The Nutrition Screening Initiative. 1994. *Incorporating Nutrition Screening and Interventions into Medical Practice: A Monograph for Physicians*.

36. Lipschitz, D.A. 1995. Approaches to the nutritional support of the older patient. *Clin. Geriatr. Med.*, 11, 715.

37. McWhirter, J.P., and Pennington, C.R. 1994. Incidence and recognition of malnutrition in hospital. *BMJ*, 308, 945.

38. Rolandelli, R.H. and Ullrich, J.R. 1994. Nutritional support in the frail elderly surgical patient. *Surg. Clin. North Am.*, 74, 79.

39. Sullivan, D.H. 1992. Risk factors for early hospital readmission in a select population of geriatric rehabilitation patients: the significance of nutritional status. *JAGS*, 40, 792.

40. Watters, J.M., and Bessey, P.Q. 1994. Critical care for the elderly patient. *Surg. Clin. N. Am.*, 74, 187.

41. Coats, K.G., Morgan, S.L., Bartolucci, A.A., and Weinsier, R.L. 1993. Hospital-associated malnutrition: A reevaluation 12 years later. *J. Am. Diet. Assoc.*, 93, 27.

42. Gallagher-Allred, C.R. 1993. Nutrition screening and early intervention: Keys to preventing malnutrition. *J. Med. Direction*, 17.

43. Fishman, P. 1994. Detecting malnutrition's warning signs with simple screening tools. *Geriatrics*, 49, 39.

44. Ryan, C., Bryant, E., Eleazer, P., Phodes, A., and Guest, K. 1995. Unintentional weight loss in long-term care: predictor of mortality in the elderly. *Southern Med. J.*, 88, 721.

45. Chandra, R. 1995. Nutrition and immunity in the elderly: Clinical significance. *Nut. Rev.*, 53, S80.

46. Chalfin, D.B. and Nasraway, S.A. 1994. Preoperative evaluation and postoperative care of the elderly patient undergoing major surgery. *Clin. Geriatr. Med.*, 10, 51.

47. Ripa, S. and Ripa, R. 1995. Zinc and the elderly. *Minerva Medica*, 86, 275.

48. Shekleton, M.E. and Litwack, K. 1991. *Critical Care Nursing of the Surgical Patient*. Philadelphia: W.B. Saunders.

49. Barrocas, A., Belcher, D., Champagne, C., and Jastram, C. 1995. Nutrition assessment practical approaches. *Clin. Geriatr. Med.*, 11, 675.

50. Kerekes, J. and Thornton, O. 1996. Incorporating nutritional risk screening with case management initiatives. *Nutr. Clin. Prac.*, 11, 95.

51. Fishman, P. 1996. Healthy people 2000: What progress toward better nutrition? *Geriatrics*, 51, 38.

52. Velanovich, V. 1991. The value of routine preoperative laboratory testing in predicting postoperative complications: A multivariate analysis. *Surgery*, 109, 236.

53. Nogues, R., Sitges-Serra, A., Sancho, J.J., Sanz, F., Monne, J., Girvent, M., Gubern, J.M. 1995. Influence of nutrition, thyroid hormones, and rectal temperature on in-hospital mortality of elderly patients with acute illness. *Am. J. Clin Nutr.*, 61, 597.

54. Sullivan, D.H. 1995. The role of nutrition in increased morbidity and mortality. *Clin. Geriatr. Med.*, 11, 661.

55. Duffy, V.B., Backstrand, J.R., and Ferris, A.M. 1995. Olfactory dysfunction and related nutritional risk in free-living elderly women. *J. Am. Diet. Assoc.*, 95, 879.

56. Harris, J.A. and Benedict, F.G. 1919. A biometric study of basal metabolism in man. Publication #279. Washington DC: Carnegie Institute.

57. Garrel, D.R., Jobin, N., and DeJonge, L.H.M. 1996. Should we still use the Harris and Benedict equations? *Nutr. Clin. Pract.*, 11, 99.

58. FAO/WHO/UNU. 1985. *Energy and Protein Requirements*. Technical Report Series #724. Geneva, Switzerland: World Health Organization.

59. Fukagawa, N.K. and Young, V.R. 1987. Protein and amino acid metabolism and requirements in older persons. *Clin. Geriatr. Med.*, 3, 329.

60. Carter, W.J. 1991. Macronutrient requirements for elderly persons. In R. Chernoff, (Ed.). *Geriatric Nutrition*. Gaithersburg, MD: Aspen Publishers, pp. 11–24.

61. Watters, J.M. and McClaran, J.C. 1996. The elderly surgical patient. *Scientific American VII. 13, 1.*

62. Cogan, M.G. 1991. *Fluid & Electrolytes: Physiology & Pathophysiology*. Norwalk, CT: Appleton & Lange.

63. Beck, L.H. 1990. Perioperative renal, fluid, and electrolyte management. *Clin. Geriatr. Med.*, 6, 557.

64. Sica, D.A. 1994. Renal disease, electrolyte abnormalities, and acid-base imbalance in the elderly. *Clin. Geriatr. Med.*, 10, 197.

2 Vitamin C in Health and Diseases of the Elderly

Marvin Cohen and Hemmi N. Bhagavan

CONTENTS

I.   INTRODUCTION

The aging process is often accompanied by chronic and degenerative illness. Evidence continues to accumulate that oxidative damage contributes to these disorders and that ascorbic acid (AA) as well as other antioxidant vitamins may modulate their prevalence and/or severity and duration. Due to the continuing interest in this area of research, an overview of current trends based on clinical and epidemiological studies has been made in this chapter, which further defines the potential of AA to improve the health and well being of the elderly.

This chapter is an extension of two earlier reviews where we discussed the importance of AA in the nutrition of the elderly and the potential benefits of AA supplementation (1,2). The term "elderly" as used in this review refers to individuals 65 years of age or older. The primary sources of information were literature searches conducted on the MEDLINE and EXCERPTA MEDICA databases for all relevant clinical studies, epidemiological studies, and review articles published between 1992 and approximately mid-1999. A small number of earlier studies omitted from the previous review have also been included. Papers were considered for inclusion in the review if either some or all of the subjects evaluated were in the elderly age category. Much of this literature describes the use of AA combined with other antioxidants and/or micronutrients. Although the effect of AA alone cannot be determined from such studies, these data provide a useful indicator of research areas of recent or current interest and may stimulate future trials that are better designed to study the effects of individual antioxidant vitamins. In addition, a small number of studies that contained no elderly subjects were included if the research area was potentially of great interest and had relevance to the elderly.

II.   ASCORBIC ACID STATUS IN FREE-LIVING ELDERLY

A.   ASCORBIC ACID DEFICIENCY OF THE ELDERLY

Studies of AA status continue to show that in some free-living populations there is a significant incidence of AA deficiency. This varied from 5 to 18.8% in two studies and was similar for men and women (3,4). A study of 309 subjects aged 60 or more found that 27% were consuming less than 67% of the RDA/RDI for AA (5). Another survey of 138 elderly subjects found a mean daily AA intake of 43.5 to 61.1 mg (6). In contrast to these findings, plasma AA levels in other elderly populations were found to be normal or above normal (7–9).

B.   AGE AND GENDER EFFECTS ON ASCORBIC ACID STATUS

Studies on gender differences in AA status continue to show that women tend to have significantly higher plasma AA levels than men, even though AA intake is similar (10–13). However, one survey of 150 Hong Kong Chinese subjects found no gender differences when compared with Western populations (14). This suggests possible racial or genetic influence, assuming all other parameters were equal. Many studies on AA status in relation to age have shown that the elderly tend to have lower plasma AA levels (15–18). A decreased intake of AA may be one factor responsible for this observation (19,20). In contrast to these findings, some studies have found no relationship between age and plasma AA levels (14,21,22). In one study, a survey of 1161 men aged 43 to 85 showed that AA intake in men 65 and older was greater than that of younger men (23), and this seems to be an exception. There are several reviews on the AA status of the elderly including those of Russell (24), Thurnham (25), Russell and Suter (26), Koehler and Garry (27), Chernoff (1995), and Ward (29). Conclusions reached by these articles include (a) the need for vitamin supplementation by the elderly may be partly due to a change in requirement due to aging and partly due to decreased intake because of chronic illness, and (b) additional studies are needed to establish whether the RDI for micronutrients in the elderly is different from the requirement for younger subjects.

C. ASCORBIC ACID STATUS IN INSTITUTIONALIZED ELDERLY

Studies of institutionalized elderly in long-term care facilities continue to show that significant proportions of the subjects examined (19–100%) have AA intakes below the RDI when compared with elderly living in other settings (30–33). Supplementing their diet with AA or AA-rich foods rapidly normalizes their AA status (34). In addition, improvements in immune function in institutionalized elderly subjects appear to be associated with AA or multivitamin/mineral supplementation (35,36). This is discussed in more detail in Section VII.

D. USE OF ASCORBIC ACID SUPPLEMENTS BY THE ELDERLY

Three surveys of elderly subjects reported that AA supplements were used by 3 to 30% of the respondents while multivitamin or vitamin/mineral combinations were used by 8.1 to 28% (37–39). A survey of 10,788 adults, approximately 20% being 65 or older, indicated that 29.7 to 34.6% of the cohort used supplements (40). A survey of 2152 adults indicated that in those aged 65 to 84, 34.4% of men and 41.1% of women used supplements containing AA (41). Reviews on the use of supplements by the elderly and other adults include those of Buchman et al. (42) and Thurman and Mouradian (1997). Although the numbers vary, it appears that a significant proportion of the elderly use AA supplements, often in combination with other nutrients. In the case of single entity AA supplements, the dosage is most often a multiple of the RDI.

III. ASCORBIC ACID AND SMOKING

Studies comparing the plasma levels of AA and other antioxidants in elderly as well as in younger smokers and nonsmokers continue to show that plasma AA levels are significantly lower in smokers, ranging from approximately 60 to 88% of the levels in the nonsmoking population (44–49). In contrast to these reports, only slightly lower plasma AA levels were found in a group of African-American women smokers when compared with nonsmokers (50). Reduced AA intake in smokers may also contribute to lower plasma AA values (51). An increased risk of hip fracture was associated with reduced AA intake in smokers (52). This was attributed to an interference with bone resorption caused by increased oxidant stress. The number of polycyclic aromatic hydrocarbon–DNA adducts in circulating mononuclear cells of smokers was inversely proportional to serum AA levels, suggesting a mechanism for the production of precancerous lesions in subjects at risk for lung cancer (53).

IV. ASCORBIC ACID STATUS AND CANCER RISK

A. ASCORBIC ACID AND INHIBITION OF CHROMOSOMAL DAMAGE

The antioxidant activity of AA has been examined in relation to whether it has an effect on chromosomal damage. In healthy subjects, a significant inverse correlation was found between mutagen sensitivity (as measured by bleomycin-induced chromosomal breaks in lymphocytes) and plasma AA levels (54). However, in one study involving subjects with oral, pharyngeal, or laryngeal cancer, no correlation was noted for these two parameters (55). A survey of subjects over a wide age range did not find any correlation between micronucleus frequency and plasma AA levels in men aged 60 to 90 (56–58). Another survey of 407 subjects found no relationship between plasma AA levels and urinary excretion of 8-hydroxy-2′-deoxyguanosine, a product of oxidative DNA damage (59). Thus, the relationship between AA status as assessed by plasma levels and risk for mutagen-induced damage is not clear. The degree of inadequacy or deficiency is an important factor. It is also possible that this is a synergistic phenomenon where the status of other antioxidants need to be considered.

Intervention studies with AA have not produced consistent results. Administration of 150 mg/day AA combined with other antioxidant micronutrients over a 4-month period reduced the incidence of spontaneous and gamma radiation-induced micronuclei in lymphocytes (60). In contrast to these results, administration of 500 mg/day AA, either alone or in combination with vitamin E, for 2 months had no effect on the urinary excretion of 8-oxo-7,8-dihydro-2′-deoxyguanosine, a product of oxidative DNA damage (61).

B. Overall Cancer Mortality and Incidence

Several studies have examined the ability of supplementation with AA as well as other micronutrients to modulate the incidence and/or mortality rate due to cancer. In a major study sponsored by the National Cancer Institute and conducted in China with 29,584 adults over a 6-year period, the results showed that daily administration of AA and molybdenum as well as other antioxidant vitamin combinations decreased overall cancer incidence (62). In another study, patients randomized to receive a cardioprotective Mediterranean-type diet showed a significantly lower incidence of cancer as well as a higher AA intake than subjects on a control diet (63). An epidemiological survey of 2974 men over a 17-year period found that overall cancer mortality was associated with low mean plasma AA levels (64). A similar long-term (24-year) follow-up of 1556 men found an inverse relationship between AA or beta-carotene intake and cancer mortality (65). However in one study, a 14-year follow up of 2112 men found no effect of AA intake on the incidence of gastrointestinal cancers (66). The majority of studies show an inverse relationship between AA status and cancer incidence and mortality. The subject of micronutrient intake and overall cancer risk has been reviewed by Goodwin and Brodwick (67).

C. Breast Cancer

Table 2.1 summarizes the results of studies published from 1991 to 1999 that examined various aspects of the relationship between AA status and breast cancer risk. In ten epidemiological studies, either no relationship or a slight but no significant effect on breast cancer risk was found as a function of AA intake (68–77). In contrast to these, a significant inverse relationship between AA intake and breast cancer risk was reported in three epidemiological studies (78–80).

Other studies have suggested that AA status may play a role in the level of risk for breast cancer. In one study that found an inverse relationship between plasma AA and plasma prolactin levels, it was concluded that this was a possible mechanism by which AA status could affect breast cancer risk (81). Lockwood et al. (82) reported that a high dose of AA combined with other antioxidants appeared to stabilize or cause an apparent partial remission of breast cancer in 32 patients. However, studies confirming these findings have not appeared in the scientific literature. Two studies found significantly reduced serum AA levels in patients with breast tumors (83,84), but it is difficult with data of this type to determine whether reduced AA status increased breast cancer risk or whether the onset of disease depleted AA reserves.

D. Colorectal Cancer

Table 2.2 summarizes the results of several studies reported during the period 1992–1998 that examined possible relationships between AA intake and colorectal cancer risk. Six epidemiological

TABLE 1.1
Studies on Ascorbic Acid (AA) Intake and Breast Cancer Risk

Reference	Subjects and Site	Results
68	1335 breast cancer patients, 10,245 controls, 8 yr. follow-up; California	No relationship between AA intake and breast cancer risk
69	18,586 postmenopausal women aged 50–107 yr., 359 breast cancer cases; New York State	No relationship between AA intake and breast cancer risk
70	515 cases of breast cancer; 1182 controls; Canada	Slight but not significant inverse relationship between AA intake and breast cancer risk
72	34,387 women aged 55–69 yr., 879 breast cancer cases, 6 yr. follow-up; Iowa	No significant relationship between AA intake and breast cancer risk
73	2569 women (528 aged 65 or more) with breast cancer, 2588 controls; Italy	No relationship between AA intake and breast cancer risk
74	4697 women followed 25 yr., 88 breast cancer cases; Finland	No relationship between AA intake and breast cancer risk
75	62,573 women aged 55–69 yr., 4.3 yr. Follow-up, 650 breast cancer patients; Netherlands	Small reduction in breast cancer risk with increasing AA intake
76	414 breast cancer patients, 420 controls; Montreal	No relationship between AA intake and breast cancer risk
77	117 postmenopausal cancer patients, 233 controls; New York State	No effect of AA intake on breast cancer risk
78	673 breast cancer patients; Canada	Dose-related inverse relationship between AA intake and breast cancer risk
79	834 breast cancer patients aged 20–69 yr., 834 controls; China	Significant inverse relationship between AA intake and breast cancer risk
80	83,234 women, 19,133 postmenopausal breast cancer patients, 14 yr. follow-up; United States	Strong inverse relationship between AA intake and breast cancer risk
81	249 women (66 postmenopausal subjects), mean age 58.3 yr.; Australia	Inverse relationship between plasma AA levels and plasma prolactin levels
82	32 breast cancer patients aged 32–81 yr., 2850 mg/day AA + other anti-oxidants × 18 mo.; Denmark	Stabilization or apparent partial remission of cancer
83	Postmenopausal women, 23 with malignant breast tumors, 20 with benign breast tumors, 20 controls; India	Significant decrease in serum AA levels in all women with tumors
84	Women aged 30–65 yr. With breast ($n = 100$) or cervical ($n = 100$) cancer, controls with benign conditions ($n = 25$) or healthy ($n = 50$); India	Significant reduction in serum AA levels in cancer patients

studies found a weak or no association between AA intake and colorectal cancer risk (85–90), while three other studies found a significant inverse relationship (91–93). Shibata et al. (68) found a significant inverse relationship only in women, while a meta-analysis of 13 case-control studies concluded that only a weak association existed between AA intake and colorectal cancer risk (94).

In healthy subjects, no relationship was found between AA intake and colonic cell thymidine labeling index (95), but in two studies of patients with adenomas or adenomatous polyps, administration of AA (750 mg/day for 1 month or 1000 mg/day for 6 months), either alone or in combination with other antioxidants, significantly decreased the thymidine labeling index in colon cells (96,97). In contrast to these data, administration of 1000 mg/day AA, either alone or combined with other antioxidants, over a 4-year period did not appear to affect the incidence of adenomas (98). Decreased AA intake or blood levels have also been found in patients with colorectal cancer (99,100), but it is not clear whether the reduced AA levels increased risk or whether the disease

TABLE 2.2
Studies on Ascorbic Acid (AA) Intake and Colorectal Cancer Risk

Reference	Subjects and Site	Results
68	1335 cancer patients, 10,245 controls, 8 yr. follow-up; California	In women, inverse association between AA intake and colon cancer risk
85	35,215 women aged 55–69 yr.; Iowa	No relationship between AA intake and colon cancer incidence
86	297 patients (mean age 63.8 yr.) with newly diagnosed adenomas, 198 patients (mean age 66.4 yr.) with recurrent adenomas, 347 controls with history of polypectomy but no current neoplasia; New York	No relationship between AA intake and risk for adenoma
87	488 subjects aged 50–74 yr.; California	Weak inverse association between AA intake and prevalence of colorectal adenomas
88	1993 colon cancer patients, 2410 controls; Utah, California, Minnesota	No association between AA intake and colon cancer risk
89	402 colon cancer patients aged 35–79 yr., 668 controls; Montreal	No relationship between AA intake and colon cancer risk
90	144 rectal cancer patients, 34,558 controls; Iowa	Slight but not significant inverse relationship between AA intake and rectal cancer risk
91, 92	1326 colon/rectal cancer patients (800 aged 60–74 yr.), 2024 controls; Italy	Inverse relationship between AA intake and colorectal cancer risk; 14% of cases attributable to low AA intake
93	112 colorectal cancer patients (54 aged 60 yr. or more), 108 controls; Spain	Significant inverse relationship between AA intake and colorectal cancer risk
94	Meta-analysis of 13 case-control studies	Weak relationship between AA intake and colon cancer risk
95	63 healthy subjects aged 35–73 yr.; California	No relationship between AA intake and colonic cell thymidine labeling index
96	20 patients (aged 40–80 yr.) with colorectal adenomas, 21 placebo controls; 1000 mg/day AA + vitamin A and vitamin E × 6 months; Italy	Significant decrease in thymidine labeling index that returned to pre-treatment levels within 6 mo. after termination of study
97	40 patients with adenomatous polyps, 20 controls, 750 mg/day AA × 1 mo.; Ireland	Significant reduction in colon cell labeling index
98	751 subjects (427 aged 60 yr. or more), administration of placebo, AA 1000 mg/day, or AA combined with beta-carotene and vitamin E × 4 yr.; New Hampshire	No effect on incidence of adenomas
99	249 patients with precancerous conditions of stomach/colorectum, 96 patients with gastric/colorectal cancer, 130 controls; Slovakia	Decreased AA blood levels in patients with precancerous conditions or cancers
100	50 patients with adenocarcinoma of colon or rectum, 50 controls; Brazil	Significantly lower AA intake in cancer patients

condition resulted in lower AA levels. This situation is not unique and is also seen with other nutrients. A review by Pappalardo et al. (101) discusses the relationship of micronutrient intake to colorectal cancer risk in more detail.

E. GASTRIC CANCER

Table 2.3 summarizes the results of several studies published between 1993 and 1998 that examined relationships between AA intake and gastric cancer risk. In five epidemiological studies, a significant

TABLE 2.3
Studies on Ascorbic Acid (AA) Intake and Gastric Cancer Risk

Reference	Subjects and Site	Results
99	249 patients with precancerous lesions of the stomach/colorectum, 96 patients with gastric/colorectal cancer, 130 controls; Slovakia	Decreased AA blood levels in patients with both precancerous conditions and cancer
102	117 gastric cancer patients (60 aged 60–80 yr.), 234 controls; Spain	Significant inverse relationship between AA intake and gastric cancer risk
103	338 gastric cancer patients (mean age 67.7 yr.), 679 controls; Sweden	Significant inverse relationship between AA intake and gastric cancer risk.
104,105	723–746 gastric cancer patients (408 aged 60 yr. or more), 2024–2053 controls; Italy	Significant inverse relationship between AA intake and gastric cancer risk; 16% of cases could be attributed to low AA intake
106	84 cancer patients (51 aged 60–73 yr.), 89 controls; Norway	Inverse association between AA intake and risk of upper gastro-intestinal tumors.
107	301 gastric cancer patients, 2581 controls; Belgium	Significant inverse relationship between AA intake and gastric cancer risk
108	59 upper digestive tract cancer patients, 34,632 controls, 7 yr. follow-up; Iowa	Slight but not significant inverse relationship between AA intake and gastric cancer
109	282 gastric cancer patients (mean age 63 yr.), 3123 controls; Netherlands	No consistent relationship between AA intake, nitrate/nitrite intake, and gastric cancer risk
110	3318 adults aged 40–69 yr. with esophageal dysplasia, 120 mg/day AA + molybdenum × 6 yr.; China	No significant reduction in prevalence of gastric dysplasia or gastric cancer
111	43 subjects with pre-cancerous gastric lesions randomized to receive 250 mg AA 3 times daily or 500 mg slow-release AA + 150 mg standard AA once daily (both combined with vitamin E and beta-carotene) × 7 days; Venezuela	Plasma AA levels increased, but no effect on gastric AA levels; attributed to high incidence of *H. pylori*

inverse relationship was found between these two parameters (102–107). In contrast to these, Zheng et al. (108) found only a slight but not significant relationship between AA intake and gastric cancer risk. In a study comparing AA intake, nitrate/nitrite intake, and gastric cancer risks, no consistent relationship was found (109). The nitrate/nitrite intake was used as an indicator of endogenous nitrosamine load. In an intervention study in which 120 mg/day AA along with molybdenum was given over a 6-year period, no significant reduction in the prevalence of gastric dysplasia or gastric cancer was observed (110).

Decreased AA blood levels were reported in patients with precancerous gastric lesions or gastric cancer, but as in other studies of this type, it is difficult to determine whether the decreased AA levels increased risk or whether the disease state depleted AA reserves (99). The potential interactions of *Helicobacter pylori* infection with gastric cancer risk were suggested in one study. Administration of AA to subjects with a high incidence of *H. pylori* infection increased plasma AA levels but had no effect on gastric AA levels (111).

F. Prostate Cancer

Table 2.4 summarizes the results of several epidemiological studies between 1992 and 1999 that examined the relationship between AA intake and prostate cancer risk. In six studies, no relationship

TABLE 2.4
Studies on Ascorbic Acid (AA) Intake and Prostate Cancer Risk

Reference	Subjects and Site	Results
68	1335 cancer patients, 1025 controls, 8 yr. follow-up; California	No relationship between AA intake and prostate cancer risk.
112	526 prostate cancer patients, 536 controls; Sweden	No relationship between AA intake and prostate cancer risk.
113	1899 middle-aged men; United States	No relationship between AA intake and prostate cancer risk, but increased overall survival over 30 yr. follow-up positively associated with AA intake.
114	232 prostate cancer cases aged 35–84 yr., 231 controls; Montreal	No relationship between AA intake and prostate cancer risk.
115	101 prostate cancer patients (mean age 71 yr.), 202 controls; Yugoslavia	No relationship between AA intake and prostate cancer risk.
116	17 yr. follow-up of 2203 men; Switzerland	No statistical difference in plasma AA levels between 30 deaths from prostate cancer and 2173 survivors.
117	175 subjects (166 aged 60 yr. or more); Uruguay	Significant inverse relationship between AA intake and prostate cancer risk.

was found for these two parameters (68,112–116), while one study found a significant inverse relationship (117). The study by Daviglus et al. (113) concluded that AA intake was positively associated with survival of prostate cancer patients over a 30-year follow-up period.

G. ORAL/PHARYNGEAL/LARYNGEAL CANCER

Table 2.5 summarizes the results of several epidemiological studies conducted between 1992 and 1999 that investigated the relationship between AA intake and the risk for oral pharyngeal or laryngeal cancer. In two studies, a significant inverse relationship was found for AA intake and cancer risk (118,119), while in three other studies, either no relationship or a slight but not significant relationship was reported (108,120,121). A study of smokeless tobacco users found a decreased AA intake in subjects with epithelial dysplasia (122). However, as in previous situations, it is difficult to determine whether decreased AA levels increased risk or whether the presence of disease depleted AA reserves.

H. OTHER CANCERS

Epidemiological studies have examined possible relationships between AA intake and cancer risk for a variety of malignancies. However, in cases where more than one study was reported, no clear consensus emerged. Either no relationship or a slight but not significant relationship was reported for malignant melanoma (123), brain cancer (124), ovarian cancer (125), and thyroid cancer (126). An apparent protective effect of AA was found with regard to gallbladder cancer, but no dose relationship was noted (127). An inverse relationship was noted between intake of AA-containing foods and the incidence of basal cell or squamous cell cancer of the skin, but no data on dietary AA intake per se were reported (128). Decreased plasma AA levels have been reported in patients with brain cancer (129) or cervical tumors (84).

In three epidemiological studies of bladder cancer, an inverse relationship between AA intake and cancer risk was found in two cases (68,130), but no relationship was found in the third study (131). In two studies of endometrial cancer, a protective effect of AA was found in one case (132), but not the other (133). Four studies of esophageal cancer found protective effects of AA in two cases (134,135), a slight but not significant effect in a third study (108) and no effect on prevalence

TABLE 5
Studies on Ascorbic Acid (AA) Intake and Oral/Pharyngeal/Laryngeal Cancer

Reference	Subjects and Site	Results
119	80 oral/pharyngeal cancer patients (aged 58–69 yr.) with primary cancers, 189 controls, 5 yr. follow-up; United States	Significant inverse relationship between AA intake and cancer risk.
120	250 laryngeal cancer patients (mean age 62.1 yr.), 250 controls; New York State	No relationship between AA intake and laryngeal cancer risk.
121	226 subjects (mean age 57.4 yr.) with precancerous oral lesions, 226 controls; India	Slight decreased cancer risk from increased AA intake, but no dose-response.
122	347 users of smokeless tobacco aged 14–77 yr.; Virginia	Decreased AA intake among users with epithelial dysplasia.
118	41 men with oral/pharyngeal cancer (mean age 64 yr.), 398 controls; Australia	Significant inverse relationship between AA intake and oral/pharyngeal cancer risk.
108	59 upper digestive tract cancers, 34,632 controls; Iowa	Slight but not significant inverse relationship between AA intake and oral/pharyngeal cancer risk.

in a fourth study (110). In five studies of lung cancer, a protective effect of AA was found in two cases (136,137), a slight but no significant effect in one case (138), and no relationship in one case (68). An epidemiological study by Lee et al. (139) concluded that AA intake was not a predictor of lung cancer location. In two studies of pancreatic cancer, a protective effect of AA was found in one case (140), while a slight but no significant effect was found in the other (68). In two studies of renal cell cancer, a protective effect of AA was found in one case (141) while a slight but no significant effect was found in the other (142). Overall, the evidence for a relationship between AA status and risk for various types of cancer is not strong.

V. ASCORBIC ACID STATUS AND CENTRAL NERVOUS SYSTEM DISORDERS OF THE ELDERLY

A. ALTERATIONS IN COGNITIVE FUNCTION

The possible implication of free radicals in the etiology of Alzheimer's disease and other dementias has led to studies examining whether AA status is a factor affecting the risk for cognitive disorders. While some studies have not found any relationship between AA or antioxidant intake and cognitive function as measured by the Mini-Mental State Examination or the Mattis Dementia Rating Scale (143–146), other studies have reported a relationship between AA intake or plasma AA levels and cognitive test performance (147–149). One study found no significant difference in plasma AA levels between Alzheimer patients and controls, but significantly lower plasma AA levels were noted in subjects with vascular dementia (150). The authors suggested that some forms of dementia may be associated with a disturbance of antioxidant balance that can be modified by supplementation.

B. PARKINSONISM

Evidence suggesting that oxidant stress may be a risk factor for Parkinsonism has led to studies investigating a possible relationship between AA intake and risk for this disease. Several epidemiological and clinical surveys did not find a protective effect of AA or other antioxidant micronutrients (151–158). In contrast to these, a survey of 342 Parkinsonism patients and 342 controls found a significant inverse association between AA intake and the risk of Parkinsonism (159). An intervention study using a levo-dopa-carbidopa–AA combination reported beneficial effects in

Parkinsonism patients, but the contribution of AA to the effects seen could not be determined (160). In another intervention study, administration of 3000 mg/day AA extended by 2 to 3 years the time when levo-dopa was needed (161). The authors suggested that the progression of Parkinsonism may be slowed by the administration of antioxidants. These results are encouraging and additional work is certainly needed in this area.

VI.   ASCORBIC ACID STATUS AND CARDIOVASCULAR DISEASE

A.   Effects of Ascorbic Acid on Plasma Lipid Oxidation

The antioxidant activity of AA has been explored in relation to whether the vitamin can affect the oxidizability of plasma lipids. Studies in this area have generally measured *in vivo* levels of oxidized low density lipoproteins (LDL) or have used an *in vitro* method to determine the lag time for LDL oxidation.

Plasma AA was inversely associated with oxidized LDL levels or plasma levels of lipid peroxides and malondialdehyde (162,163), but in one study, a survey of 207 patients undergoing coronary angiography showed no correlation between the lag time for LDL oxidation and plasma levels of AA or other antioxidants (164). A survey of 25 smokers and 26 nonsmokers concluded that plasma AA and urate levels were the most consistent determinants of serum lipid resistance to oxidation (165). A study of subjects over 60 years old found elevated levels of serum lipid peroxides (LPOs) and noted that LPO levels >4 nmol/ml depleted serum antioxidant levels (166). The authors concluded that older subjects could be at greater risk for oxidative stress. In contrast to these data, a survey of 59 healthy elderly subjects found significantly lower serum AA levels, but a reduced susceptibility for LDL oxidation (167). A significant increase in plasma AA levels associated with increased intake of fruits and vegetables did not have any effect on plasma lipids (168). The relationship of AA status to plasma lipid profile has been reviewed by Van de Vijver et al. (169).

Intervention studies appear to have produced more consistent changes in plasma lipids. Administration of 500 or 1000 mg/day AA for 4 or 12 weeks significantly reduced the susceptibility of lipids to oxidation (170,171) or reduced plasma lipid hydroperoxides or TBARS (172). In contrast to these studies, administration of 1000 mg/day AA for 4 weeks had no effect on plasma lipid oxidation but did decrease plasma malondialdehyde levels (173).

B.   Overall Cardiovascular Mortality

A survey of 728 Chinese subjects found no difference in total antioxidant capacity in plasma between individuals with and without cardiovascular disease (22), but plasma AA was only part of this measure. Two recent reviews have discussed the possible relationships of AA to the risk for cardiovascular disease. According to Lavie et al. (174), it is still premature to recommend the routine use of antioxidants for the prevention of atherosclerosis, whereas Price and Fowkes (175) concluded that the available epidemiological evidence supports a protective role for antioxidant vitamins in cardiovascular disease, but that only a weak relationship currently exists specifically for AA.

C.   Coronary Artery Disease (CAD)

Several epidemiological and clinical surveys have found an inverse relationship between AA intake and the risk for CAD (13,35,65,176–180). In contrast to these, a few studies found no relationship between AA intake and CAD risk (181–183).

Intervention studies have shown that increased AA intake or a combination of antioxidants decreased CAD progression (184), relieved angina pectoris (185), and reduced ischemic ECG events associated with surgery for CAD (186). Intravenous doses of 1000 or 2000 mg AA significantly improved flow-mediated vasodilatation in CAD patients (187,188). These latter studies suggest that increased oxidative stress may be an important mechanism for impaired endothelial function in CAD patients. Reviews on the potential of oral AA to modify CAD include those of Gaziano and Hennekens (189) and Law and Morris (190).

D. Myocardial Infarction (MI)

Several clinical/epidemiological studies have investigated possible relationships between AA status and the risk of MI. Significantly lower plasma AA levels were found in one survey of 46 subjects and 20 controls (191), and a large survey of 1605 men found a 3.5-fold increase in the incidence of MI in those with AA deficiency compared with subjects with recommended AA levels (47). In contrast to these reports, one patient survey and one epidemiological survey found no association between AA intake and MI risk (192,193).

Some studies have suggested that the antioxidant property of AA may influence the incidence of complications in MI patients. Infusion of 10 g AA over a 4-hour period decreased the incidence of post-MI ventricular ectopic beats (194). In a study of 67 patients, data showing an inverse relationship between decreasing plasma AA levels and increasing plasma malondialdehyde levels up to 24 hours after MI led the investigators to suggest that combining antioxidant and thrombolytic therapy may reduce ischemic-reperfusion injury (195). In a longer-term intervention study, administration of 600 mg/day AA and vitamin E (600 mg/day) for 14 days to 23 MI patients significantly decreased neutrophil production of oxygen-containing free radicals and significantly increased in serum AA levels (196).

E. Stroke

Several studies have examined possible relationships between AA intake and the risk of stroke. In four cases, no relationship or a slight but no significant relationship was reported either for acute stroke (177,197,198) or the earliest signs of ischemic brain damage (199). In one intervention study, administration of AA and other antioxidants had no effect on the incidence of stroke-related disability or mortality (200). In contrast to these investigations, a study of 32 patients with stroke suggested that marked decreases (51%) in plasma AA were associated with worsening clinical condition, while in those subjects with a stable or improved clinical condition, plasma AA levels did not show this pattern (201).

F. Congestive Heart Failure (CHF)

Administration of AA as an adjunct to standard therapy may improve outcome in patients with CHF. A study in 58 patients with CHF found an inverse relationship between plasma AA levels and plasma levels of lipid peroxides and malondialdehyde (163). The authors suggested that oxidative stress may be an important determinant of prognosis in CHF and that antioxidant supplements may have a therapeutic benefit. Administration of AA either intravenously or orally prolonged the beneficial effects of nitroglycerin in CHF patients (202,203). The authors suggested that oral AA supplementation may prevent the development of nitrate tolerance during long-term nitrate therapy.

G. Peripheral Vascular Disease

Dietary AA was significantly related to ankle/brachial pressure index (ABPI) only among those subjects who had ever smoked (204). However, in nonsmokers, higher baseline ABPI values were not affected by AA intake. Administration of AA for 2 years to subjects with lower limb atherosclerosis had no effect on ABPI values, although there was a slight (–3.7%) reduction in cardiovascular events/death and significantly fewer (–18.2%) serious adverse events (205).

H. Blood Pressure

Several studies have examined the possibility that reduced plasma AA levels may be a risk factor for the development of hypertension. Two epidemiological studies found an inverse relationship between plasma AA levels and systolic/diastolic pressure (206,207). Significantly reduced plasma AA levels were found in a survey of 46 subjects with hypertension or myocardial infarction when compared with controls (191). The possible contribution of oxidant stress to hypertension was suggested by studies in which significantly higher plasma malondialdehyde levels were accompanied by significantly lower plasma AA levels in hypertensives (208). However, other studies of this type have not found a reduction in total plasma antioxidant capacity, even though levels of peroxidation products may be higher in hypertensive subjects (22,209).

Intervention studies have not provided a consistent pattern on the possible modulation of blood pressure by AA. Administration of 250 to 400 mg/day AA for 4 to 16 weeks had either no effect or a slight but no significant effect on blood pressure (210–212). In contrast to these, administration of 500 mg/day AA combined with other antioxidants for 8 weeks significantly reduced systolic blood pressure in both hypertensive and normotensive subjects (213). The authors attributed the effect to an increased availability of nitric oxide, since urinary nitrite levels rose in hypertensive subjects during the treatment.

VII. ASCORBIC ACID STATUS AND THE IMMUNE SYSTEM

Several studies have examined the ability of AA to improve immune responses, particularly in populations such as the elderly, who generally have a decreased immune response and increased susceptibility to infection. In five studies, AA administration over a wide dose range (80–1000 mg/day) and variable time period (4 weeks to 12 months), either alone or combined with other antioxidants, improved immune function using several measures of immune system response (35,214–218). In contrast to these, four studies found no effect on immune responses and/or infection rate after AA administration for up to 2 years (34,219–221). Johnson and Porter (36) examined the relative effectiveness of trace minerals and vitamins in reducing infection incidence and found that only trace elements significantly reduced infection morbidity. Review articles that discuss this issue in more detail include those of Meydani (222) and Hughes (223).

VIII. ASCORBIC ACID STATUS AND DISORDERS OF VISION

A. Cataracts

The fact that vitreous humor contains very high concentrations of AA has stimulated epidemiological surveys and clinical trials to determine whether AA intake through diet or by the use of supplements would affect the incidence of disorders of vision such as cataracts in elderly subjects. Dietary AA did not appear to influence the risk for cataracts (224–226), but prolonged use of supplements (10 years or more) appeared to have a beneficial effect (224,227,228). However, other factors probably play a role, since Mares-Perlman et al. (229) reported a beneficial effect in diabetics but not in non-diabetics, and Seddon et al. (230) found a protective effect for multivitamin preparations containing AA but not for AA supplements alone. Reviews on this subject include those of Taylor et al. (231), Christen et al. (232), and Das (233).

B. Age-Related Maculopathy

Since macular degeneration of the retina may be due in part to oxidative damage, the possible value of AA in modulating risk has been examined. However, five epidemiological studies found either no relationship or a slight but no significant protective effect of dietary or supplemental AA on the risk for macular degeneration (234–238). Reviews on this subject include those of Christen (232), Christen et al. (239) and Das (233).

C. OTHER DISORDERS OF VISION

Patients with optic neuritis and with significantly reduced blood AA levels appeared to have improved vision after receiving AA intravenously (240). The authors attributed the response seen to an effect on free radicals, but no other reports of this type have appeared in the literature. Administration of AA to patients prior to trabulectomy had no effect on the outcome of the surgical procedure (241).

IX.   ASCORBIC ACID STATES AND RESPIRATORY DISORDERS

An epidemiologic survey of 77,806 women with a 10-year follow-up concluded that AA status had no relationship to the incidence of asthma (242). An epidemiologic survey of 16 male cohorts over a 25-year period showed an inverse association between incidence of chronic obstructive pulmonary disease (COPD) and intake of fruits, but not for AA or other antioxidant vitamins (243). An epidemiologic survey of 793 men with a 25-year follow-up did not find any association between AA intake and the risk for chronic nonspecific lung disorders. (244). In contrast to these data, a survey of 2633 subjects found that FEV and FVC were significantly related to AA intake, and the investigators suggested that antioxidant vitamins may modulate the incidence of COPD (245). A smaller study in 178 subjects did not find any relationship between AA intake and lung function as measured by FEV (246). In an intervention study, administration of 1000 mg/day AA together with other antioxidants for 3 weeks in smokers improved pulmonary function and significantly decreased levels of exhaled ethane (247).

X.   ASCORBIC ACID AND DIABETES

Several studies have examined whether AA could be beneficial to diabetic subjects. Infusion of AA at a rate of 148 mg/min was reported to improve glucose metabolism in subjects with NIDDM (248), but no reports confirming these results have appeared in the literature. No difference in plasma AA was found in a comparison of NIDDM patients and healthy subjects; the authors concluded that AA status was probably not a factor in the coronary or renal complications of diabetes (249). No association was found between AA intake and glycosylated hemoglobin levels in diabetics, although an inverse association was noted in non-diabetics (250). Intervention studies have reported no effect of AA on fasting glucose (212) or insulin sensitivity (251), but high (mega) doses of AA have been reported to induce hyperglycemia (252,253).

XI.   OTHER USES OF ASCORBIC ACID

Administration of cisplatin combined with other chemotherapy caused a significant decrease in plasma AA (254). While plasma antioxidant levels returned to baseline prior to the next chemotherapy cycle, this observation suggests that AA supplementation may decrease adverse effects associated with oxidative stress induced by the treatment.

Patients undergoing dialysis have significantly reduced plasma AA levels (255–257). A titration study using different doses of AA concluded that daily administration of 150 to 200 mg was sufficient to maintain normal plasma AA levels (255).

The efficacy of AA in treating immune thrombocytopenic purpura was examined in patients who received 2000 mg/day for up to 7 months (258). A slight effect on platelet counts led the author to conclude that AA was not a suitable treatment for this condition.

A nutritional survey was undertaken using 196 patients with Crohn's disease and 124 with ulcerative colitis to determine whether AA status might be a risk factor for these conditions (259). However, no AA deficiency was found in any of the subjects.

Two clinical studies investigated whether administration of AA and vitamin E prior to coronary bypass surgery would affect the incidence of post-surgical myocardial or renal tubular injury (260,261). In both studies, administration of 1000 mg AA 12 hours prior to surgery had no effect on post-surgical complications.

The ability of AA to modify the sunburn response to ultraviolet (UV) radiation exposure was examined in ten subjects (262). Administration of 2000 mg day AA and vitamin E significantly increased the minimal erythema UV dose. This suggests that AA along with vitamin E can afford protection against sunburn.

A pilot study of the efficacy of AA and bioflavonoids in treating progressive pigmented purpura was conducted in three patients. Administration of 1000 mg/day AA and rutoside for four weeks resulted in complete clearance of the skin lesions in all the subjects (263).

An epidemiological study of 2744 postmenopausal women found no effect of AA on the incidence of gallbladder disease among those who did not consume alcohol. However, a significant inverse relationship was found among drinkers. The authors suggested that the AA–alcohol interaction may be related to an effect on cholesterol metabolism (264).

A survey of 21 hospital patients 75 years or older indicated that subjects who developed pressure sores had significantly lower (50%) levels of leucocyte AA (265). These data suggest that AA supplementation in this age group may reduce the incidence of pressure sores.

The ability of AA to modulate arthritic disorders was explored in two epidemiologic studies. A survey of 502 subjects found no relationship between AA status and symptoms of various arthritic disorders (266). Another survey of 149 subjects with osteoarthritis and 49 controls found no effect of AA status on the incidence of the disorder, but an inverse relationship between AA intake and the rate of osteoarthritis progression (267). In an intervention study, 81 rheumatoid arthritis patients received a diet containing fish oil and antioxidants including 200 mg/day AA. After 6 months, a significant improvement in mobility was noted, but the contribution of the individual dietary components to this response could not be determined (268).

A study of nutrient absorption in patients with systemic sclerosis was conducted in 30 patients and 30 controls (269). Serum AA levels in patients were 58% of the control while intake of AA was 84% of control values. These data suggest that AA supplementation might be of value in this disorder.

Administration of AA may protect against some of the gastrointestinal adverse effects of aspirin. In healthy volunteers, 900 mg aspirin was administered twice daily for three days combined with placebo or AA 1000 mg twice daily (270). AA had no effect on aspirin-related gastric injury, but appeared to protect against duodenal injury.

XII. INTERACTION OF ASCORBIC ACID WITH NUTRIENTS AND DRUGS

An epidemiologic survey of 746 individuals aged 60 or more resulted in the observation that increasing AA intake was associated with increased plasma levels of vitamin E and carotenoids (271). However, the authors did not propose a mechanism for this effect.

High doses of AA appear to inhibit aspirin absorption in healthy volunteers (272). This interaction may increase aspirin-induced gastrointestinal damage in subjects at risk for this adverse effect.

XIII. ADVERSE EFFECTS OF ASCORBIC ACID

Doses of AA in the RDI range (60–100 mg/day) are generally considered free of any adverse effects, but very high (mega) doses of 1000 to 10,000 mg/day have been reported to produce some side effects. These include hematuria or crystallinuria (273,274), tubulointerstitial nephropathy

(275), hemolysis in glucose-6-phosphate dehydrogenase deficiency (276), and interference with the ability of folic acid to normalize high homocysteine levels (277). An epidemiological survey of HANES II data did not find any relationship between AA intake and the risk of kidney stones, but (in women only) an association between AA intake and elevated serum ferritin levels was noted (278). In healthy adults, administration of 1000 to 10,000 mg AA/day for 5 days increased urinary oxalate excretion by 36 µmol/l, but this was attributed to an artifact of the analytical procedure (279). The potentially adverse effect of high AA doses on plasma glucose levels is mentioned in Section X. A review of the pharmacokinetics of high doses of AA concluded that limits to gastrointestinal absorption and plasma levels did not justify the use of very high AA doses (280). The safety of AA supplements has been reviewed by Bendich and Langseth (281).

XIV. SUMMARY AND CONCLUSIONS

Many free-living elderly populations continue to have significant proportions of individuals whose AA intake is marginal or below the RDI level. AA status as assessed by plasma AA concentrations is often reduced in the elderly when compared with younger adults. Additional research is needed to more clearly define the relative contributions of reduced AA intake to the biochemical changes (e.g., increased oxidative stress) associated with aging. The use of supplementary AA together with other vitamins and minerals should be encouraged to compensate for any dietary deficiencies.

Institutionalized elderly continue to have a high percentage of subjects with insufficient AA intake. Supplemental AA provides an efficient means of quickly correcting any deficiency or inadequacy and may have additional benefits such as improving immune response.

Epidemiologic studies have generally not found a relationship between AA intake and the risk for breast or colorectal cancer. However, the available evidence on intervention studies suggests that well-designed clinical trials should be conducted to determine whether high-dose (1000–3000 mg/day) AA supplementation has an effect on the course of these diseases. Adequate plasma AA levels appear to decrease the risk for gastric cancer, presumably due to inhibition of nitrosamine formation. There is also some indication that AA may be helpful in *H. pylori* infection. Additional research is needed to further clarify the mechanism of the beneficial effects of AA supplementation. Epidemiological and clinical studies have not shown any consistent relationship between AA intake and a variety of other cancers.

Reduced plasma AA levels in most studies that surveyed smokers suggests that vitamin supplementation should be especially encouraged in this group of individuals. Increased AA intake or AA supplementation may also reduce the risk of cardiovascular disorders associated with smoking.

AA supplementation in patients on dialysis and those susceptible to pressure sores appears to have some beneficial effect and should be explored further.

The available clinical and epidemiological evidence suggests that AA intake does not significantly affect the risk for Alzheimer's disease and Parkinsonism. However, the use of high-dose AA supplementation together with other anitoxidants during the early stages of these diseases should be explored to determine whether disease progression could be delayed.

The relationship between AA intake and a variety of cardiovascular disorders (coronary heart disease, myocardial infarction, stroke, congestive heart failure) is not consistent. Supplemental AA may benefit specific subgroups of patients, but additional research with well-designed clinical trials is needed. The clinical relevance of the ability of AA to inhibit plasma lipid oxidation and the relation of this property to the clinical course of cardiovascular disease also needs additional study.

Although there is no evidence that AA absorption or utilization is impaired in the elderly, AA intake at RDI levels or above has been linked to some health benefits in this age group. The current RDI for AA is 60 mg, but some researchers have suggested that 140 mg/day is needed to saturate body tissues, which is considered desirable (282). In this context, it is important to mention the interaction and synergy among the various nutrients. In the case of AA, its function is often influenced by the status of other nutrients in the body. In intervention trials where AA was not found to be beneficial or marginal, assuming that the dose and the duration were appropriate, supplementation with other vitamins and antioxidants might have made the difference. In addition, because of multiple nutrient inadequacies, normalizing the status of just one nutrient alone may not afford any benefit.

It should be noted that this chapter is an update of our two previous reviews and is therefore confined to papers published after 1992. It is for this reason that the evidence for a beneficial effect of AA in some situations does not appear to be strong or consistent because of the omission of the earlier literature. It is suggested that the reader also refer to our previous reviews for a more comprehensive picture of the importance of AA in the health of the elderly.

ACKNOWLEDGEMENT

The assistance of Mr. Ambrish Parekh in the preparation of the manuscript is gratefully acknowledged.

REFERENCES

1. Cheng, L., Cohen, M., and Bhagavan, H.N., Vitamin C and the elderly, in *CRC Handbook of Vitamins in the Aged*, Watson, R.R., Ed., CRC Press, Boca Raton FL, 1985, 157.
2. Cohen, M., Cheng, L., and Bhagavan, H.N., Vitamin C and the elderly—an update, in *CRC Handbook of Nutrition in the Aged*, Watson, R.R., Ed., CRC Press, Boca Raton FL, 1994, 203.
3. Inelman, E.M., Jimenez, G.F., Gatto, M.R.A., Busonera, F., Giantin, V., Tamellini, F., Zanettin, P., and Enzi, G., Energetic-vitamin intake in the usual diet of a non-institutionalized elderly sample, *G. Gerontol.*, 43, 313, 1995.
4. Cid-Ruzafa, J., Caulfield, L.E., Barron, Y., and West, S.K., Nutrient intakes and adequacy among an older population on the eastern shore of Maryland: The Salisbury Eye Evaluation, *J. Am. Diet. Assoc.*, 99, 564, 1999.
5. Kim, K.K., Yu, E.S., Liu, W.T, Kim, J., and Kohrs, B., Nutritional status of Chinese, Korean, and Japanese and American elderly, *J. Am. Diet Assoc.*, 83, 1416, 1993.
6. Maisey, S., Loughridge, J., Southon, S., and Fulcher, R., Variation in food group and nutrient intake with day of the week in an elderly population, *Br. J. Nutr.*, 73, 359, 1995.
7. Kafatos, A., Diacatou, A., Labadarios, D., Kounali, D., Apostolaki, J., Vlachonikolis, J., Mamalakis, G., and Megremis, S., Nutritional state of the elderly in Anogia, Crete, Greece, *J. Am. Coll. Nutr.*, 12, 685, 1993.
8. Caperle, M., Maiani, G., Azzini, E., Conti, E.M.S., Raguzzini, A., Ramazzotti, V., and Crespi, M., Dietary profiles and antioxidants in a rural population of central Italy with a low frequency of cancer, *Eur. J. Cancer Prev.*, 5, 197, 1996.
9. Pearson, J.M., Schlettwein-Gsell, D., Van Staveren, W., and de Groot, L., Living alone does not adversely affect nutrient intake and nutritional status of 70- to 75-year-old men and women in small towns across Europe, *Int. J. Food Sci. Nutr.*, 49, 131, 1998.
10. Hercberg, S., Preziosi, P., Galan, P., Devanlay, M., Heller, H., Bourgevis, C., Potier de Courcy, G., and Cherouvrier, F., Vitamin status of a healthy French population: Dietary intakes and biochemical markers, *Int. J. Vit. Nutr. Res.*, 64, 200, 1994.
11. Heseker, H. and Schneider, R., Requirement and supply of vitamin C, E, and beta-carotene for elderly men and women, *Eur. J. Clin. Nutr.*, 48, 118, 1994.
12. Gritschneider, K., Herbert, B., Luhrmann, P., and Neuhauser-Berthold, M., Antioxidant vitamin and selenium status in an elderly population of Giessen, *Zeits. Gerontol. Geriatr.*, 31, 448, 1998.
13. Hughes, K. and Ong, C.N., Vitamins, selenium, iron, and coronary heart disease risk in Indians, Malays, and Chinese in Singapore, *J. Epidemiol. Comm. Health*, 52, 181, 1998.
14. Benzie, I.F.F., Janus, E.D., and Strain, J.J., Plasma ascorbate and vitamin E levels in Hong Kong Chinese, *Eur. J. Clin. Nutr.*, 52, 447, 1998.

15. Mezzetti, A., Lapenna, D., Romano, F., Costantini, F., Pierdomenico, S.D., De Cesare, D., Cuccurullo, F., Riario-Sforza, G., Zuliani, G., and Fellin, R., Systemic oxidative stress and its relationship with age and illness, *J. Am. Geriatr. Soc.*, 44, 823, 1996.

16. Singh, R.B., Rastogi, V., Singh, R., Niaz, M.A., Srivastav, S., Aslam, M., Singh, N.K., Moshir, M., and Postiglione, A., Magnesium and antioxidant vitamin status and risk of complications of aging in an elderly urban population, *Magnes. Res.*, 9, 299, 1996.

17. Drewnowski, A., Rock, C.L., Henderson, S.A., Shore, A.B., Fischler, C., Galan, P., Preziosi, P., and Hercberg, S., Serum beta-carotene and vitamin C as biomarkers of vegetable and fruit intakes in a community-based sample of adults, *Am. J. Clin. Nutr.*, 65, 1296, 1997.

18. Paolisso, G., Tagliamonte, M.R., Rizzo, M.R., Manzella, D., Gambardella, A., and Varricchio, M., Oxidative stress and advancing age: Results in healthy centenarians, *J. Am. Geriatr. Soc.*, 46, 833, 1998.

19. Jarvinen, R., Knekt, P., Seppanen, R., Reunanen, A., Heliovaara, M., Maatula, J., and Aromaa, A., Antioxidant vitamins in the diet: Relationships with other personal characteristics in Finland, *J. Epidemiol. Commun. Health*, 48, 549, 1994.

20. Ghadirian, P. and Shatenstein, B., Nutrient patterns, nutritional adequacy, and comparison with nutrient recommendations among French-Canadian adults in Montreal, *J. Am. Coll. Nutr.*, 15, 255, 1996.

21. Velasquez-Melendez, G, Martins, I.S., Cervato, A.M., Fornes, N.S., and Marucci, M.D.F.N., Vitamin and mineral intake of adults resident in an area of metropolitan, S. Paulo, Brazil, *Brasil Rev. Saude Publica.*, 31, 157, 1997.

22. Woo, J., Leung, S.S.F., Lam, C.W.K., Ho, S.C., Tai-Hing L., and Janus, E.D., Plasma total antioxidant capacity in an adult Hong Kong Chinese population, *Clin. Biochem.*, 30, 553, 1998.

23. Tucker, K., Spiro, A. III, and Weiss, S.T., Variations in food and nutrient intakes among older men: age and other socio-demographic factors, *Nutr. Res.*, 15, 161, 1995.

24. Russell, R.M., Micronutrient requirements of the elderly, *Nutr. Rev.*, 50, 463, 1992.

25. Thurnham, D.I., Mircronutrients: how important in old age? *Eur. J. Clin. Nutr.*, 46 (suppl. 3), 529, 1992.

26. Russell, R.M. and Suter, P.M., Vitamin requirements of elderly people: An update, *Am. J. Clin. Nutr.*, 58, 4, 1993.

27. Koehler, K.M. and Garry, P.J., Nutrition and aging, *Clin. Lab. Med.*, 13, 433, 1993.

28. Chernoff, R., Effects of age on nutrient requirements, *Clin. Geriatr. Med.*, 11, 641, 1995.

29. Ward, J.A., Should antioxidant vitamins be routinely recommended for older people? *Drugs Aging*, 12, 169, 1998.

30. Lowik, M.R.H., van den Berg, H., Schrijver, J., Odink, J., Wedel, M., and Van Houten, P., Marginal nutritional states and institutionalized elderly women as compared to those living more independently, *J. Am. Coll. Nutr.*, 11, 673, 1992.

31. Asciutti-Moura, L.S., Guilland, J.C., Fuchs, F., and Richard, D., Vitamins E, C, thiamin, riboflavin, and vitamin B-6 status of institutionalized elderly including the effects of supplementation, *Nutr. Res.*, 13, 1374, 1993.

32. Van der Wielen, R.P.J., van Heureveld, H.A E. M., De Groot, C.P.G, M., and Van Staveren, W.A., Nutritional states of elderly female nursing home residents: The effect of supplementation with a physiological dose of water-soluble vitamins, *Eur. J. Clin. Nutr.*, 49, 605, 1995.

33. Schmuck, A., Ravel, A., Coudray, C., Alary, J. Franco, A., and Roussel, A.M., Antioxidant vitamins in hospitalized elderly patients: analyzed dietary intake and biochemical states, *Eur. J. Clin. Nutr.*, 50, 473, 1996.

34. Girodon, F., Lombard, M., Gulan, P., Brunet-Lecomte, P., Monget, A.L., Hinaud, J., Preziosi, P., and Hercberg, S., Effect of micronutrient supplementation on infection in institutionalized elderly subjects: A controlled trial, *Ann. Nutr. Metab.*, 41, 98, 1997.

35. Penn, N.D., Purkins, L., Kelleher, J., Heatley, R.V., Mascie-Taylor, B.H., and Belfield, P.W., The effect of dietary supplementation with vitamins A, C, and E on cell-mediated immune function in elderly long-stay patients: a randomized controlled trial, *Age Aging*, 20, 169, 1991.

36. Johnson, M.A. and Porter, K.H., Micronutrient supplementation and infection in institutionalized elders, *Nutr. Rev.*, 55, 400, 1997.

37. Kato, I., Nomura, A.M.Y., Stemmermann, G.N., and Chyou, P.H., Vitamin supplement use and its correlates among elderly Japanese men residing in Oahu, Hawaii, *Public Health Rep.*, 107, 712, 1992.

38. Gray, S.L., Hanlon, J.T., Fillenbaum, G.G., Wall, W.E., Jr., and Bales, C., Predictors of nutritional supplement use by the elderly, *Pharmacotherapy*, 16, 715, 1996.

39. Houston, D.K., Daniel, T.D., Johnson, M.A., and Pooh, L.W., Demographic characteristics of supplement users in an elderly population, *J. Appl. Gerontol.*, 17, 79, 1998.
40. Slesinski, M.J., Subar, A.F., and Kahle, L.L., Dietary intake of fat, fiber and other nutrients is related to the use of vitamin and mineral supplements in the U.S.: The 1992 National Health Interview Survey, *J. Nutr.*, 126, 3001, 1996.
41. Mares-Perlman, J.A., Klein, B.E.K., Klein, R., Ritter, L.L., Freudenheim, J.L., and Luby, M.H., Nutrient supplements contribute to the dietary intake of middle and older-aged adult residents of Beaver Dam, Wisconsin, *J. Nutr.*, 123, 176, 1993.
42. Buchman, A.L., Vitamin supplementation in the elderly: a critical evaluation, *Gastroenterologist*, 4, 262, 1996.
43. Thurman, J.E. and Mooradian, A.D., Vitamin supplementation therapy in the elderly, *Drugs Aging*, 11, 433, 1997.
44. Duthie, G.G., Arthur , J.R., Beattie, J.A.G., Brown, K.M., Morrice, P.C., Robertson, J.D., Shortt, C.T., Walker, K.A., James, W.P.T., and Rimm, E., Cigarette smoking, antioxidants, lipid peroxidation, and coronary heart disease, *Ann. New York Acad. Sci.,* 686, 120, 1993.
45. Singh, R.B., Niaz, M.A., Bishnoi, I., Sharma, J.P., Gupta, S., Rastogi, S.S., Singh R., Begum, R., Chibo, H., and Shoumin, Z., Diet, antioxidant vitamins, oxidative stress and risk of coronary artery disease: the Peerzada prospective study, *Acta Cardiol.*, 49, 453, 1994.
46. Buiatti, E., Munoz, N., Kato, I., Vivas, J., Muggli, R., Plummer, M., Benz, M., Franceschi, S., and Oliver, W., Determinants of plasma antioxidant vitamin levels in a population at high risk for stomach cancer, *Int. J. Cancer*, 65, 317, 1996.
47. Nyyssonen, K., Parviainen, M.T., Salonen, R., Tuomilehto, J., and Salonen, J.T., Vitamin deficiency and the risk of myocardial infarction: Prospective population study of men from eastern Finland, *Br. Med. J.*, 314, 634, 1997.
48. Phull, P.S., Price, A.B., Thorniley, M.S., Green, C.J., and Jacyna, M.R., Plasma free radical activity and antioxidant vitamin levels in dyspeptic patients: Correlation with smoking and *Helicobacter pylori* infection, *Eur. J. Gastroenterol. Hepatol.*, 10, 573, 1998.
49. Liu, C.S., Chen, H.W., Li, C.K., Chen, S.C., and Wei, Y.H., Alterations of small molecular-weight antioxidants in the blood of smokers, *Chem. Biol. Interact.*, 116, 143, 1998.
50. Pamuk, E.R., Byers, T., Coates, R. J., Vann, J.W., Sowell, A.L., Gunter, E.W., and Glass, D., Effect of smoking on serum nutrient concentrations in African-American women, *Am. J. Clin. Nutr.*, 59, 891, 1994.
51. D'Avanzo, B., LaVecchia, C., Braga, C., Franceschi, S., Negri, E., and Parpinel, M., Nutrient intake according to education, smoking, and alcohol in Italian women, *Nutr. Cancer*, 28, 46, 1997b.
52. Melhus, H., Michaelsson, K., Holmberg, L., Wolk, A., and Ljunghall, S., Smoking, antioxidant vitamins, and the risk of hip fracture, *J. Bone Miner. Res.*, 14, 129, 1999.
53. Grinberg-Funes, R.A., Singh, V.N., Perera, F.P., Bell, D.A., Young, T.L., Dickey, C., Wang, L.W., and Santella, R.M., Polycyclic aromatic hydrocarbon-DNA adducts in smokers and their relationship to micronutrient levels and the glutathione-S-transferase M1 genotype, *Carcinogenesis*, 15, 2449, 1994.
54. Kucuk, O., Pung, A., Franke, A.A., Custer, L.J., Wilkens, L.R., Le Marchand, L., Higuchi, C.M., Cooney, R.V., and Hsu, T.C., Correlations between mutagen sensitivity and plasma nutrient levels of healthy individuals, *Cancer Epidemiol. Biomarkers Prev.*, 4, 217, 1995.
55. Spitz, M.R., McPherson, R.S., Jiang, H., Hsu, T.C., Trizna, Z., Lee, J.J., Lippman, S.M., Khuri, F.R., Steffen-Batey, L., and Chamberlain, R.M., et al., Correlates of mutagen sensitivity in patients with upper aerodigestive tract cancer, *Cancer Epidemiol. Biomarkers Prev.*, 6, 687, 1997.
56. Fenech, M. and Rinaldi, J., The relationship between micronuclei in human lymphocytes and plasma levels of vitamin C, vitamin E, vitamin B12, and folic acid, *Carcinogenesis*, 15, 1405, 1994.
57. Fenech, M. and Rinaldi, J., A comparison of lymphocyte micronuclei and plasma micronutrients in vegetarians and non-vegetarians, Carcinogenesis, 16, 223, 1995.
58. Fenech, M., Chromosomal damage rate, aging, and diet, *Ann. N.Y. Acad. Sci.*, 854, 23, 1998.
59. Poulsen, H.E., Loft, S., Prieme, H., Vistisen, K., Lykkesfeldt, J., Nyyssonen, K., and Salonen, J.T., Oxidative DNA damage *in vivo*: Relationship to age, plasma antioxidants, drug metabolism, glutathione-S-transferase activity, and urinary creatinine excretion, *Free Radic. Res.*, 29, 565, 1998.

60. Gaziev, A.I., Sologub, G.R., Fomenko, L.A., Zaichkina, S.I., Kosyakova, N.I., and Bradbury, R.J., Effect of vitamin-antioxidant micronutrients on the frequency of spontaneous and *in vitro* gamma-ray-induced micronuclei in lymphocytes of donors: The age factor, *Carcinogenesis*, 17, 493, 1996.

61. Prieme, H., Loft, S., Nyyssonen, K., Salonen, J.T., and Poulsen, H.E., No effect of supplementation with vitamin E, ascorbic acid, or coenzyme Q10 on oxidative DNA damage estimated by 8-oxo-7,8-dihydro-2′-deoxyguanosine excretion in smokers, *Am. J. Clin Nutr.*, 65, 503, 1997.

62. Blot, W.J., Li, J.Y., Taylor, P.R., Guo, W., Dawsey, S., Wang, G.Q., Yang, C.S., Zheng, S.F., Gail, M., and Li, G.Y., et al., Nutrition intervention trials in Linxian, China: Supplementation with specific vitamin/mineral combinations, cancer incidence, and disease-specific mortality in the general population, *J. Natl. Cancer Inst.*, 85, 1483, 1993.

63. De Lorgeril, M., Salen, P., Martin, J.L., Monjaud, I., Boucher, P., and Mamelle, N., Mediterranean dietary pattern in a randomized trial: Prolonged survival and possibly reduced cancer rate, *Arch. Intern. Med.*, 158, 1181, 1998.

64. Eichholzer, M., Stahelin, H.B., Gey, K.F., Ludin, E., and Bernasconi, F., Prediction of male cancer mortality by plasma levels of interacting vitamins: 17-year follow-up of the prospective Basel study, *Int. J. Cancer*, 66, 145, 1996.

65. Pandey, D.K., Shekelle, R., Selwyn, B.J., Tangney, C., and Stamler, J., Dietary vitamin C and beta-carotene and risk of death in middle-aged men: The Western Electric Study, *Am. J. Epidemiol.*, 142, 1269, 1995.

66. Hertog, M.G.L., Bueno de Mesquita, H.B., Fehily, A.M., Sweetnam, P.M., Elwood, P.C., and Kromhout, D., Fruit and vegetable consumption and cancer mortality in the Caerphilly Study, *Cancer Epidemiol. Biomarkers Prev.,* 5, 673, 1996.

67. Goodwin, J.S. and Brodwick, M., Diet, aging, and cancer, *Clin. Geriat. Med.*, 11, 577, 1995.

68. Shibata, A., Paganini-Hill, A., Ross, R.K., and Henderson, B.E., Intake of vegetables, fruits, beta-carotene, vitamin C, and vitamin supplements and cancer incidence among the elderly: A prospective study, *Br. J. Cancer*, 66, 673, 1992.

69. Graham, S. Zielezny, M., Marshall, J., Priore, R., Freudenheim, J., Brasure, J., Haughey, B., Nasca, P., and Zdeb, M., Diet in the epidemiology of postmenopausal breast cancer in the New York State cohort, *Am. J. Epidemiol.*, 136, 1327, 1992.

70. Rohan, T.E., Howe, G. R., Friedenreich, C.M., Jain, M., and Miller, A.B., Dietary fiber, vitamins A, C, and E, and the risk of breast cancer: a cohort study, *Cancer Causes Control*, 4, 29, 1993.

71. Rohan, T.E., Hiller, J.E., and McMichael, A.J., Dietary factors and survival from breast cancer, *Nutr. Cancer*, 20, 167, 1993b.

72. Kushi, L.H., Fee, R.M., Sellers, T.A., Zheng, W., and Folsom, A.R., Intake of vitamins A, C, and E and postmenopausal breast cancer: The Iowa Women's Health Study, *Am. J. Epidemiol.*, 144, 165, 1996.

73. Negri, E., LaVecchia, C., Franceschi, S., D'Avanzo, B., Talamini, R., Parpinel, M., Ferraroni, M., Filbert, R., Montella, M., and Falcini, F., et al., Intake of selected micronutrients and the risk of breast cancer, *Int. J. Cancer*, 65, 140, 1996.

74. Jarvinen, R. Knekt, P., Seppanen, R., and Teppo, L., Diet and breast cancer risk in a cohort of Finnish women, *Cancer Lett.*, 114, 251, 1997.

75. Verhoeven, D.T.H., Assen, N., Goldbohm, R.A., Dorant, E., Van t'Veer, P., Sturmans, F., Hermus, R.J.J., and van den Brandt, P.A., Vitamins C and E, retinol, beta-carotene, and dietary fiber in relation to breast cancer risk: A prospective cohort study, *Br. J. Cancer*, 75, 149, 1997.

76. Ghadirian, P., Lacroix, A., Perret, C., Robidoux, A., Falardeau, M., Maisonneuve, P., and Boyle, P., Breast cancer risk and nutrient intake among French Canadians in Montreal: A case-control study, *Breast*, 7, 108, 1998.

77. Ambrosone, C.B., Coles, B.F., Freudenheim, J.L., and Shields, P.G., Glutathione-S- transferase (GSTM1) genetic polymorphisms do not affect human breast cancer risk, regardless of dietary antioxidants, *J. Nutr.*, 129, 565S, 1999.

78. Jain, M., Miller, A.B., and To, T., Premorbid diet and the prognosis of women with breast cancer, *J. Nat. Cancer Inst.*, 86, 1390, 1994.

79. Yuan, J.M., Wang, Q.S., Ross, R.K., Henderson, B.E., and Yu, M.C., Diet and breast cancer in Shanghai and Tianjin, China, *Br. J. Cancer*, 71, 1353, 1995.

80. Zhang, S., Hunter, D.J., Forman, M.R., Rosner, B.A., Speizer, F.E., Colditz, G.A., Manson, J.E., Hankinson, S.E., and Willett, W.C., Dietary carotenoids and vitamins A, C, and E, and risk of breast cancer, *J. Nat. Cancer Inst.,* 91, 547, 1999.

81. Baghurst, P.A., Carman, J.A., Syrette, J.A., Baghurst, K.I., and Crocker, J.M., Diet, prolactin, and breast cancer, *Am. J. Clin. Nutr.,* 56, 943, 1992

82. Lockwood, K., Moesgaard, S., Hanioka, T., and Folkers, K., Apparent partial remission of breast cancer in "high risk" patients supplemented with nutritional antioxidants, essential fatty acids, and coenzyme Q10, *Mol. Aspects Med.,* 15 (suppl.), S231, 1994.

83. Kumar, K., Thangaraju, M., and Sachdanandam, P., Changes observed in the blood of post-menopausal women with breast cancer, *Biochem. Int.,* 25, 371, 1991.

84. Ramaswamy, G. and Krishnamoorthy, L., Serum carotene, vitamin A, and vitamin C levels in breast cancer and cancer of the uterine cervix, *Nutr. Cancer,* 25, 173, 1996.

85. Bostick, R.M., Potter, J.D., McKenzie, D.R., Sellers, T.A., Kushi, L.H., Steinmetz, K.A., and Folsom, A.R., Reduced risk of colon cancer with high intake of vitamin E: The Iowa Women's Health Study, *Cancer Res.,* 53, 4230, 1993.

86. Neugut, A.I., Horvath, K., Whelan, R.L., Terry, M.B., Garbowski, G.C., Bertram, A., Forde, K.A., Treat, M.R., and Waye, J., The effect of calcium and vitamin supplements on the incidence and recurrence of colorectal adenomatous polyps, *Cancer,* 78, 723, 1996.

87. Enger, S.M., Longnecker, M.P., Chen, M.J., Harper, J.M., Lee, E.R., Frankl, H.D., and Haile, R.W., Dietary intake of specific carotenoids and vitamins A, C, and E, and prevalence of colorectal adenomas, *Cancer Epidemiol. Biomarkers Prev.,* 5, 147, 1996.

88. Slattery, M.L., Potter, J.D., Coates, A., Ma, K.N., Berry, T.D., Duncan, D.M., and Caan, B.J., Plant foods and colon cancer: an assessment of specific foods and their related nutrients, *Cancer Causes Control,* 8, 575, 1997.

89. Ghadirian, P. Lacroix, A., Maisonneuve, P., Perret, C., Potvin, C., Gravel, D., Bernard, D., and Boyle, P., Nutritional factors and colon carcinoma: A case-control study involving French Canadians in Montreal, Quebec, Canada, *Cancer,* 80, 858, 1997.

90. Zheng, W., Anderson, K.E., Kushi, L.H., Sellers, T.A., Greenstein, J., Hong, C.P., Cerhan, J.R., Bostick, R.M., and Folsom, A.R., A prospective cohort study of intake of calcium, vitamin D, and other micronutrients in relation to the incidence of rectal cancer among postmenopausal women, *Cancer Epidemiol. Biomarkers Prev.,* 7, 221, 1998.

91. Ferraroni, M., LaVecchia, C.D., D'Avanzo, B., Negri, E., Franceschi, S., and Decarli, A., Selected micronutrient intake and the risk of colorectal cancer, *Br. J. Cancer,* 70, 1150, 1994.

92. Fernandez, E., LaVecchia, C.D., D'Avanzo, B., Negri, E., and Franceschi, S., Risk factors for colorectal cancer in subjects with family history of the disease, *Br. J. Cancer,* 75, 1381, 1997.

93. LaVecchia, C., Ferraroni, M., Mezzetti, M., Enard, L., Negri, E., Franceschi, S., and Decarli, A., Attributable risks for colorectal cancer in northern Italyd, *Int. J. Cancer,* 66, 60, 1996.

94. Howe, G.R., Benito, E., Castelleto, R., Cornee, J., Esteve, J., Gallagher, R.P., Iscovich, J.M., Deng-ao, J., Kaaks, R., and Kune, G.A., et al., Dietary intake of fiber and decreased risk of cancers of the colon and rectum: Evidence from the combined analysis of 13 case-control studies, *J. Nat. Cancer Inst.,* 84, 1887, 1992.

95. Morgan, J.W. and Singh, P.N., Diet, body mass index, and colonic epithelial cell proliferation in a healthy population, *Nutr. Cancer,* 23, 247, 1995.

96. Paganelli, G.M., Biasco, G., Brandi, G., Santucci, R., Gizzi, G., Villani, V., Cianci, M., Miglioli, M., and Barbara, L., Effect of vitamin A, C, and E supplementation on rectal cell proliferation in patients with colorectal adenomas, *J. Nat. Cancer Inst.,* 84, 47, 1992.

97. Cahill, R.J., O'Sullivan, K.R., Matthias, P.M., Beattie, S., Hamilton, H.O., and Morlan, C., Effects of vitamin antioxidant supplementation on cell kinetics of patients with adenomatous polyps, *Gut,* 34, 963, 1993.

98. Greenberg, E.R., Baron, J.A., Tosteson,T.D., Freeman, Jr., D.H., Beck, G.J., Bond, J.H., Colacchio, T.A., Coller, J.A., Frankl, H.D., and Haile, R.W., et al., A clinical trial of antioxidant vitamins to prevent colorectal adenoma, *New Eng. J. Med.,* 331, 141, 1994.

99. Beno, I., Ondreicka, R., Magalova, T., Brtkova, A., and Grancicova, E., Precanceroses and carcinomas of the stomach and colorectum: the levels of micronutrients in the blood, *Bratisl. Lek. Listy,* 98, 674, 1997.

100. Carneiro, A.B.M., Aumond, M.D., Borges, F.B., Carvalho, L., and Forones, N.M., Evaluation of dietary pattern of patients with colorectal cancer, *Gastrentologia Endosc. Dis.*, 17, 96, 1998.

101. Pappalardo, G., Guadalaxara, A., Maiani, G., Illomei, G., Trifero, M., Frattaroli, F.M., and Mobarhan, S., Antioxidant agents and colorectal carrcinogenesis: Role of beta-carotene, vitamin E, and vitamin C, *Tumori,* 82, 6, 1996.

102. Ramon, J.M., Serra-Majem, L., Cerdo, C., and Oromi, J., Nutrient intake and gastric cancer risk: a case-control study in Spain, *Int. J. Epidemiol.*, 22, 983, 1993.

103. Hansson, L.E., Nyren, O., Bergstrom, R., Wolk, A., Lindgren, A., Baron, J., and Adami, H.O., Nutrients and gastric cancer risk, *Int. J. Cancer*, 78, 415, 1994.

104. LaVecchia, C., Ferraroni, M., D'Avanzo, B., Decarli, A., and Franceschi, S., Selected micronutrient intake and the risk of gastric cancer, *Cancer Epidemiol. Biomarkers Prev.*, 3, 393, 1994.

105. LaVecchia, C., D'Avanzo, B., Negri, E., Decarli, A., and Benichou, J., Attributable risks for stomach cancer in Northern Italy, *Int. J. Cancer*, 60, 748, 1995.

106. Freng, A., Daae, L.N., Engeland, A., Norum, K.R., Sander, J., Solvoll, K., and Tretli, S., Malignant epithelial tumors in the upper digestive tract: A dietary and socio-medical case-control and survival study, *Eur. J. Clin. Nutr.*, 52, 271, 1998.

107. Kaaks, R., Tuynsi, A.J., Haelterman, M., and Riboli, E., Nutrient intake patterns and gastric cancer risk: A case-control study in Belgium, *Int. J. Cancer*, 78, 415, 1998.

108. Zheng, W., Sellers, T.A., Doyle, T.J., Kushi, L.H., Potter, J.D., and Folsom, A.R., Retinol, antioxidant vitamins, and cancers of the upper digestive tract in a prospective cohort study of postmenopausal women, *Am. J. Epidemiol.*, 142, 955, 1995.

109. Van Loon, A.J.M., Botterweck, A.A.M., Goldbohm, R.A., Brants, H.A.M., van Klaveren, J.D., and van den Brandt, P.A., Intake of nitrate and nitrite and the risk of gastric cancer: A prospective cohort study, *Br. J. Cancer*, 78, 129, 1998.

110. Taylor, P.R., Li, B., Dawsey, S.M., Li, J.Y., Yang, L.S., Guo, W., Blot, W.J., Wang, W., Liu, B.O., and Zheng, S.F., et al., Prevention of esophageal cancer: The Nutrition Intervention Trials in Linxian, China, *Cancer Res.*, 54, 2029S, 1994.

111. De Sanjose, S., Munoz, N., Sobala, G., Vivas, J., Peraza, S., Cano, E., Castro, D., Sanchez, V., Andrade, O., and Tompkins, D., et al., Antioxidants, *Helicobacter pylori*, and stomach cancer in Venezuela, *Eur. J. Cancer Prev.*, 5, 67, 1996.

112. Andersson, S.O., Wolk, A, Bergstrom, R., Giovannucci, E., Lindgren, C., Benon, J., and Adami, H.O., Energy nutrient intake and prostate cancer risk: A population-based case control study in Sweden, *Int. J. Cancer*, 68, 716, 1996.

113. Daviglus, M.L., Dyer, A.R., Persky, V., Chavez, N., Drum, M., Goldberg, J., Liu, K., Morris, D.K., Shekelle, R.B., and Stamler, J., Dietary beta-carotene, vitamin C, and risk of prostate cancer: Results from the Western Electric Study, *Epidemiology*, 7, 472, 1996.

114. Ghadirian, P., Lacroix, A. Maisonneuve, P., Perret, C., Drouin, G., Perrault, J.P., Beland G., Rohan, T.E., and Howe, G. R., Nutritional factors and prostate cancer, *Cancer Causes Control*, 7, 428, 1996.

115. Vlajinac, H.D., Marinkovic, J.M., Ilic, M.D., and Kocev, N.I., Diet and prostate cancer: a case-control study, *Eur. J. Cancer Part A*, 33, 101, 1997.

116. Eichholzer, M., Stahelin, H.B., Ludin, E., and Bernasconi, F., Smoking, plasma vitamins C, E, retinol, and carotene, and fatal prostate cancer: Seventeen-year follow-up of the Prospective Basel Study, *Prostate*, 38, 189, 1999.

117. Deneo-Pellegrini, H., De Stefani, E., Ronco, A., and Mendilaharsu, M., Foods, nutrients, and prostate cancer: A case-control study in Uruguay, *Br. J. Cancer*, 80, 591, 1999.

118. Kune, G.A., Kune S., Field, B., Watson, L.F., Cleland, H., Merenstein, D., and Vitetta, L., Oral and pharyngeal cancer, diet, smoking, alcohol, and serum vitamin A and beta-carotene levels: A case control study in men, *Nutr. Cancer*, 20, 61, 1993.

119. Day, G.L., Shore R.E., Blot, W.J., McLaughlin, J.K., Austin, D.F., Greenberg, R.S., Liff, J.M., Preston-Martin, S., and Sarkar, S. et al., Dietary factors and second primary cancers: A follow-up of oral and pharyngeal cancer patients, *Nutr. Cancer*, 21, 223, 1994.

120. Freudenheim, J.L., Graham, S., Byers, T.E., Marshall, J.R., Haughey, B.P., Swanson, M.K., and Wilkinson, G., Diet, smoking and alcohol in cancer of the larynx: A case control study, *Nutr. Cancer*, 17, 33, 1992.

121. Gupta, P.C., Hebert, J.R., Bhonsle, R.B., Murti, P.R., Mehta H., and Mehta, F.S., Influence of dietary factors on oral precancerous lesions in a population-based control study in Kerala, India, *Cancer*, 85, 1885, 1999.

122. Kaugars, G.E., Riley, W.T., Brandt, R.B., Burns, J.C., and Svirsky, J.A., The prevalence of oral lesions in smokeless-tobacco users and an evaluation of risk factors, *Cancer*, 70, 2579, 1992.

123. Kirkpatrick, C.S., White, E., and Lee, J.A.H. Case-control study of malignant melanoma in Washington State, *Am. J. Epidemiol.*, 139, 869, 1994.

124. Hu, J., LaVecchia, C., Negri, E., Chatenoud, L., Busetti, C., Jia, X., Liu, R., Huang, G., Bi, D., and Wang, C., Diet and brain cancer in adults: a case-control study in Northeast China, *Int. J. Cancer*, 81, 20, 1999.

125. Tzonou, A., Hsieh, C.-C., Polychronopoulou, A., Kaprinis, G., Toupadaki, N., Trichopoulou, A., Karakatsani, A., and Trichopoulos, D., Diet and ovarian cancer: A case-control study in Greece, *Int. J. Cancer*, 55, 411, 1993.

126. D'Avanzo, B., Ron, E., LaVecchia, C., Franceschi, S., Negri, E., and Ziegler, R., Selected micronutrient intake and thyroid carcinoma risk, *Cancer*, 79, 2186, 1997a.

127. Zatonski, W.A., LaVecchia, C., Przewozniak, K., Maisonneuve, P., Lowencels, A.B., and Boyle, P., Risk Factors for gallbladder cancer: A Polish case-control study, *Int. J. Cancer*, 51, 707, 1992.

128. Kune, G.A., Bannerman, S., Field, B., Watson, L.F., Cleland H., Merenstein, D., and Vitetta, L., Diet, alcohol, smoking, serum beta-carotene, and vitamin A in male nonmelanocytic skin cancer patients and controls, *Nutr. Cancer*, 18, 237, 1992.

129. Lee, M., Wrensch, M., and Miike, R., Dietary and tobacco risk factors for adult onset glioma in the San Francisco Bay area, *Cancer Causes Control*, 8, 13, 1997.

130. Bruemmer, B., White, E., Vaughan, T.L., and Cheney, C.L., Nutrient intake in relation to bladder cancer among middle aged men and women, *Am. J. Epidemiol.*, 144, 485, 1996.

131. Vena, J.E., Graham, S., Freudenheim, J., Marshall, J., Zielezny, M., Swanson, M., and Sufrin, G., Diet in the epidemiology of bladder cancer in western New York, *Nutr. Cancer*, 18, 255, 1992.

132. Levi, F., Franceschi, S., Negri, E., and LaVecchia, C., Dietary factors and the risk of endometrial cancer, *Cancer*, 71, 3575, 1993.

133. Negri, E., LaVecchia, C., Franceschi, S., Levi, F., and Parazzini, F., Intake of selected micro-nutrients and the risk of endometrial carcinoma, *Cancer*, 77, 917, 1996.

134. Hu, J., Nyren, O., Wolk, A. Bergstrom, R., Yuen, J., Adami, H.O., Guo, L., Li, H., Huang, G., and Xu, X., et al., Risk factors for oesophageal cancer in Northeast China, *Int. J. Cancer*, 57, 38, 1994.

135. Tzonou, A., Lipworth, L., Garidou, A., Signorello, L.B., Lagiou, P., Hsieh, C.-C., and Trichopoulos, D., Diet and risk of esophageal cancer by histologic type in a low risk population, *Int. J. Cancer*, 68, 300, 1996.

136. Candelora, E.C., Stockwell, H.G., Armstrong, A.W., and Pinkham, P.A., Dietary intake and risk of lung cancer in women who never smoked, *Nutr. Cancer*, 17, 263, 1992.

137. Yong, L.C., Brown, C.C., Schatzkin, A., Dresser, C.M., Slesinski, M.J., Cox, C.S., and Taylor, P.R., Intake of vitamins E, C, and a risk of lung cancer, *Am. J. Epidemiol.*, 146, 231, 1997.

138. Steinmetz, K.A., Potter, J.D., and Folsom, A.R., Vegetables, fruit and lung cancer in the Iowa Women's Health Study, *Cancer Res.*, 53, 536, 1993.

139. Lee, B.W., Wain, J.C., Kelsey, K.T., Wiencke, J.K., and Christiani, D.C., Association between diet and lung cancer location, *Am. J. Respir. Crit. Care Med.*, 158, 1197, 1998.

140. Ghadirian, P., Boyle, P., Simard, A., Baillargeon, J., Maisonneuve, P., and Perret, C., Reported family aggregation of pancreatic cancer within a population-based case-control study in the Francophone community in Montreal, Canada, *Int. J. Pancreatology*, 10, 183, 1991.

141. Lindblad, P., Wolk, A., Bergstorm, R., and Adami, H.O., Diet and risk of renal cell cancer, *Cancer Epidemiol. Biomarkers Prev.*, 6, 215, 1997.

142. Yuan, J.M., Gago-Dominguez, M., Castelao, J.E., Hankin, J.H., Ross, R.K., and Yu, M.C., Cruciferous vegetables in relation to renal cell carcinoma, *Int. J. Cancer*, 77, 211, 1998.

143. Jama, J.W., Launer, L.J., Witteman, J.C.M., Den Breeijen, J.H., Breteler, M.M.B., Grobbee, D.E., and Hofman, A., Dietary antioxidants and cognitive function in a population-based sample of older persons: The Rotterdam study, *Am. J. Epidemiol.*, 144, 275, 1996.

144. Kalmijn, S., Feskens, E.J.M., Launer, L.J., and Kromhout, D., Polyunsaturated fatty acids, antioxidants and cognitive function in very old men, *Am. J. Epidemiol.*, 145, 33, 1997.

145. Mendelsohn, A.B., Belle, S.H., Stoehr, G.P., and Ganguli, M., Use of antioxidant supplements and its association with cognitive function in a rural elderly cohort, *Am. J. Epidemiol.*, 148, 38, 1998.

146. Schmidt, R., Hayn, M., Reinhart, B., Roob, G., Schmidt, H., Schumacher, M., Watzinger, N., and Launer, L.J., Plasma antioxidants and cognitive performance in middle-aged and older adults: Results of the Austrian Stroke Prevention Study, *J. Am. Geriat. Soc.*, 46, 1407, 1998.

147. Ortega, R.M., Requejo, A.M., Andres, P., Lopez-Sobaler, A.M., Quintas, M.E., Redondo, M.R., Navia, B., and Rivas, T., Dietary intake and cognitive functions in a group of elderly people, *Am. J. Clin. Nutr.*, 66, 803, 1997.

148. Riviere, S., Birlouez-Aragon, I., Nourhashemi, F., and Vellas B., Low plasma vitamin C in Alzheimer patients despite an adequate diet, *Int. J. Geriatr. Psychiatry*, 13, 749, 1998.

149. Perrig, W.J., Perrig, P., and Stahelin, H.B., The relation between antioxidants and memory performance in the old and very old, *J. Am. Geriatr. Soc.*, 45, 718, 1997.

150. Sinclair, A.J., Bayer, A.J., Johnston, J., Warner, C., and Maxwell, S.R.J., Altered plasma antioxidant status in subjects with Alzheimer's disease and vascular dementia, *Int. J. Geriatr. Psychiatry*, 13, 840, 1998.

151. King, D., Playfer, J.R., and Roberts, N.B., Concentrations of vitamins A, C, and in elderly patients with Parkinson's disease, *Postgrad. Med. J.*, 68, 634, 1992.

152. Fernandez-Calle, P., Jimenez-Jimenez, F.J., Molina, J.A., Cabrera-Valdivia, E., Vazquez, A., Urra, D.G., Bermejo, F., Matallana, M.C., and Codocco, R., Serum levels of ascorbic acid (vitamin C) in patients with Parkinson's disease, *J. Neurol. Sci.*, 118, 25, 1993.

153. Logroscino, G., Marder, K., Cote, L., Tang, M.X., Shea, S., and Mayeux, R., Dietary lipids and antioxidants in Parkinson's disease: A population-based, case-control study, *Ann. Neurol.*, 39, 89, 1996.

154. Ayuso-Peralta, L., Jimenez-Jimenez, F.J., Cabrera-Valdivia, F., Molina, J.A., Javier, M.R., Almazan De Pedro-Cuesta, J., Tabernero, C., and Gimenez-Roldan, S., Premorbid dietetic habits and risk for Parkinson's disease, *Parkinsonism Relat. Disord.*, 3, 55, 1997.

155. Scheider, W.L., Hershey, L.A., Vena, J.E., Holmlund, T., Marshall, J.R., and Freudenheim, J.L., Dietary antioxidants and other dietary factors in the etiology of Parkinson's disease, *Mov. Disord.*, 12, 190, 1997.

156. De Rijk, M.C., Breteler, M.M.B., den Breeijen, J.H., Launer, L.J., Grobbee, D.E., van der Meche, F.G.A., and Hofman, A., Dietary antioxidants and Parkinson's disease: The Rotterdam study, *Arch. Neurol.*, 54, 762, 1997

157. Anderson, C., Checkoway, H., Franklin, G.M., Beresford, S., Smith-Waller, T., and Swanson, P.D., Dietary factors in Parkinson's disease: The role of food groups and specific foods, *Movement Disord.*, 14, 21, 1999.

158. Foy, C.J., Passmore, A.P., Vahidassr, M.D., Young, I.S., and Lawson, J.T., Plasma chain-breaking antioxidants in Alzheimer's disease, vascular dementia, and Parkinson's disease, *QJM Mon. J. Assoc. Phys.*, 92, 39, 1999.

159. Hellenbrand, W., Boeing, H., Rubia, B.P., Seidler, A., Vieregge, P., Nischan, P., Joey, J., Oertel, W.H., Schneider, E., and Vim, G., Diet and Parkinson's disease II: A possible role for the past intake of specific nutrients, *Neurology*, 47, 644, 1998.

160. Linazasoro, G. and Gorospe, A., Treatment of complicated Parkinson's disease with a solution of levodopa-carbidopa and ascorbic acid, *Neurologia*, 10, 220, 1995.

161. Fahn, S., A pilot trial of high-dose alpha-tucopherol and ascorbate in early Parkinson's disease, *Ann. Neurol.*, 32 (suppl.), 5128, 1992.

162. Fickl, H. Van Antwerpen, V.L., Richards, G.A., Van der Westhuyzen, D.R., Davies, N., Van der Walt, R., Van der Merwe, C.A., and Anderson, R., Increased levels of autoantibodies to cardiolipin and oxidized low density lipoproteins are inversely associated with plasma vitamin C status in cigarette smokers, *Atherosclerosis*, 124, 75, 1996.

163. Keith, M., Geranmayegan, A., Sole, M.J., Kurian, R., Robinson, A., Omran, A.S., and Jeejeebhoy, K.N., Increased oxidative stress in patients with congestive heart failure, *J. Am. Coll. Cardiol.*, 31, 1352, 1998.

164. Halevy, D., Thiery, J., Nagel, D., Arnold, S., Erdmann, E., Hofling, B., Cremer, P., and Seidel, D., Increased oxidation of LDL in patients with coronary artery disease is independent from dietary vitamins E and C, *Arterioscler. Thromb. Vasc. Biol.*, 17, 432, 1997.

165. Nyyssonen, K., Porkkala-Sarataho, E., Kaikkonen, J., and Salonen, J.T., Ascorbate and urate are the strongest determinants of plasma antioxidant capacity and serum lipid resistance to oxidation in Finnish men, *Atherosclerosis*, 130, 223, 1997.

166. Reddy, K.K., Ramachandariah, T., Kumari, K.S., Reddanna, P., and Thyagaraju, K., Serum lipid peroxides and antioxidant defense components of rural and urban populations and aging, *Age*, 16, 9, 1992.

167. Stulnig, T.M., Jurgens, G., Chen, Q., Moll, D., Schonitzer, D., Jarosch, E., and Wick, G., Properties of low density lipoproteins relevant to oxidative modifications change paradoxically during aging, *Atherosclerosis*, 126, 85, 1996.

168. Zino, S. Skeaff, M., Williams, S., and Mann, J., Randomized controlled trial of effect of fruits and vegetable consumption on plasma concentrations of lipids and antioxidants, *Br. Med. J.*, 314, 1787, 1997.

169. Van de Vijver, L.P.L., Kardinaal, A.F.M., Grobbee, D.E., Princen, H.M.G., and Van Poppel, G., Lipoprotein oxidation, antioxidants, and cardiovascular risk: the epidemiologic evidence, *Prostaglandins Leukotrienes Essent. Fatty Acids*, 57, 479, 1997.

170. Gilligan, D.M., Sack, M.N., Guetta, V., Casino, P.R., Quyyumi, A.A., Rader, D.J., Panza, J.A., and Cannon, R.O. III, Effect of antioxidant vitamins on low density lipoprotein oxidation and impaired endothelium-dependent vasodilatation in patients with hypercholesteremia, *J. Am. Coll. Cardiol.*, 24, 1611, 1994.

171. Mosca, L., Rubenfire, M., Mandel, C., Rock, C., Tarshis, T., Tsar, T., and Pearson, T., Antioxidant nutrient supplementation reduces the susceptibility of low density lipoprotein to oxidation in patients with coronary artery disease, *J. Am. Coll. Cardiol.*, 30, 392, 1997.

172. Sakuma, N., Iwata, S., Hibino, T., Tamai, N., Sasai, K., Yoshimata, T., Kamiya, Y., Kawagichi, M., and Fujinami, T., Effects of vitamin C and vitamin E on plasma levels of lipid hydroperoxides and thiobarbituric acid reactive substances in humans, *Curr. Therap. Res.*, 58, 317, 1997.

173. Wen, Y., Cooke, T., and Feely, J., The effect of pharmacological supplementation with vitamin C on low density lipoprotein oxidation, *Br. J. Clin. Pharmacol.*, 44, 94, 1997.

174. Lavie, C.J., O' Keefe, Jr., H., Mehra, M.K., and Milani, R.V., Potential role of antioxidants in the primary and secondary prevention of atherosclerosis in the elderly, *Cardiol. Elderly*, 3, 21, 1995.

175. Price, J.F. and Fowkes, F.G.P., Antioxidant vitamins in the prevention of cardiovascular disease: The epidemiological evidence, *Eur. Heart J.*, 18, 719, 1997.

176. Manson, J.E., Stampfer, M.J., Willett, W.C., Colditz, G.A., Rosner, B., Spizer, F.E., and Hennekens, C.H., A prospective study of vitamin C and incidence of coronary heart disease in women, *Circulation*, 85, 885, 1992.

177. Gey, K.F., Staehelin, H.B., and Eichholzer, M., Poor plasma status of carotene and vitamin C is associated with higher mortality from ischemic heart disease and stroke: Basel Prospective Study, *Clin. Invest.*, 71, 3, 1993.

178. Singh, R.B., Ghosh, S., Niaz, M.A., Beegum, R., Chibo, H., Shoumin, Z., and Postiglione, A., Dietary intake, plasma levels of antioxidant vitamins, and oxidative stress in relation to coronary artery disease in elderly subjects, *Am. J. Cardiol.*, 78, 142, 1233, 1995.

179. Knekt, P., Reunanen, A., Jarvinen, R., Seppanen, R., Heliovaara, M., and Aromaa, A., Antioxidant vitamin intake and coronary mortality in a longitudinal population study, *Am. J. Epidemiol.*, 139, 1180, 1994.

180. Losonczy, K.G., Harris, T.B., and Havlik, R.J., Vitamin E and vitamin C supplement use and risk of all-cause and coronary heart disease mortality in older persons: The Established Populations for Epidemiologic Studies of the Elderly, *Am. J. Clin. Nutr.*, 64, 190, 1996.

181. Rimm, E.B., Stampfer, M.J., Ascherio, A., Giovannucci, E., Colditz, G.A., and Willett, W.C., Vitamin E consumption and the risk of coronary heart disease in men, New York, *N. Eng. J. Med.*, 328, 1450, 1993.

182. Kushi, L.H., Folsom, A.R., Prineas, R.J., Mink, P.J., Wu, Y., and Bostick, R.M., Dietary antioxidant vitamins and death from coronary heart disease in postmenopausal women, *New Eng. J. Med.*, 334, 1156, 1996.

183. Mandel, C.H., Mosca, L., Maimon, E., Sievers, J., Tsai, A., and Rock, C.L., Dietary intake and plasma concentration of vitamin E, vitamin C, and beta-carotene in patients with coronary artery disease, *J. Am. Diet. Assoc.*, 97, 655, 1997.

184. Rath, M. and Niedzwiecki, A., Nutritional supplement program halts progression of early coronary atherosclerosis documented by ultra fast computed tomography, *J. Appl. Nutr.*, 48, 68, 1996.

185. McBeath, M. and Pauling, L., A case history: lysine/ascorbate related amelioration of angina pectoris, *J. Orthomol. Med.*, 8, 77, 1993.

186. Sisto, T., Paajanen, H., Metsa-Ketela, T., Harmoinen, A., Nordback, I., and Tarkka, M., Pretreatment with antioxidants and allopurinol diminishes cardiac onset events in coronary artery bypass grafting, *Ann. Thorac. Surg.*, 59, 1519, 1995.

187. Levine, G.N., Frei, B., Koulouris, S.N., Gerhard, M.D., Keaney Jr., J.F., and Vita, J.A., Ascorbic acid reverses endothelial vasomotor dysfunction in patients with coronary artery diseasea circulation, 93, 1107, 1996.

188. Ito, K., Akita, H., Kanazawa, K., Yamada, S., Terashima, M., Matsuda, Y., and Yokoyama, M., Comparison of effects of ascorbic acid on endothelium-dependent vasodilatation in patients with congestive heart failure secondary to idiopathic dilated cardiomyopathy versus patients with effort angina pectoris secondary to coronary artery disease, *Am. J. Cardiol.*, 82, 762, 1998.

189. Gaziano, J.M. and Hennekens, C.H., Vitamin antioxidants and cardiovascular disease, *Curr. Opin. Lipidology*, 3, 291, 1992.

190. Law, M.R. and Morris, J.K., By how much does fruit and vegetable consumption reduce the risk of ischaemic heart disease? *Eur. J. Clin. Nutr.*, 52, 549, 1998.

191. Srinivasan, K.N., Pugalendi, K.V., Sambandam, G., Rao, M., Krishnan, S., and Menon, V.P., Comparison of glycoprotein components, tryptophan, lipid peroxidation, and antioxidants in borderline and severe hypertension and myocardial infarction, *Clin. Chim. Acta*, 275, 197, 1998.

192. Dusinovic, S., Mijalkovik, D., Saicic, Z.S., Duric, J., Zunic, Z., Niketic, V., and Spasic, M. J., Antioxidant defense in human myocardial reperfusion injury, *J. Environ. Pathol. Toxicol. Oncol.*, 17, 281,1998.

193. Klipstein-Grobusch, K., Geleijnse, J.M., den Breeijen, J.H., Boeing, H., Hofman, A., Grobbee, D.E., and Witteman, J.C.M., Dietary antioxidants and risk of myocardial infarction in the elderly: The Rotterdam Study, *Am. J. Clin. Nutr.*, 69, 261, 1999.

194. Laskowski, H., Minczykowski, A., and Wysocki, H., Mortality and clinical course of patients with acute myocardial infarction treated with streptokinase and antioxidants: mannitol and ascorbic acid, *Int. J. Cardiol.*, 48, 235, 1995.

195. Young, I.S., Purvis, J.A., Lightbody, J.H., Adgey, A.A.J., and Trimble, E.R., Lipid peroxidation and antioxidant status following thrombolytic therapy for acute myocardial infarction, *Eur. Heart J.*, 14, 1027, 1993.

196. Herbaczynska-Cedro, K., Klosiewicz-Wasek, B., Cedro, K., Wasek, W., Panczenko-Kresowska, B., and Wartanowicz, M., Supplementation with vitamin C and E suppresses leucocyte oxygen free radical production in patients with myocardial infarction, *Eur. Heart J.*, 16, 1044, 1995.

197. Keli, S.O., Hertog, M.G.L., Feskens, E.J.M., and Kromhout, D., Dietary flavonoids, antioxidant vitamins, and incidence of stroke: The Zutphen Study, *Arch. Intern. Med.*, 156, 637, 1996.

198. Daviglus, M.L., Orencia, A., Dyer, A.R., Liu, K., Morris, D.K., Persky, V., Chavez, N., Goldberg, J., Drum, M., and Shekelle, R.B., et al., Dietary vitamin C, beta-carotene, and 30-year risk of stroke: Results from the Western Electric Study, *Neuroepidemiology*, 16, 69, 1997.

199. Schmidt, R., Hayn, M., Fazekas, F., Kapeller, P., and Esterbauer, H., Magnetic resonance imaging white matter hyperintensities in clinically normal elderly individuals, *Stroke*, 27, 2043, 1996.

200. Zorzon, M., Vitrani, B., Biasutti, E., Mase, G., and Cazzato, G., Therapy with antioxidants in acute ischemic stroke, *Nuova Riv. Neurol.*, 6, 39, 1996.

201. Chang, C.Y., Lai, Y.C., Cheng, T.J., and Hu, M.L., Plasma status of antioxidant vitamins and oxidative products in ischemic-stroke patients during early post-stroke stage, *J. Appl. Nutr.*, 49, 77, 1997.

202. Watanabe, H., Kakihana, M., Ohtsuka, S., and Sugishita, Y., Randomized, double-blind, placebo-controlled study of ascorbate on the preventive effect of nitrate tolerance in patients with congestive heart failure, *Circulation*, 97, 886, 1998.

203. Watanabe, H., Kakihana, M., Ohtsuka, S., and Sugishita, Y., Randomized, double-blind, placebo-controlled study of the preventive effect of supplemental oral vitamin C on attenuation of development of nitrate tolerance, *J. Am. Coll. Cardiol.*, 31, 1323, 1998.

204. Donnan, P.T., Thomson, M., Fowkes, F.G.R., Prescott, R.J., and Housley, E., Diet as a risk factor for peripheral arterial disease in the general population, *Am. J. Clin. Nutr.*, 57, 917, 1993.

205. Leng, G.C., Lee, A.J., Fowkes, F.G.R., Horrobin, D., Jepson, R.G., Lowe, G.D.O., Rumley, A., Skinner, E.R., and Mowat, B.F., Randomized controlled trial of antioxidants in intermittent claudication, *Vasc. Med.*, 2, 279, 1997.

206. Moran, J.P., Cohen, L., Greene, J.M., Xu, G., Feldman, E.B., Hames, C.G., and Feldman, D.S., Plasma ascorbic acid concentrations relate inversely to blood pressure in human subjects, *Am. J. Clin. Nutr.*, 57, 213, 1993.

207. Bates, C.J., Walmsley, C.M., Prentice, A., and Finch, S., Does vitamin C reduce blood pressure? Results of a large study of people aged 65 or older, *J. Hypertens.*, 16, 925, 1998.

208. Wen, Y., Killalea, S., McGettigan, P., and Feely, J., Lipid peroxidation and antioxidant vitamin C and E in hypertensive patients, *Leukemia*, 10 (suppl. 2), 210, 1996.

209. Digiesi, V., Fiorillo, C., Oliviero, C., Gianno, V., Rosetti, M., Oradei, A., Lenuzza, M., and Nassi, P., Oxidative stress and antioxidant status in essential arterial hypertension, *Eur. J. Intern. Med.*, 9, 257, 1998.

210. Lovat, L.B., Lee, Y., Palmer, A.J., Edwards, R., Fletcher, A.E., and Bulpitt, C.J., Double-blind trial of vitamin C in elderly hypertensives, *J. Hum. Hypertens.*, 7, 403, 1993.

211. Ghosh, S.K., Ekpo, E.B., Shah, I.U., Girling, A.J., Jenkins, C., and Sinclair, A.J., A double-blind, placebo-controlled parallel trial of vitamin C treatment in elderly patients with hypertension, *Gerontology*, 40, 268, 1994.

212. Miller III, E.R., Appel, L.J., Levander, O.A., and Levine, D.M., The effect of 148 antioxidant vitamin supplementation on traditional cardiovascular risk factors, *J. Cardiovasc. Risk*, 4, 19, 1997.

213. Galley, H.F., Thornton, J., Howdle, P.D., Walker, B.E., and Webster, N.R., Combination and antioxidant supplementation reduces blood pressure, *Clin. Sci.*, 92, 361, 1997.

214. Chandra, R.K., Effect of vitamin and trace-element supplementation on immune responses and infection in elderly subjects, *Lancet*, 340, 1124, 1992.

215. Bogden, J.D., Bendich, A., Kemp, F.W., Bruening, K.S., Skurnick, J.H., Denny, T., Baker, H., and Louria, D.B., Daily micronutrient supplements enhance delayed-hypersensitivity skin test responses in older people, *Am. J. Clin. Nutr.*, 60, 437, 1994.

216. Jeandel, C., Alix, E., Boulos, N.C., Constans, T., Cournot, M.P., Giraudon, F., Herbeth, B., Jean, A., Lecompte, E., and Lettre, J., et al., Biological and immunological effects of antioxidant micronutrient supplementation in elderly long-stay hospital patients, *Ann. Med. Nancy Est*, 33, 433, 1994.

217. Buzina-Suboticanec, K., Buzina, R., Stavljelnic, A., Farley, T.M.M., Haller, J., Bergman-Markovic, B., and Gorajscan, M., Aging, nutritional status and immune response, *Int. J. Vita. Nutr. Res.*, 68, 133, 1998.

218. De la Fuente, M., Fernandez, M.D., Burgos, M.S., Soler, A., Prieto, A. Miquel, J., Immune function in aged women is improved by ingestion of vitamins C and E, *Can. J. Physiol. Pharmacol.*, 76, 373, 1998.

219. Chavance, M. and Herbeth, B., Does multivitamin supplementation prevent infection in healthy elderly subjects? A controlled trial, *Int. J. Nutr. Res.*, 63, 11, 1993.

220. Galan, P., Preziosi, P., Monget, A.L., Richard, M.J., Arnaud, J., Lesourd, B., Girodon, F., Munoz-Alferez, M.J., and Bourgeois, C. et al., Effects of trace element and/or vitamin supplementation on vitamin and mineral status, free radical metabolism and immunological markers in elderly long term-hospitalized subjects, *Int. J. Vitam. Nutr. Res.*, 67, 450, 1997.

221. Girodon, F., Galan, P., Monget, A.L., Boutron-Ruault, M.C., Brunet-Lecomte, P., Preziosi, P., Amaud, J., Manuguerra, J.C., and Hercberg, S., Impact of trace elements and vitamin supplementation on immunity and infections in institutionalized elderly patients: A randomized controlled trials, *Arch. Intern. Med.*, 159, 748, 1999.

222. Meydani, S.N., Vitamin/mineral supplementation, the aging immune response, and risk of infection, *Nutr. Rev.*, 51, 106, 1993.

223. Hughes, D.A., Effects of dietary antioxidants on the immune function of middle-aged adults, *Proc. Nutr. Soc.*, 58, 79, 1999.

224. Hankinson, S.E., Stampfer, M.J., Seddon, J.M., Colditz, G.A., Rosner, B., Speizer, F.E., and Willett, W.C., Nutrient intake and cataract extraction in women: A prospective study, *Br. Med. J.*, 305, 335, 1992.

225. Vitale, S., West, S., Hallfrisch, J., Alston, C., Wang, F., Moorman, C., Muller, D., Singh, V., and Taylor, H.R., Plasma antioxidants and risk of cortical and nuclear cataract, *Epidemiology*, 4, 195, 1993.

226. Wong, L., Ho, S.C., Coggon, D., Cruddas, A.M., Hwang, C.H., Ho, C.P., Robertshaw, A.M., and MacDonald, D.M., Sunlight exposure, antioxidant status, and cataract in Hong Kong fishermen, *J. Epidemiol. Community Health*, 47, 46, 1993.

227. Sperduto, R.D., Hu, T.S., Milton, R.C., Zhao, J.L., Everett, D.F., Cheng, Q.F., Blot, W.J., Bing, L., Taylor, P.R., and Jin-Yao, L. et al., The Linxian cataract studies: Two nutrition intervention trials, *Arch. Ophthalmol.*, 111, 1246, 1993.

228. Jacques, P.F., Taylor, A., Hankinson, S.E., Willett, W.C., Mahnken, B., Lee, Y., Vaid, K., and Lahav, M., Long-term vitamin C supplement use and prevalence of early age-related lens opacities, *Am. J. Clin. Nutr.*, 66, 911, 1997.

229. Mares-Perlman, J.A., Klein, B.E.K., Klein, R., and Ritter, L.L., Relation between lens opacities and vitamin and mineral supplement use, *Ophthalmology*, 101, 315, 1994.

230. Seddon, J.M., Christen, W.G., Manson, J.E., La Motte, F.S., Glynn, R.J., Buring, J.E., and Hennekens, C.H., The use of vitamin supplements and the risk of cataract among U.S. male physicians, *Am. J. Publ. Health*, 84, 788, 1994.

231. Taylor, A., Jacques, P.F., Epstein, E.M., Relations among aging, antioxidant status and cataract, *Am. J. Clin. Nutr.*, 62 (6 Suppl.), 1439S, 1995.

232. Christen Jr., W.G., Antioxidants and eye disease, *Am. J. Med.*, 97, 145, 1994.

233. Das, A., Prevention of visual loss in older adults, *Clin. Geriatr. Med.*, 15, 131, 1999.

234. Yannuzzi, L.A., Sorenson, J.A., Sobel, R.S., Daly, J.R., DeRosa, J.T., Seddon, J.M., Gragoudas, E.S., Pulialito, C.A., Gelles, E., and Gonet, R., et al., Antioxidant status and neovascular age-related macular degeneration, *Arch. Ophthalmol.*, 111, 104, 1993.

235. West, S., Vitale, S., Hallfrisch, J., Munoz, B., Muller, D., Bressler, S., and Bressler, N.M., Are antioxidants or supplements protective for age-related macular degeneration? *Arch. Opthalmol.*, 112, 222, 1994.

236. Seddon, J.M., Ajani, U.A., Sperduto, R.D., Hiller, R., Blair, N., Burton, T.C., Farber, M.D., Gragoudas, E.S., Haller, J., and Miller, D.T., et al., Dietary carotenoids, vitamins A, C, and E, and advanced age-related macular degeneration, *J. Am. Med. Assoc.*, 272, 1413, 1994.

237. Mares-Perlman, J.A., Klein, R., Klein, B.E.K., Greger, J.L., Brady, W.E., Palta, M., and Ritter, L.L., Association of zinc and antioxidant nutrients with age-related maculopathy, *Arch. Ophthamol.*, 114, 991, 1996.

238. Christen, W.G., Ajani, U.A., Glynn, R.J., Manson, J.E., Schaumbey, D.A., Chew, E.C., Buring, J.E., and Hennekens, C.H., Prospective cohort study of antioxidant vitamin supplement use and the risk of age-related maculopathy, *Am. J. Epidemiol.*, 149, 476, 1999.

239. Christen, W.G., Glynn, R.J., and Hennekens, C.H., Antioxidants and age-related eye disease: Current and future prospects, *Ann. Epidemiol.*, 6, 60, 1996.

240. Ichibe, Y. and Ishikawa, S., Optic neuritis and vitamin C, *J. Jpn. Ophthalmol. Soc.*, 100, 381, 1996.

241. Jampel, H.D., Moon, J.I., Quigley, H.A., Barron, Y., and Lam, K.W., Aqueous human uric acid and ascorbic acid concentrations and outcome of tabeculectomy, *Arch. Ophthalmol.*, 116, 281, 1998.

242. Troisi, R.J., Willett, W.C., Weiss, S.T., Trichopoulos, D., Rosner, B., and Speizer, F.E., A prospective study of diet and adult-onset asthma, *Am. J. Respir. Crit. Care Med.*, 151, 1401, 1995.

243. Tabak, C., Feskens, E.J.M., Heederik, D., Kromhout, D., Menotti, A., and Blackburn, H.W., Fruit and fish consumption: a possible explanation for population differences in COPD mortality, *Eur. J. Clin. Nutr.*, 52, 819, 1998.

244. Miedema, I., Feskens, E.J.M., Heederik, D., and Kromhout, D., Dietary determinants of long-term incidence of chronic nonspecific lung diseases: The Zutphen study, *Am. J. Epidemiol.*, 138, 37, 1993.

245. Britton, J.R., Pavord, I.D., Richards, K.A., Knox, A.J., Wisniewski, A.F., Lewis, S.A., Tattersfield, A.E., and Weiss, S.T., Dietary antioxidant vitamin intake and lung function in the general population, *Am. J. Respir. Crit. Care Med.*, 151, 1283, 1995.

246. Dow, L., Tracey, M., Villar, A., Coggon, D., Margetts, B.M., Campbell, M.J., Holgate, S.T., Does dietary intake of vitamin C and E influence lung function in older people? *Am. J. Respir. Crit. Care Med.*, 154, 1401, 1996.

247. Do, B.K.Q., Garewal, H.S., Clements, N.C., Jr., Peng, Y.M., and Habib, M.P., Exhaled ethane and antioxidant vitamin supplements in active smokers, *Chest*, 110, 159, 1996.

248. Paolisso, G., D'Amore, A., Balbi, V., Volpe, C., Galzerano, D., Giugliano, D., Sgambato, S., Varricchio, M., and D'Onofrio, F., Plasma vitamin C affects glucose homeostasis in healthy subjects and in non-insulin-dependent diabetics, *Am. J. Physiol. Endocrinol. Metab.*, 266, E 261, 1994.

249. Leinonen, J., Rantalaiho, V., Lehtimaki, T., Koivula, T., Wirta, O., Pasternack, A., and Alho, H., The association between the total antioxidant potential of plasma and the presence of coronary heart disease and renal dysfunction in patients with NIDDM, *Free Radic. Res.*, 29, 273, 1998.

250. Shoff, S.M., Mares-Perlman, J.A., Cruickshanks, K.J., Klein, R., Klein, B.E.K., and Ritter, L.L, Glycoslated hemoglobin concentrations and vitamin E, vitamin C, and beta-carotene intake in diabetic and nondiabetic older adults, *Am. J. Clin. Nutr.*, 58, 412, 1993.

251. Sanchez-Lugo L., Mayer-Davis, E.J., Howard, G., Selby, J.V., Ayad, M.F., Rewers, M., and Haffner, S., Insulin sensitivity and intake of vitamins E and C in African-American, Hispanic, and non-Hispanic white men and women: The insulin resistance and atherosclerosis study, *Am. J. Clin. Nutr.* 68, 1224, 1997.

252. Johnston, C.S. and Yen, M.F., Megadose of vitamin C delays insulin response to a glucose challenge in normoglycemic adults, *Am. J. Clin. Nutr.*, 60, 735, 1994.

253. Branch, D.R., High-dose vitamin C supplementation increases plasma glucose, *Diabetes Care*, 22, 1218, 1999.

254. Weijl, N.I, Hopman, G.D., Wipkink-Bakker, A., Lentjes, E.G.W.M., Berger, H.M., Cleton, F.J., and Osanto, S., Cisplatin combination chemotherapy induces a fall in plasma antioxidants of cancer patients, *Ann. Oncol.*, 9, 1331 1998.

255. Descombes, E., Hanck, A.B., and Fellay, G., Water-soluble vitamins in chronic hemodialysis patients and need for supplementation, *Kidney Int.*, 43, 1319, 1993.

256. Ha, T.K.K., Sattar, N., Talwar, D., Cooney, J., Simpson, K.O., Reilly, D., and St. J. Lean, M.E.J., Abnormal antioxidant vitamin and carotenoid status in chronic renal failure, *QJM. Mon. J. Assoc. Phys.*, 89, 765, 1996.

257. Hultqvist, M., Hegbrant, J., Nilsson-Thorell, C., Lindholm, T., Nilsson, P., Linden, T., and Hultqvist-Bengtsson, U., Plasma concentrations of vitamin C, vitamin E, and/or malondialdehyde as markers of oxygen free radical production during hemodialysis, *Clin. Nephrol.*, 47, 37, 1997.

258. Jubelirer, S.J., Pilot study of ascorbic acid for the treatment of refractory immune thromocytopenic purpura, *Am. J. Hematol.*, 43, 44, 1993.

259. Wasser, T.E., Reed, J.F., Moser, K., Robson, P., Faust, L, Fink, L.L., and Wunderler, D., Nutritional assessment and disease activity for patients with inflammatory bowel disease, *Gastroenterology*, 9, 131, 1995.

260. Westhuyzen, J., Cochrane, A.D., Tesar, P.J., Mau, T., Cross, D.B., Frennaux, M.P., Khafagi, F.A., Fleming, S.J., Effect of prospective supplementation with alpha-tocopherol and ascorbic acid on myocardial injury in patients undergoing cardiac operations, *J. Thorac. Cardiovasc. Surg.*, 113, 942, 1997.

261. Westhuyzen, J., Cochrane, A.D., Tesar, P., Mau, T., and Fleming, S.J., Effect of supplementation with antioxidants (alpha-tocopherol and ascorbic acid) on markers of renal tubular injury in cardiac surgery patients, *Nephrology*, 3, 535, 1997.

262. Eberlein-Konig, B., Placzek, M., and Przybilla, B., Protective effect against sunburn of combined systemic ascorbic acid (vitamin C) and D-alpha-tocopherol (vitamin E), *J. Am. Acad. Dermatol.*, 38, 45, 1998.

263. Reinhold, U., Seiter, S., Ugurel, S., and Tilgen, W., Treatment of progressive pigmented purpura with oral bioflavonoids and ascorbic acid: an open pilot study in 3 patients, *J. Am. Acad. Dermatol.*, 41, 207, 1999.

264. Simon, J.A., Grady, D., Snabes, M.C., Fong, J., and Hunninghake, D.B., Ascorbic acid supplement use and the prevalence of gallbladder disease, *J. Clin. Epidemiol.*, 51, 257, 1998.

265. Goode, H.F., Burns, E., and Walker, B.E., Vitamin C depletion and pressure sores in elderly patients with femoral neck fractures, *Br. Med. J.*, 305, 925, 1992.

266. Jacobsson, L., Lindgarde, F., Manthorpe, A., and Akesson, B., Fatty acid composition of adipose tissue and serum micronutrients in relation to common rheumatic complaints in Swedish adults 50–70 years old, *Scand. J. Rheumatol.*, 21, 171, 1992.

267. McAlindon, T.E., Jacques, P., Zhang, Y., Hannan, M.T., Aliabadi, P., Weissman, B., Rush, D., Levy, D., and Felson, D.T., Do antioxidant micronutrients protect against the development and progression of knee osteoarthritis? *Arthritis Rheum.,* 39, 648, 1996.

268. Hansen, G.V.O., Nielsen, L., Kluger, E., Thysen, M., Emmertsen, H., Stengaard-Pedersen, K., Hansen, E.L., Unger, B., and Andersen, P.W., Nutritional status of Danish rheumatoid arthritis patients and the effects of a diet adjusted in energy intake, fish-meal, and antioxidants, *Scand. J. Rheumatol.,* 25, 325, 1996.

269. Lundberg, A.C., Akesson, A., and Akesson, B., Dietary intake and nutritional status in patients with systemic sclerosis, *Ann. Rheum. Dis.,* 51, 1143, 1992.

270. McAlindon, M.E., Muller, A.F., Filipowicz, B., and Hawkey, C.J., Effect of allopurinol, sulphasalazine, and vitamin C on aspirin induced gastroduodenal injury, Gut, 38, 518. 1996.

271. Jacques, P.F., Halpner, A.D., and Blumberg, J.B., Influence of combined antioxidant nutrients on their plasma concentrations in an elderly population, *Am. J. Clin. Nutr.,* 62, 1228, 1995.

272. Ozdener, H., Amanvermez, R., and Celik, C., The interaction of aspirin and ascorbic acid absorption in healthy young individuals, *Ondokuz Mayis Univ. Tip Derg.,* 15, 319, 1998.

273. Iwamoto, N., Kawaguchi, T., Horikawa, K., Nagakura, S., Hidaka, M., Kagimoto, T., Takatsuki, K., and Nakakuma, H., Haemolysis induced by ascorbic acid in paroxysmal nocturnal haemoglobinuria, *Lancet,* 343, 357, 1994.

274. Auer, B.L., Auer, D., and Rodgers, A.L., Relative hyperoxaluria, crystalluria and haematuria after megadose ingestion of vitamin C, *Eur. J. Clin. Invest.,* 28, 695, 1998.

275. Nakamoto, Y., Motohashi, S., Kasahara, H., and Numazawa, K., Irreversible tubulointerstitial nephropathy associated with prolonged massive intake of vitamin C, *Nephrol. Dial. Transplant.,* 13, 754, 1998.

276. Rees, D.C., Kelsey, H., and Richards, J.D.M., Acute haemolysis induced by high dose ascorbic acid in glucose-6-phosphate dehydrogenase deficiency, *Br. Med. J.,* 306, 841, 1993.

277. Mix, J.A., Do megadoses of vitamin C compromise folic acid's role in the metabolism of plasma homocysteine? *Nutr. Res.,* 19, 161, 1999.

278. Simon, J.A. and Hudes, E.S., Relation of serum ascorbic acid to serum vitamin B12, serum ferritin, and kidney stones in U.S. adults, *Arch. Intern. Med.,* 159, 619, 1581999.

279. Wandzilak, T.R., D'Andre, S.D., Davis, P.A., and Williams, H.E., Effect of high dose vitamin C on urinary oxalate levels, *J. Urol.,* 151, 834, 1994.

280. Blanchard, J., Tozer, T.N., and Rowland, M., Pharmacokinetic perspectives on megadoses of ascorbic acid, *Am. J. Clin. Nutr.,* 66, 1165, 1997.

281. Bendich, A. and Langseth, L., The health effects of vitamin C supplementation, *J. Am. Coll. Nutr.,* 14, 124, 1995.

282. Jacob, R.A., Skala, J.H., and Omaye, S.T., Biochemical indices of human vitamin C status, *Am. J. Clin. Nutr.,* 46, 818, 1987.

3 Aging and Nutritional Needs

Waithira Mirie

CONTENTS

I.   INTRODUCTION

Aging is a normal and inevitable physiological process. However, how one ages depends on the interaction between their genetic makeup and other environmental factors including nutrition. Scientific evidence shows that the effect of a lifetime's nutritional practices compound for better or worse in later life. To date, this evidence continues to accumulate supporting the essential role of proper nutrition in preventing and delaying the onset of chronic diseases in later life. Causes of these chronic diseases are complex, and dietary factors are only part of the explanation, but it is evidently clear from epidemiological studies that there is a definite relationship between diet and health. The evidence supports the observation that personal health practices, including healthful dietary practices, lead to reduced risk of chronic diseases such as cardiovascular diseases, diabetes, and some types of cancer. Chronic diseases that account for the major causes of morbidity and mortality in later life have their pathological onset years earlier. An appropriate diet can lead to gains in quality of life and health in the elderly, helping to minimize potential health problems common in this group of people. The nutritional requirements of the elderly have been addressed, but there exist gaps in knowledge of their energy and nutrient needs. This chapter will discuss the nutritional needs of the elderly, and the effect of aging on nutritional requirements. The focus of this chapter is on the Recommended Dietary Allowance (RDA) for both men and women of 51 years and above.

II. RELATIONSHIP BETWEEN NUTRITION AND AGING

Nutrition interacts with aging in a variety of ways. Most bodily functions decline as the adult ages, a number of chronic degenerative conditions increase in frequency, and the aging process compromises the body's ability to obtain nutrients (1,2). This predisposes the elderly to nutritional risk, and as a result they suffer from malnutrition, which in most cases is a consequence of disease, inadequate diet, and certain social factors.

III. PHYSIOLOGICAL CHANGES IN THE ELDERLY

In the elderly there is measurable age-related deterioration in the functioning of most systems of the body. The rate of deterioration varies greatly between different systems. The intestinal epithelium takes a slower and later deterioration because there is replacement of dead cells as opposed to heart, brain, and muscle.

The major function of the GI system is to provide the organism with nutritive substances, vitamins, minerals, and fluids. Disorders and disease occur with age and involve all levels of the GI tract. GI changes affecting digestion and absorption may affect food consumption.

In the mouth, there is a decrease in the number of taste buds with age, which reduces taste acuity, and this can perhaps lead to increased use of salt and sugar. Between 75 and 85 years, the taste buds' deterioration is 65% reduction of sensitivity to sweet and salty tastes. There is a reduction in production of saliva in the mouth, which makes it difficult to moisten certain foods and causes difficulties with swallowing.

Poor dentition impairs biting and chewing abilities. Dentures are only effective if they fit, and the elderly person's state of oral health can affect food choices and the amount consumed, since the food selected is the soft type and certain foods are eliminated. Limited variety can also contribute to nutrient deficiencies. By age 65, most elderly people of the world are reported to no longer have their natural teeth. With age, there is atrophy of both the mucosal and muscle layers of the stomach. The amounts of digestive enzymes decrease but remain adequate for digestion. There is reduced gastric acid secretion, which may predispose the older person to GI infection that could reduce the efficiency of absorption of certain nutrients. The absorption rates of certain nutrients such as iron and calcium changes with the aging process, although the intestinal villi become shorter and broader and this reduces the absorptive surface area.

There is also a loss of muscle tone throughout the alimentary tract, which slows the digestive process and causes irregularity in elimination. A decline in gastric motility can cause constipation, which may reduce both appetite and nutrient availability. Constipation in the elderly is not only due to reduction in muscle tone of the GI, but also to lessened activity, ingestion of low-fiber foods, and inadequate fluid intake.

IV. CHRONIC DISEASE FACTORS

Chronic diseases impose the need for modified diets or interfere with tolerance for foods and ability of the elderly to manage their own diets. Therapeutic drugs used to manage these diseases may decrease absorption of nutrients and may also increase requirements for certain nutrients. These include prescription or over-the-counter drugs that are commonly used by the elderly. These drugs can cause malnutrition since they alter taste, affect appetite, and interfere with absorption of nutrients.

V.   NUTRITIONAL REQUIREMENTS

A number of researches have been conducted on the effects of aging on energy requirements and energy balance. The weight of the evidence from these investigations suggests that current RDA underestimate the usual energy needs of all ages (3). The nutritional requirements of the elderly are based on studies done on young adults and extrapolated, and therefore their requirements are basically the same. In absence of data to quantify possible differences, assumptions are made that the nutrient needs of the elderly are the same as for younger people. Setting dietary standards for older people is difficult, because individual differences become more pronounced as people grow older and develop nutritional problems, chronic diseases, physiological changes, and drug interactions, which all have an impact on nutrient needs.

VI.   KILOCALORIC NEEDS

The major physiologic change occurring with age is a decrease in number of functioning cells, which results in a slowdown of metabolic processes. Energy needs decline an estimated 3% per decade due to reduced physical activity and diminished lean body mass, hence slowed basal metabolic rate (BMR). The current RDA combines all people over 50 into one group. It is suggested that energy allowance for people between 50 and 69 years of age be kept at 1.6 basal and for over 70 be reduced to 1.5 basal. Pronounced differences in energy expenditure among individuals is noted with advancing age. Studies on nutritive intakes of older people have shown many deficits in energy intake, which appears to be related to many factors such as efforts to reduce weight, poor appetite, inability to afford food, irregular meal patterns, and poor dentition. Diets low in energy are invariably low in other nutrients such as vitamin and minerals. With low energy, protein is utilized for energy instead of protein synthesis, which leads to negative nitrogen balance. Inadequate energy and nutrient intake may account for fatigue, lassitude, and lack of interest in life. This can depress activity to the extent that the need for calories is reduced, leading to weight gain, even on a low-energy intake. The RDA for energy for men between 51 and 75 years is 2000 and 2800 kilocalories and for women of the same age group is between 1400 and 2000 kilocalories. For men 76 years and above, the range is between 1650 and 2450 kcal, and for women of the same age is 1200 and 2000 kcal. Due to variation in activity patterns of individuals, the range of daily caloric output is based on variation in energy needs of ± 400 kcal at any age, emphasizing the wide range of energy intakes appropriate for any group of people (3). Energy needs may vary by as much as 200 kcal per day for men and women between 51 and 75 years, 500 kcal for men above 75 years, and 400 kcal for women of the same age per day (4).

A. PROTEINS

Protein synthesis, turnover, and breakdown decrease with advancing age. Recent data suggests that requirements for protein often do not decline and may actually increase during disease exacerbations. It is recommended that the elderly have 0.6 g protein per kilogram body weight of high-quality and 0.8 g protein per kilogram body weight of medium-quality throughout life (5). Adequate caloric intake will facilitate proper protein utilization. Studies on the nutritional status of the elderly report poor intakes of good-quality protein sources, as well as negative nitrogen balance, edema, muscular weakness, poor wound healing, and a lowered body resistance to disease. These factors have been explained in part to be due not only to low protein intake, but also to incomplete digestion poor absorption, and insufficient caloric intake. In view of this, certain authorities argue that the elderly need more protein to allow for a greater safety margin to counteract the decreased absorption and protein losses due to illness, while others recommend a lower protein intake to reduce the need to excrete protein wastes from the deamination of protein, and avoid overburdening the kidneys, which work less efficiently with age (5). Generally, 12 to 14% of total calories per day from protein is seen as sufficient.

B. CARBOHYDRATE

Carbohydrates are good sources of energy, nutrients, and fiber. Fiber should be emphasized, as it has a role in the prevention of colonic cancer, and in the management of diverticulosis and constipation. A moderate intake of fiber is appropriate for bulk and elimination, and this will not pose risk of reducing absorption of mineral elements. The American Heart Association and the American Cancer Society recommend 55 to 60% of total daily calories to come from carbohydrate sources (6).

C. FATS/LIPIDS

Fats provide a source of energy, facilitate absorption of fat-soluble vitamins, and provide essential fatty acids. Reducing fat intake may retard the development of cancer, atherosclerosis, and other degenerative diseases seen in the elderly. A diet with 30% or less of total daily calories as fat, comprising 10% or less of saturated fats, is important for elderly people. This sums up to paying attention to quantity as well as the quality and type of fat consumed. A reduction in intake of saturated fats inevitably leads to a substantial decline in cholesterol intakes, because many sources of saturated fats are also rich in cholesterol.

D. WATER

Total body fluids decline with age. The need for water to aid in absorption, metabolism, and the excretion of nutrients and metabolites should be one of the prime dietary considerations in nutrition for the elderly (6). Dehydration is a major risk for elder adults. Thirst becomes a less sensitive indicator of need for fluid as people age. The kidneys function more efficiently when there is sufficient fluid with which to eliminate the waste solids. Water also stimulates peristalsis and thus aids in preventing constipation. It is recommended that between 6 and 8 glasses of water per day or 30 ml per kilogram body weight or 1 ml per kilocalorie is sufficient.

E. VITAMINS

Studies show that older adults often omit fruits and vegetables in their diets. This predisposes them to deficiencies of vitamins. There is no evidence that vitamin requirements are reduced with advancing years. It is safe to assume that older people need all the vitamins they did in earlier years.

1. Vitamin C (Ascorbic Acid)

Vitamin C is an important water-soluble antioxidant. Specific disease processes, e.g., cataracts, disorders of the immune response, and cancer, have been linked to oxidative damage mediated by the radicals. It has an effect in protecting against free radical-mediated oxidative tissue damage (as a reducing agent). The RDA for vitamin C for both men and women is 60 mg.

2. Vitamin D

Many elder adults have Vitamin D intakes of less than half of RDA. This is partly explained to be due to limited exposure to sunlight, and the fact that aging reduces the capacity to make vitamin D and the kidneys ability to convert it to its active form. Researchers suggest that vitamin D intake greater than RDA (5 μg or 200 International Units) in supplements may be necessary to prevent bone loss and to maintain vitamin D status in older people, especially in those who engage in minimal outdoor activity.

3. Vitamin A

Tolerance for preformed vitamin A appears to decrease with age because of increased absorption and decreased uptake by the liver. vitamin A storage in the liver is maintained or increased throughout the life span. Several studies have reported normal levels of plasma vitamin (20 µg/dl) even in older adults (7). There is little reason to expect a significant incidence of vitamin A deficiency among the elderly and the present RDA should be adequate to prevent insufficiency. Carotenes are provitamin A. Vitamin A has antioxidant properties that may protect against certain epithelial cancers (9). The RDA for vitamin A is 1000 for men and 800 for women. It is recommended that most of the vitamin A requirements be obtained from carotene-containing fruits and vegetables.

4. B-Complex Vitamins

Thiamin, niacin, and riboflavin intakes are closely related to levels of energy intake. The confusional states in the elderly might be related to a deficiency of thiamin. vitamin B_{12} is one of the B-complex vitamins that has been reported to be deficient in the elderly (9). Elderly people are particularly susceptible to metabolic and physiological changes that affect B_{12}, B_6 and folate status (7). One significant change is the loss of the ability to make stomach acid. This is related to the atrophic gastritis reported in 30% of people over 65 years. The deficiency of the vitamin may occur in people above 60 years due to gastric atrophy rather than with inadequate intake. Higher intakes of vitamin B_{12} than the current RDA might therefore be appropriate. The RDA for vitamin B_{12} is 2 µg. The deficiency of vitamin B_{12}, B_6, and folate has a bearing on the neurocogniture function, as well as the nervous system (10).

Vitamin B_6 intake correlates with protein intake favoring the supply of cofactor for enzymes in amino acid utilization. The RDA for this vitamin is 2.0 mg/day for men and 1.6 mg for women. As for vitamin B_1, B_2, and B_3, the requirements are lower to correspond with lower caloric requirements.

Vitamin E is an important fat-soluble antioxidant and the requirements are largely determined by polyunsaturated fatty acid content of the diet.

F. MINERALS

There is no indication for increasing minerals in normal aging. The same adult allowances are sufficient if provided on continuing basis though a well-balanced diet.

1. Iron

Iron deficiency anemia is the most common form of nutritional anemia (12). In post-menopausal women, this is caused by chronic blood loss from disease conditions, decreased absorption due to reduced acid secretion, use of medications such as antacids, or a diet low in iron. The RDA for iron is 10 mg/day for both elderly men and women.

2. Calcium

Long-term deficiencies of calcium deplete the calcium stores of the bone required to maintain the calcium level of the blood. Calcium absorption decreases with age due to a reduction in hydrochloric acid in the stomach, and low intake of vitamin D. There is progressive loss of bone density after 25 to 30 years of age; supplementation of calcium has proven effective in reducing this loss in elderly women. Development of osteoporosis affects a big number of the elderly. This is related to dietary as well as hormonal factors. Physical exercise as well as estrogen treatment is effective in restoring bone density. The RDA for calcium is 800 mg per day (6). It has been recommended that men over 60 years and women over 50 years increase calcium intake to 1200 mg to prevent development of osteoporosis. It is also suggested that individuals with more calcium deposited in the skeleton in childhood and bigger bones at maturity are better equipped to sustain the inevitable bone loss in later life.

3. Zinc

Zinc intake declines with aging as energy intake is reduced. In addition, older adults may absorb zinc less efficiently (11). Medication may impair zinc absorption or enhance its excretion, leading to a deficiency. Phytates, phosphates, dietary fiber, and protein also impair zinc absorption. Whether loss of taste acuity by the elderly is attributable to zinc deficiency remains unclear, as some studies show that zinc therapy may not be effective in diminishing loss of taste (11). RDA for zinc for men is 15 mg and 12 mg for women (13).

VII. CONCLUSIONS

There is overall agreement on the importance of nutrition in the care of the elderly and its influence on health and well being. The elderly constitute a heterogeneous group. There is a wide variation in their abilities to ingest, digest, absorb, and utilize nutrients, and therefore it is still difficult to confidently generalize about nutritional needs. What is clear is that individualized nutritional care must be employed. Whether the RDAs are adequate for the elderly or not, they are reasonable standards against which to gauge nutrient intake. However, we must appreciate that aging brings changed nutrient needs, either increasing or decreasing.

REFERENCES

1. Wahlguist M.L., Savige G.S., Likitow W., Nutritional Disorders in the Elderly. *Med. of Australia.* October 1995 163 (7) 376–81.
2. Mirie W., Aging and Nutritional Needs. *E. Afr. Med. J.* October, 1997 74 (10) 622–4.
3. Robert S.B., Dallar G.E., Effects of Age on Energy Balance. *Am. J. Clin. Nutr.* October 1009 68 (4).
4. Schlenger J.L., Pradignac A., Grunenberger F., Nutrition of the Elderly. A Challenge between Facts and Needs. *Holm Res* 1995, 43 (1–3) 46–51.
5. Millward D.J., Fereday A., Gibson N., Pacy P.J., Aging, Protein Requirements and Protein Turnover. *Am. J. Clin. Nutr.* October 1997, 66 (4) 774–86.
6. Eschleman M.M., *Introductory Nutrition and Diet Therapy.* J. P. Lippincott 1984.
7. Wood R.J., Suter P.M., Russel R.M., Vitamin and Mineral Requirements for Elderly People. *Am. J. Clin. Nutr.* September 1995 62 (3) 493–505.
8. Marchigiano G., Osteoporosis: Primary Prevention and Intervention Strategies for Women at Risk. *Home Care Providers.* April 1997 2 (2) 76–81.
9. Ubbink J.B., Should All Elderly People Receive Folate Supplements? *Drugs and Aging.* December 1998 13 (6) 415–20.
10. Irwin H.R., Joshua W.M., Nutritional Factors in Physical and Cognitive Function of Elderly People. *Am. J. Clin. Nutr.* 1992 55.
11. Favier A., Current Aspects about the Role of Zinc in Nutrition. *Rev. Prat.* January 1993 43 (2) 146–51.
12. Geoffrey P.W., Copeman J., *The Nutrition of Older Adults.* Arnold Publishers, 13. Geoffrey P.W. *Nutrition, a Health Promotion Approach.* Edward Arnold Publishers. England, 1996; London 1995.

4 Nutrition and Elderly Cancer Patients

Loris Pironi, Enrico Ruggeri, and Federico Mecchia

CONTENTS

The nutritional status of elderly patients with cancer appears to be the result of the concomitant effects of the aging process, the aging-associated diseases and conditions, the tumor mass, the cancer therapy, and the impact of the nutritional support (Figure 4.1).

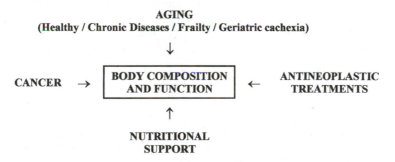

FIGURE 4.1   Factors contributing to the nutrition status of elderly patients with cancer.

I.   CHANGES IN BODY COMPOSITION AND METABOLISM IN AGING

Changes in body composition and metabolism, characterized by reduction in lean mass, total body water and bone mass, by increased fat mass, and by decreased resting energy expenditure (REE) are known to occur during aging.[1] These modifications are associated with variations in the secretion of hormones that regulate body composition.[2] Growth hormone (GH), sex hormones, and triiodothyronine (T_3) decrease. Insulin secretion decreases, and a state of insulin resistance occurs. Prolactin and cortisol secretions increase. Decreased GH, testosterone, and insulin secretion, in association with increased cortisol, are considered to account for the decreased muscle mass, whereas increased prolactin is considered to play a role in increasing fat mass. Diminished muscle mass is considered to be the main factor responsible for the decline in REE observed with age.

II.   MALNUTRITION IN THE ELDERLY

Elderly people are also at increased risk of malnutrition because of physiological, pathophysiological, psychological and socioeconomic factors associated with aging.[3] Prevalence of malnutrition has been rated as 0 to 15% in ambulatory outpatients, 5 to 12% in homebound patients with chronic diseases, 26 to 59% in institutionalized elderly persons, and 17 to 75% in hospitalized elderly patients.[4-10] The frequency of malnutrition is influenced by the clinical setting and the functional status of the patient population under study. These factors mirror the health conditions (presence of comorbidity) and the degree of frailty, a term that defines an unsteady condition between health-maintaining capacity (health functional status, availability of resources) and the emerging deficits (illness, disability, dependence on others, burden of care-givers, etc.).[11] Protein-energy malnutrition (PEM) in geriatric populations has been reported to be independently associated with increased morbidity and mortality.[12,13] On the other hand, in some disease states, the efficacy of nutritional support in reversing the risk of morbidity and mortality due to malnutrition has been demonstrated.[14-16]

In addition to PEM due to comorbidity and frailty, elderly subjects can develop a cachectic syndrome whose pathogenesis has not been clarified. This so-called geriatric cachexia is associated with anorexia and has been demonstrated to be an independent risk factor of death.[17] Geriatric cachexia seems related to increased production of the proinflammatory cytokines, tumor necrosis factor α (TNF-α, interleukin (IL)-1, IL-6, and interferon (IFN-γ), and of serotonin, which are well-known mediators of cancer cachexia as well (Table 4.1).

III.   CANCER CACHEXIA

PEM is a frequent finding in patients with cancer, mainly due to factors related to the tumor, even though a contributory role is played by antineoplastic treatments. Prevalence of PEM in cancer varies according to the type and the stage of the tumor (Figure 4.2). Incidence of weight loss was found to be greatest (83–87%) in cancer of the stomach and pancreas, intermediate (48–61%) in cancer of the colon, prostate, lung or with unfavorable non-Hodgkin lymphoma, lowest (31–40%) in non-Hodgkin lymphoma, breast cancer, sarcoma, or acute non-linphocitic leukemia.[18] PEM is not related to the histological variety of the cancer, the type of tumor spread, the tumor size, or patient age.[18]

In cancer patients, the degree of PEM is greater in the advanced stage of the disease, when it assumes the feature of cancer cachexia.[19] This syndrome is characterized by anorexia, extensive weight loss, and derangement of body composition.[19] A great proportion of weight loss is fat loss. Loss of lean body mass is smaller than that of fat mass and involves mainly the muscle proteins. The percentage of body water content increases and a state of hyperhydration appears. Decrease of visceral protein mass occurs later. Cancer cachexia is considered to be the result of decreased food intake and metabolic abnormalities characteristic of the interaction between tumor and host.

Anorexia, defined as spontaneous decline in food intake due to reduced appetite, can have various causes: effects of cytokines (TNF-α, IL-1, IL-6, and IFN-γ), disorders in central nervous system regulatory mechanisms, acquired taste disorders, nausea, vomiting and psychological problems. Food intake is regulated in the ventromedial nucleus of the hypothalamus by several neuropeptides (leptin, neuropeptide Y, insulin, galanin, endorphins, cholecystokinin) and neurotransmitters (serotonin, norepinephrin).[21] Studies on animals indicate that cancer anorexia can be due to an increase of cerebral serotonin as a consequence of the alteration of tryptophan metabolism,

TABLE 4.1

Changes in Body Composition, Metabolic Mediators and Resting Energy Expenditure (REE) in Healthy Aging, Chronic Starvation, Cancer Cachexia or Geriatric Cachexia

	Healthy Aging	Uncomplicated Starvation	Cancer Cachexia	Geriatric Cachexia
Body Composition				
Body weight	=	↓	↓↓	↓
Lean body mass	↓	=/↓	↓	↓
Fat mass	↑	↓↓	↓↓	↓
Body water	↓	↓	↑	
Protein Turnover		↓	↑	↑
Mediators				
GH	↓	↓	↓	
Insulin	↓?	↓	↑/=/↓	
	Insulin resistance		Insulin resistance	
Glucagon		↓	↑	
Cortisol	=/↓	↓	↑	
Catecholamines	↑		↑	
Triiodothyronine	=/↓?	↓	↓	
Prolactin	↑?			
Sex-steroids	↓		↓	
TNF-α		↓	↑	↑
IFN-γ			↑	
IL-1		↓	↑	↑
IL-2			↑	
IL-6		↓	↑	↑
Serotonine			↑ In brain	↑ In CSF
REE	↓	↓	↑	↑

Note: GH = Growth hormone; TNF = tumor necrosis factor; INF = interferon; IL = interleukin; CSF = cerebrospinal fluid.

the amino acid from which serotonin derives.[22] Anorexia could also depend on alterations, caused by metastasis, of the center of appetite in the lateral hypothalmus. Changes in the perception of taste have been noted, with an increase in the threshold for sweet flavors (observed in about a third of patients) and reduction in the perception of bitter taste, salt, and acid (observed less frequently).[23-25] The causes have not been clarified, but a deficit of some trace metals could be involved. General losses of taste after head and neck irradiation and development of metallic tastes following chemotherapy are due to direct damage to the taste receptors of the tongue.[26] Bernstein et al. demonstrated the development of taste aversion in children during chemotherapy, and suggested avoiding patient's favorite foods on the days of the therapy.[27]

Metabolic abnormalities involve glucose, protein, lipid, and energy metabolism.[28,29] Glucose intolerance, increased glucose production, and decreased whole body glucose utilization are the documented abnormalities of glucose metabolism. Glucose intolerance is due to insulin resistance, which results in decreased glucose disposal rate and in decreased liver glycogen synthesis.[30] Increased gluconeogenesis (liver and kidney) is sustained mainly by increased peripheral lactate production (Cori cycle) and to a lesser extent by alanine and glycerol.[31-34] Animal and human studies demonstrated that insulin resistance to carbohydrate metabolism did not affect protein metabolism, thus sparing the anabolic effect of insulin on muscle protein synthesis.[35-37] Several studies have

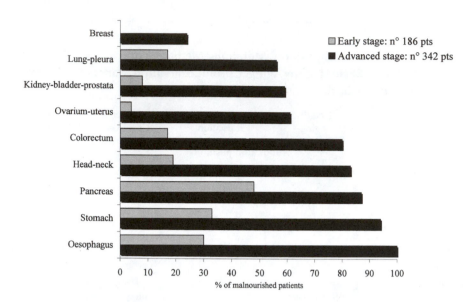

FIGURE 4.2 Frequency of malnutrition (BMI < 20) in cancer patients in different stages of the disease.

demonstrated that the tumor mass contributes in a minor extent to the overall increase in anaerobic glycolysis and lactate production.[38,39] Increased protein turnover and muscle wasting characterize protein metabolism in cancer cachexia. In cancer patients, increased whole-body protein turnover has been documented for skeletal muscle,[40-43] liver,[44] and gastrointestinal mucosa,[45] whereas heart, lung, and the kidney, appear to remain unaffected.[46-48] Muscle wasting is sustained by reduced protein synthesis[46,49] associated with normal or increased breakdown.[46,50,51] Protein loss appears to be limited to myofibrillar proteins, whereas sarcoplasmatic and extracellular proteins have been reported to be increased by approximately 25 to 30%.[52] Increased hepatic turnover is associated with a switch of protein synthesis characterized by increased synthesis of acute phase proteins and decreased visceral protein synthesis.[53-55] Cancer cachexia is associated with increased lipid mobilization from adipose tissue, decreased lipid plasma clearance, and hypertriglyceridemia. Loss of adipose tissue and hyperlipidemia are attributed both to increased lipolysis[31,56] and decreased plasma clearance of free fatty acids and VLDL (tryglycerides),[57] related to a decrease of lipoprotein lipase activity,[57,58] impaired lipogenesis,[59] and increased lipolysis,[31,60] whereas lipid oxidation does not seem to be affected.[61]

Several studies have demonstrated increased REE in cancer patients.[62] The measured REE was 4 to 40% greater than basal energy expenditure calculated by the Harris–Benedict formula.[62-66] It is suggested that increased REE contributes to weight loss, but unchanged and hypometabolic responses have also been described in 20 to 40% of patients.[64,65] Peacock et al.[67] observed that REE corrected for body cell mass was greater in noncachectic male patients with sarcoma than in healthy controls. The difference was due to both increased REE and reduced body cell mass. This result suggests that malnourished cancer patients with normal or low REE may be hypermetabolic relative to the amount of lean body mass. Furthermore, in cases of semistarvation, REE usually declines. The finding that malnourished cancer patients have normal REE may represent an abnormal adaptation to starvation. Hypermetabolism is almost entirely due to the tumor-induced alterations of host metabolism, mainly to those related to the increase of glucose turnover.[54] A smaller contribution seems to be due to the increased protein turnover. Considering that the tumor mass represents a very small percentage of body weight (less than 4 to 5%), it is unlikely that increased REE is related to tumor cell metabolism.

In tumor-bearing animals, tumor-induced anorexia and weight loss was shown to be transmittable through plasma factors.[68,69] It is assumed that cachexia is sustained by mediators of the inflammatory response, classical hormones, and other regulatory peptides (Tables 4.1 and 4.2). Early studies investigated the effects of the tumor on the hormones that regulate the host's metabolism, reporting several abnormalities. These problems can be due to either ectopic hormone syndromes or to endocrine dysfunctions, which result from the endocrine response of the host to the cancer mass. The hormone profile changes rapidly in malnourished cancer patients[70] and in animals after tumor transplantation,[71] and some of the changes are in the opposite direction to the adaptation observed in uncomplicated starvation. In malnourished cancer patients, increased 24-h urinary excretion of cortisol was observed, but plasma cortisol has been reported to be normal.[70] In tumor-bearing animals, increased plasma cortis[72] and hypertrophy of the adrenal gland not responsive to hypophysectom[73] were shown. However, no relationship was demonstrated between tumor mass and plasma corticosteroids.[74] In animals, but not in humans,[64] increased adrenaline and noradrenaline secretion, proportional to tumor mass, has been observed.[75] The role of corticosteroids and catecholamine in cancer cachexia is still uncertain, but it is considered that cortisol plays a role in insulin resistance and in impairment of glucose metabolism. Increased serum glucagon levels have been reported both in cancer patients[76] and in tumor-bearing animals.[75] In animals, hyperglucagonemia correlated with the tumor burden.[74] The decreased host insulin/glucagon ratios observed in cancer patients could contribute to the abnormalities of the glucose metabolism in cancer cachexia.[77] T_3 serum concentrations can be low in patients with cancer cachexia, a finding that is considered a normal adaptation process aimed at the conservation of energy by reducing the effect of T_3 on the REE in prolonged starvation.[78] Abnormalities in insulin secretion and function are frequent findings in cancer patients. Both low[75] and slightly increased[79] serum insulin concentrations have been reported. Recently, in both malnourished and normal nourished patients with head and neck cancer, Tayek et al. demonstrated a reduced first insulin phase response to intravenous glucose similar to that seen in type 2 diabetes.[80] Reduced insulin response correlated with reduced glucose disposal rate. As multiple regression analysis demonstrated that glucose disposal rate correlated directly with both insulin response and T_3 concentrations, a role for reduced T_3 concentration in the pathogenesis of abnormalities of glucose metabolism was also suggested. A wide range of fasting serum concentrations of growth hormone (GH) was reported in lung and colorectal cancer patients.[81] Concentrations were greater in the more malnourished patients. However, no direct correlation between GH secretion and metabolic abnormalities, such as increased hepatic glucose production, have been observed.

More recently, the role of cytokines in cancer cachexia has been investigated. Cytokines, as well as regulating the immune reaction, have a series of secondary effects on the host's metabolism. In the short term, these effects serve to move on the acute phase of the response to the tumor, sending the nutrients from the peripheral tissue to the liver for the synthesis of the acute phase proteins (C reactive protein, α-1 antitrypsin, 2-macroglobulin, etc.). The protraction of these effects in time is considered the main pathogenetic factor of both anorexia and alterations in the metabolism of nutrients, which are seen in the more advanced stages of the illness.[30] TNF-α, IL-1, IL-6, and IFN-γ have been the cytokines most extensively studied.[44,82-84] TNF-α can cause anorexia and most of the metabolic alterations observed in cancer. Intravenous administration of TNF-α produced anorexia and metabolic changes (increased glycogenolysis, increased peripheral lactate production, increased muscle protein breakdown, decreased lipoprotein lipase activity, and hypertriglyceridemia) as observed in wasting and cachectic disease states.[82,88-93] Furthermore, TNF-α can induce the production of IL-1 and IL-6.[94] In both cancer patients and tumor-bearing animals, increased TNF-α plasma levels have been shown.[95,96] In rats, the administration of anti-TNF-α attenuated cachexia induced by the implantation of tumor.[97-99] IL-1 shares most of the metabolic effects of TNF-α.[99] Some studies on animals demonstrated that IL-1 induces anorexia, loss of body protein, and a change in hepatic protein synthesis similar to that seen in cancer patients[85,86,100] (decrease of albumin and other visceral protein synthesis and increase of acute phase protein synthesis). In mice, these alterations were reverted by antibody against IL-1 receptor.[85] Jensen et al.[101] demonstrated increased IL-1 gene expression in the liver of cachectic tumor-bearing rats, but in both animals

TABLE 4.2
Metabolic Changes in Cancer Cachexia

	Changes	Suggested Mediators
• Carbohydrate Metabolism		
Serum glucose	↓ / = / ↑	
Hepatic production of glucose:	↑	
Gluconeogenesis	↑	↑ Cortisol, ↑ glucagon, TNF-α, IL-1
Glycogenolysis	↑	TNF-α
Cori cycle activity (lactate production)	↑	TNF-α
Glucose disposal and utilization	↓	Insulin resistance, ↓ FT3, TNF-α
Nonoxidative disposal	↓	
Glucose oxidation	= / ↓	
Glycogen synthesis	↓	
Glucose turnover	↑	
Glucose tolerance	↓	↓ Insulin/glucagon ratio
• Protein Metabolism		
Nitrogen balance	Negative	↑ Glucagon, TNF-α, IL-1, IL-6, IFN-γ
Muscle protein synthesis	↓	↑ Cortisol, TNF-α, IL-1, IL-6
Muscle proteolysis	↑	↑ Cortisol, TNF-α, IL-1, IL-6
Hepatic protein synthesis (acute phase proteins)	↑	TNF-α, IL-1, IL-6
Hepatic proteolysis	↑ / =	
Protein turnover	↑ / =	
Response to insulin	=	
• Lipid Metabolism		
Serum triglyceride	↑	
Fatty acid oxidation	= / ↑	
Glycerol and fatty acid turnover	↑	
Lipoprotein lipase activity	↓	TNF-α, IFN-γ, IL-1, IL-6
Lipid synthesis	↓	TNF-α, IFN-γ, IL-1
Lipolysis	↑	TNF-α, IFN-γ, IL-1, IL-6

Note: ↓ decreased; = unchanged; ↑ increased; TNF = tumor necrosis factor; INF = interferon; IL = interleukin.

and cancer patients, elevated IL-1 plasma concentrations have rarely been found.[44,96-99] Increased IL-6 is frequently detectable in serum of cancer patients (and tumor-bearing animals)[96,101-103] and IL-6 blockades reduced anorexia and weight loss in tumor-bearing animals.[102] IL-6 is considered the main factor in eliciting the acute phase protein synthesis during inflammation.[44,106,107] It is involved in muscle protein metabolism and in lipid mobilization.[108] In a rat model, Langstein et al. observed that the intraperitoneal injection of INF-γ induced anorexia and weight loss that were attenuated by the administration of anti-INF-γ antibodies.[109] Furthermore, Matthys et al. showed that the anti-INF-γ antibody administration reversed the wasting effect of Lewis lung carcinoma (INF-γ producing) in mice.[110]

Close relationships between hormonal changes and cytokines were demonstrated. In human healthy subjects, TNF-α or IL-6 infusion increases the stress hormone response.[15,111] Insulin has been shown to reduce IL-6 and IL-6 effects, whereas glucocorticoids increase cytokine effects on the acute phase response.[112]

IV. CANCER IN THE ELDERLY

Epidemiologic data shows that the aging process is associated with a growing risk for developing malignant disease.[113] The risk for cancer is 11 times greater in persons aged ≥65 years than in persons <65 years. Colorectal and lung cancers contribute to the higher incidence rate in both males and females together with prostate cancer in males and breast cancer in females. Aging is accompanied by variations in body composition and by decreases in physical function and cognitive capacity,[114] but it does not seem that these changes make cancer more aggressive in older patients. Furthermore, age per se is not considered a contraindication to antineoplastic treatment. It is assumed that there may be lower tolerance to radiotherapy and chemotherapy in the elderly patient even though no evidence has yet been reported.[115] Its seems more likely that differences in the course of the illness and in toleration of treatment between elderly and young subjects is due to the greater frequency of age-related diseases and conditions prior to the cancer diagnosis, rather than to the aging process.[116-119]

No study on cancer cachexia has clearly reported an association between patients' age and the rate and degree of PEM. Tchekmedyian et al.,[120] in a group of 218 consecutive patients with advanced cancer, observed a body weight lower than ideal body weight in 30% of 92 patients aged <65 years and in 52% of 126 patients aged ≥65 years. Furthermore, in the two groups of patients, weight loss >5% of usual body weight was present in 37% and in 47%, respectively. In a group of 492 consecutive patients with advanced cancer sent by oncologists to a nutritional team,[121] the body mass index according to Quetelet's formula (BMI, kg/m^2), weight loss as percentage of the patient's usual body weight (UBW), and weight loss during the last 6 months were assessed (Table 4.3). On the basis of the weight loss, the frequency of PEM appeared to increase with age. However, the frequency of primary tumor site localized at the gastrointestinal site was also greater in the oldest decades of age. When only the subgroup of patients with gastrointestinal cancer was evaluated, the frequency of PEM did not show any trend with age (Figure 4.3).

TABLE 4.3
Protein-Calorie Malnutrition in 490 Patients with Advanced Cancer

Primary Tumor Site

Age (Yr)	No. of Pts	M/F	Head–Neck	G.I.	Lung	Urogenital	Breast	Others
			Tumor Sites (No. % of Patients)					
≤60	143	78/65	23 (16%)	52 (36%)	21 (15%)	6 (4%)	20 (14%)	21 (15%)
61–70	158	109/49	33 (21%)	64 (40%)	28 (18%)	14 (9%)	5 (3%)	14 (9%)
>71	189	110/79	31 (16%)	101 (53%)	20 (11%)	14 (8%)	10 (5%)	13 (7%)

Frequency of Malnutrition

Age (Yr)	BMI <20		Last 6 Mo. Weight Loss ≥10%		BW ≤10% UBW	
	No. (%)	m ± sd	No. (%)	m ± sd	No. (%)	m ± sd
≤60	75 (53)	19.8 ± 4.2	82 (57)	12.5 ± 11.0	95 (66)	76 ± 8
61–70	52 (33)	21.0 ± 3.3	96 (61)	11.9 ± 10.0	118 (75)	78 ± 7
>71	92 (49)	20.3 ± 4.2	124 (66)	15.3 ± 10.2	161 (85)	75 ± 10

Note: BMI = kg/m^2; UBW = usual body weight.

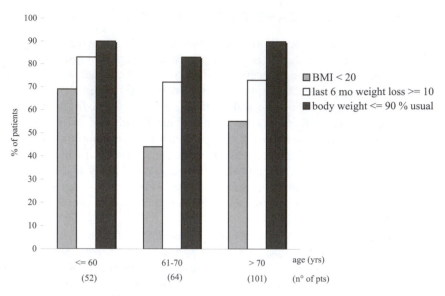

FIGURE 4.3   Protein–calorie malnutrition in 217 patients with advanced gastrointestinal cancer.

Studies on factors predicting survival demonstrated a significant correlation with nutritional parameters but not with age, both in patients undergoing antineoplastic treatments and patients with advanced cancer. DeWys et al. retrospectively analyzed the relationship between body weight loss during the last 6 months and survival in 3047 patients enrolled in a cooperative chemotherapy study.[18] They observed that a weight loss >5% was a significant prognostic factor against both survival and response to chemotherapy for a spectrum of cancers. Reuben et al. analyzed the correlation of 14 clinical symptoms with survival in 1592 patients with terminal cancer at hospice admission.[122] Performance status, measured by Karnofsky Performance Status (KPS) score, dry mouth, shortness of breath, problems eating, and weight loss had independent predictive value. Bruera et al. evaluated 61 patients with advanced cancer admitted to a palliative care unit.[123] They observed that cognitive failure, dysphagia and weight loss ≥10 kg were independently associated with poor prognosis and in a given patient predicted survival of <4 weeks with an accuracy of 74%. In an other study,[124] factors predicting survival were assessed in a group of 302 consecutive adult patients with advanced cancer admitted to a hospital-at-home program. Logistic regression analysis showed that BMI, KPS score, and daily oral energy intake were independent factors predicting length of survival (Table 4.4).

V.   THE EFFECTS OF CANCER TREATMENT ON NUTRITIONAL STATUS

Cancer treatment, both medical and surgical, can play a role in the development of PEM. Radio-therapy and chemotherapy may have acute and chronic effects on nutritional status.[125-128] During radiotherapy of the head–neck tract, patients may have anorexia, nausea, dysosmia, odynophagia, xerostomia, mucositis. Ulcers, necrosis of the jaw, trismus, and dental caries can develop after the end of the treatment. Radiotherapy of the esophagus, mediastine, or lung can cause dysphagia due to edema and ulceration of the esophagus, which occur during the treatment, and to fistulas, fibrosis, and stenosis of the esophagus, which are late complications. Acute enteritis is a common conse-quence of radiotherapy of the abdomen. It is characterized by atrophy of intestinal villi and loss of the mucosal epithelium and is associated with vomiting and diarrhea. Chronic enteritis can occur after months or even many years from the end of the treatment and has a progressive and often a very disabling course, with damage of extensive tracts of intestinal mucosa, fistulas, and bowel obstruction. The frequency of PEM due to radiotherapy varies with the site of irradiation. A

TABLE 4.4

Variables (X) Independently Associated with Survival in 3 Studies on Patients with Advanced Cancer (x = Studied Variables)

	Reuben et al.[122]	Bruera et al.[123]	Pironi et al.[125]
Sex	x	x	x
Age	x	x	
Primary tumor site	x	x	x
Metastasis	x		x
KPS scale (performance)	X	X	X
ECOG scale (performance)		X	
Pain	x	x	x
Nausea	x	x	
Anorexia	x	x	x
Dry mouth	X	x	
Dyspnea	X	x	x
Cognitive status	x	X	
Fever	x		
Hemorragie	x		
Constipation	x		
Diarrhea	x		
Bone pain	x		
Dysphagia or problems eating	X	X	
Daily oral energy intake			X
BMI			X
Weight loss:			
From UBW			x
During the last 6 months		X	x
During the last month			x
During the last 2 weeks	X		

Note: KPS = Karnofsky performance status; ECOG = Eastern Cooperative Oncology Group; BMI = body mass index; UBW = usual body weight.

significant weight loss has been documented in more than 90% of patients irradiated in the head–neck region, about 90% of patients irradiated in the abdomen, and less than 50% of those irradiated at the larynx and pelvis. The degree of weight loss is proportional to the dose of the radiation therapy and to the size of the irradiated field. The frequency and the degree of PEM due to radiotherapy have been demonstrated to be independent of the initial weight and age of the patient.[125,127,128]

Chemotherapy causes anorexia, nausea, and vomiting associated with mucositis.[128] Some drugs provoke stomatitis, gastric and duodenal ulcers, enteritis, and diarrhea. The presence of PEM seems to increase the risk of drug toxicity and animal studies suggest that malnutrition may modify the pharmacokinetics of chemotherapy drugs.

The impact of surgery on patients' nutritional status is related mainly to factors arising as a consequence of resections. Surgery of the oral–pharyngeal tract may impede the assumption of solid food for several weeks. Post-gastrectomy syndromes include early satiety from loss of gastric reservoir, dumping with malabsorption of fat and malabsorpion of iron and vitamin B_{12}. Extensive resection of the small bowel, especially if associated with resection of the ileocecal valve, results in short bowel syndrome.

VI.   THE IMPACT OF NUTRITIONAL SUPPORT ON PATIENTS UNDERGOING CANCER TREATMENT

Both parenteral nutrition (PN) and enteral nutrition (EN) are routinely used in malnourished cancer patients, in those at risk of malnutrition because of a long period of low oral intake due to diagnostic procedure and staging of the illness, or as complement treatment in those undergoing major surgery, or cycles of radiotherapy or chemotherapy that would be badly tolerated in generally debilitating conditions.[129] EN and PN have shown to be effective in stabilizing or improving the nutritional status of the malnourished cancer patient, even if the overall effect is more limited than in patients with primary PEM[129] (Table 4.5). In patients candidate to cancer treatments, nutritional support allows weight gain, increase of body fat, while increase in lean mass and visceral proteins occurs to a lesser extent. Published data suggest that perioperative artificial nutrition can be beneficial, especially preoperative support given to severely malnourished patients with cancer of the upper gastrointestinal tract.[129-131] The outcome of patients receiving only postoperative PN seems worse than that of patients receiving no nutritional support or EN because of increased rate of infections in the PN group.[132-135] It has been suggested that these results could be due to overfeeding and hyperglycemia associated with PN, which facilitate infections, rather than to the intravenous route of nutritional support. Malnourished patients with cancer of the breast or testis, or Hodgkin's disease, showed a poorer response to chemotherapy. A few studies indicated that EN may allow the completion of radiation therapy,[126,136] but both PN and EN have not been proven to improve the response and the toleration of radiotherapy and chemotherapy, as well as the survival of subjects who underwent these treatments[137-142] (Table 4.5). The effect of nutritional support on perioperative morbidity and mortality as well as on the outcome of patients undergoing radiotherapy or chemotherapy needs further studies. The design of published randomized clinical studies has many shortcomings, including heterogeneous patient population, exclusion of patients with severe malnutrition, variability of cancer therapy, suboptimal nutritional support, and inadequate sample size.

VII.   HOME ARTIFICIAL NUTRITION

Patients who have been cured from the primary cancer and who have bowel dysfunctions due to treatments (radiation enteritis, small bowel) and those who need treatments resulting in decreased food intake and bowel damage can benefit from home artificial nutrition (HAN). Nutritional therapy is not indicated in patients at the terminal stage of the disease, except for a minority (5–10%) who are at risk of death from cachexia. For these patients, home artificial nutrition programs may be indicated. The usefulness of nutritional support in advanced cancer patients is a matter of debate. The attitude to HAN in advanced cancer differs among countries for both home EN (HEN) and home PN (HPN). In HEN and HPN national registers, cancer patients are 5 to 20% in UK, 40% in the U.S., and more than 60% in Italy, most of whom are noncurable patients.[143,144] Differences seem to rely on an ethical basis, as no study has yet defined the cost–benefit and the cost-effectiveness of these different approaches. The main question is the impact of nutritional support on length and quality of life.

A 6-year-perspective survey of the practice of HAN in advanced cancer patients in an Italian health district was performed in order to evaluate the utilization rate of HAN, the length of patient survival, and the efficacy of HAN in maintaining patients at home without burdens and distress to patient and family and in improving patients' performance status.[121] Criteria for patient eligibility for HAN were hypophagia, life expectancy ≥6 weeks (clinical judgment), suitable patient and family psychophysical conditions, and verbal informed consent. During the 6-year period, 587 consecutive patients were referred by oncologists to a nutritional support team, and 164 of them were selected for HAN (135 HEN and 29 HPN) according to the eligibility criteria. Primary tumor site was in the head–neck or in the gastrointestinal tract in 78% of cases. PEM (BMI lower than normal or last 6 month weight loss ≥10%) was present in 85% of the patients. Mean (±SD) KPS

TABLE 4.5
Impact of Artificial Nutrition on Patients with Cancer

Clinical Condition	Parenteral Nutrition (PN)	Comment	Enteral Nutrition (EN)	Comment
Cancer cachexia	↑ BW ↑ FM ↑/= LBM =/↑ liver protein synthesis	Less effective than in malnourished patients without cancer	↑ BW ↑ FM ↑/= LBM =/↑ liver protein synthesis	Less effective than in malnourished patients without cancer
Preoperative	↓ mortality ↓ po complications and infections ↓ LOS	Best results obtained in malnourished patients with gastrointestinal cancer	↓ po complications vs. standard diet = po complications vs. PN	
Postoperative	= or worse outcome ↓ po complication ↑ infection rate	↑ infection rate may be related to hyperglycemia due to overfeeding with PN	↑ BW vs. PN ↓ infection rate and LOS with enhanced EN vs. standard EN	Small sample size Probably useful in malnourished patients
Chemotherapy	↑ BW in malnourished = survival = tumor response =/↓ drug toxicity ↑ infection rate	18 RCT and 2 meta-analyses	= nutritional variables = drug toxicity = tumor response = survival = quality of life	7 RCT No RCT comparing EN to PN
Radiation therapy	= survival =/↓ Rx toxicity ↑ infection rate ↑ chemotherapy during radiotherapy	4 RCT Small sample size Risk of overfeeding	↑ BW =/↓ Rx toxicity ↑ completion of therapy = tumor response = survival	7 RCT Best results obtained with EN prior to radiotherapy

Note: (↑, increased; ↓, decreased; =, unchanged); BW = body weight; FM = fat mass; LBM = lean body mass; LOS = length of stay; RCT = randomized clinical trial; po = postoperative.

From references 129–143.

score was 50 (±10). The incidence of HAN per 10^6 inhabitants was 18.4 in the first year of activity and from 33.2 to 36.9 in the following years. Incidence of HEN was four times greater than that of HPN. During the study, 158 patients (130 HEN, 28 HPN) had died because of the disease and six were on treatment. The mean (±SD) survival was 17.2 (±19.5) weeks for those on HEN and 12.2 (±8.0) weeks for those on HPN, and a total of 47 (29%) patients survived <6 weeks. The accuracy of the estimation of survival was 72%, a figure that fitted in well with those obtained using objective indexes to estimate survival in advanced cancer. Ninety-five patients had undergone 155 rehospitalizations (three for HPN complications and 152 for the disease) accounting for 15 to 23% of their survival time. Burdens due to HAN were well accepted in 76% of cases, were considered an annoyance in 18%, and were scarcely tolerated in 6%. The KPS score increased in 8% of patients, decreased in 11%, and was unchanged in the remaining 81%.

In patients with advanced cancer, the performance status decreases as the disease progresses. In malnourished patients, this negative effect may counteract the positive effect of the nutritional support. The impact of HAN on KPS of adult patients (age 64 ± 15 yr) with advanced cancer was further investigated by evaluating changes of KPS after 1 month of HAN in a group of 160 patients

(41 HPN and 119 HEN) who underwent HAN for at least 5 weeks.[145] KPS remained stable in 74% of the patients, increased in 13%, and decreased in 13%. No significant difference was observed between the HEN and the HPN subgroups. The three groups of patients (increased, unchanged, and decreased KPS) did not differ for age, sex, nutritional status, and nutritional support (kcal/kg body weight). After 1 month of HAN, body weight had increased in patients with increased KPS and had decreased in those with decreased KPS. Length of survival was significantly longer in the group of patients who had an increased KPS, suggesting that in patients with advanced cancer the performance status may improve in those in which HAN is able to improve the nutritional status and that changes of performance and nutritional status after 1 month of HAN are predictive factors of survival.

VIII.   CONCLUSIONS

Data from clinical studies suggest that aging-related body composition and function changes do not significantly interfere with nutritional status and outcome of cancer patients.

REFERENCES

1. Steen, B., Body composition and aging, *Nutr. Rev.*, 46, 45-51, 1988.
2. Roubenoff, R. and Rall, L.C., Humoral mediation of changing body composition during aging and chronic inflammation, *Nutr. Rev.*, 51, 1–11, 1993.
3. Vellas, B.J., Albarede, J.L., and Garry, P.J., Diseases and aging: patterns of morbidity with age; relationship between aging and age-associated diseases, *Am. J. Clin. Nutr.*, 55, 1225–1230, 1992.
4. McGandy, R.B., Russel, R.M., and Hartz, S.C., Nutritional status survey of healthy non-institutionalized elderly: nutrient intakes from three day diet records and nutrient supplements, *Nutr. Res.*, 6, 785–798, 1986.
5. Lipschitz, D.A., Protein calorie malnutrition in the hospitalized elderly, *Primary Care*, 9, 531–543, 1982.
6. Agarwal, N., Acevedo, F., Cayten, C.G., and Pitchomoni, C.S., Nutritional status of the hospitalized very elderly from nursing homes and privates homes, *Am. J. Clin. Nutr.*, 43, 659, 1986.
7. Patterson, B.M., Cornell, C.N., Carbone, B., Levine, B., and Chapman, D., Protein depletion and metabolic stress in elderly patients who have a fracture of the hip, *J. Bone Joint. Surg.*, 74-A, 251–60, 1992.
8. Wooton, R., Bryson, E., and Elsasser, U., Risk factors for fractured neck of femur in the elderly, *Age Aging*, 11, 160–168, 1982.
9. Bastow, M.D., Rawlings, J., and Allison, S.P., Undernutrition, hypothermia, and injury in elderly women with fractured femur: injury response to altered metabolism? *Lancet*, 1, 143–145, 1983.
10. Silver, A.J., Morley, J.E., Strome, L.S., Jones, D., and Vickers, L., Nutritional status in academic nursing home, *J. Am. Geriatr. Soc.*, 36, 487–491, 1988.
11. Rockwood, K., Fox, R.A., Stolee, P., Robertson, D., and Beattle, B.L., Frailty in elderly people: an evolving concept, *Can. Med. Assoc. J.*, 150(4), 489–495, 1994.
12. Sullivan, D.H., Patch, G.A., Walls, R.C., and Lipschitz, D.A., Impact of nutrition status and mortality in a select population of geriatric rehabilitation patients, *Am. J. Clin. Nutr.*, 51, 749–758, 1990.
13. Sullivan, D.H., Walls, R.C., and Lipschitz, D.A., Protein-energy undernutrition and the risk of mortality within 1 yr of hospital discharge in a select population of geriatric rehabilitation patients, *Am. J. Clin. Nutr.*, 53, 599–605, 1991.
14. Bostow, M., Rawlings, J., and Allison, S.P., Benefits of supplementary tube feeding after fractured neck of femur: A randomized controlled trial, *Br. J. Med.*, 287, 1589–1592, 1983.
15. Breslow, R.A., Hallfrisch, J., Guy, D.G., Crawley, B., and Goldberg, A.P., The importance of dietary protein in healing pressure ulcers, *JAGS*, 41, 357–362, 1993.
16. Delmi, M., Rapin, C.H., Bengoa, J.M., Delmas, P.D., Vasey, H., and Bonjour, J.P., Dietary supplementation in elderly patients with fractured neck of the femur, *Lancet*, 335, 1013–1016, 1990.

17. Yeh, S.S. and Schuster, M.W., Geriatric cachexia: the role of cytokines, *Am. J. Clin. Nutr.*, 70, 183–197, 1999.
18. Dewys, W.D., Begg, C., Lavin, P.T., Band, P.R., Bennett, J.M., Bertino, J.R., Cohen, M.H., Douglass, H.O. Jr., Engstrom, P.F., Ezdinli, E.Z., Horton, J., Johnson, G.J., Moertel, C.G., Oken, M.M., Perlia, C., Rosenbaum, C., Silverstein, M.N., Skeel, R.T., Sponzo, R.W., and Tormey, D.C., Prognostic effect of weight loss prior to chemotherapy in cancer patients, *Am. J. Med.*, 69, 491–497, 1980.
19. Kern, K.A. and Norton, J.A., Cancer cachexia, *J. Parenter. Enteral. Nutr.*, 12, 286–298, 1988.
20. Cohn, S.H., Ellis, K.J., Vartsky, D., Sawitsky, A., Gartenhaus, W., Yasumura, S., and Vaswani, A.N., Comparison of methods of estimating body fat in normal subjects and cancer patients, *Am. J. Clin. Nutr.*, 34, 2839–2847, 1981.
21. Rosenbaum, M., Leibel, R., and Hirsch, Obesity, *New Eng. J. Med.*, 337, 397–407, 1997.
22. Meguid, M.M., Muscaritoli, M., Beverly, J.L., Yang, Z., Cangiani, C., and Rossi-Fanelli, F., The early cancer anorexia paradigm: Changes in plasma free tryptophan and feeding indexes, *J. Parenter. Enteral. Nutr.,* 16(6), 56–59, 1992.
23. Carson, J.A.S. and Gormicam, A., Taste acuity and food attitudes of selected patients with cancer, *J. Am. Diet. Assoc.*, 70, 361–364, 1977.
24. Dewys, W.D., Changes in taste sensation and feeding behavior in cancer patients, A review, *J. Hum. Nutr.*, 32, 447–453, 1978.
25. Williams, L.R., Cohen, M.H., and Sewell, M.B., Altered taste thresholds in lung cancer, *Am. J. Clin. Nutr.*, 31, 122–125, 1978.
26. Mattes, R.D., Curran, W.J., Alavi, I., Polwlis, W., and Whittington, R., Clinical implications of learned food aversion in cancer patients treated with chemotherapy or radiation therapy, *Cancer (Philadelphia)*, 70, 192–200, 1992.
27. Bernstein, I.L., Learned taste aversion in children receiving chemotherapy, *Science*, 200, 1302–1303, 1978.
28. Heber, D., Byerley, L.O., and Tchekmedyian, N.S., Hormonal and metabolic abnormalities in the malnourished cancer patient: Effect on host-tumor interaction, *J. Parenter. Enteral. Nutr.,* 16(6), 60–64, 1992.
29. Tayek, J.A., Reduced non-oxidative glucose metabolism in cancer patients is associated with a reduced triiodothyronine hormone concentrations, *J. Am. Coll. Nutr.*, 14, 341–348, 1995.
30. DeBlaauw, I., Deutz, N.E.P., and VonMeyenfeldt, M.F., Metabolic changes in cancer cachexia, *Clin. Nutr.*, 16, 169–176, 1997.
31. Douglas, R.G. and Shaw, J.H., Metabolic effects of cancer, *Br. J. Surg.*, 77, 246–254, 1990.
32. Inculet, R.I., Peacock, J.L., Gorshboth, C.M., and Norton, J.A., Gluconeogenesis in the tumor-influenced rat hepatocyte: importance of tumor burden, lactate, insulin and glucagon, *J. Natl. Cancer Inst.*, 79, 1039–1046, 1987.
33. Lundholm, K., Edstrom, S., Karlberg, I., Ekman, L., and Schersten, T., Glucose turnover, gluconeogenesis from glycerol in cancer patients, *Cancer*, 50, 1142–1150, 1982.
34. Waterhouse, C., Jeanpretre, N., and Keilson, J., Gluconeogenesis from alanine in patients with progressive malignant disease, *Cancer Res.*, 39, 1968–1972, 1979.
35. Pisters, P.W.T. and Pearlstone, D.B., Protein and amino acid metabolism in cancer cachexia: investigative techniques and therapeutic interventions, *Crit. Rev. Clin. Lab. Sci.*, 30, 223–272, 1993.
36. Moley, J.F., Morrison, S.D., Gorschboth, C.M., and Norton, J., Body composition changes in rats with experimental cancer cachexia: Improvement with exogenous insulin, *Cancer Res.*, 48, 2784–2787, 1988.
37. Heslin, M.J., Newman, E., Wolf, R.F., Pisters, P.W., and Brennan, M.F., Effect of systemic hyperinsulinemia in cancer patients. *Cancer Res.*, 52, 3845–3850, 1992.
38. Gullino, P.M., Grantham, F.H., and Courtney, A.H., Glucose consumption by transplanted tumors in vivo, *Cancer Res.*, 27, 1031–1040, 1967.
39. Norton, J.A., Burt, M.E., and Brennan, M.F., In vivo utilization of substrate by human sarcoma bearing limbs, *Cancer*, 45, 2934–2939, 1980.
40. Waterhouse, C. and Mason, J., Leucine metabolism in patients with malignant disease, *Cancer*, 48, 939–944, 1981.
41. Norton, J.A., Stein, T.P., and Brennan, M.F., Whole body protein synthesis and turnover in normal man and malnourished patients with and without known cancer, *Ann. Surg.*, 194, 123–128, 1981.

42. Melville, S., McNurlan, M.A., Calder, A.G., and Garlick, P.J., Increased protein turnover despite normal energy metabolism and responses to feeding in patients with lung cancer, *Cancer Res.*, 50, 1125–1131, 1990.

43. Richards, E.W., Long, C.L., Nelson, K.M., Tohver, O.K., Pinkston, J.A., Navari, R.M., and Blakemore, W.S., Protein turnover in advanced lung cancer patients, *Metabolism*, 42, 291–296, 1993.

44. Fearon, K.C.H., McMillan, D.C., Preston, T., Winstanley, P., Cruickshank, A.M., and Shenkin, A., Elevated circulating interleukin-6 is associated with an acute-phase response but reduced fixed hepatic protein synthesis in patients with cancer, *Ann. Surg.*, 213, 26–31, 1991.

45. Souba, W.W., Strebel, F.R., Bull, J.M., Copeland, E.M., Teagtmeyer, H., and Cleary, K., Interorgan glutamine metabolism in the tumor bearing rat, *J. Surg. Res.*, 44, 720–726, 1988.

46. Lundholm, K., Edstrom, S., Karlberg, I., Bylund, A.C., and Schersten, T. A., Comparative study of the influence of malignant tumor in host metabolism in mice and man. Evaluation of an experimental model, *Cancer* 42, 453–461, 1978.

47. Radcliffe, J.D., Fontanez, I.N., and Morrow, S., The effect of a methylcholanthrene-induced sarcoma on the protein status of fischer rats, *Nutr. Res.*, 6, 539–547, 1986.

48. Stein, T.P., Oram Smith, J.C., Leskiw, M.J., Wallace, H.W., and Miller, E.E., Tumor-caused changes in host protein synthesis under different dietary situation, *Cancer Res.*, 36, 3936–3940, 1976.

49. Lundholm, K., Edstrom, S., Karlberg, I., Ekman, L., and Schersten, T., Metabolism in peripheral tissues in cancer patients, *Cancer Treat Rep.*, 65 (suppl 5), 79–83, 1981.

50. Heber, D., Chlebowski, R.T., Ishibashi, D.E., Herrold, J.N., and Block, J.B., Abnormalities in glucose and protein metabolism in noncachectic lung cancer patients, *Cancer Res.*, 42, 4815–4819, 1982.

51. Tessitore, L., Costelli, P., Bonetti, G., and Baccino, F.M., Cancer cachexia, malnutrition, and protein turnover in experimental animals, *Arch. Biochem. Biophys.*, 306, 52–58, 1993.

52. Clark, C.M. and Goodlad, G.A., Depletion of proteins of phasic and tonic muscles in tumor-bearing rats, *Eur. J. Cancer*, 7, 3–9, 1971.

53. Warren, R.S., Jeevanandam, M., and Brennan, M.F., Comparison of hepatic protein synthesis in vivo versus in vitro in the tumor-bearing rats, *J. Surg. Res.*, 42, 43–50, 1987.

54. DeBlaauw, I., Deutz, N.E.P., and vonMeyenfeldt, M.F., Hepatic amino acid and protein metabolism in non-anorectic, moderately cachectic tumor bearing rats, *J. Hepatol.,* 26, 396–408, 1997.

55. Warren, R.S., Jeevanandam, M., and Brennan, M.F., Protein synthesis in tumor-influenced hepatocyte, *Surgery*, 98, 275–282, 1985.

56. Devereux, D.F., Redgrave, T.G., Loda, M.F., Clowes, G.H. Jr., and Deckers, P.J., Tumor-associated metabolism in rat is a unique physiologic entity, *J. Surg. Res.*, 38, 149–153, 1985.

57. Younes, R.N., Vydelingum, N.A., Noguchi, Y., and Brennan, M.F., Lipid kinetic alterations in tumor-bearing rats: Reversal by tumor excision, *J. Surg. Res.*, 48, 324–328, 1990.

58. Vlassara, H., Spiegel, R.J., San Doval, D., and Carami, A., Reduced plasma lipoprotein lipase activity in patients with malignancy-associated weight loss, *Horm. Metab. Res.*, 18, 698–703, 1986.

59. Devereux, D.F., Redgrave, T.G., Tilton, M., Hollander, D., and Deckers, P.J., Intolerance to administered lipids in tumor-bearing animals, *Surgery*, 96, 414–419, 1984.

60. Shaw, J.H. and Wolfe, R.R., Fatty acid and glycerol kinetics in septic patients with gastrointestinal cancer. The response to glucose infusion and parenteral feeding, *Ann. Surg.*, 205, 368–376, 1987.

61. Lindmark, L., Bennegard, K., Eden, E., Svaninger, G., Ternell, M., and Lundholm, K., Thermic effect of substrate oxidation in response to intravenous nutrition in cancer patients who lose weight, *Ann. Surg.*, 204, 628–636, 1986.

62. Macfie, J., Burkinshaw, L., Oxby, C., Holmfield, J.H., and Hill, G.L., The effect of gastrointestinal malignancy on resting metabolic expenditure, *Br. J. Surg.*, 69, 443–446, 1982.

63. Bozzetti, F., Pagnoni, A.M., and Del Vecchio, M., Excessive caloric expenditure as a cause of malnutrition in patients with cancer, *Surg. Gynecol. Obstet.*, 150, 229–234, 1980.

64. Dempsey, D.T., Feurer, I.D., Knox, L.S., Crosby, L.O., Buzby, G.P., Mullen, J.L., Energy expenditure in malnourished gastrointestinal cancer patients, *Cancer*, 53, 1265–1273, 1984.

65. Knox, L.S., Crosby, L.O., Feurer, I.D., Buzby, G.P., Miller, C.L., and Mullen, JL., Energy expenditure in malnourished cancer patients, *Ann. Surg.*, 197, 152–162, 1983.

66. Shaw, J.H.P., Humberstone, D.M., and Wolfe, R.R., Energy and protein metabolism in sarcoma patients, *Ann. Surg.*, 207, 283–289, 1988.

67. Peacock, J.L., Inculet, R.I., Corsey, R., Ford, D.B., Rumble, W.F., Lawson, D., and Norton, J.A., Resting energy expenditure and body cell mass alterations in noncachectic patients with sarcoma, *Surgery* 102, 465–472, 1987

68. Kern, K.A. andNorton, J.A., Cancer cachexia, *J. Paren. Enter. Nutr.*, 12, 286–298, 1988.

69. Illig, K.A., Maronian, N., and Peacock, J.L., Cancer cachexia is transmissible in plasma, *J. Surg. Res.*, 52, 353–358, 1984

70. Drott, C., Svaninger, G., and Lundholm, K., Increased urinary excretion of cortisol and catecholamines in malnourished cancer patients, *Ann. Surg.*, 208, 645–650, 1988.

71. Besedovsky, H.O., del Rey, A., Schardt, M., Sorkin, E., Normann, S., Baumann, J., and Girard, J., Changes in plasma hormone profiles after tumor transplantation into syngeneic and allogeneic rats, *Int. J. Cancer*, 36, 209–216, 1985

72. Lawson, D.H., Richmond, A., Nixon, D.W., and Rudman, D., Metabolic approaches to cancer cachexia, *Ann. Rev. Nutr.*, 2, 277–301, 1982.

73. Ball, H.A. and Samuels, L.T., Adrenal weights in tumor bearing rats. *Proc. Soc. Exp. Biol. Med.*, 38, 441–443, 1938.

74. Inculet, R.I., Peacock, J.L., Gorschboth, C.M., and Norton, J.A., Gluconeogenesis in the tumor-influenced rat hepatocyte: importance of tumor burden, lactate, insulin, and glucagon, *J. Natl. Cancer Inst.*, 79, 1039–1046, 1987.

75. Tessitore, L., Costelli, P., and Baccino, F.M., Humoral mediation for cachexia in tumor bearing rats, *Br. J. Cancer*, 67, 15–23, 1993.

76. Permert, J., Larsson, J., Fruin, A.B., Tatemoto, K., Herrington, M.K., von Schenck, H., and Adrian, T.E., Islet hormone secretion in pancreatic cancer patients with diabetes, *Pancreas*, 15, 60–68, 1997.

77. Bartlett, D.L., Charland, S.L, and Torosian, M.H., Reversal of tumor-associated hyperglucagonemia as treatment for cancer cachexia, *Surgery*, 118, 87–97, 1995.

78. Persson, H., Bennegard, K., Lundberg, P.A., Svaninger, G., and Lundholm, K., Thyroid hormones in conditions of chronic malnutrition. A study with special reference to cancer cachexia, *Ann. Surg.*, 45, 201–52, 1989.

79. Richards, E.W., Long, C.L., Nelson, K.M., Pinkston, J.A., Navari, R.M., Geiger, J.W., Gandy, R.E., and Blakemore, W.S., Glucose metabolism in advanced lung cancer patients, *Nutrition*, 8, 245–251, 1992.

80. Tayek, J.A. and Katz, J., Glucose production, recycling, Cori cycle and gluconeogenesis in humans with and without cancer: Relationship to serum cortisol concentration, *Am. J. Physiol.*, 272, E476–484, 1997.

81. Tayek, J.A. and Bresel, J.A., Failure of anabolism in malnourished cancer patients receiving growth hormone, *J. Clin. Endocrinol. Metabol.*, 80, 2082–2087, 1995.

82. Flores, E., Bistran, B., Pomposelli, J., Dinarello, C., Blackburn, G., and Istfan, N., Infusion of tumor necrosis factor/cachectin promotes muscle catabolism in the rat, *J. Clin. Invest.*, 83, 1614–1622, 1989.

83. Tracey, K.J., Wei, H., Manogue, K.R., Fong, Y., Hesse, D.G., Nguyen, H.T., Kuo, G.C., Beutler, B., Cotran, R.S., and Cerami, A., Cachectin/tumor necrosis factor induces cachexia, anemia and inflammation, *J. Exp. Med.*, 167, 1211–1227, 1988.

84. Tracey, K.J., Loery, S.F., and Fahey, T., III., Cachectin/tumor necrosis factor induces lethal shock and stress hormone response in the dog, *Surg. Gynecol. Obstet.*, 164, 415–422, 1987.

85. Gelin, J., Moldawer, L.L., Lonnroth, C., Sherry, B., Chizzonite, R., and Lundholm, K., Role of endogenous tumor necrosis factor alpha and interleukin 1 for experimental tumor growth and the development of cancer cachexia, *Cancer Res.*, 51, 415–421, 1991.

86. Fong, Y., Moldawer, L.L., Marano, M., Wei, H., Barber, A., Manogue, K., Tracey, K.J., Kuo, G., and Fischman, D.A., Cerami. Cachectin/TNF or Il-1 alpha induces cachexia with redistribution of body proteins, *Am. J. Physiol.*, 256, R659–665, 1989.

87. Greenberg, A.S., Nordan, R.P., McInttosh, J., Calvo, J.C., Scow, R.O., and Jablons, D., Interleukin 6 reduces lipoprotein lipase activity in adipose tissue of mice in vivo and in 3T3.L1 adipocytes: A possible role for interleukin 6 in cancer cachexia, *Canc. Res.*, 52, 4113–4116, 1992.

88. Fried, S.K. and Zencher, R., Cachectin/tumor necrosis factor decreases human adipose tissue lipoprotein lipase mRNA levels, synthesis, and activity, *J. Lipid. Res.*, 30, 1917–1923, 1989.

89. Zechner, R., Newman, T.C., Scherry, B., Cerami, A., and Breslow, J.L., Recombinant human cachectin/tumor necrosis factor but not interleukin-1 alpha downregulates lipoprotein lipase gene expression at the transcriptional level in mouse 3T3-L1 adipocytes, *Mol. Cell. Biol.*, 8, 2394–2401, 1988.

90. Evans, D.A., Jacobs, D.O., and Wilmore, D.W., Effects of tumor necrosis factor on protein metabolism, *Br. J. Surg.*, 80, 1019–1023, 1993.

91. Sakurai, Y., Zhang, X.J., and Wolfe, R.R., Short-term effects of tumor necrosis factor on energy and substrate metabolism in dogs, *J. Clin. Invest.*, 91, 2437–2445, 1993.

92. Starnes, H.F. Jr., Warren, R.S., Jeevanandam, M., Gabrilove, J.L., Larchian, W., Oettgen, H.F., and Brennan, M.F., Tumor necrosis factor and the acute metabolic response to tissue injury in man, *J. Clin. Invest.*, 82, 1321–1325, 1988.

93. Van der Poll, T., Romijn, J.A., Endert, E., Borm, J.J., Buller, H.R., and Sauerwein, H.P., Tumor necrosis factor mimics the metabolic response to acute infection in healthy humans, *Am. J. Physiol.*, 261, E457–465, 1991.

94. Broukaert, P., Spriggs, D.R., and Demetri, G., Circulating inerleukin 6 during a continuous infusion of tumor necrosis factor and interferon gamma, *J. Exp. Med.*, 169, 2257–2262, 1989.

95. Balkwill, F., Osborne, R., Burke, F., Naylor, S., Talbot, D., Durbin, H., Tavernier, J., and Fiers, W., Evidence for tumor necrosis factor/cachectin production in cancer, *Lancet* (ii), 1229–1232, 1987.

96. Nakazaki, H., Preoperative and postoperative cytokine in patients with cancer, *Cancer*, 70, 709–713, 1992.

97. Costelli, P., Carbo, N., Tessitore, L., Bagby, G.J., Lopez-Soriano, F.J., Argiles, J.M., and Baccino, F.M., Tumor necrosis factor alpha mediates changes in tissue protein turnover in a rat cancer cachexia model, *J. Clin. Invest.*, 92, 2783–2789, 1993.

98. Sherry, B.A., Gelin, J., Fong, Y., Marano, M., Wei, H., Cerami, A., Lowry, S.F., Lundholm, K.G., and Moldawer, L.L., Anticachectin/tumor necrosis factor-a antibodies attenuate development of cachexia in tumor models, *FASEB J.*, 3, 1956–1962, 1989.

99. Tracey, K.J., Vlassara, H., and Cerami A. Cachectin/tumor necrosis factor. *Lancet*, (i), 1122–1126, 1989.

100. Jensen, J.C., Buresh, C.M., and Fraker, D.L., Enhanced hepatic cytokine gene expression in cachetic tumor bearing rats, *Surg. Forum*, 41, 469, 1990.

101. Smith, B.K., Conn, C.A., and Kluger, M.J., Experimental cachexia: Effects of MCA sarcoma in the Fischer rat, *Am. J. Phisiol.*, 265, E376–384, 1993.

102. Strassmann, G., Fong, M., Kenney, J.S., and Jacob, C.O., Evidence for the involvement of interleukin 6 in experimental cancer cachexia, *J. Clin. Invest.*, 89, 1681–1684, 1992.

103. Falconer, J.S., Fearon, K.C.H., Plester, C.E., Ross, J.A., and Carter, D.C., Cytokines, the acute phase response, and resting energy expanditure in cachetic patients with pancreatic cancer, *Ann. Surg.*, 219, 325-331, 1994.

104. Strassman, G., Masui, Y., Chizzonite, R., and Fong, M., Mechanism of experimental cancer cachexia. Local involvment of Il-1 in colon-26 tumor, *J. Immunol.*, 150, 2341–2345, 1993.

105. Grande, F., Anderon, J.T., and Keys, A., Changes of basal metabolic rate in man in semistarvation and refeeding, *J. Appl. Physiol.*, 12(2), 230–238, 1958.

106. Bereta, J., Kurdowska, A., Koj, A., Hirano, T., Kishimoto, T., Content, J., Fiers, W., Van Damme, J., and Gauldie, J., Different preparations of natural and recombinant human interleukin 6 similarly stimulate acute phase protein synthesis and uptake of alpha-aminoisobutiryric acid by cultured rat hepatocites, *Int. J. Biochem.*, 21, 361–366, 1989.

107. Geiger, T., Andus, T., Klapproth, J., Hirano, T., Kischimoto, T., and Heinrich, P.C., Induction of rat acute-phase proteins by interleukin 6 in vivo, *Eur. J. Immunol.*, 18, 717–721, 1988.

108. Roubenoff, R., Harris, T.B., Abad, L.W., Wilson, P.W., Dallal, G.E., and Dinarello, C.A., Monocytes cytokine production in an elderly population. Effect of age and inflammation, *J. Gerontol. A Biol. Sci. Med. Sci.*, 53, M20–26, 1998.

109. Langestein, H.N., Doherty, G.M., Fraker, D.L., Buresh, C.M., and Norton, J.A., The role of gamma-interferon and tumor necrosis factor alpha in an experimental rat model of cancer cachexia, *Cancer Res.*, 51, 2302–2306, 1991

110. Matthys P, Heremans H, Opdenakker G, and Billiau A. Anti-interferon-gamma antibody treatment, growth of lewis lung tumors in mice and tumor associated cachecxia, *Eur. J. Cancer*, 27, 182–187, 1991.

111. Stouthard, J.M., Romijn, J.A., Van der Poll, T., Endert, E., Klein, S., Bakker, P.J., Veenhof, C.H., and Sauerwein, H.P., Endocrinologic and metabolic effects of interleukin-6 in humans, *Am. J. Physiol.*, 286, E813–819, 1995.

112. Baumann, H. and Gauldie, J., The acute phase response, *Immunol Today*, 15, 74–80, 1994.

113. Yancik, R., Epidemiology of cancer in the elderly, current status and projections for the future, *RAYS* (suppl to N.1), 3–9, 1997

114. Vellas, B.J., Albarede, J., and Garry, P., Diseases and aging: patterns of morbidity with age; relationship between aging and age associated diseases, *Am. J. Clin. Nutr.*, 55, 1225S–1230S, 1992.

115. Fentiman, I.S., Tirelli, U., Monfardini, S., Schneider, M., Festen, J., Cognetti, F., and Aapro, M.S., Cancer in the elderly: Why so badly treated? *Lancet*, 325, 1020–1022, 1990.

116. Havlik, R.J., Yancik, R., Long, S., Ries, L., and Edwards, B., The National Institute on Aging and the National Cancer Institute SEER collaborative study on comorbidity and early diagnosis of cancer in the elderly, *Cancer*, 74, 2101–2106, 1994.

117. Balducci, L. and Lyman, G.H., Cancer in the elderly: Epidemiologic and clinical implications. In: Balducci L., *Cancer in the Elderly-part 1, Clin. Geriat. Med.*, 13 (1), 1–14, 1997.

118. Coebergh, J.W.W., Significant trends in cancer in the elderly, *Eur. J. Cancer*, 32A(4), 569–571, 1996.

119. Stariano, W.A. and Ragland, D.R.. The effect of comorbidity on 3-year survival of women with primary breast cancer, *Ann Intern Med*, 120, 104–110, 1994.

120. Tchekmedyian, N.S., Zahyna, D., Halpert, C., and Heber, D., Clinical aspects of nutrition in advanced cancer, *Oncology* 49(suppl 2), 3–7, 1992.

121. Pironi, L., Ruggeri, E., Tanneberg, M.D., Giordani, S., Pannuti, F., and Miglioli, M., Home artificial nutrition in advanced cancer, *J. R. Soc. Med.* 90, 597–603, 1997.

122. Reuben, D.B., Mor, V., and Hiris, J., Clinical symptoms and length of survival in patients with terminal cancer, *Arch. Intern. Med.*, 148, 1586–1591, 1988.

123. Bruera, E., Miller, J.M., Kuehn, N., MacEachern, T., and Hanson, J., Estimate of survival of patients admitted to a palliative care unit: a prospective study, *J. Pain Symptom. Manage.*, 7, 82–86, 1992.

124. Pironi, L., Ruggeri, E., Martoni, A., Morselli-Labate, A.M., Pannuti, F., Barbara, L., Miglioli, M., of short-term survival of patients with advanced cancer: An objective prognostic score, *Ital. J. Gastro-enterol.*, 27 (suppl 1): 206–207, 1995

125. Chencharick, J.D. and Mossman, K.L., Nutritional consequences of radiotherapy of head and neck cancer, *Cancer*, 51, 811–815, 1983

126. Daly, J.M., Hearne, B., Dunaj, J., LePorte, B., Vikram, B., Strong, E., Green, M., Muggio, F., Groshen, S., and DeCosse, J.J., Nutritional rehabilitation in patients with advanced head and neck cancer receiving radiation therapy, *Am. J. Surg.*, 148, 514–520, 1984.

127. Donaldson, S.S., Nutritional consequences of radiotherapy, *Cancer Res.*, 37, 2407–2413, 1997.

128. Donaldson, S.S. and Lenon, R.A., Alterations of nutritional status: impact of chemotherapy and radiation therapy, *Cancer*, 43, 2036–2052, 1979.

129. Klein, S., Kinney, J., Jeejeebhoy, K., Alpers, D., Hellerstein, M., Murray, M., and Twomey, P., Nutrition support in clinical practice: review of published data and recommendations for future research directions, *J. Paren. Enter. Nutr.*, Vol. 21, No. 3, 133–156, 1997.

130. Muller, J.M., Brenner, U., Dienst, V., and Pichlmaier, H., Preoperative parenteral feeding in patients with gastrointestinal carcinoma, *Lancet*, 1, 68–71, 1982.

131. Heatley, R.V., Williams, R.H., and Lewis, M.H., Preoperative intravenous feeding; a controlled trial, *Postgrad. Med. J.*, 55, 541–554, 1979.

132. Klein, S. and Koretz, R.L., Nutrition support in patients with cancer: what do the data really show? *Nutr. Clin. Pract.*, 9, 91–100, 1994.

133. Ghavimi, F., Shils, M.E., Scott, B.F., Brown, M., and Tamaroff, M., Comparison of morbidity in children requiring abdominal radiation and chemotherapy, with and without total parenteral nutrition, *J. Pediatr.*, 101, 530–537, 1982.

134. Harrison, L.E., Hochwald, S.N., Heslin, M.J., Berman, R., Burt, M., and Brennan, M.F., Early postoperative enteral nutrition improves peripheral kinetics in upper gastrointestinal cancer patients undergoing complete resection: A randomized trial, *JPE N*, 21(4), 202–207, 1997.

135. Shirabe, K., Matsumata, T., Shimada, M., Takenaka, K., Kawahara, N., Yamamoto, K., Nishizaki, T., and Sugimachi, K,. A comparison of parenteral hyperalimentation and early enteral feeding regarding systemic immunity after major hepatic resection: The results of a randomized prospective study, *Hepato-Gastroenterology*, 43(13), 205–209, 1997.

136. Hunter, A.M., Nutrition management of patients with neoplastic discure of the head and neck treated with radiation therapy, *Nutr. Clin. Prac.,* 11(4), 157–169, 1996.

137. Klein, S., Simes, J., and Blackburn, G.L., Total parenteral nutrition and cancer clinical trials, *Cancer*, 58, 1378–1386, 1986.

138. McGeer, A.J., Detsky, A.S., and O'Rourke, K., Parenteral nutrition in cancer patients undergoing chemotherapy: A meta analysis, *Nutrition*, 6, 233–240, 1990.

139. Solassol, C., Joyeux, H., Astruc, B., Fourtillan, J.B., Hazane, C., Saubion, J.L., and Jalabert, M., Complete nutrients mixtures with lipids for total parenteral nutrition in cancer patients, *Acta. Chir. Scand. Suppl,* 498, 151–154, 1980.

140. Kinsella, T.J., Malcom, A., Bothe, A. Jr., Valerio, D., and Blackburn, G.L., Prospective study of nutritional support during pelvic irradiation, *Int. J. Radiat. Oncol. Biol. Phys.*, 7, 543–548, 1981.

141. Valerio, D., Overett, L., Malcom, A., and Blackburn, G.L., Nutritional support for cancer patients receiving abdominal and pelvic radiotherapy: A randomized prospective clinical experiment of intravenous versus oral feeding, *Surg. Forum.,* 29, 145–148, 1978.

142. Donaldson, S.S., Wesley, M.N., Ghavimi, F., Shils, M.E., Suskind, R.M., and DeWys, W.D., A prospective randomized clinical trial of total parenteral nutrition in children with cancer, *Med. Pediatr. Oncol.,* 10, 129–139, 1982.

143. Elia, M., An international prospective on artificial nutritional support in the community, *Lancet*, 345, 1345–1349, 1995.

144. Pironi, L. and Tognoni, G., Cost benefit and cost effectiveness analysis of home artificial nutrition: Reappraisal of available data, *Clin. Nutr.*, 14 (suppl), 87–91, 1995.

145. Pironi, L., Ruggeri, E., Paganelli, F., Pannuti, F., and Miglioli, M., Impact of home artificial nutrition (HAN) on performance status in advanced cancer, *Clin. Nutr.*, 18 (suppl 1), 52, 1999.

Section II

Undernutrition: Role in Longevity

5 Trace Element Requirements of the Elderly

S.A. Udipi, P. Ghugre, H. Hoskote, and K. Kenjle

CONTENTS

I. INTRODUCTION

Trace elements are defined as those elements that make up no more than 0.01% of the dry weight of the body.[1] Ultratrace elements are those elements with an established, estimated, or suspected requirement, generally indicated by micrograms. At least 18 elements could be considered ultratrace elements: aluminum, arsenic, boron, bromide, cadmium, chromium, fluoride, germanium, iodide, lead, lithium, molybdenum, nickel, rubidium, selenium, silicon, tin, vanadium, manganese and cobalt.[2]

The quality of the experimental evidence for nutritional essentiality varies widely for the ultratrace elements[1] and may not be complete for all of them. Criteria for defining an element as essential are:

- It occurs in the natural environment.
- It is present in physiological amounts in the normal diet.
- It is present in body tissues at relatively constant concentrations.
- It is found in the newborn and/or maternal milk.
- Withdrawal produces similar structural and physiological abnormalities in different species and these are reversed or prevented by addition of the element to the diet.
- A biochemical function(s) is associated with the element.[1]

The evidence for the essentiality of iodide, manganese, molybdenum, and selenium is substantial and noncontroversial, since specific biochemical functions have been defined for them.[2] Evidence is compelling also for elements like arsenic, silicon, nickel, and vanadium, although their essentiality is based on circumstantial evidence.[3]

In this context, the four trace elements discussed herein are: manganese, vanadium, molybdenum and silicon.

A. MANGANESE

Manganese (Mn) is the 12th-most-common element in the earth's crust. It can assume 11 different oxidation states—from –3 to +7—but in living tissues it is found in the +2, +3 and +4 oxidation states. Mn^{5+}, Mn^{6+}, Mn^{+7}, as well as other complexes of higher oxidation states, are generally unrecognized in biological materials. Typically found in compounds with a coordination number 6 and lacking octahedral coordination complexes, Mn tends to form very tight complexes with other substances. As a result, its free plasma and tissue concentrations tend to be extremely low.[4]

1. Metabolism

Absorption of Mn from diet is very low. On the basis of ^{54}Mn retention, it has been estimated that adult humans absorb 5.9(4.8% of ingested Mn.[5] Absorption apparently decreases with increasing Mn intake. As the *Neuro Toxicol.* Mn intake increased from 1.5 to 100 (g/g in rats, the absorption declined from 29% to 2%.[6] Ingested Mn^{2+} is thought to be converted into Mn^{3+} in the duodenum, which is absorbed equally well throughout the small intestine.[7] However, the actual mechanism of Mn absorption is not clearly established. In rats, Mn absorption declined linearly with time when the element was perfused at concentrations ranging between 0.0125–1.00mM. Moreover, Mn absorption during perfusion at a 2:1 ratio of ligand (histidine and citrate) to Mn was three times greater than in the absence of any ligand, thus indicating that intestinal Mn absorption could be a rapidly saturable process probably mediated by a high-affinity, low-capacity active transport system.[8] On the other hand, diffusion has also been implicated because studies with brush border membrane vesicles indicated that mucosal transport of Mn occurs through a nonsaturable simple diffusion process. It appears that both the processes might be involved and operate simultaneously, with apical to basolateral Mn uptake and transport being strictly concentration-dependent and basolateral apical being saturable.[7]

Relatively few dietary ingredients have a major effect on Mn absorption, however, the interaction between Mn and iron (Fe) is strong. Increased Fe in the diet depresses Mn absorption and increased dietary Mn interferes with Fe metabolism. In a recent study, it was shown that interaction of ferritin status and dietary Mn content affected [54]Mn absorption and biological half-life. Absorption was greatest in subjects with low ferritin concentration when they were consuming the low Mn diet and was least in subjects with high ferritin concentration.[9] Finley et al.[10] found that men absorbed significantly less [54]Mn than women and these differences were related to iron status. Similarly, in patients with varying iron stores and subjected to duodenal perfusion with Mn, the rate of Mn absorption was found to increase in Fe deficiency. The enhanced Mn absorption was inhibited by iron.[6] A hypothesis explaining the interaction between Mn and Fe is that Mn may be recognized by Fe transport mechanism and consequently be absorbed with Fe. Therefore, factors that up-regulate Fe absorption (such as low Fe stores) also may increase Mn absorption, and factors affecting Fe absorption may also regulate Mn. Therefore, Mn absorption may be substantially increased under some dietary conditions.[11]

In addition to variable absorption, Mn homeostasis is controlled by biliary excretion, which represents the major route of excretion of Mn. Mn-deficient rats were found to conserve Mn by a dramatic reduction in biliary Mn excretion and secreted only 0.7% as much Mn in bile as did Mn-repleted rats. However, the large reduction in biliary Mn secretion was not complete enough to prevent 50–80% reductions in tissue Mn concentrations. It appears that variations in biliary manganese secretion and intestinal absorption are more apt to effectively maintain constant tissue Mn concentration when variations in intakes are less extreme.[12] Also, mucosal tissue has been proposed to play a role in Mn homeostasis by sequestering Mn, which is subsequently lost with sloughing of intestinal mucosa.[13] Thus, given the central importance of hepatic Mn metabolism, anything that impairs liver function could conceivably depress Mn excretion and increase the retention of Mn within the body.[11]

Absorbed Mn is complexed with albumin and transported to the liver, the key organ in Mn metabolism. In the liver, Mn is found in both rapid- and slow-exchanging pools. The former is the precursor of biliary Mn, while the latter serves as a source of Mn for the liver as well as transferrin-bound Mn. Transferrin and (-2 macroglobulin have been proposed as the proteins responsible for transporting Mn to peripheral tissues.[13]

Although little is known about the uptake of Mn by cells at the tissue level, more is known regarding its transport in the central nervous system (CNS). It enters the brain from the blood either across the cerebral capillaries and/or the cerebrospinal fluid (CSF). At normal plasma concentration, the former appears to be the primary route, while at high plasma concentration and upon acute bolus injections of Mn, the transport across the choroid plexus predominates. When rats were chronically exposed to high Mn levels, the elevation of Mn in all selected areas of brain–the striatum, substantia nigra, hippocampus and frontal cortex–was similar in magnitude to that in CSF rather than plasma, thus indicating that the Mn within CSF may serve as a "sink" for Mn deposition in brain tissues.

The chemical form in which Mn is transported across the blood–brain barrier (BBB) still remains controversial. Facilitated diffusion, active transport, transferrin (Tf)-dependent mechanisms are all likely to be involved. Non-protein-bound Mn enters the brain more rapidly than Tf-bound Mn. Since albumin or α_2 macroglobulin are excluded from transport across the BBB, Mn bound to these plasma-binding proteins does not cross the BBB, unless the integrity of the BBB is compromised.

At physiological Mn blood concentration, it is postulated that Mn transport across the BBB occurs both as Mn^{2+} and as Tf-Mn conjugate. Both appear to be saturable transporters. There is much theoretical and some experimental evidence to suggest that Tf functions prominently in Mn transport across the BBB. When complexed with Tf, Mn is exclusively present in the trivalent oxidation state, with two metal ions tightly bound to each Tf molecule. At normal plasma Fe concentrations (0.9–2.8 μg/ml), normal iron binding capacity (2.5–4 μg/ml) and normal Tf concentration in plasma, (3 mg/ml), with two metal-ion-binding sites per molecule, of which 30% are occupied by Fe^{3+}, Tf has available 50 μmol of unoccupied Mn^{3+} binding sites per litre. Since Tf receptors are present on the surface of the cerebral capillaries, it has been suggested that Mn enters the endothelial cells complexed with Tf. Mn is then released from the complex in the endothelial cell interior by endosomal acidification and the apo-Tf-Tf complex is returned to the luminal surface. Mn released within the endothelial cells is subsequently transferred to the abluminal cell surface for release into the extracellular fluid. The endothelial Mn is delivered to brain-derived Tf for extracellular transport and subsequently taken up by neurons, oligodendrocytes, and astrocytes for usage and storage. Further, it has been shown that intravenous administration of ferric-hydroxide dextran complex significantly inhibited Mn brain uptake, and high Fe intakes reduced CNS Mn concentrations, thus indicating a relationship between Fe and Mn transport.

Besides these saturable transport systems (Tf-Mn conjugates and Mn^{2+}), a third transport system for Mn represents a leak pathway, presumably via circumventrical organs or choroid plexus. As the plasma Mn concentration increases, Mn transport via all the pathways increases. However, since the capacity of saturable transport system is limited, the leak-pathways become the predominant mode of Mn transport at high blood concentrations.[4,14] Within the CNS, Mn accumulates primarily in the astrocytes. The uptake of Mn into astrocytes is facilitated by a specific membrane-transport protein. Mn transport kinetic data exhibit saturation kinetics, competition by related substrates, and a probable counter-transport mechanism. As long as the concentration of Mn^{2+} in normal peripheral blood is less than 0.1μM and the level of free Mn^{2+} in blood is less than 0.02μM, the uptake on Mn^{2+} by astrocytes will increase as a linear function of concentration for a considerable range of Mn values. A number of cations affect astrocytic Mn^{2+} transport. Zn^{2+} inhibits the initial rate of Mn^{2+} uptake, but overall increases total Mn^{2+} accumulation, whereas Cu^{2+} increases both the initial rate and the total amount of accumulated Mn^{2+}. Therefore, increased Cu^{2+} and/or Zn^{2+} may lead to increased steady-state levels of Mn in the astrocytic cytoplasm, in turn altering the activity of an Mn-sensitive enzyme such as glutamine synthase.[4,14]

Within cells, manganese is found predominantly in mitochondria such as liver, kidney, and pancreas, which have relatively high Mn concentrations. In contrast, plasma Mn is extremely low.[7] There are no storage forms for Mn. Bone contains substantial quantities of Mn, however, there is no mechanism for releasing the mineral from bone. Thus, bone Mn is considered as passive storage, as it is released only as a result of normal bone turnover or in situations of accelerating bone resorption such as a sub-optimal calcium intake.[13]

Manganese is almost totally excreted in feces (92%) with only trace amounts in urine.

2. Functions

Manganese is considered essential throughout the life span because of its known function in mammalian enzyme systems, both as an integral part of metalloenzymes and as an enzyme activator. The enzymes that can be activated by Mn are numerous and include hydrolases, kinases, decarboxylases, transferases, lyases, oxidoreductases, lyases, and ligases. Most enzymes activated by Mn–except glycosyltransferases and possibly xylosyltransferase, which are Mn specific–can also be activated by other metals, especially Magnesium. In contrast to the many Mn-activated enzymes, there are only a few Mn metalloenzymes, namely arginase, pyruvate carboxylase, glutamine synthetase, and Mn superoxide dismutase.[7]

a. Antioxidant activity

Mn is one of the essential elements, which can protect against oxidative damage. *In vitro* experiments indicated that Mn scavanged superoxide radicals at nanomolar concentrations whereas hydroxyl radicals were scavanged at mocromolar concentrations.[15] A critical function attributable to Mn is the mitochondrial enzyme superoxide dismutase (SOD) that catalyzes the disproportion-ation of superoxide (O_2^-), the univalent reduction product of dioxygen. SOD functions in mito-chondrial oxygen radical metabolism, catalyzing the formation of hydrogen peroxide from reactive oxygen species.[4] Therefore, Mn deficiency could damage mitochondrial membrane by depressing the activity of Mn-SOD. Little work has been done to assess Mn-SOD activity in humans, however, a number of investigators have reported depressed activity of the enzyme in Mn-deficient animals. Zidenberg-Cherr et al.[16] reported significantly lower activity of Mn-SOD and higher mitochondrial lipid peroxidation in Mn-deficient rats than in Mn-sufficient rats. Similarly, it was demonstrated that dietary Mn could protect against *in vivo* oxidation of heart mitochondrial membrane. Mn-deficient rats had more conjugated dienes in the heart mitochondria than the Mn-adequate rats.[17] Further, it appears that the effect of Mn deficiency on tissue Mn-SOD activity is highly variable, as Mn deficiency had no effect on conjugated diene formation in liver mitochondria, heart microsomes or liver microsomes.

Besides maintaining mitochondrial membrane in the heart, Mn is also required for normal cell structure in the optic nerve[18] and cornea.[19] Mn has been also shown to perform biological functions in the retina. Photoreceptor cells of rats fed a Mn-deficient diet for 12 months showed karyopy-knosis-like changes of nuclei and a decrease in size and number of outer segments. When Mn deficiency was prolonged up to 18 months, there was a complete loss of photoreceptor cells. Deficiency for 30 months resulted in total loss of neural cells, and Muller-like cells proliferated.[20] Damage of photoreceptor cells could be attributed to decreased antioxidant action due to lower levels of Mn-SOD.

In addition to the detrimental effect on membrane integrity, altered levels of Mn-SOD have been implicated in multistage carcinogenesis in both rodents and humans. Mn-SOD activity has been reported to be low or absent in tumor cells when compared with their appropriate normal-cell counterparts in both rodents and humans. An increased amount of SOD has been shown to be protective against cancer. The addition of exogenous SOD has led to the inhibition of oncogenic transformation induced by X-ray both *in vitro* and *in vivo*. Elevation of Mn-SOD levels in tumor cells to those found in normal cells resulted in reversion of the malignant phenotype.[21] However, further work is required to investigate the association between low dietary intake of Mn and increased cancer susceptibility.

b. Carbohydrate metabolism

Mn plays an important role in carbohydrate metabolism. Enzymes—pyruvate carboxylase and phosphoenol pyruvate carboxykinase (PEPCK)—involved in gluconeogenesis require Mn for opti-mal function. No significant losses in the activity of pyruvate carboxylase have been reported during Mn deficiency, as Mn is replaced by magnesium.[16] However, low activities of PEPCK have been reported in Mn-deficient rats, although functional significance of this reduction has not been fully characterized.[22] Mn-deficient animals often exhibit a diabetic response to oral glucose challenges characterized primarily by impaired insulin production. Experiments conducted by Keen et al.[22] on Sprague Dawley rats strongly suggest a role for Mn in regulation of insulin transcription and/or in insulin mRNA turnover. These findings are consistent with reports that Mn is also involved in regulating the expression of other pancreatic genes such as amylae.[23]

c. Integrity of cartilage

Mn plays an important role in proteoglycan biosynthesis, which is essential for the integrity of cartilage. Mn deficiency results in reduction in cartilage polysaccharide content as well as qualitative changes in size and distribution of the polysaccharides.[13] One of the first structural abnormalities that was recognized to be a potential consequence of Mn deficiency was perosis in chickens, a disorder characterized by shortened and thickened limbs, curvature of the spine, and swollen and enlarged joints. Bone defects similar to those observed in birds also occur in rats and mice fed Mn-deficient diets during early development. These bone abnormalities have been largely ascribed to a reduction in proteoglycan synthesis secondary to a reduction in the activities of several Mn-dependent glycosyl transferases. These enzymes are needed for the synthesis of proteoglycan chondroitin sulphate side chains. Skeletal abnormalities in animals are characteristics of Mn deficiency, which could be attributed to decreased glycosyltransferase activity.[21] Further Mn deficiency has also been shown to reduce the activity of glycosyltransferase and concentration and composition of glycosaminoglycan (GAG) in rat aortas. Chondroitin were decreased by 38 and 36% respectively.[24] It appears that Mn is involved in arterial GAG metabolism and changes in its concentration and composition could affect arterial wall integrity and subsequently cardiovascular health.

Altered metabolism of insulin-like growth factor (IGF) has been observed in rats during chronic Mn deficiency. The deficient animals displayed lower circulating concentration of IGF-1 and insulin despite having significant elevations in circulating somatotropin concentration relative to the control group.[25] These alterations could contribute to the growth and bone abnormalities observed in deficient animals. Mn deficiency has also been reported to result in impaired osteoblast and osteoclast activities, suggesting that abnormal rate of bone growth and remodeling may also contribute to the bone deformities.

d. Development of brain

Mn is an essential trace metal required for development and functioning of the brain. This metal is a necessary component of glutamine synthetase (GS), an astrocyte-specific enzyme. GS contains 8 Mn ions per octamer and accounts for approximately 80% of total Mn in the brain. Astrocytes remove extracellular glutamate by a Na^+-dependent mechanism. In the presence of ammonia, glutamate is metabolized to glutamine by GS, maintaining $[glutamate]_0$ at $0.3\mu M$. Studies have suggested that divalent Mn or the ratio between Mn^{2+} and Mg^{2+} play a role in regulating GS.[4,14] Astrocytes are some of the neuroglial cells of the central nervous system. A reciprocal relationship exists between neurons and neuroglial cells and this association is vital for mutual differentiation, development, and functioning of these cells. Therefore, perturbations in glial cell function, as well as glial metabolism of chemicals to active intermediates, can lead to neuronal dysfunction.[26]

Recently, it has been demonstrated that Mn is released with neurotransmitters into the extracellular space during stimulation with high K^+. Mn ions may be involved in the processes dynamically coupled to the electrophysiological activity of neuronal axons. Therefore, it may be important to study the role of Mn as a functioning factor in association with synaptic transmission.[27]

Mn thus appears to be essential for optimal enzyme and membrane transport system function in all mammalian tissues and its essentiality is critical throughout the life span.

3. Deficiency

Although Mn deficiency has been observed in many species of animals, there is little evidence of its deficiency in humans. It has not been reported in free-living populations, as Mn is widely distributed in variety of foods.[28] However, a limited number of studies have reported symptoms from consuming experimental diets deficient in Mn.

Doisy et al.[29] described a case of a man who was fed a semipurified diet deficient in vitamin K and Mn (0.35 mg Mn/d) for 4 months. He developed dermatitis, decreased levels of clotting protein, weight loss, depressed growth of hair and nail, hypocholesterolemia, and slight reddening of the hair. Subsequent to the appearance of these symptoms, it was realized that Mn had been omitted from his diet. The subject responded to a mixed hospital diet, but no supplementation with Mn alone was tried.

Another possible case of Mn deficiency in humans was reported.[30] Young men fed a diet containing only 0.11 mg of Mn per day for 39 days exhibited decreased serum cholesterol, which did not respond to short-term Mn supplementation for 10 days. A fleeting dermatitis, Milliaria crystallina, developed in five out seven subjects at the end of depletion but disappeared on repletion. However, the sample size was very small.

Evidence is accumulating that Mn deficiency may be present in select populations. It has been reported in patients on long-term parenteral nutrition when the solutions were low in Mn content.[6]

Post-menopausal women supplemented with Mn maintained spinal bone density, however trace-mineral supplement also included zinc and copper.[31]

Modest supplementation of iron can result in lowering of lymphocyte Mn-SOD activity in humans.[32] In view of high frequency of iron supplementation by some groups, it is worthwhile finding out the incidence of Fe-supplementation-induced reductions in Mn status–especially in the elderly.

In addition, Mn deprivation may contribute to disease processes. Low dietary Mn and/or low blood and tissue Mn have been associated with osteoporosis, diabetes, epilepsy, atherosclerosis, and impaired wound healing.[7] Arnaud et al.[33] assessed Mn status after an acute episode of myocardial infarction. Plasma and erythrocyte Mn remained unchanged during the 2 weeks after the infarction, however, a decrease of erythrocyte Mn with age was noted. The results suggested that plasma and erythrocyte Mn do not indicate myocardial damage. The observed progressive decrease of Mn status in the elderly could be one of the risk factors for development of cardiovascular diseases. Nonetheless, Mn status in the elderly merits further attention.

4. Toxicity

In humans, Mn toxicity is recognized as a serious health hazard resulting in multiple central nervous system abnormalities. Overload or breakdown of homeostatic control of Mn leads to increased delivery to the brain, with neurotoxic consequences that appear to lie on a dose-related continuum of nervous-system dysfunction. Lower levels of Mn exposure have been associated with increased risk for sub-clinical, neurological signs consistent with early manganism. On the far end of the continuum, where Mn exposures are highest, a syndrome characterized by severe psychiatric symptoms including ataxia and disturbances of libido is present. The toxicity results in persistent damage to the extra-pyramidal system, giving rise to symptoms similar to Parkinson's disease, which include tremors, bradykinesia, abnormal gait, and dystonia. Clinical signs include elevated whole-blood Mn and urine and fecal Mn.[34] The symptoms of Mn toxicity appear very slowly over a period of several months or years. Although the course and degree of Mn intoxication can vary greatly, manganism is generally considered to have two to three phases. The first is characterized by non-specific symptoms such as asthenia, anorexia, apathy, headaches, hypersomnia, spasms, weariness of the legs, and irritability. These symptoms can occur independent of clinical neurologic signs. The second stage is characterized by signs of basal ganglia dysfunction and may include expressionless face, speech disturbance, altered gait, and fine tremor. In the final stage, muscular rigidity, staggering gait, and fine tremor are present.[35,36]

It has been suggested that older people may be more susceptible to the effects of Mn than a younger population.[34,35] Mergler et al.,[34] in their community-based study, observed Mn–age interaction for certain motor tasks, with the poorest performance observed among those > 50 years. Mn inhibits synaptosmal uptake of dopamine under *in vitro* conditions. Mn inhibition of terminal dopamine uptake could have potentially toxic effects. It appears that such inhibition is age-dependent, as it has not been observed in synaptosomes isolated from neonatal rats and such animals do not develop neurotoxicity.[37] This could partially answer the age-dependent variability, however higher vulnerability to Mn because of age needs further research.

A number of etiological factors have been recognized in Mn toxicity. Most cases in humans have been linked to the exposure of individuals to high levels of airborne Mn (>1mg/m^3).[22] Sources of environmental exposure of Mn include emissions from metallurgical processing and mining operations as well as toxic dumpsites that may contaminate groundwater, soil, and air. Mn-containing seed protectants and foliar fungicides, used on a variety of fruits and vegetables, present a risk through spraying and groundwater contamination. A relatively recent source of environmental pollution by Mn is from the use of methylclopentadienyl manganese tricarbonyl (MMT) as an anti-knock agent added to gasoline. There is evidence that levels of airborne Mn are higher in areas with higher traffic density.[34] In Greece, progressive increases of Mn concentration in drinking water were associated with a progressively higher prevalence of neurological signs of chronic Mn poisoning. However, a cross-sectional study of two cohorts in Germany separated on the basis of Mn levels in well water, found no significant difference in any neurological measure.[38] Further, Mergler et al.,[34] in their community-based study, showed that blood Mn levels greater than 7.5 µg/litre were significantly associated with changes in coordinated upper limb movements and poor learning and recall.

Mn toxicosis due only to excessive dietary intake of the element has not been reported,[22] however, it is possible that Mn obtained via food may accumulate in the body under special conditions. Reports have shown that Mn toxicosis can arise in individuals with impaired biliary function.[21] As dietary Mn is normally cleared by the liver, it is hypothesized that hepatic dysfunction could lead to Mn overload and account for the MRI abnormalities seen in patients with chronic liver diseases.[39]

Further, total parenteral nutrition bypasses the normal homeostatic mechanisms of the liver and gut. Hypermanganesemia, neurological symptoms and Mn deposition in the brain on MRI scanning have been reported in patients receiving long-term parenteral nutrition.[40,41] There appears to be a need to administer lower doses of Mn during parenteral nutrition.

The unique combination of low dietary intake of calcium and magnesium together with high concentrations of aluminium and Mn in drinking water, has been proposed as a factor in the incidence of amyotrophic lateral sclerosis and Parkinsonian dementia in specific areas of the western Pacific. These metal–metal interactions may lead to unequal distributions of aluminium and Mn in bones and the central nervous system, resulting in neural degeneration.[42]

The biochemical mechanisms underlying Mn toxicity are complex, and possibly a number of metabolic dysfunctions together account for Mn neurotixicity. Mn may produce its effects through glutamate excitotoxicity. Sustained increases in glutamate are neurotoxic, presumably by persistent interactions with N-methyl-D-aspartate (NMDA) receptors and a resulting sustained influx of calcium ions. It has been shown that Mn produces changes consistent with NMDA excitotoxic lesions.[36]

At higher concentrations, Mn can be neurotoxic by generating the free radicals.[43] Mn-induced dopamine auto-oxidation has been suggested as a possible mechanism, although its significance is unknown, due to the direct antioxidant property of Mn.[37]

Neuron loss and gliosis in the globus pallidus are hallmarks of human and experimental manganism in primates. The globus pallidus is characterized by a high rate of oxidative phosphorylation. Mn accumulates within mitochondria and is associated with an inhibition of oxidative phosphorylation and decreased ATP synthesis. Mn is transported out of mitochondria via the slow Na^+- independent efflux mechanism, but inhibits Ca^{2+} efflux, thereby poising the mitochondria for promoting a Ca^{2+} permeability transition, collapsing the mitochondrial membrane potential and decreasing both oxidative phosphorylation and intra mitochondrial glutathione (GSH). The lowered GSH content would be expected from the altered NADPH/NADP ration induced by defective mitochondrial function. These metabolic dysfunctions ultimately lead to reduced energy status, increased lipoperoxidation, and abnormal $[Ca^{2+}]$. Accelerations of neurotoxicity ensue through the activation of an excitotoxic state consequent upon mitochondrial dysfunction.[37]

5. Dietary Requirements

Mn is essential for life, however, there are few reported cases of Mn deficiency in humans. Because of this lack of information, a Recommended Dietary Allowance (RDA) has not yet been suggested for Mn in humans. Instead, the estimated safe and adequate daily dietary intake (ESADDI) has been put forward by the National Research Council, as shown in Table 5.1.[7]

TABLE 5.1
Estimated Safe and Adequate
Daily Dietary Intakes (ESADDI)
for Mn for Various Age Groups

| Age (Years) | ESADDI for Mn | |
	μmol/day	Mg/day
Infants 0–0.5	5.5–10.9	0.3–0.6
Infants 0.5–1	5.5–18.2	0.3–1.0
Children 1–3	18.2–27.3	1.0–1.5
Children 4–6	27.3–36.4	1.5–2.0
Children 7–10	36.4–54.6	2.0–3.0
Adolescents 11–18	36.4–91.0	2.0–5.0
Adults	36.4–91.0	2.0–5.0

Reference: No. 7.

These values are based on the reasoning that most dietary intakes fall into this range and do not result in deficiency or toxicity signs. However, there are number of shortcomings in the approach used to determine the ESADDI:

- Values have been set in the absence of good biomarkers and have been based on typical intakes of Mn and on data from short-term balance studies.
- Approach ignored the impact of bioavailability.
- Entire body of literature on balance and regression studies using the factorial approach was not considered.[44,45]

Separate ESADDI have not been recommended for the elderly, whose Mn requirements may be different from those for younger individuals because:

- Mn is a component of mitochondrial SOD and thus is involved in the metabolism of free radicals. Oxidative stress is associated with a number of degenerative diseases common among older people.
- Mn is essential for the integrity of cartilage. Its supplementation, along with Cu and Zn, has been shown to maintain spinal bone density in postmenopausal women. It appears that low Mn intake may be associated with osteoporosis.
- Fe supplements are commonly recommended to the elderly. Interactions between Fe and Mn may compromise Mn status if dietary intake of the latter is low.

In view of this, ESADDI of Mn may need further modification.

In contrast to the paucity of substantiated reports of Mn deficiency, there are many reports of Mn toxicity in humans. Most of these are cases of acute toxicity, primarily in miners who inhale Mn-laden dust. Therefore, the Environmental Protection Agency (EPA) has established the reference dose for Mn (the amount of Mn that can be safely consumed on a daily basis over the course of a lifetime) at 0.14 mg Mn/kg/d or 10 mg Mn/d for a 70-kg individual. EPA officials thought that a separate standard was required for Mn in drinking water because of the greater bioavailability of Mn in water than in food. Based on epidemiological studies in Greece, EPA estimated the lowest-observable-adverse-effect level (LOAEL) for Mn in water to be 4.2 mg Mn per day or 0.06 mg Mn/kg/d.[21,44,45] Thus, on the basis of very limited data, these standards suggest that individuals consuming the amount of Mn recommended by the ESADDI (5mg Mn/d) could consume excessive amounts of Mn (> 4.2 mg Mn/d) if most of the Mn came from water. This may be a matter for concern, especially among older people, who are more susceptible to the neurotoxic effects of Mn. There appears to be lack of consensus and overlap between the reference dose of Mn put forward by the EPA and the ESADDI suggested by the National Research Council.

There is a need to develop alternative approaches, such as the response of reliable biomarkers to changes in Mn status. Potential indices for assessing the effects of Mn under conditions of deficiency and excess in humans may include concentrations of plasma Mn, mononuclear blood cell Mn, and lymphocyte Mn-SOD activity. For toxicity, a magnetic resonance image (MRI) showing Mn deposition may be the best indicator.[45]

6. Sources

Unrefined cereals, nuts, leafy vegetables, and tea are major contributors of daily dietary Mn. Indian diets high in foods of plant origin supply, on average, 8.3 mg of Mn/day, whereas highly refined hospital diets in the U.S. supply a range less than 0.36–1.78 mg Mn/day. Similarly, Mn intakes of adults consuming self-selected diets in Canada, New Zealand, and the U.S. have been reported to be 3.1, 2.7, and 2.9 mg respectively.[6] The average daily dietary intake of Mn by Austrians tested at 12 different locations was found to be 4.69 mg (range 4.39–5.66 mg).[46] The FDA's Total Diet Study estimated a mean daily Mn intake of 2.7 and 2.2 mg for adult men and women respectively.[28] Thus, reported mean intakes of Mn throughout the world are less than the reference dose of 10 mg/day.

Fruits and vegetables are a rich source of Mn, and vegetarian diets may contain considerably higher amounts of Mn. However, there are no definitive data suggesting any problems when dietary intake surpasses the reference dose. Biochemical and physiological changes were not observed in two separate studies when young women were fed 15 mg of supplemental Mn/d (providing a total intake of approx. 18 mg/d) for 126 days and 9.5 mg Mn/d for 56 days.[21] Further, cereals and green vegetables, which are important dietary sources of Mn, also contain significant amounts of Fe. Therefore, their impact on Mn status will be limited because of the interaction between Mn and Fe.[38]

Mn exposure from dietary sources may be exacerbated by factors that either increase its absorption or reduce its excretion.

B. Vanadium

Vanadium, atomic number 23, is a transition element whose necessity for humans has not been firmly established. Interest in vanadium has increased since 1977, with the finding on ion transport pathways and that it inhibits ATPases.[7] However, the physiological essentiality of vanadium in the regulation of these ion pumps was not established. Since the 80s, the role of vanadium as an active pharmacological substance, both *in vivo* and *in vitro,* has been the subject of study. Absence of vanadium may adversely affect growth as well as the animal's ability to deal with experimental stress, toxins, or carcinogens,[47] although its essentiality is still inconclusive.[48] The evidence for the possible essentiality of vanadium has appeared only since 1987.[7]

The effects of vanadium compounds on a wide variety of biological systems are of interest, especially its regulatory capabilities.

1. Chemistry

Vanadium is multivalent, can exist in oxidation states from −1 to +5, and forms polymers frequently. Under physiological conditions (pH 3–7, aerobic solution, ambient temperature) the chemical species includes vanadate, a mixture of $[HVO_4]^{2-}$, $[HVO_4]^-$ and vanadyl, and VO^{2+}. In higher animals, tetravalent and pentavalent states are apparently the most important forms. The tetravalent vanadyl cation, VO^{2+} behaves like a simple divalent aquo ion and completes with Ca^{2+}, Mn^{2+}, Fe^{2+}, etc. for ligand-binding sites.[7] Vo^{2+} easily complexes with proteins. Thus, *in vivo*, like other metal ions, it is complexed with molecules associated with iron, such as transferrin or ferritin, albumin in plasma, hemoglobin in erythrocytes, glutathione or other low-molecular-weight compounds intracellularly.[47] Complexation with such proteins stabilizes vanadate against oxidation.

Vanadate also complexes with cis-diols and those substances that result in its being a phosphate transition state analog. Vanadyl binds to 2-amino acids, nucleic acids, phosphates, phospholipids, glutathione, citrate, oxalate, lactate, ascorbate etc.[49] Thus, vanadate competes with phosphate in many biochemical processes.[48]

Vanadium is easily reduced by ascorbate, glutathione, or NADH. In cells like adipocytes, vanadate enters through nonspecific anionic channels and is reduced and complexed by glutathione. The predominant form in extracellular fluids is vanadate (VO_{-3}, V^{+5}) and inside the cell vanadyl (VO^{2+}, V^{+4}) respectively.[49]

In biologic systems, three types of behavior can be predicted for vanadium.[50]

1. As vanadate, it competes at the active sites of phosphate-transport proteins, phosphohydrolases, and phosphotransferases.
2. As vanadyl, it competes with other transition metal ions for binding sites on metalloproteins and for small ligands such as ATP.
3. Vanadium participates in redox reactions within the cell, particularly with relatively small molecules that can reduce vanadate non-enzymatically, e.g. glutathione.

The potential for redox interplay increases the versatility of vanadium in the biological milieu. Although vanadium may not play an essential role in normal mammalian metabolism, it has a potential therapeutic role at pharmacological concentrations. Vanadium has potential as a complementary approach to the management of diabetes for insulin resistance and insulin deficiency.[51,52] Enhanced glucose uptake, oxidation, and synthesis; protein tyrosine phosphorylation, potassium uptake, decreased triglyceride hydrolysis, and protein degradation were demonstrated *in vitro*.[49]

2. Metabolism

Although most foods contain less than 1 ng of vanadium per gram of the material, food is the major source of vanadium. Lungs also absorb vanadium (V_2O_5).[53]

Most orally ingested vanadium is not absorbed and it is predominantly excreted through the feces. Studies indicate that generally 1% of vanadium ingested through the diet is absorbed, and, more often than not, the amount does not exceed 5%. However, under some conditions, rats have been observed to absorb more than 10%. Thus, it cannot be assumed that the poor absorption of this element is uniform under all conditions.[48,50]

Most ingested vanadium is transformed to VO^{2+} in the stomach, in which form it passes through the duodenum. Vanadate can enter cells through phosphate or other anion transport systems. VO_{3-} is absorbed 3 to 5 times more effectively than VO^{2+}. The percentage of ingested vanadium absorbed may depend on the form, the rate at which it is transformed into VO^{2+}, and the effect of other dietary components. Substances such as EDTA, ascorbic acid, chromium, protein, and ferrous iron can reduce vanadium toxicity.[50]

The homeostatic mechanisms for clearance of ingested or injected vanadium from the blood stream are efficient. It is retained in highest amounts in the kidney, liver, testes, bone, and spleen. The tissues normally contain less than 10 ng v/g fresh weight. Most of the excessive retained (exogenous) vanadium is deposited in bone.

Urinary excretion accounts for one-third to almost half of an intravenous dose of [48]V within 96 hours with 9–10% being found in the feces of rats. A significant portion may also be excreted through bile.[50,54] Binding of the vanadyl ion to iron-containing non-heme proteins is of significance. High- and low-molecular-weight complexes, one of which may be transferrin, have been detected in urine. Although no reference values are established, values around 1 n mol/l for blood and serum and approximately (10 n mol/l for urine may be considered tentative normal values in persons without occupational exposure to vanadium. In Belgium, concentrations of 0.014-0.222 ng/ml of serum in adults were observed.[55] In Czechoslovakia, 0.024–0.226 ng/ml of whole blood was observed in non-exposed children. In potentially exposed children, the range of concentrations was similar, although the mean value was almost twice that of the non-exposed children.[48]

Vanadium serves as a cofactor for several halogen peroxidases and may be important in regulation of thyroxine deiodinase. High-iodine diets have been found to exacerbate the effects of vanadium deprivation in rats.[53]

3. Functions and Mode of Action

For a nutrient to be recognized as essential, its deficiency has to be linked to a well-documented pathology. Studies in animals suggest that vanadium may play a role in reproduction. Vanadium deficiency has been observed to result in abortion, perinatal mortality, bone abnormalities, and changes in thyroid metabolism.

The potential role of vanadium in thyroid metabolism may possibly be explained by nutrients such as iodide, iron, and sulfur containing amino acids that interact with vanadium and that are important for thyroid function. In experimental studies, vanadium was found to influence metabolism of protein, chloride, iodide, chromium, iron, copper, ascorbic acid, and riboflavin.[52]

The basic mechanism underlying the biological role of vanadium could be related to its effect on bioenergetic processes such as phosphorylation/dephosphorylation and activation/ deactivation of several important enzymes such as Na K-ATPases, Ca-ATPase, Mg-ATPase and myosin-ATPase, which are inhibited by vanadium. Vanadate's close resemblance to phosphate enables it to inhibit many of the enzymes involved in phosphate metabolism and in phosphorylation and dephosphorylation.[52]

Iodoperoxidase and bromoperoxidase facilitate formation of carbon–halogen bonds. Thyroid peroxidase, which is a good example of a haloperoxidase in rats, has been shown to be affected by vanadium deprivation.[3]

Vanadium may exert a complex regulatory effect on levels and activity of cAMP through activation of tyrosine kinase and protein kinase c-mediated processes. Thus, a broad range of functions that result from the role of cAMP in hormonal interactions may be affected.[52]

4. Pharmacological Role/Function

a. Insulin-mimetic effects

Initial studies on cell homogenates showed that vanadium has insulin-like effects. It stimulates glucose uptake, glycogen synthesis, and glucose oxidation in adipocytes, hepatocytes, and skeletal muscle. In diabetic animals, oral vanadate treatment partially or completely restored liver and muscle activities of enzymes involved in glycolysis and glycogenesis such as glucose kinase, phosphoenolpyruvate carboxykinase, pyruvate kinase, and glycogen synthase. These effects were not secondary to a restoration of normal plasma glucose levels. Treatment *in vivo* has been consistently and reproducibly associated with a decrease in plasma insulin, apparently enhanced peripheral insulin sensitivity, and lowered insulin demand. Clinical trials of vanadium compounds in IDDM (Type I) and NIDDM (Type II) human subjects have yielded positive results—improved insulin sensitivity, decreased fasting-glucose concentration as well as hepatic-glucose production.[53,56] Decrease in glycosylated hemoglobin were also observed.[57]

Lipid pathways were affected in specific tissues such as inhibition of lipolysis, stimulation of lipogenesis in adipocytes in animals,[56] and a decline in plasma free fatty acid concentrations in humans.[56] Hepatic and skeletal muscle insulin sensitivity was improved in NIDDM but not in obese subjects.[56]

Organic complexes of vanadium have been found to be superior to inorganic vanadate or vanadyl (at significantly lower doses).

b. Other biological effects

- Other effects that have been observed include (in animals) a digitalis-like action on the cardiovascular system, increased diuresis, and excretion of sodium possibly through inhibition of sodium reabsorption. This natruretic effect of vanadium may be reversible.
- Vanadium compounds may behave as antioxidants.
- In rats, vanadium feeding with sucrose lowered systolic blood pressure by 11–16% of the sucrose-fed value, decreased angiotensin II significantly (25–60% of the sucrose-fed value), and a 61–76% of increase in endothelin-1 level.[58]
- Vanadium may have an antineoplastic role. Ammonium monovanadate before initiation, or throughout initiation and the promotional period, significantly reversed alterations in haematological indices. Observations suggest that vanadium may offer protection against DENA-mediated rat liver carcinogenesis.[59]

However, the levels at which vanadium has demonstrated these effects are relatively high (1-2 mg/kg/day in humans and 0.1 and 0.7 m mol/kg/day in animals). This may be at least 50 to 100 times more than the habitual daily dietary intakes of humans. The amount used in the clinical studies indicates that this element is being used as nutraceutical.

5. Deficiency

Deficiency of vanadium has been difficult to establish because of its ubiquitous nature and its very low requirement by animals. Also, the diets used in early studies on deprivation had wide variations in their contents of other nutrients such as protein, sulphur, amino acids, ascorbic acid, iron, copper, and others that can affect vanadium.[50] The amount of vanadium supplemented in these diets was also high. Efforts have been made to characterize a consistent set of deficiency signs for animals.

In vanadium-deprivation studies on goats, animals receiving 2 ng vanadium per gram of diet compared with controls fed 10 µg vanadium per gm of diet, showed higher abortion rate and produced less milk during the first 56 days of lactation. Forty percent of the newborn goats born to vanadium-deprived mothers died between days 7 and 91 of life, compared with a mortality of only 9% newborns in the vanadium-supplemented group. Also, the vanadium-deprived animals had developmental skeletal deformations in the forelegs and forefoot tarsal joints. In addition, biochemical alterations such as elevated serum creatinine and β-lipoproteins and depressed blood glucose levels have been observed.

In rats, vanadium deprivation resulted in impaired reproduction—decreased fertility and increased perinatal mortality. These alterations were observed only in the fourth generation of vanadium-deprived animals. Changes were also seen in thyroid weight. Vanadium deficiency significantly increased packed cell volume in chicks.[60] Vanadium deprivation in chicks led to depressed growth, elevation in haematocrit, and plasma cholesterol, as well as adversely affected bone development.

The effects of vanadium deprivation on growth and skeletal abnormalities may be related to the element's role in thyroid functions. Thyroid hormones affect bone formation and hypothyroidism can reduce bone formation and resorption. Thyroid hormones may also enhance the production of somatomedins, which regulate cartilage growth and maturation.

Rats fed less than 100 ng vanadium per gram of diet exhibited poor growth, higher plasma and bone iron, as well as higher hematocrits than controls.

In animals, at least, vanadium appears to be essential. However, in humans, its broad pharmacological activity *in vitro* and *in vivo* point to its biological importance, but do not clearly provide the evidence for its essentiality.[52]

6. Sources

Foods rich in vanadium include shellfish, mushrooms, parsley, and black pepper. Fresh fruits and vegetables are poorer sources of vanadium,[55] containing 1 to 5 ng/g. Whole grains, sea foods, meat, and dairy products contain 5 to 30 ng/g.[17] Normal diets have been found to supply 118–393 nmol of V per day.[1] Daily intakes may vary widely. Nine institutional diets supplied 12.4-30.1 μg of vanadium/day, with an average of 20 μg[6]. In the UK, average dietary intakes of 13 μg per day were observed. In the USFDA's Total Diet Study of daily intakes of vanadium for eight age-sex groups, intakes of 6.2 to 18.3 μg were observed.

Most diets supply 15 μg/day and the content does not exceed 30 μg/day.[50] The highest intakes observed are in the range of 60 μg/day.[61]

7. Requirements

A daily intake of 10 μg/day will probably meet vanadium requirements. Average basal and normative requirements cannot be set, because requisite data are not available. Toxicity effects have been observed at levels 10 to 100 times the amount normally present in the diet. Uthus et al.[3] have recommended that, for ultratrace elements such as vanadium, for which very little information is available, the term "estimated daily dietary intake" be used. These authors suggested that the EDDI should be 10–20 μg. The postulated need by humans can be met by typical diets.[55]

8. Toxicity

Vanadium is also a major trace element in fossil fuels. Their combustion is a significant source of this ultratrace element in the environment. It is also widely used in steel and chemical industries. Mining and milling of vanadium-bearing ores and combustion of fossil fuels result in high levels of respirable vanadium particles/fuels in the workplace. Vanadium exposure has been linked to lung cancer.[2] Occupational exposure is common in petrochemical, mining, steel, and utilities industries.

Vanadium is relatively toxic. The threshold for toxicity apparently is near 10–20 mg/day or 10–20 μg/g of diet in both animals and humans.[48] A variety of signs of vanadium toxicity exist because they vary with species and dosage. Consistently observed toxic effects include depressed growth, elevated organ vanadium, diarrhea, depressed food intake, and death. Gastrointestinal disturbances and green tongue were observed in humans given 13.5 mg for 2 months followed by 22.5 mg for 5 months. In another study, signs of toxicity were observed on intakes of 4.5–18 mg/day for 6 to 10 weeks. In a supplementation study for treatment of NIDDM, transient mild effects such as mild nausea, diarrhea, and cramps were observed on intakes of approximately 23.5 mg vanadium/day in the form of vanadyl sulfate.[55]

Recent studies in experimental animals suggest that several toxic effects may occur.

- Significant reduction in general activity and learning in rats.[62]
- Vanadate (V^{+5}) and Vanadyl (V^{+4}) may be reproductive and developmental toxins in mammals.[49]
- Hepatoxicity and nephrotoxicity have also been observed. Vanadium, like some other metals, tends to accumulate in the kidney, often leading to nephrotoxicity. The effects observed in rats include hypokalemic distal renal tubular acidosis, enhanced renal peroxidation, increased urinary excretion of solutes and water, inhibition of Na^+-K^+-ATPase and organic ion accumulation, natriuresis, diuresis, and vasoconstriction.

- Vanadate and vanadyl ions induce mutagenic and genotoxic effects. These ions make chemical complexes that have the property of inhibiting or increasing the activity of enzymes participating in DNA and RNA synthesis. Effects observed include cytotoxicity, increase in cellular differentiation, and gene expression alterations.[63]
- Vanadium exposure has been associated with inflammatory changes in the upper and lower respiratory tracts as well as changes in pulmonary function. In rats, vanadium compounds increased mRNA levels for cytokines in bronchoalveolar lavage cells in a dose-dependent manner.[64]

In vanadium-plant workers, there is evidence to suggest that inhaled V_2O_5 induces bronchial hyper responsiveness and asthma.[65]

The nephrotoxic effects of vanadate were found to be more severe in adult rats. Morphologic changes in the kidney were more pronounced with age. These findings are of concern, especially if vanadium compounds are to be used in treatment of diabetic patients. Vanadium has prooxidant activity and higher intakes may increase selenium requirements. In rats, vanadium administration led to increased lipid peroxidation in brain cells, and concurrent selenium treatment prevented the oxidative effect. The prooxidant activities of vanadium fumes may induce inflammatory changes in eye conjunctiva as well.

In animals fed high dietary vanadate, tissue vanadium was markedly elevated, especially in kidney, bone and liver.[52]

The dosages required for therapeutic action are far in excess of estimated daily dietary intakes. At present, inadequate information limits the possibility of suggesting requirements—especially for the elderly. It is first necessary to seek answers to questions such as how much vanadium humans need. How much of the dietary vanadium is absorbed and utilized? Does aging reduce the ability of various organs to metabolize—especially to eliminate the element? Although this ultratrace element has biological potential, its nutraceutical role should be viewed separately from dietary requirements.

C. MOLYBDENUM

Molybdenum (Mo) is an essential trace metal for every form of life. It is an active cofactor for a number of enzymes. The evidence for essentiality of Mo is noncontroversial, since specific biochemical functions have been defined for it. However, deficiency of Mo has yet to be unequivocally identified in humans in the general population.[50]

The first evidence for essentiality of this element was provided by the finding that Mo in the enzyme xanthine oxidase (dehydrogenase) was involved in the conversion of tissue purines to uric acid.[6]

Its radioisotope, [99]Mo, may be released in significant amounts as a consequence of accidents in nuclear power plants or nuclear medicine installations.[66] In Chernobyl, about 6% of the total activity released within the first 10 days was due to [99]Mo.[67] It is used with activities in nuclear medicine in ^{99m}Tc generators, with its mishandling leading to contamination.[67] The biokinetics and metabolism of Mo have been widely studied in ruminants. Severe diseases are caused by an imbalance in the concentrations of molybdenum, copper, and sulfur in their forage.[68]

1. Chemistry

Mo is a transition element. Its ability to exist in a number of different oxidation states explains its remarkable catalytic activity and its action as an electron transfer agent in oxidation reduction reactions.[7,69] Mo is the main constituent of the cofactor of enzymes such as xanthine oxidase, sulfite oxidase, and aldehyde oxidase. The cofactor is molybdopterin, a substituted pterin to which Mo is bound by two sulfur atoms.[6] Molybdenum-cofactor-containing enzymes catalyze the transfer of an oxygen atom, ultimately derived from or incorporated into water, to or from a substrate in a 2-electron redox reaction.

In the oxidized form of molybdoenzymes, molybdenum is probably present in the 6+ state. The enzymes are probably first reduced to the 5+ state during electron transfer. However, other oxidation states have been found in reduced enzymes. Mo-containing enzymes catalyze basic metabolic reactions in the nitrogen, sulfur, and carbon cycles,[7] Mo is present at the active site of enzymes as a cofactor containing a pterin nucleus. With the exception of the nitrogenase cofactor, molybdenum is incorporated into proteins as the molybdenum cofactor that contains a mononuclear molybdenum atom coordinated to the sulfur atoms of a pterin derivative molybdopterin.[70] Although the function of the molybdopterin ligand has not yet been conclusively established, interactions of this ligand with the coordinated metal are sensitive to the oxidation state, indicating that the molybdopterin may be directly involved in the enzymatic mechanism.[70]

Almost all Mo in liver is present as this cofactor, with almost 60% in sulfite oxidase and xanthine oxidase. In addition to the molybdenum cofactor and "enzymatic" Mo, the other important form of Mo is the molybdate ion (MoO_4^{2-}), which is the main form in blood and urine.

2. Metabolism

Mo is readily absorbed from foods. Werner et al.[69] observed that the pattern of intestinal Mo absorption may be different from that of other essential trace metals like iron or cobalt. Small amounts of up to 1mg Mo are completely absorbed. With higher doses up to 5mg, there is only a slight reduction in absorption. Compared with aqueous solution, where $\geq$ 90% is absorbed, Mo in black tea is less well absorbed, probably because of binding by polyphenols.

Mo from labeled cress and a labeled composite meal was less well absorbed than from aqueous solutions, suggesting that there may be inhibitory factors in the composite meal.[69] When Mo was given with a solid meal, intestinal absorption was less than 50% of the administered amount.

In seven healthy subjects, when high amounts of [100]Mo were administered, i.e., 50 µg Mo per kg body weight (equivalent to 3–5 mg) as ammonium molybdate in coffee, intestinal absorption ranged from 35% to 96%.[5] Thus, variable amounts of Mo appear to be absorbed, influenced by various factors.

Studies were conducted on human subjects for prolonged periods by Turnlund et al.[71,72] wherein the natural Mo content of the daily diet was kept constant at levels ranging from 22 µg to 1500 µg. At different junctures, dietary Mo was replaced by an analogous mass of [100]Mo. The intestinal absorption was high, between 88% and 93%, depending on the mass of total dietary Mo. As the amount of dietary Mo increased from 22 µg, 120 µg and then 1500 µg, respectively; the amount of the 33 µg of Mo excreted rose from 13 µg (39%) to 28 µg (85%) and 31 µg (94%). Thompson and coworkers[73] studied Mo metabolism in four young, healthy male volunteers given five dietary levels of Mo ranging from 22 to 1470 µg/day. These studies indicated that diffusion was the major absorptive mechanism, with the concentration of the Mo being rate-limiting.

It has been suggested that, at low concentrations, absorption of this element is active and carrier mediated. However, when absorption was studied over a 10-fold range of concentrations, the *in vivo* absorption rates were essentially unchanged, indicating that the absorption may be occurring by diffusion. It is possible that Mo is transported by both diffusion and by active transport. At high concentrations, the active transport mechanism may contribute much less to the movement of Mo.[7]

Molybdenum is transported loosely attached to erythrocytes in blood. Mo tends to bind specifically to α_2-macroglobulin. Organs that retain the highest amount of Mo are the liver and kidneys. The compartment with the longest retention time is the skeleton, which accounts for 10% of the systemic Mo. The remaining Mo is distributed among the liver (25%), kidney (5%) and "other tissues" (60%).[67,74]

The liver takes up Mo and tends not to release it, unlike the kidney and gastrointestinal tract. Supplemental Mo is found predominantly in the liver 24 hours after infusion. The kidney and spleen also constitute fast turnover tissues, although the kinetics of disappearance are different from the liver's.[73]

Very little Mo is found in muscle or brain.[73] However, Nakagawa[75] observed in a murine model, senescence-accelerated mouse prone 10 (SAMP 10), that Mo levels in the brain increased with age as compared with the control. It is possible that abnormal metabolism of Mo as well as zinc, copper, manganese, rubidium, and neurotransmitters may cause the senescence acceleration of SAMP 10.

Mo is excreted either through urine or into feces through the intestines. Mo in systemic circulation is transferred to the kidney, the bladder, and to the storage in approximate ratios of 100:50:7. The stored Mo is excreted with an approximate ratio urine; feces equal to 2:1. Significant amounts of Mo are also excreted in bile.

Urinary excretion rather than absorption is the major site of homeostatic regulation. In most animal species, retention of Mo is low and more or less complete excretion occurred during the first 2 weeks after single exposure. Elevated intakes of Mo result in rapid attainment of balance and no progressive accumulation.[73] Urinary excretion is reported to be very fast. The ratio between urinary and fecal excretion may be 8:1.[67]

Concentrations of Mo in serum and blood are normally very low, from 2 to 12 nmol/l ranging over four orders of magnitude.[6] Levels in urine are 11 to 88 (g per 24 hours.[1] Paschal et al.[74] observed that Mo was detectable in 99.8% of samples of urine obtained from U.S. residents. Mo concentrations ranged up to 688 µg/l, the 95th percentile concentration being 168 µg/l.

Defects in liver function, whether induced by infection, tumors, or drugs are frequently accompanied by elevation in serum Mo. Elevated blood Mo has also been observed in uremia, rheumatic disorders and cardiovascular diseases.[6]

On the whole, further data is required to derive reliable estimates of Mo status in normal individuals.[6]

3. Functions

Molybdoenzymes catalyze hydroxylation of various substrates. Aldehyde oxidase oxidizes and detoxifies various pyrimidines, purines, pteridines, and related compounds. Xanthine oxidase catalyzes the transformation of hypoxanthine to xanthine and the latter to uric acid. Sulfite oxidase catalyzes the transformation of sulfite to sulfate.

Mo may be involved in stabilizing the steroid-binding ability of unoccupied steroid receptors. *In vitro*, Mo has been found to protect the glucocorticoid receptor against inactivation. It is possible that this ultratrace element affects the glucocorticoid receptor because it mimics an endogenous compound called "modulator."[7]

There are some reports in the literature from South Africa and China that a high incidence of esophageal cancer may be linked to deficiency of Mo. In rats, 2 or 20 µg Mo/g of diet inhibited esophageal and stomach cancer following administration of N-nitrososarcosine ethyl ester. At concentrations of 10 mg/l in drinking water of rats, Mo was found to inhibit mammary carcinogenesis induced by N-nitroso-N-methylurea.

In humans, some studies suggest that Mo may have an anticariogenic effect. Teeth accumulate Mo and dental enamel is relatively rich in Mo. However, further studies are required to conclusively state where Mo plays a preventive role in dental caries.[6]

Similarly, it has been noted that, for development of Keshan's disease, coexisting Mo deficiency with Selenium deficiency is necessary. However, in areas where the disease is endemic, high content of Mo has been observed for rice, wheat, and soya as well as in the tissue and hair of subjects. The role of Mo in development of Keshan's disease still remains to be elucidated.[6]

4. Toxicity

Toxicity has been considered to be of greater concern than deficiency for Mo.[45] Mo intake in the general population depends on the soil and water content of a particular region. Few humans have been exposed to high intakes of Mo except in cases of industrial exposure, although high intakes of up to 10–15 mg/day have been observed in India and Russia. In some parts of Turkey, Mo content of water is high.

Intakes of 10–15 mg/d may lead to gout-like symptoms along with high blood concentrations of Mo, uric acid, and xanthine oxidase.[45] Occupational exposure to Mo may occur, for, example, in molybdenum-roasting plants. In Armenia, elevated serum Mo values and abnormally high activities of xanthine dehydrogenase were associated with elevated concentrations in blood and urine.[6]

High levels of Mo intake are suspected of interfering with copper metabolism and may result in gout-like symptoms in humans.[73] In cattle, it was observed that Mo supplementation lowered copper (Cu) storage in the liver. Excess dietary Mo might induce Cu deficiency. Also, a low Mo concentration of normal copper content in forage might predispose sheep to Cu toxicity. Sulfur renders both Cu and Mo biologically unavailable and only in the presence of dietary sulfur does Mo lower copper availability. When all three are present, cupric tetrathiomolybdate, a highly insoluble complex, is formed. Absorption of thiomolybdate and subsequent formation of $CuMoS_4$ in the blood of ruminant animals, accounts for the high concentration of blood copper that is not bioavailable.[76]

There are some reports about a possible relationship between Mo concentrations in soils, diet, and tumor incidence.[77] Mo intoxication is accompanied by a wide range of symptoms, some of which may be linked to induction of a secondary deficiency of copper. Typical features of acute, uncomplicated molybdenosis include defects in osteogenesis, possibly caused by deranged phosphorus metabolism, leading to skeletal and joint deformities, spontaneous subepiphyseal features, and mandibular exostoses. Alkaline phosphatase activity and the proteoglycan content of cartilage are decreased.[6] Extrapolation of data from other species suggests that, in humans, high intakes observed in China and Russia may promote thiomolybdate formation and, in turn, induce systemic antagonistic effects on copper utilization. In nonhuman species, Mo intoxication inhibits synthesis of "active" sulfate (phosphoadenosine phosphosulfate), and estrus as well as inducing interstitial testicular degeneration, possibly through effects on estrogen- and androgen-receptor activities. However, the extent to which these can extrapolated to humans needs to be determined.[6]

The role of xanthine oxidase in oxidative stress needs to be considered. This enzyme normally functions as a dehydrogenase. However, when it reacts with oxygen, it initiates the production of a series of highly reactive oxygen-rich free radicals.[6] Free radicals have been associated with tissue damage and consequently with a variety of diseases such as diabetes mellitus, atherosclerosis, cancer etc. Excess Mo has been associated with tissue damage due to free radicals.

Mo may be one of the metals released from prostheses and implants. Increased concentrations of alloy materials have been found in blood and tissues of patients in whom devices have failed. It is possible that sensitivity reactions could be established with further destruction of the implant.[2]

5. Dietary Considerations and Requirements:

There is enough evidence to indicate that Mo is essential. However, deficiencies of this element due to inadequate dietary intake have not been unequivocally identified in humans. This is probably because it is ubiquitous and because of the low levels of intake required. Also, estimates of daily intake vary considerably, in part, due to the difficulty in estimating dietary Mo accurately. Also, there are extreme regional variations in soil, availability of Mo, and the extent to which Mo is present in food crops. Foods such as milk and milk products, dried legumes, organ meats like liver and kidney, and cereals are good sources of the element. Nonleguminous vegetables, fruits, sugar, and fish are poor sources.[7]

However, vegetation grown on soil derived from shales, mineralized granites, and some peats tend to have higher Mo content. This may lead to Mo toxicity in farm livestock and possibly to threshold Mo toxicity in humans. Similarly, industrial pollution may also lead to high Mo content of crops grown near and around Mo-processing plants.[6]

Intakes of 0.076 to 0.24 mg/d have been reported.[45] Earlier reports indicated that usual dietary intakes of Mo were 0.1 to 0.46 mg/d. However, intakes as high as 856 µg have been observed. In Japan, median intakes of 250 µg/day have been reported, with a mean of 255 ± 67 µg/day.[78]

Holzinger and Coworkers[79] investigated the Mo consumption in 1988, 1992, and 1996, in 14 test groups of persons with mixed diets. The Mo intakes of adults with mixed diets increased significantly from 1988 to 1996. Intake differed among locations and the kind of diet. Intakes of vegetarians were higher—179 µg/d among females and 170 µg/d among males compared with 89 µg/d and 100 µg/d respectively for subjects on mixed diets from the two sexes. The average intake of Mexican men was 208 µg/d, which was higher than the average of German men (162 µg/d). In France, the Mo intake has been estimated to be 275 µg/d.[80]

An international survey of dietary trace element intakes was conducted with rigorous analytical control under the supervision of the IAEA. Carried out in 11 countries, the study suggests that the average Mo intake is approximately 100 µg/day for adults.[6]

In breast-fed infants, typical Mo intakes ranged from 0.1 to 0.5 µg per kg of body weight per day. These intakes were lower than the previous recommendation of the World Health Organization (WHO) (2 µg Mo/kg body weight) and the U.S. National Academy of Sciences (30–60 µg Mo/day). However, in the Philippines and India, high Mo content in breast milk has been observed.

In children between weaning and 3 years of age, Mo intakes were higher—5–7 µg/kg body weight. Thereafter, intakes appeared to be lower, namely 1.5–3 µg/kg of body weight. Intakes by adolescents and adults appeared to be in a similar range.

However, Asian diets may contain more Mo partly because of predominantly vegetarian diets. Intakes on data from New Zealand and Switzerland suggest that dietary intakes may be relatively low.

Recently, Biego et al.[80] observed average intakes in France to be 275 µg/day. These values are higher than the intakes of 120 µg/day in Finland estimated by Vario and Koivistoinen, but in the range of intakes (80–350 µg) in the USA, determined by Winston. These researchers estimated that about 39% of total Mo intake was contributed by vegetables, about half that by cereals, milk, and dairy products respectively. Fruits contributed 10%, canned foods 10%, and non-vegetarian foods a little less than 30%.

6. Deficiency

Molybdenum deficiency has not been observed under usual conditions, although rare deficiencies have been reported. True molybdenum deficiency has not been achieved in experimental animals.[81] A case of Mo deficiency has been observed in a patient on long-term TPN. Symptoms observed were irritability leading to coma, tachycardia, tachypnea, and night blindness. Biochemical abnormalities were found including hypermethioninemia, increased urinary xanthine and sulfite, and decreased urinary uric acid and sulfate, as would be seen in xanthine oxidase deficiency. Supplementation with 300 µg/Mo per day led to dramatic decrease of these abnormal metabolites in the urinary content and the capacity to tolerate TPN.[81]

Two young adults with Crohn's disease maintained on TPN after ideal resection had extensive losses of trace minerals, including molybdenum, from the intestinal tract. Parenteral infusion of 500 µg of ammonium molybdate, equivalent to 225 µg of molybdenum, increased uric acid levels in plasma and urine of these patients.[6]

Although these two reports provide some evidence regarding the essentiality of Mo, the data are highly inadequate in terms of determining human requirements.

Studies in animals that indicate the importance of Mo have been summarized in Table 5.2.

TABLE 5.2
Effects of Low Mo Diets in Animals

Animal Model	Effects Observed
Goats	↓ conception rates
	Poor fetal survival
Chicks	↑ embryonic mortality
	Abnormal growth and development
Older birds	Skeletal lesions
	Osteolytic changes in the femoral shaft
	Lesions in overlying skin
Rats	Abnormally low xanthine oxidase/dehydrogenase activities in
	liver and intestinal mucosa and sulfite oxidase activity in liver

Possibly the copper content of the commercial diet fed was high and inclusion of low levels of Mo in the diet abolished the problems observed in chicks. It appears, therefore, that Mo deficiency alone may be a benign condition and therefore asymptomatic,[81] since signs have been observed only when antagonism is involved.

Further, there are no established indices of Mo status because of lack of cases of Mo deficiency.[45]

Reduced activities of the enzyme sulfite oxidase and xanthine oxidase are found in a syndrome in which children have mental retardation, dislocation of the lenses in the eyes, and xanthinuria. Both enzymes require a molybdenum cofactor. Inheritance is autosomal recessive.[2] Urinary output of sulfite, S-sulfocysteine, thiosulfate, and decreased urinary output of sulfate has been observed.[77]

7. Requirements

Normal health and development can apparently be maintained on quite low Mo intake. An intake of approximately 0.4 µg Mo per kg of body weight can be regarded as the average basal requirement. The RDI for adults is 0.78–2.61 µmol or 75–250 µg, although there is very little data to support these estimates.[7]

The lowest levels of intake at which toxicity occurs is likely to be 0.14–0.20 mg Mo per kg of body weight.

In young men, the Mo requirement has been estimated to be 0.025 mg/day, based on experiments, since no adverse effects were observed on a diet supplying 0.022 mg/day. However, long-term studies are required to conclusively state that this level of intake will be adequate and safe. Freeland-Graves and Turnlund[45] have suggested that, if an upper recommendation is to be made, intakes of 0.5 mg/d may be associated with no apparent risks.

There are no studies on Mo in relation to aging and current data is inadequate to extrapolate and derive tentative estimates other than the level of intakes recommended for young men.

D. SILICON

Silicon (Si) occupies a unique position among the trace elements, being, next to oxygen, the most prevalent element on earth. It is not found free in nature but occurs chiefly as the oxide and silicates. Orthosilicic acid $[Si(OH)_4]$, formed by hydration of the oxide, is soluble in water in amounts up to about 120 ppm. Above 120 ppm, super saturation causes dehydration and polymerization into complex, less soluble forms. Asbestos, tremolite, the feldspars, clays, and micas are a few of the silicate minerals.[6]

1. Chemistry

The chemistry of silicon is similar to that of carbon, its sister element. Silicon forms silicon–silicon, silicon–carbon bonds. Thus, organo-silicon compounds are analogues of organo-carbon compounds. However, substitution of silicon for carbon, or vice versa, in organo compounds results in molecules with different properties, because silicon is larger and less electronegative than carbon.

Silicon is ubiquitous in water, foods, and animal and plant tissues. In animals, it is found both free and bound. Silicic acid probably is the free form. The bound form has never been rigorously identified. It might be present in biologic material as a silanolate, an ether (or esterlike) derivative of silicic acid. Bridges of R_1-O-Si-O-R_2 or R_1-O-Si-O-Si-O-R_2 possibly play a role in the structural organization of some mucopolysaccharides or collagen.[7]

2. Metabolism

Little is known about the metabolism of silicon. It appears that a form of dietary silicon determines the extent of absorption. Some dietary forms are well absorbed, as indicated by high daily urinary excretion of the element, wherein almost 50% of daily silicon intake was recovered in the urine. In a study, humans absorbed only about 1% of a large single dose of an alumino-silicate compound compared with more than 70% of a single dose of methylsilanetriol salicylate.[7] Absorption of silicon is also affected by age, sex, and hormonal status, especially with reference to hormonal secretions of the adrenal and thyroid glands.[82] However, the mechanisms involved in intestinal absorption and blood transport of silicon are not known. In plasma, silicon appears to exist almost entirely in the undissociated form as monomeric silicic acid, $[Si(OH)_4]$. Silicon is largely found in connective tissues in the aorta, trachea, tendon, bone, and skin. Silicon-containing granules are also found in mitochondria of normal rat kidney, liver, and spleen. It has been shown that silicon concentrations in human arteries decrease with increasing age and with the onset of atherosclerosis. A combination of large intravenous and oral doses of silicon reduced the incidence and severity of atherosclerosis in cholesterol-fed rabbits. Several reports independently confirmed a decline in silicon with age in some animal tissues, but its causes and possible relevance to the aging process remain unknown.[6] The kidney is the main excretory organ for silicon, almost entirely by glomerular filtration. Thus, it is mainly eliminated via urine, where it possibly exists as magnesium-orthosilicate. Renal insufficiency is invariably associated with increased plasma silicon levels, which tend to rise in parallel with the increase in serum creatinine levels.[83]

3. Functions

The essential function of silicon has been independently demonstrated by two groups of researchers in two species of experimental animals. Growth stimulation of rats following administration of silicon was observed only when low-silicon (< 5 µg of silicon/g of diet) synthetic rations based on crystalline amino acids were fortified with 250–500 µg of silicon/g of diet. However, regardless of dietary composition, all other experiments in which silicon deficiency has been induced have demonstrated the importance of the element for the normal development of connective tissue and bone in chickens and rats,[6] where its primary effect is on matrix formation.[83]

Silicon influences bone formation by affecting cartilage composition and ultimately cartilage calcification. Silicon is localized in the active growth areas or the osteoid layer. It is present in high concentration in mitochondria of metabolically active osteogenic cells in the bones of young mice. In silicon-deficient animals, hexosamine (glycosaminoglycans) and collagen concentration in the bone are depressed, but macromineral composition is not markedly affected.[3]

The role of silicon in bone formation is possibly to facilitate the formation of glycosaminoglycan and collagen components, as it is a constituent of the enzyme prolylhydroxylase.[6] Silicon deficiency decreases ornithine aminotransferase, which is also involved in collagen formation.[7] Additionally, silicon may play a role with phosphorus in the organic phase in the series of events leading to calcification.[3] Further, silicon may also have a structural role as a component of glycosaminoglycans and glycosaminoprotein complexes in which silicon is believed to occur as silanolate in muco-polysaccharides, linking different polysaccharides in the same polysaccharide chain or linking acid mucopolysaccharides to protein. The postulated structures of such links have still to be identified.

a. Silicon–mineral interaction

The physiologic interaction of two or more mineral ions can have significant effects on health. The interrelationships between Si and Fe and Si and Al have recently gained interest and could have important health implications.

b. Si–Fe interaction

Silicon has been shown to facilitate iron absorption and transport. Jia et al.[84] conducted an experiment in rats using two dietary levels of silicon (1 and 500 mg/kg of diet), iron (35 and 187 mg/kg of diet) and ascorbic acid (1 and 900 mg/kg of diet) to identify interactions among these nutrients. Results revealed that supplemental silicon in conjunction with the higher dietary iron level prevented the plasma-iron decreasing effect observed for the higher level of iron in the absence of silicon. Further, in the absence of ascorbic acid, silicon also increased iron concentration in the liver. Although not very clear, the mechanism involved could be explained as follows.

High dietary iron inhibits copper and zinc absorption. Both copper and zinc increase the synthesis of ceruloplasmin, a copper-containing ferroxidase that oxidizes, Fe^{2+} to Fe^{3+} to facilitate iron transportation and distribution among the tissues. It appears that the release of iron from liver and mucosal cells into the plasma also requires the action of ferroxidase. Thus, copper and zinc inadequacy prompted by excess dietary iron could cause impairment of iron utilization. However, if Fe^{3+} formed a complex with silicic acid and this complex aided iron absorption in its Fe^{3+} form, it could be expected that the impairment of iron transportation caused by copper and/or zinc inadequacy would be ameliorated by silicon supplementation. Ascorbic acid is a potent reducing agent that reduces Fe^{3+}, chelates Fe^{2+}, and increases iron absorption. However, the accompanying reduction in copper absorption, the resulting lower blood-ceruloplasmin concentrations, and subsequent decrease in Fe^{3+} for incorporation into transferrin may prevent efficient portal transport of absorbed iron. Therefore, the absorbed iron would remain in mucosal cells and would eventually be excreted as those cells are sloughed.

Further, Si–Fe interaction appears to be pH dependent, as indicated in an experimental study on rats, where it was shown that the supplementation of 500 mg silicon per kg of diet increased plasma-iron concentration in rats fed the acidic diets but not in rats fed the basic diet.[85]

The lower iron status associated with elevated amounts of supplemental iron, mediated through an iron-imposed copper inadequacy, may have important implications where iron supplementation is often practiced. However, exacerbation of this effect by ascorbic acid and amelioration by silicon needs further research.

c. Si–Al interaction

At present, it is well established that an increased level of both aluminum and silicon are associated with senile plaques in Alzheimer's disease (AD), resulting in final formation of alumino-silicates in the brain. However, it has also been shown that dissolved silicon is an important factor in limiting the absorption of dietary aluminum.[86] The intestinal absorption of aluminum differs according to its chemical structures, as well as coexistent substances such as maltose, citric acid, silicon, and hydrogen-ion-concentration exponent.[87] It has been reported that silicic acid protects against aluminum toxicity in biota by probable formation of hydroxyl-aluminosilicates. Belles et al.[86] examined the influence of supplementing silicon in the diet on tissue aluminum retention in rats exposed to oral aluminum. Aluminum concentration in various regions of the brain, liver, bone, spleen, and kidney were significantly lower in the groups exposed to 59 and 118 mg silicon/L than in the control group. Significant reduction in the urinary aluminum levels in the experimental groups was also observed. The effect of silicon could be due to a sequestration of the metal, which promotes aluminum excretion and reduces tissue aluminum accumulation. Because silicic acid is a very weak acid, it interacts only with metals that are basic. Aluminum is basic at physiological pH. Strong and specific interaction of silicic acid with aluminum suggest the protective role of silicon. The chemical affinity of silicic acid for aluminum has been shown to reduce the bioavailability of aluminum in studies of human gastrointestinal absorption.[88]

AD will be a serious health problem in countries where the proportion of elderly people is showing rapid increase. High intake of aluminum seems to be one of the risk factors. Silicon appears to effectively prevent gastrointestinal aluminum absorption and thus may play an important role in protecting against the neurotoxic effects of aluminum, especially when its intake is high. It has been demonstrated in a case control study in eight regions of England and Wales that any risk of AD from Al in drinking water at a concentration below 0.2 mg per litre is small and silicon has no protective role.[89]

4. Deficiency Signs

Signs of silicon deficiency have not been defined for humans. Most of the silicon deficiency in chickens and rats indicates aberrant metabolism of connective tissue and bone. Chicks fed a semisynthetic, silicon-deficient diet exhibit skull structure abnormalities associated with depressed collagen content, and long-bone abnormalities characterized by small, poorly formed joints and defective endochondral growth. Tibias of silicon-deficient chicks exhibit depressed contents of articular cartilage, water, hexosamine, and collagen. In rats, bone hydroxyproline is decreased, plasma amino acid and bone mineral compositions are altered, and femur alkaline and acid phosphatase are decreased by silicon deprivation. However, growth of the rats is not markedly affected.[3,7]

5. Toxicity

The general manifestations of silicon toxicity are collectively described as silicosis. In humans, silicon is essentially nontoxic when taken orally. Magnesium trisilicate, an over-the-counter antacid, has been used by humans for more than 40 years without obvious deleterious effects. Other silicates are food additives used as anticaking or antifoaming agents.[7]

However, certain chemical forms of silicon are toxic if inhaled or ingested in large amounts. Antioxidant enzymes including dismutase, catalase, and glutathione peroxidase were reduced in rats given high amounts of sodium metasilicate in drinking water (1–2 mg silicon/ml).[3] Similarly, carcinogenic effects of asbestos fibers have caused serious public-health problems where some forms of asbestos have been used extensively in construction projects in the past.[6] There is evidence that, following exposure to crystalline silica, the release of several proinflammatory cytokines contributes to the induction of unbalanced inflammatory reactions leading to lung fibrosis.[90] It was also confirmed that *in vivo* exposure of rats to silica significantly increases nitric oxide production by broncho laveolar lavage cells, a population of cells that includes alveolar macrophages.[91]

Since the kidney is the main excretory organ for silicon, renal patients often have high plasma-silicon levels and are thus at risk for development of silicon-related toxicity. Two dialysis patients with markedly elevated plasma-silicon levels (3,849 and 2,350 μg/L) had painful nodular skin eruptions and aberrant hair growth, characterized as perforating folliculitis on skin biopsy, which is compatible with known effects of organosilicon compounds in man and animals. One of the patients also exhibited hypercalcemia, with low PTH, vitamin D and plasma aluminum levels. Similarly, serum calcium levels correlated weakly with plasma-silicon levels in 30 dialysis patients with moderately elevated plasma silicon ($> 10 \pm 53$ μg/L) indicating that silicon may affect calcium metabolism. It appears that silicon may play a role in the neurotoxicity and bone disease of dialysis, however, further research is required to confirm these findings.[83]

6. Sources

Foods of plant origin contain more silicon than those of animal origin. Whole grasses and cereals may contain 3–6% silica. The richest sources of silicon are unrefined grains of high-fiber content, and cereal products. Most foods of plant origin contain the element in amounts roughly proportional to their fiber content. Normally, refining reduces the silicon content of foods. Silicate additives used in prepared foods could increase the total content of silicon, however, its bioavailability from these additives may be low. The silicon content of drinking water and beverages made using it shows geographic variation as silicon is high in hard-water and low in soft-water areas.[3,6,7]

Thus, dietary silicon intake of humans varies greatly and is determined by the proportion of vegetable vs. animal foods and unrefined vs. refined or processed foods consumed. The factors governing the biological availability of silicon have not been adequately defined.

7. Requirements

The specific biochemical function of silicon is unknown, but animal studies strongly suggest that it is required by humans. However, at present, it is difficult to postulate adequate dietary intake as no appropriate human data is available and usable animal data is limited. Rats fed about 4.5 mg silicon/kg diet, mostly as the very bioavailable sodium metasilicate, did not differ from rats fed about 35 mg silicon/kg diet. Both prevented the silicon-deficiency signs exhibited by rats fed about 1 mg silicon/kg diet. Thus, based on animal data, if dietary silicon is highly available, the human requirement for silicon is in the range of 2–5 mg/d. However, much of the silicon found in most diets probably is not absorbable or as available as sodium metasilicate. Significant amounts occur as aluminosilicate and silica from which silicon is not readily available. Therefore, the recommended intake of silicon may have to be higher than the estimated requirement.[3,7]

The calculated silicon content of the FDA total diet was 19 mg/d for women and 40 mg/d for men. A human balance study indicated that the oral intake of silicon was in the range of 21–46 mg/d. The average British diet supplies 31 mg silicon per day. These findings suggest that an EDDI of 20–50 mg is appropriate.[3]

Further, a silicon intake of 1.07 to 1.25 mmol (30–35 mg) per day was suggested for athletes on the basis of balance data. This intake was 0.18 to 0.36 mmol (5–10 mg) higher than that for non-athletes.[7] However, silicon intake has not been suggested for the elderly. It has been shown that factors such as aging and low estrogen status apparently decrease the ability to absorb silicon.[3] Oral doses of silicon reduced the incidence and severity of atherosclerosis in rabbits that were fed cholesterol. The silicon concentrations in human arteries decreased with increasing age and with the onset of atherosclerosis.[6] Thus, silicon appears to have a role in atherosclerosis. In recent years, various studies have related elevated concentrations of aluminum in drinking water to an increased incidence of Alzheimer's disease and cognitive impairment associated with aging. A high intake of silicic acid could limit the aluminum absorption from drinking water and/or other dietary sources in the alkaline environment of the intestine, thereby protecting against the neurotoxic effects of aluminum.[86] In view of this, further work is required to establish the importance of silicon in the elderly and suggest its requirements.

ACKNOWLEDGEMENT

The authors acknowledge the financial support given by UGC under DSA Phase II for the preparation of this paper.

REFERENCES

1. Taylor, A. Detection and monitoring of disorders of essential trace elements. *Ann. Clin. Biochem.* 33: 486-510, 1996.
2. Nielson, F.H. Should dietary guidance be given for mineral elements with beneficial actions or suspected of being essential. *J. Nutr.* 126(9S): 2377S-2385S, 1996.
3. Uthus, E.O. and Seaborn, C.D. Deliberations and evaluations of the approaches, end points and paradigms for dietary recommendations of the other trace elements, *J. Nutr.* 126: 2452S-2495S, 1996.
4. Aschner, M. Manganese Homeostasis in the CNS. Environmental Research Section A 80, 105–109, 1999.
5. Greger, J.L. Dietary standards for manganese: overlap between nutritional and toxicological studies *J. Nutr.* 128: 368 S–371 S, 1998.
6. WHO, Trace Elements in Human Nutritional Health, 1996.
7. Nielson, F.H. Ultra Trace Elements. In Shils, M.E, J.A. Olson, M. Shike, and R.C. Ross (Eds). *Modern Nutrition in Health and Disease* 9th ed. Williams and Wilkins pp. 283–304, 1998.
8. Garcia Aranda, J.A, R.A. Wapni and F. Lifshitz. In-vivo intestinal absorption of Mn in rats, *J. Nutr.* 113: 2601–2607, 1983.
9. Finley, J.W. Mn absorption and retention by young women is associated with serum ferritin concentration. *Am. J. Clin. Nutr.* 70: 37–43 1999. Abstract.
10. Finley J.W., P.E. Johnson, and LuAnn K. Johnson. Sex affects Mn absorption and retention by humans from a diet adequate in Mn. *Am. J. Clin. Nutr.* 60: 949–955, 1994.
11. Finley, J.W. and Davis C.D. Manganese deficiency and toxicity: Are high or low dietary amounts of Mn cause for concern? *BioFactors* 10: 15–24 (1999).
12. Malecki, E.A, Radzanowski, G.M., Radzanowski, T.J. Gallaher, D.D. and Greger, J.L. Billiary manganese excretion in conscious rats is affected by acute and chronic Mn intake but not by dietary fat. *J. Nutr.* 126: 489–498, 1996.
13. Leech, R.M. and Harris, E.D. Manganese. In: B.L. O'Dell and R.A. Sunde (Eds.) *Handbook of Nutritionally Essential Mineral Elements.* Marcel Dekker Inc. New York, 1997. pp. 335–355.
14. Aschner, M., Vrana, K.E. and Zheng, W. Manganese uptake and distribution in the central nervous system (CNS). *Neurotoxicology* 20(2–3): 173–180, 1999.
15. Hussain S. and Ali, S. F. Manganese scavenges superoxide and hydroxyl radicals: an *in vitro* study in rats. *Neutrosci. Lett.* 261 (1–2): 21–24, 1999. Abstract.
16. Zidenbert–Cherr, S., Keen, C.L., Lonnerdal, B., and Hurley, L.S. Superoxide dismutase activity and lipid peroxidation in the rat: Developmental correlations affected peroxidation in the rat: Developmental correlations affected by Mn deficiency. *J. Nutr* 117: 2498–2504, 1983.
17. Malecki, E.A. and Greger, J.L. Mn protects against heart mitochondrial lipid peroxidation in rats fed high levels of polyunsaturated fatty acids. *J. Nutr.* 126: 27–33, 1996.
18. Gong H. and Amemiya T. Optic nerve changes in Mn-deficient rats. *Ext. Eye Res.* 68 (3): 313–320, 1999(a). Abstract.
19. Gong, H. and Amemiya, T. Corneal changes in Mn-deficient rats. Cornea 18(4): 472–82, 1999(b). Abstract.
20. Gong, H. and Amemiya, T. Ultra structure of retina of Mn-deficient rats. *Invest. Ophthalmol. Vis. Sci.,* 37 (10): 1967–1974, 1996. Abstract.
21. Finley, J.W. and Davis C.D. Manganese deficiency and toxicity: Are high or low dietary amounts of Mn cause for concern? *BioFactors* 10: 15–24 (1999).
22. Keen, C.L., Ensunsa. J.L., Watson. M.H., Baly. D.L., Donovan. S.M., Monaco. M.H. and Clegg. M.S. Nutritional aspects of Mn from Experimental Studies. *Neuro Toxicol.* 20(2–3): 213–224, 1999.
23. Dietary Mn deficiency on rat pancreatic amylase mRNA levels *J. Nutr.* 120: 1228–1234, 1990.
24. Ying, Y.P. and Klimis, T.J. Effects of dietary Mn on arterial glycos aminoglycan metabolism in Sprague–Dawley rats. Biological Trace Element Research 64 (1): 275–288, 1998. Abstract.
25. Clegg, M.S., Donovan, S.M., Monaco, M.H., Baly, D.L., Ensunsa, J.L. and Keen C.L. The influence of Mn deficiency on serum IGF-1 and IGF binding proteins in male rats. *Proc. Soc. for Exper. Biol. and Med.* 219(1): 41–47, 1998. Abstract.
25. Aschner, M., Allen, J.W., Kimelberg, H.K., LoPac, R.M. and Streit, W.J. Glial cells in neurotoxicity development. *Annu. Rev. Pharmacol. Toxicol..* 39: 153–173, 1999(b).

27. Takeda, A., Ishiwatari, S., and Okada, S. Manganese uptake into rat brain during development and aging. *J. Neurosci. Res.* 56: 93-98, 1999.

28. Pennington, A.T., Young, B.E., Wilson, D.B., Johnson, R.D. and Vanderveen, J.E. Mineral content of foods and total diets—the selected mineral in foods survey 1982–1984 *JADA* 86: 876–891, 1986.

29. Doisy, E.A. Jr. Micronutrient controls of biosynthesis in clotting proteins and cholesterol. Trace substances in environmental health, 6: 193-199, 1992 cf. WHO. Trace Elements in Human Nutrition and Health 1996.

30. Friedman, B.J., Freeland-Graves, J.H., Balis, C.W., Behmardi, F., Shorey-Kutschke, R.L., Wittis, R.A., Croshy, J.B., Trickkett ,P.C., and. Houston, S.D. Manganese balance and clinical observations in young men fed a Mn-deficient diet. *J. Nutr.* 117: 133-143, 1987.

31. Strause, L., Saltman, P., Smith, K.T., Bracker, M. and Andon, M.B. Spinal bone loss in postmenopausal woman supplemented with calcium and trace minerals *J. Nutr.* 124: 1060–1064, 1994.

32. Davis, C.D. and Greger, J.L. Longitudinal changes of manganese-dependent superoxide dismutase and other indexes of manganese and iron status in women. *Am. J. Clin. Nutr.* 55: 747-752, 1992.

33. Arnaud, J., Bourlard, P., Denis, B., and Favier, A. Plasma and erythrocyte Mn concentrations: influence of age and acute myocardial infarction. *Biological Trace Element Research* 53: 129-136, 1996.

34. Mergler, D., Baldwin, B. M., Belanger, S., Larribe, F., Beuter, A., Bowler, R., Panisset, M., Edwards, R., Geoffroy, A., Sassine, M., and Hudnell, K. Mn neurotoxicity, a continuum of dysfunction: results from a community based study. *Neuro Toxicol.* 20 (2–3): 327–342, 1999.

35. Mergler, D. and Baldwin, M. Early manifestations of Mn neurotoxicity in humans: an update. *Environ. Res.* 73: 92-100, 1997.

36. Mc Millan. A brief history of the neurobehavioral toxicity of Mn: Some unanswered questions. *Neuro Toxicol.* 20(2-3)–499-508, 1999.

37. Verity, M.A. Manganese neurotoxicity: a mechanistic hypothesis. *Neuro Toxicol.* 20 (2–3): 489–498, 1999.

38. Baldwin, M., Mergler, D., Larribe, F., Belanger, S., Tardif, R., Bilodean, L., and 39.Hudnell, K. Bio-indicator and exposure data for a population based study of Mn. *NeuroToxicol.* 20(2–3) 343–354, 1999.

39. Houser, R.A., Zesiewicz, T.A., Martinez, C., Rosemurgy, A.S., and Olanow, C.W. Blood Mn correlates with brain magnetic resonance imaging changes in patients with liver disease. *Can. J. Neurol. Sci.* 23 (2): 95–98, 1996. Abstract.

40. Fell J.M., Reynolds A.P., Meadows N., Khan K., Long S.G., Quaghebeur G., Taylor W.J. and Milla P.J. Mn toxicity in children receiving long-term parenteral nutrition *Lancet* 347: 1218–1221, 1996.

41. N. Reynolds, Blumsohn A., Baxter J.P., Houston G. and Pennington C.R. Mn requirement and toxicity in-patients on home parenteral nutrition. *Clinical Nutrition* 17(5): 227–230, 1998.

42. Goyer R.A. Toxic and essential metal interactions. *Annu Rev. Nutr.* 17: 37-50, 1997.

43. Hussain, S. and A.S. Ali. Mn scavenges superoxide and hydroxyl redicals: an invitro study in rats. *Neurosci Leth.* 261(1-2): 21-24, 1999.

44. Gregor, J.L. Dietary Standards for Manganese: Overlap between nutritional and toxicological studies. *J. Nutr.* 128: 368S–371S, 1998.

45. Freeland-Graves, J.H. and Turnlund, J.R. Deliberations and evaluation of the approaches, endpoints and paradigms for Mn and Mo dietary recommendations. *J. Nutr.* 126: 2435S–2440S, 1996.

46. Wilplinger, M., Zochling, S., and Pfannhauser, W. An analysis of Mn supply in Austria on the basis of a selected diet. *Food Res. and Technol.* 208 (4): 251–253, 1999. Abstract.

47. De la Torre, A., Granero, S., Mayayo, E., Corbella, J., and Domingo, J.L. Effect of age on vanadium nephrotoxicity in rats, *Toxcol. Lettr.* 105: 75:82; 1999.

48. Nielson, F.H. Vanadium. In O'Dell, B.L. and Sunde, R.A., Eds. *Handbook of Nutritionally Essential Mineral Elements.* Marcel Dekker Inc. New York, Chapter 22, 1997.

49. Domingo, J.L. Vanadium: A review of the reproductive and developmental toxicity. *Reprod. Toxicol.* 10(3): 175-182, 1996.

50. Nielson, F.H. *UltraTrace Elements in Modern Nutrition in Health and Disease.* Vol. I Shils, M. E., Olson, J. A., and Shike, M. Lea and Febiger. Chapter 22 pp. 282–286, 1994.

51. Thompson, K.H.; McNeill, J.H.; Orvig, C. Vanadium compounds as insulin mimics. *Chem. Rev.* 99(9): 2561-2571, 1999.

52. Badmaev, V., Prakash, S., Majeed, M. Vanadium: A review of its potential role in the fight against diabetes. *J. Alt. Complement. Media,* 5(3): 273-291, 1999.

53. Barceloux, D.G. Vanadium. *J. Toxicol. Clin. Toxicol.* 37(2): 265-278, 1999. Abstract.

54. Thompson, K.H. Vanadium and diabetes, *Biofactors*, 10: 43-51, 1999.

55. Sabbioni, E., Kueera, J., Pietra, R., Vesterberg, O., A critical review on normal concentrations of vanadium in human blood, serum and urine. *Sci. Total Environ.* 188(1): 49-58, 1996. Abstract.

56. Thompson, K.H., McNeill, J.H., Orvig, C. Vanadium compounds as insulin mimics. *Chem. Rev.* 99(9): 2561-2571, 1999.

57. Halberstam, M., Cohen, N., Shlimovich, P., Rossetti, L., and Shamoon, H. Oral vanadyl sulphate improves insulin sensitivity in NIDDM but not in obese non-diabetic subjects. *Diabetes* 45: 659-666, 1996.

58. Shi, S.J., Preuss, H.G., Abernethy, D.R., Li, X., Jarrell, S.T., and Andrawis, N.S. Elevated blood pressure in spontaneously hypertensive rats consuming a high sucrose diet is associated with elevated angiotensin II and is reversed by vanadium. *J. Hypertens.* 15(8): 857-62; 1997. Abstract.

59. Bishayee, A., Karmarkar, R., Mandal, A., Kundu, S.N., and Chatterjee, M. Vanadium-mediated chemoprotection against chemical hepato carcinogenesis in rats: haematological and histological characteristics. *Eur. J. Cancer Prev.* 6(2): 58–70, 1997. Abstract.

60. Nielson, F.H., Ollerich, D.A. Studies on vanadium deficiency in chicks. *Fed. Proc.* 32: 929, 1973.

61. Barceloux, D.G. Vanadium. *J. Toxicol. Clin. Toxicol.*, 37(2): 265-78, 1999. Abstract.

62. Sanchez, D.J., Colomina, M.T., Domingo, J.L. Effects of vanadium on activity and learning in rats. *Physiol. Behav.* 63(3): 345-50, 1998. Abstract.

63. Altamirano-Lozano, M. Genotoxic effects of vanadium compounds. *Invest Clin.* 39 Suppl., 1:39-47, 1998. Abstract.

64. Pierce, L.M., Alessandrini, F., Godleski, J.J., Paulauskis, J.D. Vanadium–induced chemokine mRNA expression and pulmonary inflammation. *Toxicol. Appl. Pharmacol.* 138(1): 1-11, 1996. Abstract.

65. Irsigler, G.B., Visser, P.J., Spangenberg, P.A., Asthma and chemical bronchitis in vanadium plant workers. *Am. J. Ind. Med.* 35(4): 366-374, 1999. Abstract.

66. Giussani, A., Roth, A., Werner, E., Greim, H., Cantone, M.C., and de Bartolo, D.A. A biokinetic model for molybdenum radionuclides: New experimental results. *Radiation Protection Dosimetry* 79(1-4): 367-370, 1998.

67. Guissani, A., Cantone, M.C., de Bartolo, D., Roth, P., Werner, E. A revised model of molybdenum biokinetics in humans for application in radiation protection. *Health Physics* 75(5): 479-486, 1998.

68. Cantone, M.C., de Bartolo, D., Guissani, A., Hansen, C.H., Roth, P., Schramel, P., Wendler, I., Werner, E., and Nisslin, F. Stable tracers for tracer kinetic investigations of molybdenum: intrinsic and extrinsic tagging. In *Trace Elements in Man and Animals–9: Proc. of the 9th Int. Symp. on Trace Elements in Man and Animals.* Fischer, P.W.F., L'Abbé, M.R., Cockell, K.A., Gibson, R.S. NRC Research Press, Ottawa, Canada pp. 267–269.

69. Werner, E., Giussani, A., Geinrichs, U., Roth, P., Greim, H. Biokinetic studies in humans with stable isotopes as tracers. Part 2. Uptake of molybdenum from aqueous solutions and labelled foodstuffs. *Isotopes Environ. Health. Stud.* 34: 297-301, 1998.

70. Kisker, C., Schindelin, H., and Rees, D.C. Molybdenum-cofactor-containing enzymes: structure and mechanism. *Ann. Rev. Biochem.* 66: 233-267, 1997.

71. Turnlund, J.R., Keyes, W.R., and Pfeiffer, G.L., Molybdenum absorption, excretion and retention studied with stable isotopes in young men at five intakes of dietary molybdenum *Am. J. Clin. Nutr.* 62: 790-796, 1995.

72. Turnlund, J.R., Keyes, W.R., and Pfeiffer, G.L., Molybdenum absorption, excretion and retention studied with stable isotopes in young men at five intakes of dietary molybdenum *Am. J. Clin. Nutr.* 62: 790-796, 1995.

73. Thompson, K.H., Scott, K.C., Turlund, J.R. Molybdenum metabolism in men with increasing molybdenum intakes: changes in kinetic parameters. *J. Appl. Physiol.* 81(3): 1404-1409, 1996.

74. Paschal, D.C., Ting, B.G., Morrow, J.C., Pirkle, J.L., Jackson, R.J., Sampson, E.J., Miller, D.T., and Coldwell, K.L. Trace metals in urine of United States residents: reference range concentrations. *Environ. Res.* 76(1): 53-59, 1998.

75. Nakagawa, N. Studies on changes in trace elements of brain related to aging. *Hokkaido Igaku Zasshi* 73(2): 181-199, 1998. Abstract.

76. O'Dell, B.L. Paper 16: The concept of trace element antagonism: The Cu-Mo-S Triangle (Dick, 1952–1954) *J. Nutr.* 127(5 Suppl) 1045S–1047S, 1997.

77. Guissani, A., Hansen, C., Niisslin, F., and Werner, E. Application of Mo absorption in humans. *Int. J. Mass Spectrometry Ion Processes.* 148: 171-178, 1995.

78. Shimbo, S., Hayase, A., Murakami, M., Hatai, I., Higashikawa, K., Moon, C.S., Zhang, Z.W., Watanbe, T., Iguchi, H., and Ikeda, M. Use of a food composition database to estimate daily dietary intake of nutrient or trace elements in Japan, with reference to its limitation. *Food Additives and Contaminants* 13(7): 775-786, 1996.

79. Holzinger, S., Anke, M., Rohrig, B., and Gonzalez, D. Molybdenum intake of adults in Germany and Mexico. *Analyst* 123(3): 447-450, 1998. Abstract.

80. Biego, G.H., Joyeux, M., Hartemann, P., Debry, G. Daily intake of essential minerals and metallic micropollutants from foods in France. *Sci. Total Environ.* 217(1-2): 27-36, 1998. Abstract.

81. Rajgopalan, K.V. Molybdenum: An essential trace element in human nutrition. *Ann. Rex. Nutr.* 8: 401-427, 1988.

82. Udipi, S.A. and Vaidya, A.B. Trace element requirements in the elderly. In Watson, R.R. (Ed). *Handbook of Nutrition in the Aged, 2nd Edition*, CRC Press London, pp. 363–384, 1994.

83. Saldanha, L.F., Gonick, H.C., Rodriguez, H.J., Marmelzat, J.A., Repique, E.V. and Marcus, C.L. Silicon related syndrome in dialysis patients, *Nephron*, 77: 48-56, 1997.

84. Jia, X., Emerick, R.J. and Kayongo-Male, H. Biochemical interactions among silicon, iron, and ascorbic acid in the rat. *Biol. Trace Elem. Res.*, 59: 123-131, 1997.

85. Jia, X., Emerick, R.J., and Kayongo-Male, H. The pH dependence of silicon-iron interaction in rats. *Biol. Trace Elem. Res.*, 59: 113-122, 1997.

86. Belles, M. Sanchez, D.J., Gomez, M., Corbella, J., and Domingo, J.L. Silicon reduces aluminum accumulation in rats: Relevance to the aluminum hypothesis of Alzheimer Disease, *Alzheimer Disease and Associated Disorders*. 12(2): 83-87, 1998.

87. Uchida, H. and Nagai, M. Intakes and health effects of aluminum, is aluminum a risk factor for Alzheimer Disease? *Nippon Koshu Eisei Asshi*, 44(9): 671-81, 1997. Abstract.

88. Bellia, J.P., Birchall, J.D., and Roberts, N.B. The role of silicic acid in the renal excretion of aluminum, *Ann. Clin. Lab. Sci.* 26: 227-233, 1996.

89. Martyn, C.N., Coggon, D.N., Inskip, H., Lacey, R.F. and Young, W.F. Aluminum concentrations in drinking water and risk of Alzheimer's disease. *Epidemiology* 8(3): 281-286, 1997. Abstract.

90. Huaux, F., Louahed, J., Hudspith, B., Meredith, C., Delos, M., Repauld, J.C., and Lison, D. Role of interleukin–10 in the lung response to silica in mice. *Am. J. Respir. Cell. Mol. Biol.*, 18(1): 51-59, 1998. Abstract.

91. Huffman, L.J., Judy, D.J., and Castranova, V. Regulation of nitric oxide production by rat alveolar macrophage in response to silica exposure. *J. Toxicol. Environ. Health*, 53(1): 29-46, 1998. Abstract.

6 Early Undernutrition: Good or Bad for Longevity?

Avan Aihie Sayer and Cyrus Cooper

CONTENTS

I.   INTRODUCTION

The effects of nutritional manipulation in early life are profound and far reaching. Immediate alterations in growth and development are matched by long-term changes in aging and lifespan. It is well recognized that postweaning diet restriction in a number of species results in reduced aging and prolonged lifespan. However, the long-term effects of earlier diet restriction on aging remain little explored. The few studies in this area suggest that preweaning diet restriction may have an opposite effect, and now there is growing epidemiological evidence that human undernutrition in early life is associated with detrimental structural and functional consequences in the long term. In this chapter, we summarize the findings from animal diet restriction studies and human epidemiological studies investigating the long-term effects of undernutrition in early life.

II.   POSTWEANING DIET RESTRICTION

The well-documented beneficial effects of postweaning diet restriction on aging include the prolongation of life span, a reduced incidence of various age-related diseases, and the attenuation of structural and functional changes associated with age. The first studies were done on rodents as early as 1917,[1,2] where restriction of total energy intake was found to prolong life. Subsequent diet restriction studies have confirmed extension of mean and median lifespan as well as beneficial effects on other population mortality characteristics such as mortality rate doubling time.[3] A further consistent finding with postweaning diet restriction has been the reduction in certain age-related processes and diseases.[4] These include organ-specific effects such as an attenuated decline in structure and function of bone,[5] muscle,[6] connective tissue,[7] kidney,[8] endocrine pancreas,[9] and thymus,[10] together with more generalized effects occurring at the cellular and molecular level.[11] There have also been reports of a reduced decline in complex higher functions such as learning and motor coordination.[12] Both age-related nephropathy[13] and tumors[14] occur less frequently in diet-restricted rats.

All these studies have utilized diets sufficient to avoid malnutrition, but otherwise a variety of dietary manipulations have been found effective.[15-17] These include variable reduction in protein, fat, carbohydrate, and calorie intake implemented over differing periods of time after weaning. There is some evidence for a dose–response relationship between the severity and duration of reduced feeding and prolongation of life,[18] but this has not been a consistent finding.[19]

Mechanisms remain speculative partly because of the wide range of physiological changes associated with diet restriction. Initial suggestions that the effects were mediated through reduced growth have been reviewed since diet restriction was shown to have similar effects even when initiated in postmaturational life.[19] Similarly, the proposal that diet restriction slowed metabolic rate and thereby slowed aging have been disproved in studies showing that prolonged lifespan is not associated with a lower metabolic rate per unit lean body mass.[20] Possible cellular mechanisms include alteration in free radical production, changes in protein turnover, or altered gene expression. It also remains possible that the differences in survival between diet-restricted and freely fed animals may be due to detrimental effects associated with unrestricted food and overeating.

Since the early work in rodents, these studies have been replicated in a number of different species, most recently primates.[21] However, whether the findings are applicable to humans is not known. There has been just one controlled study of diet restriction and longevity in humans and in this the intervention was not instituted until late life.[22] Healthy subjects over 65 years of age living in a religious institution for the aged were either given a balanced diet containing 2,300 calories on odd days and 1 l of milk with 500 g fruit on even days or given balanced diet every day. Those given the restricted diet spent significantly less time in an infirmary than controls and six died compared with 13 fed more, but this difference was not statistically significant.

III.   PREWEANING DIET RESTRICTION

Although postweaning diet restriction has been extensively investigated, the effect of the same intervention prior to weaning has been little studied.[23] The few existing gerontological studies suggest an opposite effect. One very early study on mice showed that alteration of diet shortly after birth sufficient to slow growth resulted in reduced lifespan,[24] and recently a study in which prenatal protein restriction was followed by a normal postnatal diet demonstrated that the lifespan of the offspring was shortened.[25] Other work has focused on age-related processes. One study showed that maternal diet restriction resulted in progeny with permanent stunting of growth, anemia, and reduced resistance to hypothermia[26] and another demonstrated earlier age-related hemoglobin decline in the offspring.[27] Further research found that reduction of nutrition in prenatal and early postnatal life resulted in increased age-associated enzymes in the liver and kidney[28] and in the 1970s this led to the first clear proposal that diet restriction in the earliest stages of life might be associated with accelerated aging.[29] Although the relevance of considering developmental influences on aging and lifespan has not gone unrecognized,[30] these ideas have not been taken up widely in gerontological research. However, more evidence comes from the field of fetal physiology, where studies have been developed to investigate the long-term effects of undernutrition in prenatal life. The process whereby early environmental factors such as nutrition acting at a critical period of development in early life can have lasting or lifelong importance is called "programming."[31] Research into programming has shown that reducing protein in the diet of pregnant animals can cause permanent age-related alterations in the offspring such as raised blood pressure,[32] impaired insulin response to glucose,[33] reduced secretion of growth hormone[34], lower bone mineral content,[35] reduced thymus size[36] with impaired immune function,[37] and poorer performance on learning tasks.[38] Other changes include degenerative changes in the lung[39] and kidney.[40]

The direct effect of prenatal and early postnatal undernutrition on aging has been little explored in humans. One observational study considered racial differences in renal and hepatic histologic aging between Japanese and Caucasian people. Increased aging changes were seen in the Japanese specimens, and it was suggested that this might be explained by the relatively low protein diet taken by the Japanese throughout life.[41] Another study observed an association between poor early diet and worse cognitive function in children, but whether this persisted into later life was not ascertained.[42]

The evidence from these limited studies suggests an opposite effect of prenatal and early postnatal diet restriction. Undernutrition prior to weaning appears to be associated with faster aging and decreased lifespan.[23] Considerable support for this theory is now emerging from large-scale epidemiological studies linking poor early nutrition and growth with adverse long-term effects in humans. These are described below.

IV.　FETAL AND INFANT ORIGINS OF ADULT DISEASE

Much research into chronic disease etiology has focused on genetic and adult lifestyle factors. However, their failure to fully explain many common diseases[43] has caused renewed interest in the early environment and programming. Coronary heart disease is an example of a condition that requires further explanation because identified risk factors have proven insufficient to explain either geographical or temporal trends. For example, the rates are highest in the industrial northern areas of the U.K. and lowest in the more affluent southeast. Yet the steep increase in coronary heart disease this century has been attributed to rising prosperity. Furthermore, at an individual level, the traditional risk factors such as smoking and cholesterol levels have only been of limited value in predicting individuals who will be affected.

The first move away from the conventional adult lifestyle model of coronary heart disease (CHD) came in the 1970s with the results of a study showing that CHD rates correlated with past infant mortality in 20 Norwegian counties. It was suggested that a poor standard of living in childhood and adolescence was a risk factor for CHD.[44] However, this idea was not developed until a further geographic study showed that differences in CHD death rates in different parts of England and Wales paralleled past differences in death rates among newborn babies.[45] One proposed explanation was that poor early social conditions causing high infant mortality were linked with poor adult lifestyles, which themselves caused CHD. However, the nature of such a link remained obscure. It was unlikely to be cigarette smoking, because the distribution of deaths from lung cancer was very different from that of past infant mortality. Likewise, differences in dietary fat consumption did not follow that of past infant mortality. The likely explanation was therefore felt to be that adverse environmental influences in childhood associated with poor living standards directly increased susceptibility to the disease. This idea was pursued using detailed maternal and infant records preserved in England and Wales. Neonatal mortality could be distinguished from postneonatal mortality, and CHD in adults was found to be closely linked to neonatal rather than postnatal mortality. High neonatal mortality is associated with low birth weight and poor maternal physique and health. Therefore, for the first time, a geographical link was discovered between poor fetal growth, poor maternal state, and high death rates from CHD in adult life. Temporal trends are also relevant. Infant mortality has fallen dramatically this century, yet CHD continued to rise until the early 1980s. These opposing trends are best reconciled by postulating two groups of causes of CHD, one linked to poor living standards and acting in infancy, and the other associated with prosperity and adult lifestyle.[46]

Support for this hypothesis has come from innovative retrospective cohort studies in individuals. These were carried out in areas of England where birth records had been stored from the early part of the century. The studies showed that low early weight[47] and thinness or shortness[48] at birth were associated with raised death rates from coronary heart disease in later life. These relationships held true in men and women and were specific. For example, there was no relationship between birth weight or weight at 1 year and deaths from lung cancer.[49] Independent associations were also demonstrated between poor early growth and increased CHD risk factors including blood pressure,[50] plasma fibrinogen,[51] serum cholesterol,[52] impaired glucose tolerance,[53] left ventricular mass,[54] and arterial compliance,[55] as well as CHD morbidity.[56] These relationships were independent of length of gestation. A high placental to birth weight ratio was found to be a particularly strong predictor of raised blood pressure.[57] The relationships between birth weight and blood pressure, as well as glucose tolerance, have been replicated in children,[58,59] and the work on adults has been repeated in other countries including the U.S.A.,[60] Sweden,[61] and India.[62] Other chronic degenerative disorders linked to poor early growth include non-insulin-dependent diabetes,[63] chronic obstructive pulmonary disease,[64] and osteoporosis.[65]

It has been suggested that the associations between early life and adult disease occur because individuals whose growth was impaired in utero and infancy continue to be exposed to an adverse environment in adult life, and this later environment is responsible for the effects attributed to programming. However, the relationships described above are independent of social class and are strong, graded, and specific. Furthermore, their replication in different populations strongly supports a causal explanation. It has also been proposed that the link between poor early growth and adverse adult outcomes is genetic. However, there is longstanding evidence that genetic factors are not the major determinants of early growth. For example, in cross breeding experiments using Shire horses and Shetland ponies, the offspring of the Shire mares were much larger than those of the Shetland mares, despite similar genotypes.[66] Intergenerational studies have shown that birth weight is largely determined by maternal, not paternal, weight.[67,68] Also, recent embryo transfer experiments[69] and ovum donor studies[70] have shown that the maternal environment contributes more than genetic constitution to birth weight.

The most important determinant of early growth is nutrition and the fetal origins hypothesis proposes that fetal undernutrition programs the long-term adverse sequelae of small size at birth. This is consistent with the findings of adverse effects on aging in preweaning diet restriction animal studies.

V.   EARLY UNDERNUTRITION AND AGING IN MAN

People who are small at birth and during infancy experience higher rates of age-related diseases such as coronary heart disease and as a consequence have a shorter lifespan. For example, among 10,000 British men, those who had below average birth weight and weighed less than 8.2 kg at 1 year had 4 years' less expectation of life than those with above average birth weight who reached 12.25 kg at 1 year.[49] The relationship between poor early growth and aging processes, however, had not been explored until a recent epidemiological study.[71]

This study was carried out in North Hertfordshire, U.K., where birth and infant records dating back to the early part of the century were available. 1428 men and women born between 1920 and 1930 with records of early weight were traced. Of these, 824 agreed to home interview by one of four nurses, and information on medical and social history, including smoking and drinking habits, was obtained. Social class was defined from occupation. After interview, 717 attended a local clinic for measurement of current size, grip strength, skin thickness, eye examination, and a hearing test. Statistical analyses were used to quantify the relationship between birth weight, weight at 1 year, and each of the aging measures. Lower weight at 1 year was associated with reduced grip strength, thinner skin, increased lens opacity, and worse hearing (Table 6.1).[71] Adult grip strength was significantly related to birth weight as well as weight at 1 year such that those in the lowest birth weight group had a grip strength 12% less than those in the highest group (Figure 6.1).

This work provides preliminary evidence that human aging processes may be influenced by nutrition in early life. The aged phenotype may be viewed as the result of intrinsic and extrinsic exposures, starting at conception and occurring throughout life, and the corresponding response in terms of regeneration and repair (the lifelong exposure-response model of aging). It follows that early nutrition may influence aging in a number of ways (Figure 6.2). Early nutrition directly affects growth. This is mediated through endocrine factors released into the circulation and by paracrine peptide growth factors, such as insulin-like growth factor 1 (IGF-1), acting locally. Undernutrition in fetal life may be associated with permanent stunting of growth[26] and could therefore affect aging by setting a lower peak from which age-related decline will occur. Nutrition in early life also affects the setting of the glucose, insulin, IGF-1 and growth hormone axis,[72] and undernutrition appears

TABLE 6.1

The Association Between Early Weights and Age-Related Outcomes Adjusted for Age and Sex

Early Weight		Mean Lens Opacity Score (LOCS III)*		Aging Hearing Threshold (dBA)[a]		Outcome (No.) Grip Strength (kg)		Skin Thickness (mm)	
At Birth									
[g]	[lb]								
≤2500	[≤5.5]	2.27	(16)	24.4	(16)	28.5	(16)	1.19	(16)
–2950	[–6.5]	2.36	(94)	29.3	(93)	30.3	(95)	1.27	(95)
–3400	[–7.5]	2.38	(224)	29.2	(231)	31.0	(231)	1.24	(231)
–3860	[–8.5]	2.38	(205)	28.7	(217)	32.2	(217)	1.24	(217)
–4310	[–9.5]	2.29	(84)	28.4	(89)	32.5	(89)	1.22	(89)
>4310	[>9.5]	2.36	(32)	28.8	(35)	32.4	(35)	1.25	(35)
Multiple regression[b]		$p = 0.71$		$p = 0.97$		$p = 0.01$		$p = 0.32$	
At 1 Year									
[kg]	[lb]								
≤8.16	[≤18]	2.67	(26)	33.6	(26)	29.8	(26)	1.20	(26)
–9.07	[–20]	2.40	(1.33)	29.4	(134)	30.7	(134)	1.22	(134)
–9.98	[–22]	2.33	(198)	29.3	(209)	31.1	(211)	1.24	(211)
–10.89	[–24]	2.37	(187)	29.1	(194)	31.6	(194)	1.25	(194)
–11.79	[–26]	2.33	(70)	26.5	(77)	32.6	(77)	1.25	(77)
>11.79	[>26]	2.24	(41)	24.8	(41)	34.2	(41)	1.25	(41)
Multiple regression[b]		$p = 0.003$		$p = 0.008$		$p = 0.02$		$p = 0.19$	
All		2.36	(655)	28.8	(681)	31.5	(683)	1.24	(683)
Standard deviation		1.21		1.6		10.1		0.18	

[a] Logarithms used in analysis therefore means geometric.

[b] Adjusted for age, sex, current social class, social class at birth, and height.

Source: Aihie Sayer, A., Cooper, C., Evans, J.R., Rauf, A., Wormald, R.P.L., Osmond, C., and Barker, D.J.P., Are rates of ageing determined in utero? *Age Aging*, 1998;27:579-583.

to be associated with higher circulating glucose levels. Both proteins and nucleic acids are modified by reducing sugars in a process called nonenzymatic glycosylation. The extent of the modification is dependent on both sugar concentration and length of exposure; higher sugar concentration and extended exposure lead to the formation of larger amounts of glycosylation end products. This process is of particular relevance to long-lived molecules and is associated with altered function as well as structure.[73] It has been proposed that such changes are relevant to aging as well as diabetes in causing features such as increased atherosclerosis, cataracts, and cross-linkage of collagen.

The ability to respond to deleterious exposures is increasingly recognized as an important determinant of aging. The responses include repair and replacement of damaged molecules and cells. The disposable soma theory proposes that the avoidance of aging with perfect repair and regeneration processes does not occur because the energy requirements would jeopardize reproduction and therefore not be of evolutionary benefit.[74] There is some evidence that both repair and regeneration are maximal in embryonic and fetal life. At this early stage, these processes are regulated by peptide growth factors, which are widely synthesized and act within the local tissue environment. The insulin-like growth factors (IGFs) and transforming growth factors (TGFs) are thought to be of prime importance in cellular maintenance.[75] Many cells continue to express growth

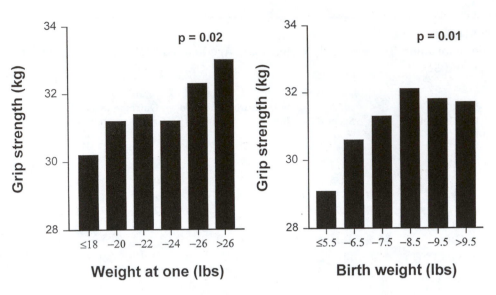

FIGURE 6.1 Grip strength in 628 men and women aged 64–74 years according to weight at one year and birth weight.

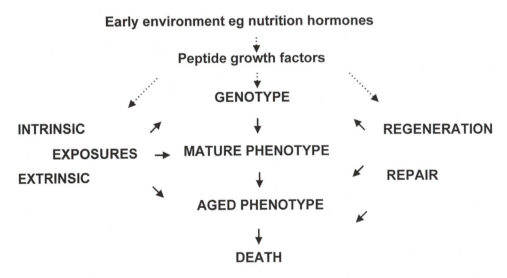

FIGURE 6.2 The lifelong exposure-response model of aging illustrating how aging could be affected by nutrition in early life.

factors even after differentiation, suggesting that growth factors continue to be involved in cell function in later life. There is some evidence that chronic early undernutrition permanently reduces IGF production,[76] and this could be the mechanism by which it has long-term effects on aging.

Further support for a long-term influence of early nutrition on repair and aging comes from the North Hertfordshire study. The systems in which aging was related to early growth shared the feature of having a high proportion of long-lived molecules or cells.[77] For example, the lens contains crystallins that, once formed, are never turned over.[78] They are synthesized in the outer cortex of the lens and gradually are moved to the center as new crystallins are formed. The center of an adult lens therefore contains molecules formed in utero. The cochlea of the ear contains long-lived collagen molecules and hair cells that, like brain cells, are not replaced.[79] Muscle and skin contain large amounts of collagen as well as elastin, which also has a very slow turnover. Long-lived molecules and cells are particularly dependent on efficient repair systems to maintain their integrity.

At present, the mechanisms for the nutritional programming of aging remain speculative. However, work is under way to investigate molecular repair mechanisms and their relationship to early growth and nutrition. Markers of DNA repair capacity including HPRT mutation rate, telomere length, DNA strand breaks, and mitochondrial DNA deletions will be measured in a large molecular epidemiological study based in Hertfordshire.[71]

VI. CONCLUSION

Evidence from animal interventional studies and human observational studies of nutrition and growth supports the notion that the effect of undernutrition on aging is critically dependent on the stage at which it is imposed. Early undernutrition occurring in prenatal or infant life appears to be associated with increased aging and a reduction in lifespan. This contrasts with the well-recognized beneficial effects of postweaning diet restriction. Possibly the switch in effect occurs when development is largely complete. Recognition that the timing of the nutritional intervention is critical is relevant to understanding the mechanisms underlying the effects of diet restriction on aging and lifespan. Furthermore, the demonstration of a relationship between early undernutrition and increased human aging may help future development of effective anti-aging strategies.

This work now needs to be taken forward. The effects of preweaning diet restriction can be explored more fully in animal models. Further epidemiological studies, including follow-up of the North Hertfordshire cohort, will allow exploration of how early nutrition and growth relate to the rate of aging with investigation of molecular and cellular mechanisms of repair.

REFERENCES

1. Osborne, T.B., Mendel, L.B., and Ferry, E.L., The effect of retardation of growth upon the breeding period and duration of life of rats, *Science*, 1917;45:294-295.
2. McCay, C.M., Crowell, M.F., and Maynard, L.A., The effect of retarded growth upon the length of lifespan and upon the ultimate body size, *J. Nutr.*, 1935;10:63-79.
3. Neafsey, P.A., Longevity hormesis, a review, *Mech. Aging Dev.*, 1990;51:1-31.
4. Berg, B.N., Nutrition and longevity in the rat. I. Food intake in relation to size, health, and longevity, *J. Nutr.*, 1960;71:242-254.
5. Kalu, D.N., Hardin, R.R., Cockerham, R., Yu, B.P., Norling, B.K., and Egan, J.W., Lifelong food restriction prevents senile osteopenia and hyperparathyroidism in F344 rats, *Mech. Aging Dev.*, 1984;26:103-112.
6. McCarter, R. and McGee, J., Influence of nutrition and aging on the composition and function of rat skeletal muscle, *J. Geron.*, 1987;42:432-441.
7. Everitt, A.V., Porter, B.D., and Steele, M., Dietary, caging, and temperature factors in the aging of collagen fibers in rat-tail tendon, *Gerontol.*, 1981;27:37-41.
8. Hayashida, M., Yu, B.P., Masoro, E.J., Iwasaki, K., and Ikeda, T., An electron microscopic examination of age-related changes in the rat kidney: The influence of diet, *Exp. Gerontol.*, 1986;21:535-553.
9. Reaven, E.P. and Reaven, G.M., Structure and function changes in the endocrine pancreas of aging rats with reference to the modulating effects of exercise and calorie restriction, *J. Clin. Invest.*, 1981;68:75-84.
10. Weindruch, R.H. and Suffin, S.C., Quantitative histologic effects on mouse thymus of controlled dietary restriction, *J. Gerontol.*, 1980;35:525-531.
11. Yu, B.P., Putative interventions. In: Masoro, E.J., Ed. *Handbook of Physiology*, Section 11, Aging. New York: Oxford University Press, 1995;619-621.
12. Ingram, D.K., Weindruch, R., Spangler, E.L., Freeman, J.R., and Walford, R.L., Dietary restriction benefits learning and motor performance of aged mice, *J. Gerontol.*, 1987;42:78-81.

13. Saxton, J.A. Jr. and Kimball, G.C., Relation of nephrosis and other diseases of albino rat to age and to modifications of diet, *Arch. Pathol.*, 1941;32:951-965.
14. Ross, M.H. and Bras, G., Tumor incidence patterns and nutrition in the rat, *J. Nutr.*, 1965;87:245-260.
15. Young, V.R., Diet as a modulator of aging and longevity, *Fed. Proc.*, 1979;38:1994-2000.
16. Berg, B.N. and Simms, H.S., Nutrition and longevity in the rat. II. Longevity and onset of disease with different levels of food intake, *J. Nutr.*, 1960;71:255-263.
17. Berg, B.N. and Simms, H.S., Nutrition and longevity in the rat. III. Food restriction beyond 800 days, *J. Nutr.*, 1961;74:23-37.
18. Nolen, G.A., Effect of various restricted dietary regimens on the growth, health, and longevity of albino rats, *J. Nutr.*, 1972;102:1477-1494.
19. Yu, B.P., Masoro, E.J., and McMahon, A., Nutritional influences on aging of Fischer 344 rats. I. Physical, metabolic, and longevity characteristics, *J. Gerontol.*, 1985:40:657-670.
20. McCarter, R., Masoro, E.J., and Yu, B.P., Does food restriction retard aging by reducing the metabolic rate? *Am. J. Physiol.*, 1985;248:E488-E490.
21. Roth, G.S., Ingram, D.K., and Lane, M.A., Slowing aging by caloric restriction, *Nat. Med.*, 1995;1:414-415.
22. Vallejo, E.A., La dieta de hambre a dias alternos en la alimentacion de los viejos, *Rev. Clin. Exp.*, 1957;63:25.
23. Aihie Sayer, A. and Cooper, C., Undernutrition and aging, *Gerontol.*, 1997;43:203-205.
24. Brailsford, Robertson T., and Ray, L.A., On the growth of relatively long lived compared with that of relatively short lived animals, *J. Biol. Chem.*, 1920;42:71-77.
25. Hales, C.N., Desai, M., Ozanne, S.E., and Crowther, N.J., Fishing in the stream of diabetes: From measuring insulin to the control of fetal organogenesis, *Biochem. Soc. Trans.*, 1996;24:341-350.
26. Chow, B.F. and Lee, C.-J., Effect of dietary restriction of pregnant rats on body weight gain of the offspring, *J. Nutr.*, 1964;82:10-18.
27. Kahn, A.J., Embryogenic effect on postnatal changes in hemoglobin concentration with time, *Growth*, 1968;32:13-22.
28. Roeder, L.M., Effect of the level of nutrition on rates of cell proliferation and of RNA and protein synthesis in the rat, *Nutr. Rep. Int.*, 1973;7:271-288.
29. Roeder, L.M. and Chow, B.F., Maternal undernutrition and its long term effects on the offspring, *Am. J. Clin. Nutr.*, 1972;25:812-821.
30. Finch, C.E., *Longevity, Senescence and the Genome.* Chicago: University of Chicago Press, 1990.
31. Lucas, A., Programming by early nutrition in man. In: Bock, G.R. and Whelen, J., Eds. *The Childhood Environment and Adult Disease.* Chichester, U.K.: John Wiley, 1991;38-55.
32. Langley, S.C. and Jackson, A.A., Increased systolic blood pressure in adult rats induced by fetal exposure to maternal low protein diets, *Clin. Sci.*, 1994;86:217-222.
33. Swenne, I., Crace, C.J., and Milner, R.D.G., Persistent impairment of insulin secretory response to glucose in adult rats after limited periods of protein-calorie malnutrition early in life, *Diabetes*, 1987;36:454-458.
34. Stephan, J.K., Chow, B., Frohman, L.A., and Chow, B.F., Relationship of growth hormone to the growth retardation associated with maternal dietary restriction, *J. Nutr.*, 1971;101:1453-1458.
35. Roach, H., Langley-Evans, S., and Cooper, C., Protein deficiency during pregnancy affects skeletal development in the offspring, *J. Bone Min. Res.*, 1999; 14 (suppl 1): S394.
36. Winick, M. and Noble, A., Cellular response in rats during malnutrition at various ages. *J. Nutr.*, 1966;89:300-306.
37. Chandra, R.K., Interactions between early nutrition and the immune system. In: Bock, G.R. and Whelen, J., Eds. *The Childhood Environment and Adult Disease.* Chichester, U.K.: Wiley, 1991:77-92.
38. Caldwell, D.R. and Churchill, J.A., Learning ability in the progeny of rats administered a protein-deficient diet during the second half of gestation, *Neurol.*, 1967;17:95-99.
39. Matsui, R., Thurlbeck, W.M., Fujita, Y., Yu, S.Y., Kida, K., Connective tissue, mechanical and morphometric changes in the lungs of weaning rats fed a low protein diet, *Pediat. Pulmonol.*, 1989;7:159-166.
40. Zeman, F.J., Effects of maternal protein restriction on the kidney of the newborn young of rats, *J. Nutr.*, 1968;94:111-116.

41. Tauchi, H., Effect of nutritional state on the aging process of the human organs, *Mech. Age Devel.*, 1972;1:111-116.
42. Lozoff, B., Nutrition and behavior, *Am. Psychol.*, 1989;44:231-236.
43. Oliver, M.F., Doubts about preventing coronary heart disease, *BMJ*, 1992;304:393-394.
44. Forsdahl, A., Are poor living conditions in childhood and adolescence an important risk factor for arteriosclerotic heart disease? *Brit. J. Prev. Soc. Med.*, 1977;31:91-95.
45. Barker, D.J.P. and Osmond, C., Infant mortality, childhood nutrition and ischaemic heart disease in England and Wales, *Lancet*, 1986;1:1077-1081.
46. Osmond, C., Coronary heart disease mortality trends in England and Wales 1952–1991, *J. Public Health Med.*, 1995;17:404-410.
47. Barker, D.J.P., Winter, P.D., Osmond, C., Margetts, B., and Simmonds, S.J. Weight in infancy and death from ischaemic heart disease, *Lancet*, 1989;ii:577-580.
48. Barker, D.J.P., *Mothers, Babies and Health in Later Life*. Edinburgh: Churchill Livingstone, 1998.
49. Osmond, C., Barker, D.J.P., Winter, P.D., Fall, C.H.D., and Simmonds, S.J., Early growth and death from cardiovascular disease in women, *BMJ*, 1993;307:1519-1524.
50. Barker, D.J.P., Osmond, C., Golding, J., Kuh, D., and Wadsworth, M.E.J., Growth in utero, blood pressure in childhood and adult life, and mortality from cardiovascular disease, *BMJ*, 1989;298:564-567.
51. Barker, D.J.P., Meade, T.W., Fall, C.H.D., Lee, A., Osmond, C., and Phipps, K. et al., Relation of fetal and infant growth to plasma fibrinogen and factor VII concentrations in adult life, *BMJ*, 1992;304:148-152.
52. Fall, C.H.D., Barker, D.J.P., Osmond, C., Winter, P.D., Clark, P.M.S., and Hales, C.N., Relation of infant feeding to adult serum cholesterol concentration and death from ischaemic heart disease, *BMJ*, 1992;304:801-805.
53. Hales, C.N., Barker, D.J.P., Clark, P.M.S., Cox, L.J., Fall, C., and Osmond, C. et al. Fetal and infant growth and impaired glucose tolerance at age 64, *BMJ*, 1991;303:1019-1022.
54. Vijayakumar, M., Fall, C.H.D., Osmond, C., and Barker, D.J.P., Birth weight, weight at one year, and left ventricular mass in adult life, *Brit. Heart. J.*, 1995;73:363-367.
55. Martyn, C.N., Barker, D.J.P., Jesperson, S., Greenwald, S., Osmond, C., and Berry, C., Growth in utero, adult blood pressure and arterial compliance, *Brit. Heart J.*, 1995;73:116-121.
56. Fall, C.H.D., Vijayakumar, M., Barker, D.J.P., Osmond, C., and Duggleby, S., Weight in infancy and prevalence of coronary heart disease in adult life, *BMJ*, 1995;310:17-19.
57. Barker, D.J.P., Bull, A.R., Osmond, C., and Simmonds, S.J., Fetal and placental size and risk of hypertension in adult life, *BMJ*, 1990;301:259-262.
58. Law, C.M., de Swiet, M., Osmond, C., Fayers, P.M., Barker, D.J.P., Cruddas, A.M., and Fall, C.H.D., Initiation of hypertension in utero and its amplification throughout life, *BMJ*, 1993;306:24-27.
59. Law, C.M., Gordon, G.S., Shiell, A.W., Barker, D.J.P., and Hales, CN., Thinness at birth and glucose tolerance in 7-year-old children, *Diab. Med.*, 1995;12:24-29.
60. Rich-Edwards, J., Stampfer, M., Manson, J.E., Rosner, B., Hankinson, S.E., and Colditz, G.A. et al., Birth weight and risk of cardiovascular disease in a cohort of women followed up since 1976, *BMJ*, 1997;315:396-400.
61. Leon, D.A., Koupilova, I., Lithell, H.O., Berglund, L., Mohsen, R., and Vagero, D., Failure to realise growth potential in utero and adult obesity in relation to blood pressure in 50 year old Swedish men, *BMJ*, 1996;312:401-406.
62. Stein, C.E., Fall, C.H.D., Kumaran, K., Osmond, C., Cox, V., and Barker, D.J.P., Fetal growth and coronary heart disease in South India, *Lancet*, 1997;348:1269-1273.
63. Lithell, H.O., McKeigue, P.M., Berglund, L., Mohsen, R., Lithell, U.B., and Leon, D.A., Relation of size at birth to non-insulin dependent diabetes and insulin concentrations in men aged 50-60 years, *BMJ*, 1996;312:406-410.
64. Barker, D.J.P., Godfrey, K.M., Fall, C., Osmond, C., Winter, P.D., and Shaheen, S.O., The relation of birthweight and childhood respiratory infection to adult lung function and death from chronic obstructive airways disease, *BMJ*, 1991;303:671-675.
65. Cooper, C., Cawley, M., Bhalla, A., Egger, P., Ring, F., and Morton, L. et al., Childhood growth, physical activity, and peak bone mass in women, *J. Bone Min. Res.*, 1995;10:940-947.

66. Walton, A. and Hammond, J., The maternal effects on growth and conformation in Shire horse-Shetland pony crosses, *Proc. Roy. Soc. Lond. B.*, 1938;125:311-335.

67. Morton, N.E., The inheritance of human birth weight, *Ann. Hum. Genet.*, 1955;20:125-134.

68. Carr Hill, R., Campbell, D.M., Hall, M.H., and Meredith, A., Is birth weight determined genetically? *BMJ*, 1987;295:687-689.

69. Walker, S.K., Hartwich, K.M., and Seamark, R.F., The production of unusually large offspring following embryo manipulation: concepts and challenges, *Theriogenology*, 1996;45:111-120.

70. Brooks, A.A., Johnson, M.R., Steer, P.J., Pawson, M.E., and Abdalla, H.I., Birth weight: nature or nurture? *Early Human. Devel.*, 1995;42:29-35.

71. Aihie Sayer, A., Cooper, C., Evans, J.R., Rauf, A., Wormald, R.P.L., Osmond, C., and Barker, D.J.P., Are rates of aging determined in utero? *Age Aging*, 1998;27:579-583.

72. Iglesias-Barreira, V., Ahn, M.-T., Reussens, B., Dahri, S., Hoet, J.J., and Remacle, C., Pre- and postnatal low protein diets affect pancreatic islet blood flow and insulin release in adult rats, *Endocrinology*, 1996;137:3797-3801.

73. Lee, A.T. and Cerami, A., Modifications of proteins and nucleic acids by reducing sugars: possible role in aging. In: Schneider, E.L. and Rowe, J.W., Eds. *Handbook of the Biology of Aging*, 3rd ed. San Diego: Academic Press, 1990:116-130.

74. Kirkwood, T.B.L. and Wolff, S.P., The biological basis of aging, *Age Aging*, 1995;24:167-171.

75. Han, V.K.M. and Fowden, A.L., Paracrine regulation of fetal growth. In: Ward, R.H.T., Smith, S.K., and Donnai, D., Eds. *Early Fetal Growth and Development*. London: RCOG Press, 1994:275-291.

76. Owens, J.A., Endocrine and substrate control of fetal growth: Placental and maternal influences and insulin-like growth factors, *Reprod. Fert. Dev.*, 1991;3:501-517.

77. Sell, D. and Monnier, V.M., Aging of long-lived proteins: Extra-cellular matrix (collagens, elastins, proteoglycans) and lens crystallins. In: Masoro, E.J., Ed. *Handbook of Physiology*, Section 11, Aging. New York: Oxford Univeristy Press, 1995.

78. Harding, J., *Cataract Biochemistry, Epidemiology and Pharmacology*. London: Chapman and Hall, 1991.

79. NIH Consensus Development Conference. Noise and hearing loss. National Institutes of Health, 1990.

7 Assessment of Nutritional Status in the Older Adult

Adele Huls

CONTENTS

I. NUTRITIONAL INADEQUACIES

Aging has replaced birth rate as the most important population issue in developed countries.[1] Yet we don't have a clear picture of adequate nutritional requirements in the healthy older adult. We do know many elders are malnourished and that nutrition plays a key role in keeping the human body functional. An inadequate supply of a given nutrient(s) to body cells and tissues leads to clinical symptoms of malnutrition. Nutrient inadequacies may result from a lack of food availability (primary deficiency) or be conditioned from an increase in requirement, a reduction in absorption or availability, a reduction in storage facilities, or inadequate intakes (secondary deficiencies).[2]

If nutrient availability to body tissues continues to be inadequate, stores are reduced and body dimensions may be affected. Levels of the nutrient or its products fall in body fluids and tissues. The result is altered enzyme activity (biochemical lesions), altered rates of protein and other metabolically active compound production, and changed efficiency of dietary energy utilization (protein-energy malnutrition). Organ dysfunction and biophysical defects lead to functional consequences. Early tissue changes represent the subclinical stage of nutritional disease. The next stage is the appearance of clinical symptoms and signs of dietary deficiency (i.e., weakness and lethargy with anemia).[3,4] A consequence of this last stage could be premature decline in the older adult.

Functional decline is not equally distributed in the older population, nor is the rate of decline. For some people in this heterogeneous group the rate of decline is slow. Genetic factors and lifestyle habits affect adaptive capacity (one's ability to overcome or effectively cope with injury) and functional reserve (percentage of an organ required to perform adequately) and may contribute to the lifespan of the oldest old. Healthy elderly individuals have a high threshold for acquiring disease and a slow rate of disease progression, according to the theory of James Fries.[5] In addition, healthier lifestyles and medical advances have the potential of compressing morbidity, mortality, and disability into a relatively short period of infirmity,[5] delaying the onset of chronic diseases by about 10 years.[6] Nutrition is one modifiable factor in healthier lifestyles.

0-8493-2228-6/01/$0.00+$.50
© 2001 by CRC Press LLC

A study of healthy elderly people who received an ordinary vitamin–mineral supplement or a placebo for 1 year resulted in approximately half as many infections and improved levels of T cells in the supplemented group.[7] This suggests some older adults have diets deficient in one or more nutrients or that nutrient requirements are higher in some older adults.

Malnutrition in older persons is associated with the development of frailty and physical, cognitive, and affective functional status decline. Approximately 16% of the U.S. population 65 years and over ingest fewer than 1,000 calories per day, which is incompatible with maintaining nutritional status.[8] Malnutrition is a serious problem in the elder population. As compared with younger people, individuals over the age of 70 consume one third fewer calories and 40% of subjects over the age of 70 are significantly underweight.[9] Both independently living and institutionalized elderly have been found to have energy intakes below the Recommended Dietary Allowance (RDA). For example, in the independent living population, one third of the energy intakes of the subjects were below the RDA; minerals and vitamins were below the RDA in up to 50%, with blood levels being subnormal in 10 to 30%.[10] Of the institutionalized subgroup of U.S. older adults, 30 to 50% were found to be substandard in body weight, mid-arm muscle circumference, and serum albumin level indicative of protein-calorie malnutrition.[10] Blood values were frequently found to be low in both water-soluble and fat-soluble vitamins.[10]

II. FUNCTIONAL DECLINE

Poor nutritional status may lead to sarcopenia, the age-related loss of muscle mass.[11] Sarcopenia is a direct cause of age-associated loss of muscle strength.[12] Inadequate dietary protein intake (amount recommended is 25% above the mean for young subjects) may be an important sarcopenia cause.[12] With age, resting energy expenditure decreases resulting in decreased energy needs (as a consequence of declines in muscle mass and physical activity). Reduced strength, another consequence of decline in muscle mass, contributes to reductions in mobility.[9] Physical functional dependency also affects the ability to prepare or eat meals, increasing the risk of further nutritional status decline. At very low levels of intake, resting metabolism and voluntary physical activity decrease. Maintaining mobility is the key to preventing unnecessary nursing home placement.[13] Rudman et al.[14] found functional impairment directly related to death and death inversely related to body weight as a percentage of ideal. A loss of physical functional mobility has been associated with a 50% mortality rate within 6 to 12 months among nursing home patients.[15] Decline in functional status in the 75 and over adult (high-risk) population can be expected within 6 months as an adverse effect of unrecognized, untreated, or untreatable nutritional status decline.

A decline in cognitive and affective function is also associated with poor nutrition. Nutritional status is associated with both dementia (cognitive functional decline) and depression (affective functional decline), which are often found to coexist in the geriatric population. Folate, vitamin B_6, and vitamin B_{12} deficiencies may specifically affect metabolism and cause depressive disorders and dementia.[16-20] Depression and weight loss are often intertwined and may be related to locus of control.[21,22] More than 60% of patients with clinical depression experience anorexia and weight loss.[23] Depression is both a cause and effect of poor nutritional status.[23] Microcytic anemias (iron deficiency) as well as deficiencies of thiamin and riboflavin have been related to cognitive performance and neuropsychological function.[24]

III. THE CHALLENGE

New research on the impact of nutrition has revealed that many problems that have been attributed to aging are really due to suboptimal diets and nutrient intakes. Achieving adequate nutrient, energy, and protein intakes becomes a very important challenge with advancing age. Recent research suggests current Recommended Dietary Allowances (RDAs) for calcium, vitamin D, vitamin B_6, folic acid, and vitamin B_{12} for the older adult are higher than for middle-aged adults in the face of decreasing energy needs.[25] Protein requirements are now thought to be greater for the older adult.[26] Protein requirements increase even more with injury or stress factors.

To compound the situation, research has found the threshold at which the risk of death increased in the older adult population occurred within the conventional "normal range" for albumin (< 4 g/dl), cholesterol (< 160 mg/dl), and hematocrit (< 41%) and subnormal findings are often ignored.[14,20]

The relationship between cholesterol levels and mortality risk, as well as between weight and mortality risk, appears to be U- or J-shaped in elders. Risk is increased at the lower as well as the upper ranges of cholesterol and relative body weight levels.[27] Low cholesterol levels (130 mg/dl) in nursing home residents[28] were associated with an eightfold greater risk of dying and high cholesterol levels (around 255 mg/dl) with a sevenfold greater risk of death.

Medicine has focused primarily on diagnosis and treatment.[29] It is now recognized that 75% of our health and life expectancy after age 40 is modifiable through changes in lifestyle, environment, and nutrition.[30]

IV. OBSERVE INDICATOR TRENDS

Geriatric nutrition professionals need to observe trends in client's nutritional indicators and where a negative trend is seen, provide interventions early in the decline trajectory. Basic indicators, readily available in the medical records of most clients, are first-line clues to nutritional status. They help guide the practitioner in making recommendations for further testing and suggestions for interventions. In this chapter, some of those readily available or easily attainable nutritional indicators will be stressed as they lead to clues that may clarify causes of malnutrition or, if necessary, suggest further more-specific and costly testing.

The basic indicators of nutritional status we will review include biochemical tests such as albumin, total lymphocyte count, cholesterol, hemoglobin; anthropometric measures such as mid-arm circumference and muscle area, height and weight to calculate body mass index as well as percentage of usual body weight and percentage of ideal body weight, and triceps and subscapular skinfolds; clinical observations in the nutrition physical examination; and the use of a subjective as well as objective nutritional assessment tools. The nutritional assessment tool that will be introduced in this chapter, the Mini Nutritional Assessment (MNA), is validated specifically for use with the older adult and can be completed by the client in less than 5 minutes with the nutrition professional then measuring mid-arm and leg circumferences.[31]

The first indicator of nutritional status, albumin, the major protein of human plasma, reflects visceral body protein stores and decline as a precursor to sarcopenia. Albumin is synthesized by the liver, at the rate of about 12 g/day.[32] Rate of biosynthesis is determined by dietary protein intake, ambient temperature, and plasma colloidal oncotic pressure near the site of synthesis.[33] Serum albumin levels below 3.5 g/dl suggest possible visceral protein depletion if there is no infection present.[34]

Total lymphocyte count (TLC) reflects immunocompetence. B and T lymphocytes synthesize antibodies and act in cell-mediated immunity.[35] Lymphocyte proliferation and maturation are affected in protein-energy malnutrition. Deficiencies of vitamins A, B_6, C, zinc, and iron also affect immunocompetence.[36] TLC falls especially with protein malnutrition.[37] TLCs are interpreted by Grant[37] as follows: values between 1200 and 2000/mm³ associated with mild depletion, between 800 and 1199 associated with moderate depletion, and >800 associated with severe depletion.

Total cholesterol reflects response to nutritional depletion as hypocholesterolemia in the older adult. Cholesterol is synthesized in many tissues of the body. Approximately half of the body's cholesterol is synthesized and the remainder is provided by the usual diet. Cholesterol is the precursor of all other steroids in the body including sex hormones, corticosteroids, bile acids, and vitamin D.[38] Low cholesterol levels are correlated with increased mortality in the long-term care setting. Hypocholesterolemia is directly related to body weight as percentile of standard, serum albumin, hemoglobin, hematocrit, and ability to walk and feed oneself[39] and death.[28,40] Hypercholesterolemia, on the other hand, is related to coronary heart disease.

Hemoglobin reflects hematologic response to protein and energy intake. Hematologic response increases hemoglobin levels when lean body mass increases.[41] Lipschitz et al.[42] evidence that declines in hemoglobin levels with aging are not a consequence of the aging process but may be caused by protein deprivation. Hemoglobin transports oxygen from the lungs to peripheral tissues and transports carbon dioxide and protons from the peripheral tissues back to the lungs for excretion. Common anemias (reductions in the amount of red blood cells or of hemoglobin in the blood) result from impaired hemoglobin synthesis (i.e., in iron deficiency) or impaired erythrocyte production (i.e., vitamin B_{12} or folate deficiency).[43]

Anthropometric measures of nutrition include mid-arm muscle area (MAMA), triceps skinfold, (TSF) and subscapular skinfold (SSF). MAMA, usual body weight (UBW), and ideal body weight (IBW) percentiles reflect somatic protein mass (primarily skeletal muscle). Skeletal muscle accounts for the greatest protein turnover. Negative nitrogen balance may be the consequence of increased protein breakdown (inadequate calorie or protein intake) or of decreased protein synthesis (decreased protein intake). If caloric expenditure is known to be greater than caloric intake, it can be assumed that nutritional status is deteriorating.

TSF and SSF are reflective of body fat mass. Each is highly correlated with estimates of body fat in elderly individuals.[44] Many older adults experience an unintentional weight loss by not meeting their energy requirements.[45] Anthropometric measures to identify trends over time are important to differentiate normal differences in body builds from unintentional skeletal muscle or weight losses.

The physical signs of malnutrition reflect nutritional deficiencies. Practitioners trained to perform a nutrition physical examination are taught to identify these physical signs of malnutrition, well outlined by Hammond.[46] Tissues that proliferate rapidly are most likely to manifest signs of nutrient deficiency.[47] Clinical signs of manifestations of nutritional depletion are evident at a late stage of being actively malnourished. However, few new tests are yet available for micronutrient status assessment and the tests that are available are often too costly to be routinely run, so clinical physical examination remains of great importance.[3] When combined with other data, knowledge acquired from the nutrition physical examination is invaluable and leads to a comprehensive nutrition assessment.[46]

The MNA[31] is a subjective and objective assessment reflective of nutritional status that includes anthropometric, general, dietary, and self-perception areas. Anthropometric measures relate to protein-calorie intakes. The general area, an assessment of lifestyle, medications, psychological factors, mobility, and skin condition, both affects and is affected by nutritional status. The dietary area evaluates number of meals, food and fluid intake, and autonomy of eating, all of which affect the outcome and adequacy of nutrient intake. The self-perception assessment area involves self-perception of health and nutrition, which influences and is affected by nutritional status. The 1998 revision of the MNA, the MNA short form (MNA-SF),[48] has six questions that are answered and scored to determine if it is necessary (11 points or below indicating malnutrition is possible) to go on and answer and score the other 12 assessment questions. If all the questions are answered, the scores from the screening and assessment questions are totaled to give a malnutrition indicator score (less than 17 points, malnourished; 17 to 23.5 points, at risk of malnutrition). It is a tool that can be used in any setting to identify and refer those at risk to the nutrition professional.

Any nutritional assessment parameters used by nutrition professionals (biochemical, anthropometric, clinical observation, or screening/assessment tools) that are considered to be abnormal are indicators or clues to health problem areas of the client. It is then the responsibility of the professional to make recommendations for intervention to help prevent or slow the progress of or reverse the area of decline.

V. EARLY DIAGNOSIS AND TREATMENT

Physical, cognitive, and affective functional status decline can be both caused by and the cause of malnutrition. Diagnosing of malnutrition early in the decline trajectory and determination of the etiology of the problem are important to successful reversal or slowing of the decline. Often environmental or lifestyle changes can help a person gain more independence. Tools for measuring functional status decline help to objectively recognize problems in the vicious cycle of malnutrition and in loss of independence.

The Tinetti Balance and Gait Evaluation,[49] Physical Self Maintenance Test (PSMT),[50] and Instrumental Activities of Daily Living (IADL)[50] are measures of physical functional status. Physical function decline results from gait and balance disorders, the inability to perform activities of daily living, or the inability to adapt to the environment.

Physical function decline as reflected by decline in gait and balance can be measured using the Tinetti Evaluation. The Tinetti Evaluation identifies and quantifies gait and balance, a physical function necessary for mobility. When one loses mobility, often anorexia of aging becomes a problem, and it becomes very difficult to meet nutritional needs.

Physical function decline as reflected by decline in ability to perform activities of daily living (ADLs) can be measured using the PSMT. ADLs include activities needed to sustain independent living (bathing, dressing, toileting, transferring, continence, and feeding).[51] ADLs are usually lost in the opposite order in which they were learned with inability to feed oneself often affecting nutritional status.

A decline in physical function, as reflected by decreased ability to adapt to the environment, can be measured using the IADL scale. The IADL scale measures ability to perform household chores, activities implying mobility and cognitive activities.[51] Loss in ability to perform IADLs lead to dependence and inability to live in one's own home alone. IADLs most related to nutritional status include meal preparation, shopping, and transportation.

Affective functional decline is reflective of depression. The Geriatric Depression Scale (GDS)[52] is a well recognized measure of affective functional status. Depression is a prevalent and treatable condition associated with increased mortality in older adults living in community populations and nursing homes.[53-55] Research suggests folate[16] and vitamin B_{12}[19] deficiency may play a primary role in depression.

A decline in cognitive functional status is the most common important disturbance in mental status.[56] The California Verbal Learning Test (CVLT)[57] and the Mini-Mental State Exam[58] are tools that can be used to measure cognitive functional status. Other less formal methods of checking cognitive status include making change with coins, telling the time on a clock, and questions as to time and place. Nutritional causes of cognitive functional decline include deficiencies of thiamin, riboflavin, niacin, pyridoxine, vitamin B_{12}[59] and iron.[60] With decline in cognitive function, modification of environment, lifestyle, and nutritional factors become very difficult or are accomplished only because of the interventions of others. In the case of nutritional cognitive function decline, treatment of the nutritional deficiency can improve cognition. Other dementias may not be reversible.

VI. MODIFY INDUCIBLE GENES

Medicine is built on the principle of the deterministic nature of genes and how health is controlled by them. We are now beginning to recognize that gene expression can be modified. Determining our health as we age is a consequence of how we care for and thus modify the expression of inducible genes (genes sensitive to environmental, lifestyle, and nutritional factors).[61,62] Nutritional demands in excess of nutrient intakes predict hidden consequences that may have negative functional status effects.[60] Functional status decline is often preventable. Changes in functional status over time are inevitable but need not be premature or due to reversible or preventable nutritional deficiency.

Timely nutritional assessments by nutrition professionals who are aware of or can obtain measures of a client's nutritional parameters over time are able to identify nutritional declines as early on as possible, allowing interventions to be started while the condition may still be reversible. Client nutritional "trends" are important to the holistic nutritional picture and to the treatment of each individual.

REFERENCES

1. Olshansky, S.J., Carnes, B.A., and Cassel, C.K., The aging of the human species, *Sci. Am.*, 1993;268:46-52.
2. Berg, R.L. and Cassells, J.S., *The Second Fifty Years: Promoting Health and Preventing Disability.* Washington, DC: National Academy Press; 1990.
3. McLaren, D.S., *A Colour Atlas and Text of Diet-Related Disorders.* 2nd ed. London: Mosby-Europe; 1992.
4. Sheldon, H., *Boyd's Introduction to the Study of Disease.* 10th ed. Philadelphia: Lea & Febiger; 1988.
5. Perls, T.T., The oldest old, *Sci. Am.*, 1995;272:70-75.
6. Fries, J.F., Strategies for reduction of morbidity, *Am. J. Clin. Nutr.*, 1992;55:1257S-1262S.
7. Chandra, R.K., Effect of vitamin and trace-element supplementation on immune responses and infection in elderly subjects, *Lancet.*, 1992;340:1124-1127.
8. Morley, J.E. and Miller, D.K., Malnutrition in the elderly, *Hosp. Pract.*, 1992;27:95-116.
9. Lipschitz, D.A., Nutrition and health in the elderly, *Curr. Opin. Gastroenterol.*, 1991;7:277-283.
10. Abbasi, A.A. and Rudman, D., Undernutrition in the nursing home: Prevalence, consequences, causes and prevention, *Nutr. Rev.*, 1994;52(4):113-122.
11. Evans, W.J., What is sarcopenia? *J. Gerontol.*, 1995;50A:5-8.
12. Evans, W.T. and Cyr-Campbell, D., Nutrition, exercise, and healthy aging, *J Am Diet Assoc.*, 1997;97:632-638.
13. Blocker, W.P., Maintaining functional independence by mobilizing the aged, *Geriatrics.*, 1992;42:42-56.
14. Rudman, D., Mattson, D.E., Nagraj, H.S., Caindec, N., Rudman, I.W., and Jackson, D.L., Antecedents of death in the men of a veterans administration nursing home. *J. Am. Geriatr. Soc.*, 1987;35:496-502.
15. Kemper, P. and Christopher, M.H., Lifetime use of nursing home care, *New Engl. J. Med.*, 1991;234:595-600.
16. Bottiglieri, T., Folate, Vitamin B12, and neuropsychiatric disorders, *Nutr. Rev.*, 1996;54:382-390.
17. Stampfer, M.J., Malinow, R., and Willett, W.C., et al. A prospective study of plasma homocyst(e)ine and risk of myocardial infarction in U.S. physicians, *JAMA*, 1992;268:877-881.
18. Rosenberg, I.H. and Miller, J.W., Nutritional factors in physical and cognitive functions of elderly people, *Am. J. Clin. Nutr.*, 1992;55:1237S-1243S.
19. Bell, I.R., Edman, J.S., and Miller, J., et al. Relationship of normal serum vitamin B-12 and folate levels to cognitive test performance in subtypes of geriatric major depression, *J. Geriatr. Psych. Neurol.*, 1990;3:98-105.
20. Goodwin, J.S., Goodwin, J.M., and Garry, P.J., Association between nutritional status and cognitive functioning in a healthy elderly population, *JAMA*, 1983;249:2917-2921.
21. Morley, J.E., Letters to the editor: The strange case of an older woman who was cured by being allowed to refuse therapy, *J. Am. Geriatr. Soc.*, 1993;41:1012-1013.
22. Morley, J.E. and Kraenzle, D., Causes of weight loss in a community nursing home, *J. Am. Geriatr. Soc.*, 1994;42:583-585.
23. Nutrition Screening Initiative. *Nutrition Interventions Manual for Professionals Caring for Older Adults.* Washington, DC: Nutrition Screening Initiative; 1992.
24. Tucker, D.M., Penland, J.O., Sandstead, H.H., Milne, D.B,, Heck, D.G., and Klevay, L.M., Nutritional status and brain function in aging, *Am. J. Clin. Nutr.*, 1990;52:93-102.
25. Russell, R.M., New views on the RDAs for older adults, *J. Am. Diet. Assoc.*, 1997;97:515-518.
26. Campbell, W.W., Crin, M.C., Dallal, G.E., Young, V.R., and Evans, W.J., Increased protein requirements in elderly people: New data and retrospective reassessments, *Am. J. Clin. Nutr.*, 1994;60:501-509.

27. Hazzard, W.R., Dyslipoproteinemia. W.R. Hazzard, E.L. Bierman, J.P. Blass, W.H. Ettinger Jr., and J.B. Halter, Eds. *Principles of Geriatric Medicine and Gerontology.* 3rd ed. New York: McGraw Hill; 1994:855-866.
28. Frisoni, G.B., Franzoni, D., Rozzini, R., Ferrucci, L., Boffelli, S., and Trabucchi, M., A nutritional index predicting mortality in the nursing home, *J. Am. Geriatr. Soc.,* 1994;42:1167-1172.
29. Bland, J.S., The use of complementary medicine for healthy aging, *Alternative Ther. Health Med.,* 1998;4:42-48.
30. Murray, C.J.L. and Lopez, A.D., Alternative projections of mortality by cause 1990-2020: Global burden of disease, *Lancet.,* 1997;349:1498-1504.
31. Guigoz, Y., Vellas, B., and Garry, J.P., Mini Nutritional Assessment: A practical assessment tool for grading the nutritional state of elderly patients, *Facts Res. Gerontol.,* 1994;Suppl. 2:15-59.
32. Harfenist, E.J. and Murray, R.K., Plasma proteins, immunoglobulins, and blood coagulation, Murray, R.K., Granner, D.K., Mayes, P.A., and Rodwell, V.W., Eds. *Harper's Biochemistry.* 23rd ed. Norwalk, CT: Appleton & Lange; 1993:665-687.
33. Heymsfield, S.D. and Williams, P.J., Nutritional assessment by clinical and biochemical methods, M.E. Shils and V.R. Young, Eds. *Modern Nutrition in Health and Disease.* 7th ed. Philadelphia: Lea & Febiger; 1988:817-860.
34. Rosenberg, I.H., Nutrition and aging. W.R. Hazzard, E.L. Bierman, J.P. Blass, W.H. Ettiger Jr., and J.B. Halter, Eds. *Principles of Geriatric Medicine and Gerontology.* New York: McGraw-Hill; 1994:49-59.
35. Murray, R.K., Red & white blood cells. Murray, R.K., Granner, D.K., Mayes, P.A., and Rodwell, V.W., Eds. *Harper's Biochemistry.* 23rd ed. Norwalk, CT: Appleton & Lange; 1993:688-703.
36. Chandra, R.K., Immunocompetence is a sensitive and functional barometer of nutritional status, *Acta. Paediatr. Scand.,* 1991;374:129-132.
37. Grant, J.P., Nutritional Assessment by body compartment analysis, *Handbook of Total Parenteral Nutrition.* 2nd ed. Philadelphia: Saunders; 1992:15-47.
38. Mayes, P.A., Cholesterol synthesis, transport, and excretion. Murray, R.K., Granner, D.K., Mayes, P.A., and Rodwell, V.W., Eds. *Harper's Biochemistry.* 23rd ed. Norwalk, CT: Appleton & Lange; 1993:266-278.
39. Rudman, D., Mattson, D.E., and Nagraj, H.S., et al. Prognostic significance of serum cholesterol in nursing home men, *JPEN.,* 1988;12:155-158.
40. Verdery, R.B. and Goldberg, A.P., Hypercholesterolemia as a predictor of death: A prospective study of 224 nursing home residents, *J. Gerontol.,* 1991;46:M84-89.
41. Torun, B. and Chew, F., Protein-energy malnutrition, Shils, M.E., Olson, J.A., Shike, M., Eds., *Modern Nutrition in Health and Disease.* 8th ed. Philadelphia: Lea & Febiger; 1994:950-976.
42. Lipschitz, D.A., Anemia. Hazzard, W.R., Bierman, E.L., Blass, J.P., Ettinger, W.H., Jr., and Halter, J.B., Eds., *Principles of Geriatric Medicine and Gerontology.* 3rd ed. New York: McGraw-Hill; 1994:741-747.
43. Rodwell, V.W., Proteins: Myoglobin and hemoglobin. Murray, R.K., Granner, D.K., and Mayes, P.A., et al., Eds. *Harper's Biochemistry.* 23rd ed. Norwalk, CN: Appleton-Lange; 1993:49-59.
44. Roche, A.F., Siervogel, R.M., Chumlea, W.C., and Webb, P., Grading body fatness from limited anthropometric data, *Am. J. Clin. Nutr.,* 1981;34:2831-2838.
45. Gray-Donald, K., Payette, H., Boutier, V., and Page, S., Evaluation of the dietary intake of homebound elderly and the feasibility of dietary supplementation, *J. Am. Coll. Nutr.,* 1994;13:277-284.
46. Hammond, K.A., The nutritional dimension of physical assessment, *Nutrition,* 1999;15:411-419.
47. Alpers, D.H., Stenson, W.F., and Bier, D.M., *Manual of Nutritional Therapeutics.* 3rd ed. Boston: Little, Brown; 1995.
48. Rubenstein, L.Z., Harker, J., Guigoz, Y., and Vellas, B., Comprehensive Geriatric Assessment (CGA) and the MNA: An overview of CGA, nutritional assessment, and development of a shortened version of the MNA. Nestle Nutrition Workshop Series Clinical and Performance Programme, Vol. 1: *Mini Nutritional Assessment (MNA): Research and Practice in the Elderly*; Nestec Ltd.; Lausanne, Switzerland. Basel: S. Vevey & A.G. Karger; 1999.
49. Tinetti, M.E., Performance oriented assessment of mobility problems in elderly patients, *J. Am. Geriatr. Soc.,* 1986;34:119-126.

50. Lawton, M.P. and Brody, E.M., Assessment of older people: Self-maintaining and instrumental activities of daily living, *Gerontologist.,* 1969;9:179-186.
51. Finch, M., Kane, R.L., and Philp, I., Developing a new metric for ADLs, *J. Am. Geriatr. Soc.,* 1995;43:877-884.
52. Yesavage, J.A., Brink, T.L., and Rose, T.L., et al. Development and validation of a geriatric depression scale: A preliminary report, *J. Psychiatr. Res.,* 1983;17:37-49.
53. Rovner, B.W., German, P.S., Brant, L.J., Clark, R., Burton, L., and Folstein, M.F., Depression and mortality in nursing homes. *JAMA,* 1991;265:993-996.
54. Snowdon, J., The prevalence of depression in old age, *Int. J. Geriatr. Psych.,* 1990;5:141-144.
55. Bruce, M.L. and Leaf, P.J., Psychiatric disorders and 15-month mortality in a community sample of older adults, *Am. J. Public Health,* 1989;79 :727-730.
56. Lachs, M.S., Feinstein, A.R., and Cooney, L.M., et al., A simple procedure for general screening for functional disability in elderly patients, *Ann. Intern. Med.,* 1990;112:699-706.
57. Delis, D.C., Kramer, J.H., Kaplan, E., and Ober, B.A., *The California Verbal Learning Test Manual.* Research Ed. ed. New York: Psychological Corporation, 1987.
58. Folstein, M.F., Folstein, S.E., McHugh, P.R., "Mini-Mental State" a practical method for grading the cognitive state of patients for the clinician, *J. Psychiatr. Res.,* 1975;12:189-198.
59. Bender, D.A., B vitamins in the nervous system, *Neurochem. Int.,* 1984;6:297-321.
60. Underwood, B.A., Micronutrient malabsorption: Is it being eliminated? *Nutrition Today,* 1998;33: 121-129.
61. Berdanier, C.D., Ed., *Nutrients and Gene Expression: Clinical Aspects.* Boca Raton, FL: CRC Press; 1996.
62. Baeurle, P.A., Ed., *Inducible Gene Expression. Part I: Environmental Stresses and Nutrients.* Boston: Birkhauser; 1994.

8   Bone Loss, Body Mass Index, and Fracture Histories in an Arizona Elderly Population

William A. Stini

CONTENTS

I.   INTRODUCTION

The condition generally referred to as osteoporosis has become widely recognized as a major health problem in most of the industrialized nations. The reasons for increasing awareness of this condition are several. First, the number of people living long enough to experience age-related bone loss increased dramatically during the 20th century. For instance, life expectancy in the U.S. has increased from about 46 years, sexes combined, in 1900 to more than 76 years at present. Consequently, the total number of at-risk years for age-related bone loss has undergone a substantial increase. In fact, the comparison of life expectancies at birth understates the number of years at risk, since the predicted age of death at age 50 now exceeds 79.3 years. Bone density usually peaks sometime between the late 20s and the 30s and remains stable until sometime around age 50, when first evidence of osteopenia, or loss of bone density, is often detected. Therefore, increases in the conditional probability of survival beyond age 50 have the effect of steadily increasing the proportion of the population at risk for osteoporosis. The impact of the changing demographic profile is further enhanced by the fact that the life expectancies have increased more rapidly for women than for men. In the U.S. in 1996, life expectancy at birth was 79.3 years for women and 72.5 years for men (1). In that same year, the predicted age at death for individuals who had attained the age of 50 years was 81.5 years for women and 77.1 years for men.

This disparity in life expectancies has particular relevance to the incidence of osteoporosis, since female bone loss begins earlier than male. Type I, or *postmenopausal*, osteoporosis is a condition peculiar to women. In Type I osteoporosis, the decline in estrogen production that initiates menopause is associated with a 1- to 3-year period of rapid bone loss. The phase of rapid bone loss is then followed by a sustained period of more-gradual loss that may eventually result in *senile*, or Type II osteoporosis. Since the average age of menopause in the U.S. is about 50 years, this sequence of rapid followed by more gradual bone loss may persist for 30 years or more.

It has recently been estimated (2) that osteoporosis is a major public health threat for 28 million Americans, 80% of whom are women. Ten million Americans are now believed to have osteoporosis and 18 million more have low bone density and are therefore at increased risk for fractures. On the basis of these statistics it is predicted that one out of every two women and one in eight men over the age of 50 years will experience an osteoporosis-related fracture during their lifetimes. Osteoporosis is responsible for 1.5 million fractures annually in the U.S., incurring an estimated cost of $14 billion.

As will be shown in the following discussion of longitudinal monitoring of bone mineral status conducted in Arizona, the result of 30 years of unmitigated bone loss is almost always osteoporosis as clinically defined. Although the situation is different for men, they are also subject to bone loss of the Type II or *senile* form. However, since the onset of bone loss is usually later in men and the rate of loss more gradual, bone density low enough to be considered clinically significant occurs much later. Moreover, male peak bone density is substantially greater than female, with the result that even after bone loss begins, it takes longer for bone density to decline to a level that would warrant a diagnosis of osteoporosis.

The endocrinological events that precipitate bone loss in males differ from those in females. The interaction of the sex steroids and the other hormones involved in the regulation of calcium metabolism is complex and sensitive to a variety of environmental factors. Among these factors are nutrition, exercise, medications, concurrent disabilities, stress-inducing conditions, and, in females, reproductive histories. The 16-year longitudinal study of bone density status conducted in Sun City and Tucson, Arizona from 1982 to 1998 addressed a number of issues concerning the relationships of certain of these environmental factors and bone loss in a large population of healthy retirees of both sexes.

II.   MATERIALS AND METHODS

The Arizona Bone Density Study was initiated in 1982. The first cohort of subjects was drawn from the Volunteer Association of the Walter O. Boswell Memorial Hospital in Sun City Arizona. These subjects were, by and large, retirees. Most owned their own homes and were financially independent. Almost all were of European ancestry. In order to broaden the demographics of the study, a second cohort was recruited from residents of publicly subsidized retirement housing in Tucson, Arizona. These subjects were, on the average, less affluent than those from Sun City. Also, most of the Tucson subjects had been Arizona residents for a longer period of time, often since birth, and roughly 30% of them were of Hispanic origin as compared with less than 5% in Sun City. A small sample of African-American subjects was also recruited in Tucson. From the outset, more women than men were recruited in both the Sun City and Tucson populations. This sampling bias reflected the belief, prevalent at the time, that osteoporosis was primarily a condition affecting women.

From 1982 through 1998, data were collected annually at both Sun City and Tucson. Since the average age of the subjects of the first cohort was 70 years, and the loss of subjects for various reasons could be expected, new subjects were added each year. By the end of 1998, the total sample was 5475 (4121 women and 1354 men). Of this sample, 173 subjects (126 women and 47 men) participated for 10 years or more. Over the course of the study, subjects from several rural communities in Pinal County Arizona (Casa Grande, Eloy, and Florence) had been incorporated in the study population, as had subjects enrolled in wheat bran fiber and piroxicam colon cancer prevention clinical trials conducted in Sun City and Tucson.

The primary objective of the study was to monitor changes in bone density over time. However, other changes were monitored as well. Height and weight were measured on each occasion for all subjects, and bioelectric impedance assessments of body composition were conducted on a sample of 451 (277 men and 174 women) who were enrolled in the wheat bran fiber and piroxicam clinical trials. Alkaline phosphatase levels and concentrations of serum calcium and other minerals were also determined through the analysis of blood samples from these subjects. On each occasion, all subjects were requested to complete questionnaires containing questions about bone fracture histories, medications, stress-inducing experiences, exercise patterns, milk consumption, and use of dietary supplements. On the occasion of their first visit, women were asked to complete an additional questionnaire concerning age at menarche and menopause and reproductive and breast feeding histories.

Annual scans of the left radius were conducted using single-beam photon absorptiometry (Lunar Radiation SP-1 and SP-2 Bone Densitometers). While both dual-photon (DPA) and dual-energy X-ray (DEXA) instruments provide more information about clinically sensitive areas such as the lumbar spine and the femoral neck, the objective of comparing serial measurements of cortical bone density was satisfactorily achieved using the single photon devices. The portability of the single photon device was a major consideration in its favor, because, to reach the target populations of the Arizona study, it was necessary to set up the equipment at a number of sites in several cities and in rural areas. Change in cortical bone density over time can be measured with a high degree of accuracy at the radial site using single-beam photon absorptiometry. Since cortical bone makes up more than 80% of the total bone mass of the adult, the SPA scanning of this bone as a surrogate for whole-body scanning yields useful results.

Within this limited context, SPA bone scans are a highly reliable method for effecting valid assessments of cortical bone density. When suitable safeguards are taken to assure that all scans are taken at precisely the same site, the method is ideal for the monitoring of bone density change through serial measurements. Thus, when used as a research method for a large sample, mixed longitudinal study of bone density change it is a very powerful tool. However, its clinical use as a predictor of fractures at sites where trabecular bone is more abundant cannot be recommended. Since the objectives of the present study did not include estimates of trabecular bone density or changes thereof, the advantages of SPA methodology considerably outweighed its disadvantages. Results of a comparative study involving subjects drawn from the Arizona Bone Density Study yielded a correlation of 89% between the values for whole-body bone density attained by DEXA measurement and the values for bone density of the distal one-third site of the radius attained through SPA measurement (3). An additional advantage of the SPA method is that the highly collimated photon stream emitted by its 200 mC ^{125}I source produces a very low radiation dose for the subject, and its low scatter minimizes the risk of radiation to both subjects and investigators.

The measurement of stature to the nearest millimeter was done using a freestanding field anthropometer with the subject shoeless. Weight in kilograms was taken using a portable medical scale. The same anthropometrist took each of these measurements on each scanning occasion throughout the study. Body mass index was calculated using the equation: BMI = wt (kg)/ ht (m).[2] More than 14,000 records of these measurements as well as bone scan reports, human subjects' consent forms, and questionnaires remain on file in the Biological Anthropology Laboratory at the University of Arizona.

III.   RESULTS

Table 8.1 shows the values for bone density and body mass index arranged by 5-year categories for a sample of 4036 women and 1264 men for whom complete records are available. The values that appear in this table represent those obtained at each subject's final examination. In some instances, this may be the last of 16 such measurements and in others, it is the first and only one. The values shown in this table therefore represent a purely cross-sectional database.

As the values in Table 8.1 indicate, average cortical bone density declines steadily from age 50 onward in women. The relatively small sample of men in the 50- to 55-year age group would appear to experience a sharp decrease in bone density, but it is probable that the apparent

TABLE 8.1
Bone Density and Body Mass Index Values by Age Category

| | Bone Density (BMD)[a] | | | | | | Body Mass Index (BMI)[b] | | | |
| | Women | | | Men | | | Women | | Men | |
AGE	n	BMD	S.D.	n	BMD	S.D.	BMI	S.D.	BMI	S.D.
< 50	369	0.6591	0.063	50	0.7803	0.056	25.79	6.47	26.12	5.01
50–55	142	0.6532	0.065	20	0.7468	0.091	27.36	7.74	29.30	7.44
55–60	202	0.6188	0.072	38	0.7553	0.086	26.97	5.94	27.58	4.49
60–65	332	0.5908	0.088	84	0.7502	0.087	26.17	5.41	27.40	4.02
65–70	684	0.5585	0.087	208	0.7279	0.089	26.16	5.12	26.91	3.72
70–75	808	0.5295	0.094	286	0.7157	0.088	25.79	4.73	26.70	4.07
75–80	708	0.4946	0.087	295	0.7054	0.083	25.34	4.59	26.91	4.16
80–85	497	0.4773	0.091	183	0.6763	0.100	24.94	4.45	25.17	2.89
85–90	246	0.4512	0.097	81	0.6341	0.128	24.31	4.02	24.21	2.84
90–95	69	0.4161	0.080	18	0.5817	0.135	23.58	3.42	24.72	3.12
>95	11	0.3966	0.100	1	0.4106	–	23.26	4.22	23.30	–

[a] Bone density is calculated in g/cm^2.
[b] Body Mass Index = weight (kg)/height (m)^2.

acceleration of bone density decrease is an artifact of small sample size in this age group. Succeeding age groups exhibit a rate of decline similar to that seen in the values for women. The decline in bone density in both sexes is sufficient to dispel the widely held notion that bone density decrease is primarily a women's problem. However, the lower average bone densities experienced by women throughout early adulthood make them susceptible to bone fractures at an earlier age than men.

Figure 8.1. Shows the relationship of bone density to age for 5180 individuals, sexes combined. The "best fit" regression equation for this nonlinear relationship is $y = a - bx^3$. Figure 8.2. Shows the same relationship restricting the analysis to the female sample of 3942 individuals. Again, the relationship is nonlinear, with the best-fit equation being $y = a - bx^2$. The relationship of bone density values to age for the male sample of 1238 individuals (Figure 8.3) is also nonlinear, with the same best fit equation as the combined sex sample. However the value of the intercept (a) is approximately .700 for the women while it is about .800 for males, reflecting the sex difference in peak bone density. The slopes (b) for all of these curves are negative. Comparison of the slopes for male vs. female values clearly shows the steeper rate of decline in bone density experienced by women.

Although sample size for the male subjects in the over-50 age group is small (50) and contains only one individual in the 95 to 100 age group, BMI values are informative when all age groups are compared. For instance, the highest values for both sexes occur in the 50 to 55-year age group. The decline in BMI from age 50 to age 95 is quite similar in both sexes. However, the observed change in BMI may not accurately reflect the more significant changes occurring in body composition. This relationship will be examined in a later section. Figure 8.4 shows the relationship of body mass index values to age for the entire sample of 5180 individuals of both sexes. The nonlinear regression equation that best fits this relationship is $y = a - bx^3$. Figures 8.5 and 8.6 show the BMI/age relationships for females and males, respectively. As in the case of the bone density values, the slopes of these regressions are all negative.

In Figure 8.7, which represents the nonlinear regression of bone density on BMI, the slope is positive, the best fit equation being $y = a + b/x^2$. However, when estimates of percent lean body mass obtained using the bioelectric impedance method were regressed on BMI, the slope was negative (Figure 8.8), while the slope for percent body fat was positive (Figure 8.9). These

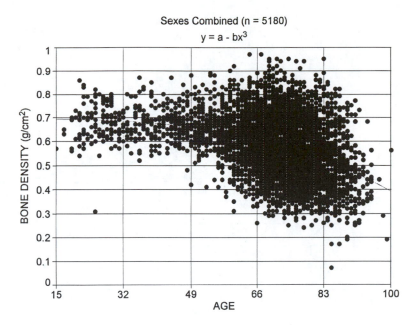

FIGURE 8.1 Bone density by age.

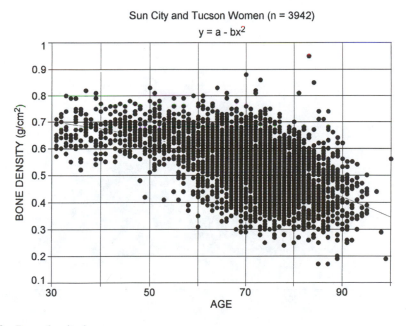

FIGURE 8.2 Bone density by age.

relationships reflect the degree to which the proportions of lean as opposed to adipose tissue affect BMI values.

Bone density values obtained through single SPA are expressed as grams of bone mineral per square centimeter of area. However, these values can be used to estimate the three-dimensional configuration of the radial diaphysis, and, by applying certain assumptions, the cross-sectional areas of the cortex and medullary cavity can be estimated. The method used in making these estimates is described in detail elsewhere (4). Normal remodeling of the diaphysis of long bones such as the

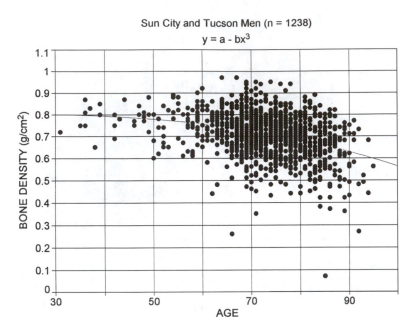

FIGURE 8.3 Bone density by age.

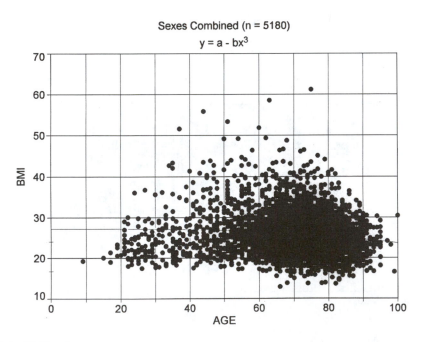

FIGURE 8.4 BMI and age.

radius usually involves resorption at the endosteal surface and appositional growth at the subperiosteal surface. With increasing age, the deposit of new bone at the subperiosteal surface declines
while resorption at the endosteal surface continues. The result is a thinning of the cortex. In its
earlier stages, the increased cross sectional area of the diaphysis may confer an advantage in
withstanding torsional stress. However, thinning of the cortex eventually leads to increased vulnerability to fractures produced by buckling of the cortex. Therefore, estimation of changes in the

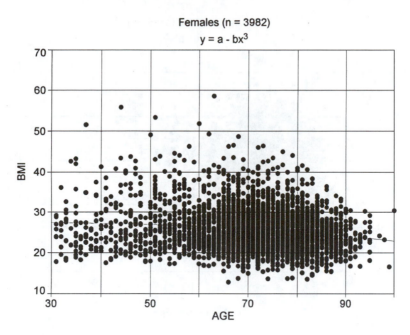

FIGURE 8.5 BMI and age.

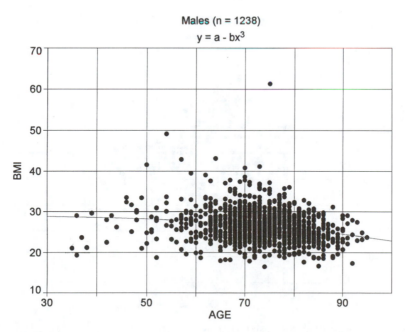

FIGURE 8.6 BMI and age.

ratio of cortical area to total cross sectional area (PCA) of the radius provides a useful means of estimating the risk of fracture in the radius. Table 8.2 shows the average initial and final values for PCA for women and men.

As can be seen from the values for PCA in Table 8.2, women enter the postmenopausal period with PCA values as high or higher than those of men. However, they are already experiencing a decline in cortical area in the 50- to 55-year age interval, while men show little change until the

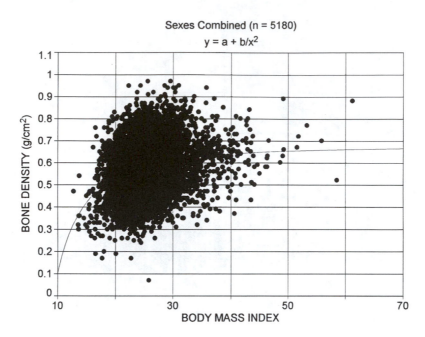

FIGURE 8.7   Bone density as related to body mass index.

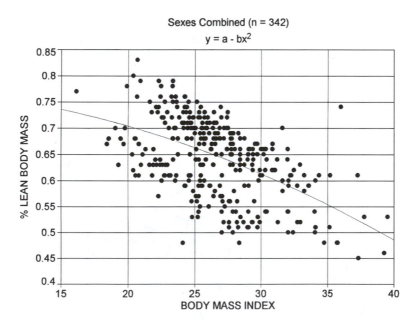

FIGURE 8.8   Relationship of percent lean body mass to BMI.

65- to 70-year interval. Because of the differences in age of onset and rate of decrease in PCA, initial values for men in the 80- to 85-year age group are higher than those for women in the 65- to 70-year age group. The rate of loss in the later years of life, however, is very similar in both sexes.

As the regression line shown in Figure 8.7 shows, there is a positive correlation between body mass index and cortical bone density. The relationships between body mass index and PCA at various ages are shown in Table 8.3. In Table 8.3, BMI values conventionally used to assign the

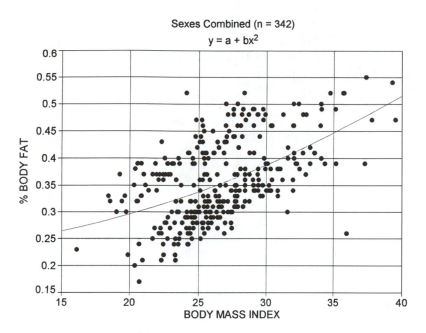

FIGURE 8.9   Relationship of percent body fat to BMI.

TABLE 8.2
Initial and Final Percent Cortical Area,
Sexes Compared

	Women		Men	
Age	Initial PCA	Final PCA	Initial PCA	Final PCA
50–55	64.6	63.5	61.0	61.0
55–60	59.5	58.6	59.3	59.1
60–65	58.0	57.4	59.1	59.1
65–70	54.5	53.3	58.0	57.3
70–75	52.4	50.5	57.9	56.6
75–80	49.0	47.0	57.4	55.7
80–85	48.7	45.5	54.8	52.8
85–90	46.0	43.1	54.3	49.8
90–95	42.6	39.1	50.4	45.9

designations "obese" (BMI > 28.0), and "excessively lean" (BMI < 20.0) were applied to average values in the 10-year age categories 60–70, 70–80, and 80–90 to assess the relationship between extreme BMI values and PCA. Along with the aforementioned decline in PCA with age, the PCA values for subjects of both sexes with high BMI values are seen to be substantially higher than for those with low BMI values.

When the values for PCA, bone mineral content, and bone density for subjects drawn from the low BMI ($n = 370$) and high BMI ($n = 1228$) categories are compared, the differences for all three of these indicators of bone fracture risk are highly significant ($p < .0001$). This is true of all age categories whether calculated by sex or with sexes combined. Analysis of variance to test the relationship of PCA to BMI at all ages yields an F value of 91.9 ($p < .0001$) sexes combined.

TABLE 8.3
PCA Values in Three Age Groups and by
BMI Category

	Female	Male
Age Group 60–70		
Average BMI	26.1	26.7
Average PCA	54.6 ($n = 928$)	57.9 ($n = 212$)
PCA (BMI > 28)	56.9 ($n = 288$)	58.7 ($n = 62$)
PCA (BMI < 20)	50.4 ($n = 60$)	54.5 ($n = 5$)
Age Group 70–80		
Average BMI	25.6	26.8
Average PCA	48.9 ($n = 1423$)	56.2 ($n = 418$)
PCA (BMI > 28)	51.2 ($n = 348$)	56.7 ($n = 147$)
PCA (BMI < 20)	45.8 ($n = 115$)	52.9 ($n = 12$)
Age Group 80–90		
Average BMI	24.8	24.8
Average PCA	44.7 ($n = 732$)	51.9 ($n = 250$)
PCA (BMI > 28)	47.8 ($n = 144$)	53.6 ($n = 36$)
PCA (BMI < 20)	41.4 ($n = 86$)	45.1 ($n = 15$)

Separate analyses of variance for the male and the female samples yield F values of 15.5 and 65.9, respectively, both also significant at the $p < .0001$ level.

Normative bone density values, developed from a number studies conducted in various geographic areas of the U.S., are consistently higher than the averages for each age group for both sexes in the Arizona study. When the mean percent of the national normative values for Arizona subjects is compared with their mean BMI values, a t-test yields a two-tailed significance $< .0001$, similar to the level of significance for the comparison of means for body mass index and percent of peak bone density.

All subjects filled out questionnaires that contained questions about fracture histories. Although there was often some doubt about the bone fractured, the response level to this question was high, and the locations indicated usually made it possible to assign the fracture to such broad categories as "hip," "thigh," "leg," "arm," "rib," and so on. Fractures associated with automobile accidents were excluded from analysis. Of the 3939 records containing usable fracture histories, 1066 individuals (878 women and 188 men) reported at least one fracture. The relationship between bone density and fracture histories was equivocal for the male subjects before the age of 80 but was highly significant in the 80 to 90 year age group. However, as can be seen in Table 8.4, there is an increasingly clear relationship in the female subjects with increased age.

Analysis of variance of bone density values within and between the fracture history categories yields F values of 0.389 (n.s.) for the 50 to 60 age group; $F = 9.828$ ($p = .003$) for the 60 to 70 age group; $F = 16.14$ ($p < .0001$) for the 70 to 80 age group; and 12.2 ($p < .0001$) for the 80 to 90 age group. These values reflect the age of occurrence of first and subsequent fractures the subjects reported. The average age of occurrence of the first fracture for women was 64.4 years. The average age at which men experienced their first fracture was 62.7 years. Of the 301 individuals (268 women and 33 men) reporting a second fracture, the average age of occurrence was 70 years for women and 67.8 years for men. A third fracture was reported by 102 women, with an average age of occurrence of 72.2 years. Only three men reported a third fracture, the average age being 68.3 years.

TABLE 8.4
Bone Densities of Women with Different Fracture Histories

Age Group	No Fractures		1 Fracture		> 1 Fracture		Percent[a]
	n	BMD	n	BMD	n	BMD	
50–60	192	.6366	17	.6393	3	.6217	9.4
60–70	435	.5732	152	.5509	37	.5233	30.2
70–80	635	.5203	340	.4998	102	.4809	41.0
80–90	291	.4823	244	.4454	102	.4335	54.3

[a] Percentage of women in each age group reporting one or more fractures

IV. DISCUSSION

The major objectives of the Arizona Bone Density Study were

(1) to record actual changes in bone density over time
(2) to identify other changes in body composition occurring as a part of the aging process
(3) to compare the loss of bone density experienced by the most-vulnerable component of the Arizona population, women, with that reported in other populations

A. OBSERVED BONE LOSS

The rate of bone loss observed in both sexes in the Arizona population was greater than that derived from normative values used for diagnostic purposes. This is true whether the comparison is with the cross-sectional mean values shown in Table 8.1, or with averaged longitudinal values. In order to make the last-mentioned comparison, only individuals who were scanned five times during the 5-year period represented by their age group were included. Thus, the decline in bone density recorded women in the 50- to 55-year age group who had been scanned at ages 50, 51, 52, 53, and 54 was calculated by subtracting the bone density value observed at age 54 from that observed at age 50. While reducing the sample size substantially, this procedure made it possible to compare averages derived from individual experience with averages derived from a local population and a national one. In some age groups, the longitudinal data are inadequate to permit meaningful statistical comparisons, but most age groups are sufficiently well represented to provide indicators of similarity and differences. The results of this comparison are shown in Table 8.5, where sample sizes for the cross-sectional and longitudinal components of the Arizona population are entered in parentheses.

As can be seen by comparison of the values in Table 8.5, the rate of density decrease for Arizona subjects is more rapid than national normative values would predict at most ages. Bone density values are also lower for both sexes and all age groups. Following the convention that values above 90% of peak bone density can be considered normal, Arizona average values remain within the normal category until the 55 to 60 age group, by the 65 to 70 age group, average values have declined to less than 80% of peak density, and by ages 75 to 80 are below 70% of peak density, a level usually considered diagnostic of osteoporosis. Average values for men do not fall below the 90% level until the 65- to 70-year age group and below the 80% level after age 85. However, the longitudinal data indicate that male bone loss actually exceeds female in a number of age categories. Because of their greater peak bone density, men are less vulnerable to osteoporosis than women, but are clearly not immune to bone loss.

TABLE 8.5
Rates of Bone Density Loss Derived from Normative, Cross-Sectional, and Longitudinal Values

	Women			Men		
Ages	Standard	Cross-Sectional	Longitudinal	Standard	Cross-Sectional	Longitudinal
50–55	.0106	.0059 (142)	.0594 (7)	.0335	.0335 (20)	.0420 (1)
55–60	.0405	.0344 (202)	.0366 (16)	.0305	.0000 (38)	.0790 (2)
60–65	.0250	.0280 (332)	.0366 (15)	.0199	.0051 (84)	.0310 (1)
65–70	.0378	.0323 (684)	.0445 (68)	.0145	.0223 (208)	.0352 (13)
70–75	.0297	.0290 (808)	.0363 (147)	.0435	.0122 (286)	.0296 (32)
75–80	.0292	.0349 (708)	.0427 (163)	.0065	.0103 (295)	.0431 (50)
80–85	.0384	.0173 (497)	.0544 (165)	.0048	.0291 (183)	.0384 (58)
85–90	.0287	.0261 (246)	.0532 (77)	.0648	.0422 (81)	.0838 (29)
90–95	.0181	.0351 (69)	.0576 (25)	.0331	.0524 (18)	.1226 (5)

B. CHANGES IN BODY COMPOSITION

The widely used estimate of body composition, Body Mass Index is one obvious measure of change that merits careful attention. However, BMI values can be misleading. For instance, young individuals with high lean body mass (LBM) to total body mass (TBM) ratios will exhibit higher BMI values than those with normal amounts of total body fat (TBF). This is because the LBM compartment of TBM is of higher density. In fact the Seri equations used to calculate TBF and LBM by comparison of a conventional measure of weight with one taken with the subject immersed in water are based on the specific gravity values for TBF and LBM. As can be seen from the regression lines in Figures 8.8 and 8.9, in the age groups represented in the Arizona population, increasing BMI is negatively correlated with increased LBM and positively correlated with TBF. These results are consistent with those reported by Kehayias et al. (5) in their analysis of total body potassium (Table 8.6). These investigators estimate a decline of total body potassium (TBK) of 7.2 mgK/kg body weight/year in women, and 9.2 mgK/kg/yr in men. The steady decline in TBK is closely related to a decline in intracellular fluid (ICF) mass and therefore cell number. Cell number is directly related to basal metabolic rate. Therefore, the decline in TBK is a measure of the decline in required energy intake associated with increasing age. An average daily energy intake of 1910 kcal was reported for the 1303 individuals of both sexes (average age 66.2 years) who completed that Wheat Bran Fiber Colon Cancer Prevention study.

Another way of estimating energy requirements is to calculate body surface area (SA) using height and weight values. This is the most commonly used method of estimating BMR. When the male and female values for surface area are compared for a total of 3858 women and 1166 men, the female average SA is 1.71 m^2 and the male average is 1.95 m^2. Since the same values, height and weight, are used to derive both BMI and SA it is expected that BMI and SA would be highly correlated, as indeed they are, ($r = 0.838$ for women and 0.781 for men). Also expected would be a decline in SA with age. Surface area is negatively correlated with age in both sexes, (–0.166 for women and –0.249 for men). All of these correlations are significant at the 0.01 level (two-tailed test). Perhaps more interesting is the high positive correlation between percentage of body fat and surface area, and negative correlations between percentage of lean tissue and surface area, ($r = 0.761$ for women and $r = 0.644$ for men), derived from bioelectric impedance values for 128 women and 214 men participating in the Wheat Bran Fiber study.

The two-compartment method of estimating body composition through hydrostatic weighing has long been considered the "gold standard" of body composition analysis. However, the components of the lean tissue compartment are more variable with respect to mass and density than are

TABLE 8.6
Age Changes in Body Mass Index and Total Body Calcium in Women and Men

Age	Women				Men			
	BMI	TBK(g)	TBK/Ht	TBK/Wt	BMI	TBK(g)	TBK/Ht	TBK/Wt
20–29	22.8	101.4	0.62	1.67	24.8	164.5	0.92	2.06
30–39	23.6	98.7	0.60	1.59	25.0	145.6	0.83	1.90
40–49	25.3	96.4	0.58	1.41	27.6	148.3	0.84	1.72
50–59	27.5	95.8	0.59	1.35	28.4	146.1	0.83	1.68
60–69	24.3	85.2	0.53	1.36	25.3	128.2	0.74	1.70
70–79	26.6	79.8	0.51	1.24	25.6	120.2	0.69	1.56
80–89	23.6	72.3	0.46	1.26	26.3	106.8	0.64	1.46

Source: Kehayias, J.J., Fiataione, M.A., Hang, Z., Roubenoff, R. 1997. Total body potassium and body fats: relevence to aging, *Am. J. Clin. Nutr.*, 66:904–100. With permission.

those of the adipose compartment. This is especially true of the portion of LBM represented by bone, which is much denser than skeletal muscle but has lower energy requirements. Thus, the impact of declining bone density will be more significant from the perspective of LBM than from that of BMR. The nonlinear relationship between bone density and BMI can clearly be seen in Figure 8.7, where the best fit regression equation is $y = a + b/x^2$. The decline in bone density with age, as seen in Figures 8.1 to 8.3, is clearly more precipitous than the decline in BMI with age, as seen in Figures 8.4 to 8.6.

The implications of this disparity raise questions about the appropriateness of using BMI values to estimate energy requirements in older populations although the decline in TBK with age indicates a steady decline in basal metabolic rate. It should come as no surprise that weight control is often a problem during late middle age, when the proportion of fat to lean tissue is rising, in consequence of decreases in both skeletal muscle mass and bone density. Even maintenance of a constant body weight can mask substantial accumulation of fat when the increase is offset by loss of both high-density bone mineral and metabolically active skeletal muscle. By the same token, the early stages of bone density decline often go undiagnosed, since there are no obvious indications of bone density decrease in the absence *in vivo* monitoring using sophisticated instrumentation.

C. Bone Loss among Women: A Comparison

Osteoporosis has long been recognized as a problem faced by postmenopausal women. The values for bone density obtained from Arizona women provide clear evidence of a progressive decrease that continues from age 50 through all age groups up to age 100. Moreover, the decline recorded in Table 8.1, based on cross-sectional analysis of data from 4086 women, is confirmed by longitudinal analysis of 683 women for whom at least five consecutive scans were obtained. In some of these cases, as many as 16 consecutive scans were on record. As cited in an earlier section, both the cross-sectional and longitudinal comparisons with normative values indicate that the Arizona women are experiencing more bone density loss than would be predicted. This observation raises questions about the possibility that environmental factors are implicated in the Arizona pattern. A number of possible environmental factors, including nutrition, exercise, sunshine exposure, and concurrent physical disabilities are all currently under investigation, but a detailed discussion of this aspect of the study is beyond the scope of the current discussion.

Comparison of the Arizona pattern of bone loss with that reported from other populations will allow this aspect of the study to focus on specific environmental factors. The importance of calcium intake is one such factor. Comparison with Chinese populations reporting sharply differing dietary patterns provides an opportunity to approach the question of the importance of dietary calcium intakes in the maintenance of bone density in women. Table 8.7 shows comparisons of bone densities of Arizona women, whose average daily calcium intake is 853 mg/day with five populations of Chinese women living in different environmental settings and consuming substantially differing amounts of calcium, dairy products, protein, and carbohydrates, reported by Hu et al. (6,7).

TABLE 8.7
Comparison of Bone Mineral Content and Density of Arizona and Chinese Populations

Age Group	Arizona (n = 2250)	Xianghuangqi (n = 143)	Tuoli (n = 175)	Jiexiu (n = 165)	Cangxi (n = 180)	Changli (n = 164)
			BMC (g/cm)			
35–44 (125)[a]	.846 (0.11)[b]	1.010 (0.12)	0.910 (0.15)	0.910 (0.14)	0.860 (0.15)	0.860 (0.16)
45–54 (247)	.823 (0.10)	0.980 (0.15)	0.860 (0.19)	0.820 (0.13)	0.780 (0.09)	0.830 (0.11)
55–64 (506)	.769 (0.13)	0.770 (0.16)	0.730 (0.14)	0.690 (0.14)	0.710 (0.09)	0.690 (0.12)
65–74 (1372)	.695 (0.13)	0.680 (0.10)	0.650 (0.14)	0.610 (0.12)	0.620 (0.12)	0.580 (0.08)
			BMD (g/cm²)			
35–44 (125)	.666 (0.06)	0.810 (0.09)	0.770 (0.06)	0.770 (0.06)	0.740 (0.09)	0.760 (0.06)
45–54 (247)	.655 (0.06)	0.750 (0.11)	0.690 (0.10)	0.700 (0.09)	0.690 (0.07)	0.720 (0.07)
55–64 (506)	.603 (0.08)	0.590 (0.10)	0.610 (0.11)	0.580 (0.11)	0.600 (0.06)	0.600 (0.10)
65–74 (1372)	.542 (0.09)	0.520 (0.06)	0.540 (0.10)	0.520 (0.10)	0.530 (0.08)	0.500 (0.07)

[a] Arizona n [b] Std. dev.

Note: Measured at the distal one third site on the radius by single photon absorptiometry.

Two of the Chinese communities sampled were pastoralists, although the women in one of them (Tuoli) only drank milk tea with meals and consumed no other dairy products. In the other pastoral community (Xianghuangqi), dairy products were an important component of the diet of both sexes. The Tuoli community resides in a plateau region of Xinjiang Autonomous Region and is of the Kazak minority population. The people of Xianghuangqi are Mongolian and live in a high plateau region of the Neimongol Autonomous Region. The remaining three communities, all of the Han majority group, consume little or no milk or other dairy products. These populations reside in Jiexiu (a plains area in Shanxi Province), Cangxi (a mountainous area in Sichuan Province), and Changle (a coastal area in Fujian Province). The people of Changle, living on the coast, have access to seafood, which is a regular part of their diet, along with pork and other animal products. The people of Jiexiu and Cangxi, on the other hand, are predominantly vegetarian.

Of particular interest in this comparison is the high bone densities reported in the Chinese populations in the youngest age group, all of whom exhibit values superior to those of Arizona women of comparable age. However, the Arizona women have the highest values beyond age 65.

V. CONCLUSIONS

In the U.S., post-menopausal women are the segment of the population most susceptible to osteoporosis-related fractures. These fractures are often nontraumatic, and the incidence of mortality within a year after a nontraumatic hip fracture is on the order of 20 to 25%. Even when fatality does not result, there is a high risk of long-term incapacity. Chrischilles et al. (8) estimate that osteoporosis-related fractures will lead to long-term dependency for 6.7% of American women, with an additional 7.8% requiring nursing home care for an average of 7.6 years. For osteoporosis-related fractures at all sites, the overall risk has been estimated at 40% (9).

Osteoporosis is becoming recognized as a worldwide problem of increasing significance, particularly for women. Among the countries for which high incidences have been reported are Finland, (10), France (9), Hong Kong, (11), Italy, 12), Japan, (13), Poland, (14), Switzerland, (15). and Taiwan (16). As monitoring for osteoporosis becomes increasingly common, it can be predicted that most of the world's population either is or soon will be affected by what might quite properly be designated an epidemic of osteoporosis-related fractures. The exceptions might be found in areas where life expectancy, especially that of women, remains low. Clearly, osteoporosis is predominantly a condition associated with aging. In fact, the probability of its occurrence rises to better than 90% in people surviving beyond age 90.

The widespread occurrence of osteoporosis-related fractures might be viewed as expression of an intrinsic human attribute; the loss of bone density in advanced age being an inevitable component of the aging process. The reason for the dramatic increase in its occurrence we are now observing is that more people are living sufficiently long for its deleterious effects to become manifest in the form of fractures. When life expectancies averaged less than 50 years few women lived long enough to experience the decline in estrogen production associated with Type I osteoporosis. If reproductive life had been completed, not much time elapsed before death occurred. Even when women lived well past menopause, long enough to experience significant bone loss, fractures and the complications following them had no effect on their reproductive success. In terms of selective pressure, even when osteoporosis occurred, it was irrelevant, a situation consistent with the establishment of an antagonistic pleiotropy.

Men, who usually are not subject to the relatively abrupt decline in gonadal hormone production that characterizes menopause in women, experience bone density decreases later than women, as can be seen by comparison of male and female bone densities shown in Table 8.1 (4,17,18,19). Since men achieve greater bone densities, on the average, than women in early adulthood, the loss that does eventually occur takes longer to reach clinically significant levels. Although men do not experience the clear-cut end of reproductive life that menopause represents for women, sexual activity does decline, and few men father children in their eighth and ninth decades of life, a time when a significant loss of bone density occurs in most men. Thus, selective pressure associated with the loss of bone density is modest for both sexes, and its genetic determinants can accumulate in the gene pool. Although bone density decreases occur in both sexes, the pattern is different. Women experience loss of trabecular bone at a rate approximating 1% per year in the early postmenopausal years, followed by loss of cortical bone at a slower rate for the remainder of life. The rate of loss for most men is more gradual, and significant loss usually begins in the 60s. Also, the remodeling associated with bone loss is more pronounced in women.

Using a criterion of bone density more than two standard deviations below the young normal value as diagnostic of osteoporosis, Melton and Riggs (20) found 45% of a Minnesota sample of Caucasian women over 50 years of age at risk at one or more sites. Of these subjects, 32% had low values in the lumbar spine, 29% in the proximal femur and 26% in the mid-radius. Associated with these observed risk values is a lifetime probability of 40% of experiencing a fracture at one of these sites (9). Other investigators, including Chrischilles et al. (8), calculate the risk at 54%. They estimate that osteoporosis-related fractures will cause 6.7% of American women to become dependent on the help of others to conduct the basic activities of daily living, while an additional 7.8% will require nursing home care for an average of 7.6 years.

It has been estimated that hip fractures alone are responsible for medical expenses in excess of $10 billion annually in the U.S. This cost is likely to increase as the number of women over the age of 50 years increases. Nevertheless, some clinicians argue that bone mass assessments should be limited to women approaching menopause or who have significantly impaired ovarian function (22). With female life expectancy at birth in the U.S. now approaching 80 years, age-related causes of morbidity such as osteoporosis promise to become a major source of concern for future generations. Bone loss, once it begins, seems to continue throughout life and may even accelerate after the age of 70 (23). Vertebral crush fractures, another debilitating consequence of osteoporotic bone loss will also become more common as the aging population increases. The incidence of this form of fracture is currently 17.1/10,000 per year for Caucasian women compared with 9.9/10,000 for Caucasian men. For African-American women, the incidence is 3.7/10,000, and for African-American men 2.5/10,000, (24).

Observations of familial tendencies toward early bone loss are frequently cited but, until recently, the mechanisms underlying such tendencies have proven elusive. Small, slender women with a light complexion have generally been regarded as typifying the high-risk individual. For the most part, this constellation of traits has proven to be indicative of high risk, and twin studies support the contention that there is a genetic basis for this risk. In recent studies, some of the factors involved in the attainment of low peak bone density, the major risk factor for osteoporosis, have been identified (8,22-33).

Tokita et al. (34) studied pairs of monozygotic and dizygotic female twins to isolate genetically determined differences in the synthesis and degradation of Type I collagen related to low bone density. Spotila et al. (35) focused their study on the coding sequence for Type-I procollagen in osteogenesis imperfecta patients, identifying several mutations in these sequences. Cassella et al. (36) found abnormalities in the Type I collagen fibrils of osteogenesis imperfecta patients that they believe affect the formation and stability of the bone mineral associated with it.

It has been estimated that 46 to 62% of the variance in bone mineral density has a genetic basis (37). Associations between low bone density, osteoporotic fractures, and inherited variation in the vitamin D receptor have been reported by Norman and Collins (38), Eisman et al. (39) and Morrison et al. (40). The existence of genetically determined variation in the human vitamin D receptor (VDR) raises the possibility that natural selection at the VDR locus has produced different allele frequencies in different human populations. Mundy (41) suggests that polymorphism in the vitamin D receptor accounts for up to 75% of the genetic variation in bone density in Caucasian women in Australia. Identification of allelic variation at the vitamin D receptor locus and the relationship of certain alleles at this locus to excessive bone loss provides a promising lead for the identification of one genetic determinant of osteoporotic tendencies. Reproductive histories of women of different vitamin D receptor genotypes can be compared for evidence of differential reproductive success associated with different genotypes. The fact that calcium supplementation has yielded so little success in preventing osteoporosis is closely related to the poor calcium absorption efficiency, seldom exceeding 40%, in the human intestine. One of the major physiological roles played by vitamin D is the facilitation of calcium absorption through direct interaction with the DNA of intestinal epithelial cells resulting in the synthesis of calbindin, the protein that transports calcium across the gut wall. Despite the ready availability of vitamin D supplements in the U.S., there is still strong evidence that vitamin D deficiency is common among older Americans, (42).

With age, the long bones of the appendages increase in cross-sectional area. Since bone mineral is being lost while this increase is occurring, bone density declines if for no other reason than that the same amount of (or less) bone mineral is distributed over a greater area. This happens in both sexes, but more pronouncedly in women (4). In addition, since women start the process with less bone mineral, expanding the area over which it is distributed will affect bone density sooner than it will in men. The process is one in which bone is resorbed from the inner surface of the long bone (endosteal resorption), while at the same time, new bone is being added to its outer surface (periosteal apposition). The net result is an expansion of the medullary cavity and a thinning of the cortex. This thinning of the cortex is the clinically significant component of the remodeling process.

In its early stages, expansion of the cross-sectional area may actually increase the bone's ability to resist bending stress. This is because the mass of mineral present possesses greater resistance to bending stress if it lies farther from a line passing through the center of the diaphysis (shaft). This improves strength for the same reason that a metal tube has greater resistance to torsional forces than a rod of the same mass (43–46). But this holds true only up to a point, beyond which the metal tube or the long bone's diaphysis is susceptible to buckling. In the case of bone, such buckling results in fracture.

The familiar Colle's fracture of the distal radius is one example of such a fracture. It is often the result of an attempt to break the force of a fall with the hands, with the result that the wrist is twisted or bent while weight is being placed on it. Colle's fractures are very common in postmenopausal women.

Bone remodeling, as important as it is in the thinning of the cortex of long bones, is not the major cause of senile osteoporosis. Outright loss of bone mineral is far more important. The reason for loss of bone mineral is the change in bone mineral turnover that occurs later in life. Bone is a dynamic tissue that is continually exchanging calcium and phosphorus. Even in the densest area of cortical bone, the system of lacunae and canaliculae that permit communication between osteocytes and the vascular system serve to exchange the constituents of bone mineral on an ongoing basis. There is considerable variation in the rate of exchange occurring in different parts of the skeleton, with the most rapid turnover in the trabecular bone, which may be totally exchanged in some bones every 3 to 4 years. The slowest turnover in cortical bone may be as much as 10 years. Many factors, including the stresses the bone experiences, influence the turnover rate. Lack of weight-bearing stress, for instance, can lead to bone mineral loss due to lack of stimulation of osteoblast activity while osteoclasts continue to resorb bone.

For reasons not yet understood, turnover that would maintain constant bone density in early adulthood is altered with age so that osteoblastic bone formation fails to keep pace with osteoclastic bone resorption. Endocrine factors are clearly implicated in this disruption of the orderly replacement of bone mineral, but there appears to be more involved than a simple reduction in the production of estrogens or testosterone. Although higher levels of calcium intake and physical activity have both been shown to be positively correlated with bone mass and turnover in women (47), it is not clear that the relationship is any different in men than in women. Reduced activity levels late in life probably play a role in the onset of senile osteoporosis, but the pattern of change in bone density does not appear to parallel directly changes in activity level, especially in the very active segment of the aging population. Moreover, the fact that women lose bone earlier and more rapidly than men is not consistent with changes in activity patterns characteristic of males as opposed to females in later life if bone loss is to be explained on the basis of reduced activity levels.

Overall loss of fat-free body mass, which is an important factor in human aging (48), is associated with loss of bone mineral, and it is likely that both are influenced by such factors as changed endocrine status, nutritional patterns, concurrent illnesses, and activity levels. It is highly unlikely that any single factor will be identified that will explain fully the majority of cases of bone mineral loss, since so many aspects of physiological homeostasis have the potential to alter bone mineral turnover. However, the maintenance of calcium homeostasis, the oldest and most critical function of bone, will always receive the highest priority in the turnover of bone mineral. Endogenous or exogenous factors that cause serious disruption of normal blood calcium concentration will evoke a prompt and vigorous response.

Nulliparity has been suggested as a risk factor for osteoporosis (49). However, Kroger et al.'s study found only a weak statistically significant correlation between parity and femoral BMD. Multiple parity may also trigger an adaptive response in the mother for increased calcium absorption at critical times such as pregnancy and lactation. Contrary to conventional wisdom, multiple parity may serve as a bone protection mechanism rather than one causing calcium loss. Results from the longitudinal bone density study in Arizona suggest this possibility (50,51). Elderly women who had two or more children and who breastfed show higher bone mass at the distal radius site than those in their age-cohort who had two or fewer births.

Resorption of trabecular bone is thought to be the result of decreased estrogen release during lactation (52,53), increased parathyroid hormone secretion, and increased synthesis and conversion of calcitriol (53,54). The net result of all these changes is an increase in calcium resorption through stimulation of osteoclasts (55), which also involves suppression of osteoblast paracrine function that lowers interleukin-1 levels. These adjustments maintain serum calcium levels at or near normal throughout lactation (56). After weaning, when estrogen levels return to normal, recovery of bone mineral is quite rapid (52,53).

This rapid recovery is remarkable under any circumstances, but becomes truly impressive when calcium intake is low. The efficiency of absorption necessary to support rapid replacement of lost bone density at a calcium intake of 300 mg per day must substantially exceed 50%, a level not reported in any physiological state. Much remains to be learned about the mechanisms that make this possible. From an evolutionary perspective, the selective advantage gained through rapid repletion of bone mineral following lactation seems quite clear. If another pregnancy occurs, and calcium intake is chronically low, the need to restore lost bone would conflict with the demands of another fetus. Both mother and fetus would be at risk, and reproductive success would be compromised.

The capacity to withdraw calcium from bone when estrogen levels decline during lactation, and the capacity to restore lost bone rapidly when estrogen levels return to normal after weaning, allow frequent pregnancy and lactation even when calcium intake is low. The mechanism that permits the system to work is adjustment of calcium absorption efficiency and/or reduction of the amount of calcium secreted into the gut. The low efficiency of absorption that normally prevails when calcium intake is high avoids kidney damage associated with excessive urinary calcium excretion. It would be useful to determine to what extent the absorption efficiency curve is influenced by early experience.

If chronically low calcium intakes prevail throughout growth, development, and adulthood, does developmental acclimatization result in higher efficiency throughout life? There is evidence to suggest that this is indeed the case (57). Comparison of bone densities of women in Arizona, whose daily calcium intake averages nearly 800 mg per day with those of women from five districts in China show that Chinese bone density values do not differ appreciably from those reported in Arizona. In the Chinese populations, average daily calcium intakes range from a high of 724 mg per day at Xianghuangqi to 369 mg at Tuoli, 359 mg at Jiexiu, 328 mg at Cangxi, and 230 mg at Tangle. Clearly, adjustments in absorption efficiency are implicated in the capacity of Chinese women to maintain normal bone density with such low calcium intakes. The fact that the Chinese women had nearly twice as many children on the average would also indicate that they had been able to resorb and restore bone mineral effectively when the stringent demands of pregnancy and lactation required it.

When bone densities and reproductive histories and fracture histories of the Arizona women were examined, evidence was found suggesting that pregnancy and lactation occurring early in life are associated with greater bone density and fewer fractures later in life (50,51). This observation raises the possibility that the experience of pregnancy and lactation, during which calcium absorption efficiency is substantially improved, may have a carry-over effect that extends up to menopause and possibly beyond.

Despite the ability of Chinese women to maintain bone density while ingesting low-calcium diets, and the possible benefits in absorption efficiency they may derive from repeated pregnancy and lactation, osteoporosis is emerging as a major health problem in Hong Kong (11) and in Taiwan (16), as life expectancies increase. Just as in the U.S. and other Western countries, the system that functions so effectively in youth seems prone to failure later in life. The apparent universality of this aspect of human senescence raises the possibility that it is part of our evolutionary heritage. If this indeed turns out to be the case, osteoporosis may eventually be added to the list of antagonistic pleiotropies that are suspected to underlie many facets of human senescence. In the case of osteoporosis, the early advantages of a low calcium absorption efficiency that protects kidney function and mechanisms to adjust absorption efficiency at critical junctures in reproductive life have sufficient impact on reproductive success to have high selective value. Many genes may be involved in the maintenance of this functional adaptation. Allelic variation in vitamin D receptors associated with different levels of calcium absorption have already been reported (38, 60–65).

REFERENCES

1. United Nations. 1997. *World Statistics Pocketbook and Statistical Yearbook*. Geneva, United Nations.
2. National Institutes of Health. 1998. Osteoporosis Overview. http://www.osteo.org/osteo.htm Washington D.C. Osteoporosis and Related Bone Diseases-National Resource Center.
3. Chen, Z., Lohman, T.G., Stini, W.A., Ritenbaugh, S., and Aiken, M., Fat or lean tissue mass: which one is the major determinant of bone mineral mass in healthy post-menopausal women? *J. Bone Mineral Res.,* 12:144-151.
4. Stini, W.A., Stein, P., and Chen, Z., 1992. Bone remodeling in old age: longitudinal monitoring in Arizona, *Am. J. Hum. Biol.,* 4:47-55.
5. Kehayias, J.J., Fiatarone, M.A., Hong, Z., and Roubenoff, R., 1997. Total body potassium and body fat: relevance to aging, *Am. J. Clin. Nutr.,* 66:904-10.
6. Hu, J.F., Zhao, X.-H., and Jia, J.-B., 1993a. Dietary calcium and bone density among middle-aged and elderly women in China, *Am. J. Clin. Nutr.,* 58:219-27.
7. Hu, J.F., Zhao, X.-H., Parpia, B., and Campbel, T.C., 1993b. Dietary intake and urinary excretion of calcium and acids: a cross-sectional study of women in China, *Am. J. Clin. Nutr.,* 58:398-406.
8. Chrischilles, E.A., Butler, C.D., Davis, C.S., and Wallace, R.B., 1991. A model of lifetime osteoporosis impact, *Arch. Int. Med.,* 151(10):2026-32.
9. Audran, M.J., 1992. Epidemiology, etiology, and diagnosis of osteoporosis. Current opinion, *Rheumatology,* 4:394-401.
10. Tuppurainen, M., Honkanen, R., Kroger, H., Saarikoski, S., and Alhava, E., 1993. Osteoporosis risk factors, gynaecological history and fractures in perimenopausal women — the results of the baseline postal enquiry of the Kuopio Osteoporosis Risk Factor and Prevention Study, *Maturitas,* 17(2):89-100.
11. Lau, E.M. and Cooper, C., 1993. Epidemiology and prevention of osteoporosis in urbanized Asian populations, *Osteoporosis Int.* 3 Suppl. 1:23-6.
12. Mazzuoli, G.F., Gennari, C., Passeri, M., Acca, M., Camporeale, A., and Pioli, G., 1993. Hip fracture in Italy: epidemiology and preventive efficacy of bone-active drugs, *Bone,* 14 Suppl 1:S81-4.
13. Fujita, T., 1994. Anti-osteoporotic programs in Japan. Nippon Rinsho – *Jpn. J. Clin. Med.,* 52:2448-53.
14. Miazgowski, T., Napierala, K., Czekalskin, S., Krzysztalkowski, A., and Ogonowski, J., 1993. Prevalence and risk factors of osteoporosis in a population sample of Szczecin residents over 50 years of age, *Polski Tygodnik Lekarski,* 48 Suppl 3:13-5.
15. Nydegger, V., Rizzoli, R., Rapin, C.H., Vasey, H., and Bonjour, J.P., 1991. Epidemiology of fractures of the proximal femur in Geneva: Incidence, clinical and social aspects, *Osteoporosis Int.,* 2(1):42-7.
16. Shaw, C.K., 1993. An epidemiologic study of osteoporosis in Taiwan, *Ann. Epidemiol.* 3(3):264-71.
17. Stini, W.A., 1990. "Osteoporosis": etiologies, prevention, and treatment, *Yearb. Phys. Anthrop.,* 33:151-94.
18. Stini, W.A., 1994. Comparison of Chinese and Arizona bone densities, *Collegium Antropologicum,* 18:155-63.
19. Stini, W.A., Chen, Z., and Stein, P., 1994. Aging, bone loss, and body mass index in Arizona retirees, *Am. J. Hum. Biol.,* 6:43-50.
20. Melton, L.J. 3rd and Riggs, R.L., 1987. Epidemiology of age-related fractures. In: LV Avioli, Ed. *The Osteoporotic Syndrome.* (2nd ed.) New York: Grune and Stratton. pp 1-30.
21. Melton, L.J. 3rd, Chrischilles, E.A., Cooper, C., Lane, A.W., and Riggs, B.L., 1992. Perspective. How many women have osteoporosis? *J. Bone Min. Res.,* 7(9):1005-10.
22. Lindsay R. 1994. Bone mass measurement for postmenopausal women. *Osteoporosis Int.* 4 Suppl 1: 39-41.
23. Kanis, J.A. and Adami, S.. 1994. Bone loss in the elderly, *Osteoporosis Int.,* 4 Suppl 1:59-65.
24. Jacobsen, S.J., Cooper, C., Gottlieb, M.S., Goldberg, J., Yahnke, D.P., and Melton, L.J. 3rd., 1992. Hospitalization with vertebral fracture among the aged: A national population-based study, 1986-1989. *Epidemiology* 3(6):515-18.
25. Baran, D.T., 1994. Magnitude and determinants of premenopausal bone loss, *Osteoporosis Int.,* 4: Suppl 1 31-34.
26. Christiansen, C., 1994. Postmenopausal bone loss and the risk of osteoporosis, *Osteoporosis Int.* 4 Suppl. 1:47-51.

27. Cormier, C., 1994. Epidemiology, diagnosis, and treatment of osteoporosis, *Current Opinion in Rheumatology,* 6(3):329-35.

28. Johnston, C.C., Jr. and Slemenda, C.W., 1994. Peak bone mass, bone loss and risk of fracture, *Osteoporosis Int.,* 4 Suppl. 1:43-5.

29. Lappe, J.M., 1994. Bone fragility: assessment of risk and strategies for prevention, *J. Obst. Gynecol. Neonatal Nurs.,* 23(3):260-8.

30. Nakajima, T., 1994. A study of bone mineral density in postmenopausal and senile osteoporosis with vertebral fractures in female, *Nippon Ika Daigaku Zasshi* (Journal of the Nippon Medical School) 61:190-9.

31. Riis, B.J., 1994. Premenopausal bone loss: fact or artifact? *Osteoporosis Int.,* 4 Suppl 1:35-7.

32. Seeman, E., 1994. Reduced bone density in women with fractures: Contribution of low peak bone density and rapid bone loss, *Osteoporosis Int.* 4 Suppl 1:15-25.

33. Stracke, H., Renner, E., Knie, G., Leidig, G, Minne, H., and Federlin, K., 1993. Osteoporosis and bone metabolic parameters in dependence upon calcium intake through milk and milk products, *Europ. J. Clin. Nutr.,* 47(9):617-22

34. Tokita, A., Kelly, P.J., Nguyen, T.V., Qi, J.C., Morrison, N.A., Risteli, J., Sambrook, P.N., and Eisman, J.A., 1994. Genetic influences on type I collagen synthesis and degradation: further evidence for genetic regulation of bone turnover, *J. Clin. Endocrinol. Metab.,* 78:1461-6.

35. Spotila, L.D., Colige, A., Sereda, L., Constantinou-Deltas, C.D., and Whyte, M.P., et al., 1994. Mutation analysis of coding sequences for type I procollagen in individuals with low bone density, *J. Bone. Min. Res.,* 9(6):923-32.

36. Cassella, J.P., Barber, P., Catterall, A.C., and Ali, S.Y., 1994. A morphometric analysis of osteoid collagen fibril diameter in osteogenesis imperfecta, *Bone,* 15:329-34.

37. Krall, E.A. and Dawson-Hughes, B., 1993. Calcium and bone metabolism *J. Bone Min. Res.* 8:1-9.

38. Norman, A.W. and Collins, E.D. 1994. Correlation between vitamin D receptor allele and bone mineral density, *Nutr. Rev.,* 52(4):147-9.

39. Eisman, J.A., Kelly, P.J., Morrison, N.A., Pocock, N.A., Yoeman, R., Birmingham, J., and Sambrook, P.N., 1993. Peak bone mass and osteoporosis prevention, *Osteoporosis Int.* 3 Suppl. 1: 56-60.

40. Morrison, N.A., Yoeman, R., Kelly, P.J., and Eisman, J.A., 1992. Contribution of trans-acting factor alleles to normal physiological variability: vitamin D receptor gene polymorphism and circulating osteocalcin, *Proc. Nat. Acad. Am.,* 89:6665-9.

41. Mundy, G.R., 1994. Boning up on genes, *Nature,* 367:216-217.

42. Jacques, P.F., Felson, D.T., Tucker, K.L., Mahnken, B., Wilson, P.W.F., Rosenberg, I.H., and Rush D. 1997. Plasma 25-hydroxyvitamin D and its determinants in an elderly population sample, *Am. J. Clin. Nutr.,* 66:929-36.

43. Lanyon, L.E., 1981. Locomotor loading and functional adaptation in limb bones, *Symp. Zoolog. Society,* 48:305-29.

44. Lanyon, L.E. and Ruben, C.T., 1985. Functional adaptation in skeletal structures. In: M. Hildebrand, et al. Eds. *Functional Vertebrate Morphology* Cambridge MA: Harvard University Press. pp 1-25.

45. Lazenby, R.A., 1990a. Continuing periosteal apposition 1: Documentation, hypotheses, and interpretation, *Am. J. Phys. Anthrop.,* 82:451-72.

46. Lazenby, R.A., 1990b. Continuing periosteal apposition II: The significance of peak bone mass, strain equilibrium, and age-related activity differentials for mechanical compensation in human tubular bones, *Am. J. Phys. Anthrop.,* 82:473-84.

47. Suleiman, S., Nelson, M., Li, F., Buxton-Thomas, M., and Moniz, C., 1997. Effect of calcium intake and physical activity level on bone mass and turnover in healthy, white, postmenopausal women, *Am. J. Clin. Nutr.,* 66:937-43.

48. Morais, J.A., Gougeon, R., Pencharz, P.B., Jones, P.J.H., Ross, R., and Marliss, E.B., 1997. Whole-body protein turnover in the healthy elderly, *Am. J. Clin. Nutr.,* 66:880-9.

49. Kroger, H., Tuppurainen, M., Honkanen, R., Alhave, E., and Saarikoski, S., 1994. Bone Mineral Density and Risk Factors for Osteoporosis — A population-based study of 1600 perimenopausal women, *Calcif. Tissue Int.,* 55:1-7.

50. Galloway, A., 1988. *Long Term Effects of Reproductive History on Bone Mineral Content in Women.* Doctoral Dissertation, Department of Anthropology, University of Arizona.

51. Maxwell, D.B.S. and Huxley, A.K., 1995. Effects of breastfeeding on osteoporotic fracture. (abstract) *Am. J. Phys. Anthrop.,* Suppl. 22.

52. Sowers, M.F., Corton, G., Shapiro, B., Jannauseh, M.L., Crutchfield, M., Smith, M.L., Randolph, J.F., and Hollis, B., 1993. Changes in bone density with lactation, *JAMA,* 269:3130-35.

53. Speroff, L., Glass, R.H., and Kase, N.G., 1994. *Clinical Gynecologic Endocrinology and Infertility.* 9th Ed. Baltimore, MD, Williams and Wilkins, pp. 251-89.

54. Fallon, M.D. and Schwann, H.A., 1990. Metabolic and other nontumorous disorders of bone. In: J.M. Kissane, Ed., *J.M. Anderson's Pathology*, 9th ed., vol. 2. St. Louis, Mo: C.V. Mosby. pp. 1929-2017.

55. Pacifici, R., 1992. Is there a causal role for IL-1 in postmenopausal bone loss? *Calcif. Tissue Res.,* 50:295-9.

56. Kent, G.N., Price, R.I., Gutteridge, D.H., Smith, M., Allen, J.R., Bhagat, C.I., Barnes, M.P., Hickling, C.J., Retallack, A.W., Wilson, S.G., Devlin, R.D., Davies, C., and St. John, A., 1990. Human lactation: forearm trabecular bone loss, increased bone turnover, and renal conservation of calcium and inorganic phosphate with recovery of bone mass following weaning, *J. Bone Min. Res.,* 5(4):361-9.

57. Allen, L.H., 1982. Calcium bioavailability and absorption: A review, *Am. J. Clin. Nutr.,* 35:783-808.

60. Norman, A.W., Nemere, I., Muralidharan, K.R., and Okamura, W.H., 1992. 1 beta (OH)$_2$-vitamin D$_3$ is an antagonist of 1alpha, 25 (OH)$_2$-vitamin D$_3$ stimulated transcaltachia (the rapid hormonal stimulation of intestinal calcium transport), *Biochem. Biophys. Res. Comm.,* 189(3):1450-6.

61. Norman, A.W., Okamura, W.H., Farach-Carson, M.C., Allewaert, K., and Branisteanu, D., et al..1993a.Structure-function studies of 1,25-dihydroxyvitamin D$_3$ and the vitamin D endocrine system. 1,25-dihydroxy-pentadeuterio-previtamin D$_3$ (as a 6-s-cis analog) stimulates nongenomic but not genomic biological responses, *J. Biol. Chem.,* 286(19):13811-9.

62. Norman, A.W., Sergeev, I.N., Bishop, J.E., Okamura, W.H., 1993b. Selective biological response by target organs (intestine, kidney, and bone) to 1,25-dihydroxyvitamin D$_3$ and two analogues, *Cancer Res.,* 53(17):3935-42.

63. Norman, A.W., Bouillon, R., Farach-Carson, M.C., Bishop, J.E., Zhou, L.X., et al. 1993c. Demonstration that 1 beta, 25-dihydroxyvitamin D$_3$ is an antagonist of the nongenomic but not genomic biological responses and biological profile of the three A-ring diastereomers of 1 alpha, 25-dihydroxyvitamin D$_3$, *J. Biol. Chem.,* 268 (27):20022-30.

64. Norman, A.W. and Collins, E.D., 1994. Correlation between vitamin D receptor allele and bone mineral density, *Nutr. Rev.,* 52(4):147-9.

65. Farach-Carson, M.C., Abe, J., Nishii, Y., Khoury, R., Wright, G.C., and Norman, A.W., 1993. 22-Oxacalcitriol: dissection of 1, 25 (OH)2 D$_3$ receptor-mediated and Ca^{2+} entry-stimulating pathways, *Am. J. Physiol.,* 265 (5 pt 2):F705-11.

66. Dormanen, M.C., Bishop, J.E., Hammond, M.W., Okamura, W.H., Nemere, I., and Norman, A.W., 1994. Nonnuclear effects of the steroid hormone 1 alpha, 25 (OH)2- vitamin D$_3$: Analogs are able to functionally differentiate between nuclear and membrane receptors, *Biochem. Biophys. Res. Comm.,* 201(1):394-401.

9 Gender Differences in Nutritional Lifestyles in the Aged

Katsumi Kano and Satoshi Toyokawa

CONTENTS

I. INTRODUCTION

Life expectancy at birth is an important health index indicating health condition in a community. At present, the Japanese life expectancy is the longest in the world. According to a recent document (1998), life expectancy in Japan is 77.01 years for males and 83.59 years for females with a difference of 6.58 years between the sexes.[1] Almost without exception, life expectancy for females is longer than that for males.

In Japan, there are more than 10,000 persons aged 100 or older, and the females account for about 80%. The reasons are considered to be as follows: (1) a female has two X-chromosomes, which make them biologically dominant, (2) females have more opportunities to receive health examinations at young ages because of pregnancy and delivery, (3) females have a lifestyle with relatively less involvement in drinking, smoking, driving, and risky sports, (4) females use medical facilities at a higher frequency, (5) physical load due to labor and mental load in females are relatively less. The difference of life expectancy between males and females in developed countries is higher than that in developing countries. One of the main reasons is considered to be because the main causes of death are infectious diseases in developing countries and chronic noninfectious diseases in developed countries, including cancers, ischemic heart disease, cerebrovascular disease, diabetes, cirrhosis of the liver, and so on. Generally, these death rates are higher in males.[2-4] Many epidemiologic studies have clarified that dietary habits are deeply associated with these diseases.[5]

II. GENDER DIFFERENCE OF DIETARY HABITS IN THE AGED

Thus, we investigated dietary habits in subjects who were selected randomly from an area representative of disease patterns in our country and a high proportion of the aged. Gender differences were also investigated.[6] Besides items related to dietary habits, other items such as smoking and exercise were also investigated. Among the investigation items, there were the seven health habits by Breslow[7] and the 12-point precautions for cancer prevention proposed by National Cancer Center (Japan).[8] Table 9.1 shows the results of the items related to dietary habits in subjects aged 60 or older. The frequency of the item "One or more fruits are eaten daily" was significantly higher in

TABLE 9.1
The Gender Difference of Dietary Habits in the Aged

	Items	Sex	Age[a] 60–69 yrs [% (n)]	70 + yrs [% (n)]
1.	The meal times are always constant.	M	84.3 (43)	89.5 (34)
		F	80.3 (53)	59.6 (28)
2.	Breakfast is sometimes omitted.	M	11.8 (6)	5.3 (2)
		F	9.1 (6)	8.5 (4)
3.	Meals other than breakfast are sometimes omitted.	M	9.8 (5)	2.6 (1)
		F	10.8 (7)	10.6 (5)
4.	The meal is eaten slowly and enjoyably.	M	66.0 (34)	63.2 (24)
		F	69.7 (46)	80.9 (38)
5.	I eat moderately, not excessively.	M	78.4 (40)	86.8 (33)
		F	86.2 (57)	80.8 (38)
6.	I eat any foods, without likes or dislikes.	M	88.2 (45)	86.8 (33)
		F	80.3 (53)	80.9 (38)
7.	Main foods such as rice or bread are always taken at each meal.	M	84.3 (43)	89.5 (34)
		F	86.4 (57)	91.5 (43)
8.	Animal protein foods such as meat, fish, or egg are taken at each meal.	M	82.4 (42)	78.9 (30)
		F	68.2 (45)	76.6 (36)
9.	One or two vegetable foods are taken at each meal.	M	96.1 (49)	94.7 (36)
		F	90.9 (60)	91.5 (43)
10.	Green and yellow vegetables are taken daily.	M	68.6 (35)	71.1 (27)
		F	65.2 (43)	78.7 (37)
11.	Oily foods such as the fat part of meat are avoided.	M	66.7 (34)	65.8 (25)
		F	69.7 (46)	72.3 (34)
12.	One bottle of milk or yogurt is taken daily.	M	50.0 (26)	47.4 (18)
		F	59.1 (39)	59.6 (28)
13.	One or more fruits are taken daily.	M	56.9 (29)	57.9 (22)
		F	78.8 (52)	85.1 (40)
14.	Seaweed such as laver, tangle, or wakame seaweed are taken twice or three times a week.	M	90.2 (46)	86.8 (33)
		F	97.0 (64)	95.7 (45)
15.	Plant protein foods such as soybeans and tofu are taken daily.	M	70.0 (36)	71.1 (27)
		F	77.3 (51)	70.2 (33)
16.	Vegetable oil is used mainly as a seasoning.	M	88.2 (45)	94.7 (36)
		F	81.8 (54)	89.4 (42)
17.	The amount of oil, sugar, or salt used as seasonings is one or two spoons daily.	M	52.0 (27)	50.5 (23)
		F	59.1 (39)	57.4 (27)
18.	Seasoning is light.	M	58.8 (30)	63.2 (24)
		F	65.2 (43)	74.5 (35)
19.	I remember to eat foods containing calcium.	M	76.0 (39)	68.4 (26)
		F	72.7 (48)	59.6 (28)
20.	I remember to eat foods containing rich fibers.	M	78.4 (40)	73.7 (28)
		F	75.8 (50)	72.3 (34)
21.	I do not eat scorched food, if possible.	M	62.8 (32)	68.4 (26)
		F	72.7 (48)	72.3 (34)
22.	I do not eat musty foods.	M	72.6 (37)	81.6 (31)
		F	84.9 (56)	80.9 (38)

TABLE 9.1 (CONTINUED)
The Gender Difference of Dietary Habits in the Aged

			Age[a]	
			60–69 yrs	70 + yrs
	Items	Sex	[% (*n*)]	[% (*n*)]
23.	Hot foods are eaten after being cooled.	M	68.0 (35)	71.1 (27)
		F	63.6 (42)	72.3 (34)
24.	I do not eat sweet foods daily.	M	31.4 (16)	36.8 (14)
		F	45.4 (30)	63.8 (30)
25.	I drink alcohol moderately daily.	M	39.2 (20)	39.5 (15)
		F	4.6 (3)	2.1 (1)
26.	I drink a large amount of alcohol daily.	M	19.6 (10)	7.9 (3)
		F	1.5 (1)	0.0 (0)

[a] M = male, F = female.

females. Fruits can prevent gastric cancer[9] and contain a high level of flavonoids that contributing to lowering the death rate from ischemic heart disease.[10] Seaweed is related to intake of dietary fibers and can contribute to the prevention of both colon and rectal cancer.[11] Since our country is an island, we eat seaweed such as lavers, tangles, and wakame seaweed frequently. There was no gender difference in eating seaweed. Generally, Japanese take a large amount of salt, 13 g or more per day on average, which is pointed out to be associated with a high incidence of cerebrovascular disease in Japanese.[12] There were no gender differences in the intake of salt. As for the items proposed by National Cancer Center (Japan), "I do not eat scorched food if possible" and "I do not eat musty foods," their gender difference has not been reported. We also obtained similar results in this study. As for the item, "Oily foods such as the fat part of meat are avoided," such avoidance is effective to prevent ischemic heart disease and cerebrovascular disease[13] and its gender difference was not seen. As expected, the frequency for the item "I drink alcohol moderately daily" was higher in males than in females. Marmot et al. stated that the death rate of males drinking at an intermediate level is low.[14] Doll et al. also reported that alcohol intake reduces ischemic heart disease.[15] Apparently, an unhealthy habit in males is excessive drinking in addition to smoking. The frequency for the item "I drink a large amount of alcohol daily" was significantly higher in males than females. Excessive drinking is a factor to induce liver cancer, and the incidence of liver cancer that appears to be induced by drinking is high.[16] Excessive drinking is a factor in hypertension and it is reported that cerebrovascular disease in Japanese males is caused mainly by a large amount of drinking.[17,18] Belloc et al. stated that chronic diseases are associated with heavy drinking.[13] The habit of drinking large amounts in males is said to influence their health adversely. Berkman and Breslow compared two groups, namely a group that maintained the seven health habits including control of smoking and drinking, management of sleeping time, exercise amount, and body weight, and intake of breakfast and snacks, and another group that did not maintain such habits.[7] They proved that there was a large difference in the death rate. When this was seen in life expectancy, it became clear that the males aged 45 who had only three or less favorable lifestyle habits had 11 years shorter life expectancy than the males of the same age having six or more good health habits. The group having unhealthy lifestyle is apparently inferior in terms of health degree and their death rate is influenced very adversely. In this study, we investigated the gender difference in the items related to dietary habits of the items based on the seven health habits by Breslow. As for control of body weight, obesity is an etiology for many diseases,[19] and it is thus important to maintain an appropriate body weight for preventing chronic noninfectious diseases related to lifestyles. A cause of obesity is excessive eating.[20] There were no gender differences in terms of the items, "I eat moderately, not excessively" and "I do not eat sweet foods daily."

In the 12-point precautions for cancer prevention, there are many items related to dietary habits. As for the gender difference of the incidence of cancer, the incidence in males is higher than that in females. The clear gender difference of the incidence was assumed to be due to the difference of lifestyles. The females had better lifestyles than males. Differences are mainly related to smoking and drinking and the adverse effect of smoking is pointed out in many studies.[21,22]

In females, since bone density reduces and fractures occur easily after menopause, to prevent the loss of bone density, it is necessary to take sufficient calcium.[23] Although females were expected to have higher concern about intake of calcium than males, no difference was found.

The results from this investigation were similar to those from the nationwide nutrition survey in Japan.[24] There was no clear gender difference in terms of dietary habits, except for drinking. The reason is assumed to be because both elderly males and females are likely to eat at home, and the contents of foods are similar and the concern about their health is high in both males and females. On the other hand, as for drinking, because there is an apparent gender difference, starting at young ages, and because drinking tends to be habitual, its difference is considered not to be lessened at older age.

Popkins et al. investigated the changes of food intake over 10 years, using records of meals for 3 days in the aged of 65 or older by Nationwide Food Consumption Survey (NFCS) carried out in 1977 and 1988 in the U.S.[25] According to the survey, the consumption of beef, pork, chicken, fish with low fat, milk, milk products with low fat, and whole grain breads has increased, while the consumption of beef, pork, whole milk, milk products with high fat, refined breads, and eggs have decreased.

However, consumption of desserts containing high fat that supplies energy, butter and margarine as fat sources, and dietary fiber foods such as fruits, vegetables, and grains has changed only slightly over 10 years. It is found that the shift in foods is moderate. No great gender difference was found in the tendency of food intake. However, in 1977, many females had already reduced the intake of whole milk and increased the intake of milk with low fat and no milk. The males tended to follow the same pattern. As for food intake, females tend to precede males in terms of change.

III. GENDER DIFFERENCE OF DIETARY HABITS IN THE AGED OF 100 OR OLDER

Professor Shoji Kondo of Public Health at Tohoku University conducted field surveys at more than 1000 villages in Japan and investigated the conditions of long life.[26] The results are as follows:

1. Villagers with unbalanced diets and a large number of meals suffer from premature senility and have a short life.
2. Fish or soybeans are always eaten in villages where residents have an average lifespan.
3. Vegetables are always eaten in large amounts in villages with average lifespan. Specifically, there are many villagers with long lifespans who eat carrots and pumpkins frequently.
4. The life expectancy is short in villages having residents who do not eat vegetables sufficiently.
5. There are only a few cerebrovascular disease cases and many residents with long lifespans in villages where seaweed is always eaten.

This report was not conducted using an epidemiologic method and is based on subjective impressions by the professor himself. Although it is not scientific, strictly speaking, the report is richly indicative. Subsequently, in a survey for about 1000 elderly persons in Japan, it was clarified that these persons take protein foods at a higher frequency than average and that their preferences for some types of protein foods differ (Table 9.2).[27] In the survey for the aged of 100 or older, as for meats, the answer "dislike" was shown in 13.3% of males and 24.6% of females, and the rate of "like" was the lowest among the foods. That is, the intake of meats is considered less than those of the other foods. The integrated results are identical to those from the survey in the persons with a long life. As for the results to what extent vegetables or seaweed are liked or disliked, the rate of "dislike" in females was very low, 2.8% and 2.4%, respectively, and that in males was slightly higher, 4.4% for vegetables, and 2.2% for seaweed. The rate of "dislike" for seaweed is less among the foods. As such, the aged of 100 or older are fond of vegetables and seaweed. The fact is interesting because it is compatible for the condition of the intake of dietary fibers as well as supply of vitamins and minerals.

TABLE 9.2
The Gender Difference of Food Preference in the Aged of 100 or Older

Kinds of Foods	Sex	Likes [% (n)]	Fair [% (n)]	Dislikes [% (n)]	Unknown [% (n)]
Meats	M	49.2 (82)	37.6 (68)	13.3 (24)	
	F	33.7 (279)	40.9 (339)	24.6 (204)	0.7 (6)
Fish	M	62.4 (113)	32.6 (59)	5.0 (9)	
	F	53.0 (439)	37.3 (309)	8.3 (73)	0.8 (7)
Eggs	M	58.6 (106)	38.1 (69)	3.3 (6)	
	F	52.8 (437)	41.3 (342)	5.2 (43)	0.7 (6)
Soybean products	M	60.2 (109)	38.1 (69)	1.1 (2)	0.6 (1)
	F	53.7 (445)	37.7 (312)	7.9 (65)	0.7 (6)
Vegetables	M	63.5 (115)	32.0 (58)	4.4 (8)	
	F	67.0 (555)	29.5 (244)	2.8 (23)	0.7 (6)
Seaweed	M	55.2 (100)	42.5 (77)	2.2 (4)	
	F	52.5 (435)	44.1 (365)	2.4 (20)	1.0 (8)

Male (M)181, Female (F)828

In our survey of the aged of 100 or older, the gender difference is not great, and we find that they maintain a balanced diet with multiple kinds of foods.[28] Other findings are as follows: (1) salt is taken moderately, (2) they are not overweight, (3) they move their bodies frequently and do not eat meats frequently and do not smoke. They have hobbies that stimulate curiosity, and they are optimistic.

IV.   DIETARY HABITS IN SINGLE MALE ELDERLY PERSONS

In the aged, generally, females live longer than males and there is a high likelihood that the male will live together with his spouse. Even if a female becomes single, she will have fewer problems in dietary life than the male.[29] However, problems may occur when the male becomes single. Charlton investigated three points, the intake of nutrients from meals and dietary life, standard for selecting foods, and necessity of nutrition education activities.[30] The subjects were 66 males aged 70 to 93 (mean age, 78.9), among whom 33 males were the members of a lunch club and the remaining 33 males were elderly persons living in nursing homes.

The results showed that the intakes of nutrients other than dietary fibers were almost appropriate and the intake of energy was lower than the expected daily mean necessary amount in 47% of the subjects. The intake did not reach even two thirds in 9% of the subjects. As for the standard for selecting foods, 39.4% of the subjects, the largest portion, answered "tastiness," followed in order by wide availability, being healthy, easy cooking, and cost. Nutrition information was obtained mainly from mass media, physician, dietitian, and nurse in 77.3% of the subjects, and parents and friends in 56.1% of the subjects (multiple answers in any cases). However, only half of the subjects received benefit from nutritional education. From these results, it was concluded that, generally, aged males living alone were in insufficient nutritional condition, but that they knew the role of meals in their health. Therefore, although further nutritional education is necessary, it is a difficult subject because this age group does not accept it easily.

REFERENCES

1. HWSA, *Health and Welfare Statistics in Japan 1999*, Health and Welfare Statistics Association, 1999.
2. Kano, K. and Yamaguchi, S., A study on gender differences in death rates by causes, *Medicine and Biology*, 102, 151, 1981.
3. Kano, K. and Yamaguchi, S., Studies on sex differences in mortality rates from major causes in urban and rural areas, *Human Ecology and Race Hygiene*, 46, 149, 1980.
4. Lopez, A.D., Sex differentials in mortality, *WHO Chron.*, 38, 217, 1984.
5. Miller, D.L. and Farmer, R.D.T., *Epidemiology of Diseases*, Blackwell Scientific Publications, 1982.
6. Saito, T., Sakuragi, C., Ueji, M., Takahashi, H., and Kano, K., Gender differences in lifestyles of the middle-aged and the elderly — a study in Satomi village, Ibaraki, Japan, *Jpn. J. Public Health*, 44, 803, 1997.
7. Berkman, L. F. and Breslow, L., *Health and Way of Living: The Alameda County Study*, Oxford University Press, New York, 1983.
8. National Cancer Center (Japan), *12-Point Precautions for Cancer Prevention*, Foundation for Promotion of Cancer Research,1998.
9. Burr, M.L. and Holliday, R.M., Fruit and stomach cancer, *J. Hum. Nutr. Diet.*, 2, 273, 1989.
10. Hertog, M.G., Kromhout, D., Aravanis, C., Blackburn, H., Buzina, R., Fidanza, F., Giampaoli, S., Jansen, A., Menotti, A., and Nedeljkovic, S., et al., Flavonoid intake and long-term risk of coronary heart disease and cancer in the seven countries study, *Arch. Int. Med.*, 155, 381, 1995.
11. Hoshiya Y., Sekine T., and Sasaba T., A case-control study of colorectal cancer and its relation to diet, cigarettes, and alcohol consumption in Saitama Prefecture, Japan, *Tohoku J. Exp. Med.*, 171, 153, 1993.
12. Ueshima, H., Tanigaki, M., Iida, M., Shimamoto, M., Konishi, M., and Komachi, Hypertension, salt, and potassium, *Lancet*, 8218, 504, 1981.
13. Belloc, N. B. and Breslow, L., Relationship of physical health status and health practices, *Prev. Med.*, 1, 409, 1972.
14. Marmot, M.G., Rose, G., and Shipley, M.J., Alcohol and mortality, a U-shaped curve, *Lancet,* 8220, 580, 1981.
15. Doll, R., Peto, R., Hall, E., Wheatley, K., and Gray, R., Mortality in relation to consumption of alcohol, 13 years' observation on male British doctors, *Br. Med. J.*, 309, 911, 1994.
16. Rogers, A.E. and Cornner, N.W., Alcohol and cancer, *Adv. Exp. Med. Biol.*, 473, 1986.
17. Ueshima, H., Ohsaka, T., and Asakura, S., Regional differences in stroke mortality and alcohol consumption in Japan, *Stroke*, 17, 19-24, 1986.
18. Kiyohara, Y., Kato, I., Iwamoto, H., Nakayama, K., and Fujishima, M., The impact of alcohol and hypertension on stroke incidence in a general Japanese population. The Hisayama Study, *Stroke*, 26, 368, 1995.
19. Lee, I., Manson, J. E., Hennekens, C.H., and Paffenbarger, R. S., Body weight and mortality — a 27-year follow-up of middle-aged men, *JAMA*, 270, 2823, 1993.
20. Garrow, J.S., Is obesity an eating disorder? *J. Psychosom. Res.*, 32, 585, 1988.
21. Fletcher, C.M. and Horn, D., Smoking and health, *WHO Chron.*, 24, 345, 1970.
22. U.S. Department of Health Education and Welfare, *Smoking and Health, a Report of the Surgeon General*, 1979.

23. Holbrook, T.L., Barrett-Connor, E., and Wingard, D.L., Dietary calcium and risk of hip fracture:14-year prospective population study, *Lancet*, 8619, 1046, 1988.

24. The Current Situation of National Nutrition (Japan), 1998. Daiichi-Shutsuppan, 1998.

25. Popkin, B.M., Haines, P.S., and Patterson, R.E., Dietary changes in older Americans, 1977–1987, *Am. J. Clin. Nutr.*, 55, 823, 1992.

26. Kondo, S., *Villages with the Long Life or with the Short Life in Japan*, Sun Road Publication, 1972.

27. Tomabechi, K., A survey of dietary life in the aged of 100 or older, *Databook of Food, Nutrition & Health*, 1982, 99, Ishiyaku Publisher, 1983.

28. Watanabe, T., Matsuo, J., and Kano, K., An epidemiologic study on health life of individual lifestyles in the aged of 100 or older, *Jpn. J. Public Health*, 30, 35, 1983.

29. Davis, M.A., Randall, E., Forthofer, R.N., Lee, E.S., and Margen, S., Living arrangements and dietary patterns of older adults in the United States, *J. Gerontol.*, 40, 434, 1985.

30. Charlton, K.E., The nutrient intake of elderly men living alone and their attitude toward nutrition education, *J. Hum. Nutr. Diet.*, 10, 343, 1997.

10 Undernutrition: A Factor of Accelerated Immune Aging in Healthy and Diseased Aged Persons

Bruno M. Lesourd

CONTENTS

Immune aging has been extensively studied in past years. It is well known that aging has stronger influences on cell-mediated immunity than on humoral immunity (1,2) and fewer effects on non-specific (i.e., macrophage functions) immunity (3). The immune system is a body-wide system under permanent renewal and producing millions of immune cells daily. Immune cell renewal is further increased in infectious disease, from which recovery depends on the respective rate of cell divisions between the invading microorganism and the immune (lymphocytes) cells. Therefore, the immune system is a major user of nutrients, in particular macronutrients and also micronutrients involved in DNA, RNA, and protein synthesis; the nutrient need is highly increased during illness. It is well known that undernutrition has a strong influence on the immune system at all ages, but mainly in growing and aged human beings (1,3-4). Undernutrition is a common symptom in diseased elderly: the prevalence of protein-energy malnutrition (PEM), which is linked to immunodeficiency (1), varies between from 30 to 60% in the hospitalized elderly and from 1 to 5% in the home-living elderly (5–7). In addition, micronutrient deficiencies are also quite common in home-living, self-sufficient elderly: 5 to 10% for folic acid, 15 to 40% for zinc, 6 to 16% for vitamin B_6, all micronutrients for which deficiency is associated with lower immune responses (8–10). This review mainly focuses on the influence of undernutrition in home-living elderly at a stable stage and after disease occurrence, focusing mainly on such influence on cell-mediated immunity (CMI), for which age-related changes are far more important. In addition, the influence of undernutrition in diseased patients will be briefly described.

I.   IMMUNE AGING

Age is associated with changes in T (11,12) and B-cell (13) subsets, and those changes are the main explanation of changes in CMI functions.

A.   Changes in T Lymphocyte Subsets

There is an age-related decrease in new T lymphocyte generation, which depends on the thymus involution that starts after puberty and is almost complete by age 60. Therefore, lymphocyte numbers decrease in peripheral blood with age (12,14). Nevertheless, this change is nonsignificant in very healthy young olds (65–80 years), selected by specific criteria for healthiness (Table 10.1) (15,16) and similar very healthy nonagenarians (Table 10.2 and 10.3) while it is significant in young unhealthy elderly (12, 14; Table 10.1). This shows the influence of the clinical (and nutritional) status on immune responses of the elderly. The age-related thymic function decrease leads, in peripheral blood, to decreased numbers of mature T cells (CD3+ lymphocytes), which are replaced by less mature T lymphocytes (CD2+CD3–) and/or (NK) (CD57+) cells with lower proliferative capacity (11,12,14,17; Table 10.2). When the decrease of CD3+ lymphocyte is important, there is also an increase in CD2+CD4–CD8– T cells (12) which reflects that the produced T cells are very immature. It as been postulated (12) that such very immature T cells are produced not in the thymus but in another primary immune organ, perhaps in the liver as shown in aged mice (18).

TABLE 10.1
Absolute Counts of T Cell Subsets in Peripheral Blood of Very Healthy and in Frail Healthy Elderly Subjects

	Young Adults (25–34 Years of Age) (n = 50)		Young Elderly (65–85 Years of Age) (n = 30)		Old Elderly (>90 Years of Age) (n = 16)		Frail Young Elderly (70–85 Years of Age) (n = 46)	
	Mean	SD	Mean	SD	Mean	SD	Mean	SD
Age (years)	28.8	3.4	79.4	5.4	94.5	3.4	78.8	6.4
Albumin (g/l)	43.3	2.9	42.1	4.0	41.4	3.5	37.3	3.8
Lymphocytes (/mm³)	2230	460	1970	580	1830*	650	1720**	450
CD2+ (/mm³)	2005	320	1800**	410	1600**	470	1505***‡	420
CD3+ (/mm³)	1880	270	1580**	330	1340**‡	370	1230***‡	290
CD2+CD3– (/mm³)	130	120	215*	230	250*	230	280**	240
CD2+CD4–CD8– (/mm³)								
CD57+ (/mm³)	200	130	450***	180	430**	205	470**‡	210
CD4+ (/mm³)	1250	215	1130*	250	990*	260	820***‡‡	270
CD8+ (/mm³)	670	145	440***	180	390***	210	380***	190
CD45 RA (/mm³)	1180	310	630***	210	420***‡‡	200	450***‡	220
CD45 R) (/mm³)	840	205	1180***	390	1160***	470	1070*	490

Note: Healthy young adults and elderly of different ages and health status were selected according to the SENIEUR protocol (86) and added criteria (14,15). CD45 RA, memory T lymphocytes; CD45 RO, naive T lymphocytes. Mean values were significantly different from those for the young adults; *$p < 0.05$, **$p < 0.01$, ***$p < 0.001$. Mean values were significantly different from those for the young elderly: ‡$p < 0.05$, ‡‡$p < 0.05$.

TABLE 10.2

Functions from Peripheral Phytohemaglutinin-Stimulated T Lymphocytes of Very Healthy and Frail Elderly Subjects

	Young Adults (25–34 Years of Age) ($n = 42$)	Young Elderly (65–85 Years of Age) ($n = 37$)	Old Elderly (>90 Years of Age) ($n = 16$)	Frail Young Elderly (70–85 Years of Age) ($n = 42$)
Age in years	28.7 ± 3.9	79.3 ± 4.9***	93.9 ± 3.3***	78.4 ± 6.3***
Albumin (g/l)	43.4 ± 2.9	42.2 ± 3.9	41.2 ± 3.8	37.1 ± 3.3**‡
C-reactive protein (mg/l)	<6	<6	<6	12.7 ± 11.4**‡
Lymphocyte Proliferation				
PHAp: 1 µg/10^6 cells				
³H thymidine (10³ cells)	145 ± 41	109 ± 28	78 ± 31**	53 ± 35***‡‡
% CD25+ cells at 72 hours	64.4 ± 6.9	58.6 ± 7.3	43.6 ± 8.7**‡	31.8 ± 10.2***‡‡
***In Vitro* Cytokine Release After 22–24-Hour Cultures**				
IL2 (ng/ml)	2.12 ± 0.33	1.69 ± 0.35	1.18 ± 0.46***‡	1.13 ± 0.39***‡
IL6 (ng/ml)	1.35 ± 0.15	1.78 ± 0.23*	1.98 ± 0.33***	1.48 ± 0.41

Note: Healthy young adults and elderly of different ages and health status were selected according to the SENIEUR protocol (86) and added criteria (14,15). Mean values were significantly different from those for the young adults; *$p < 0.05$, **$p < 0.01$, ***$p < 0.001$. Mean values were significantly different from those for the young elderly: ‡$p < 0.05$, ‡‡$p < 0.05$.

TABLE 10.3

Functions from Peripheral Lipopolysaccharide-Stimulated Monocytes of Very Healthy and Frail Elderly Subjects

	Young Adults (25–34 Years of Age) ($n = 39$)	Young Elderly (65–85 Years of Age) ($n = 33$)	Old Elderly (>90 Years of Age) ($n = 16$)	Frail Young Elderly (70–85 Years of Age) ($n = 29$)
Age in years	28.8 ± 3.9	79.2 ± 4.7***	93.9 ± 3.3***	81.3 ± 6.7***
Albumin (g/l)	43.4 ± 2.8	42.3 ± 3.8	41.2 ± 3.8	37.3 ± 3.6**‡
C-reactive protein (mg/l)	<6	<6	<6	11.4 ± 10.8**‡
Interleukin 1 (ng/ml)				
³Spontaneous Release	N.D.	0.2 ± 1.2	0.2 ± 1.2	0.9 ± 1.7*‡
LPS stimulated cultures (3 µg/10^6 cells)	2.8 ± 2.0	2.6 ± 2.3	2.5 ± 2.4	1.8 ± 1.3**‡
Interleukin 6 (ng/ml)				
³Spontaneous Release	N.D.	N.D.	N.D.	0.17 ± 0.13***‡
LPS stimulated cultures (3 µg/10^6 cells)	1.24 ± 0.32	1.48 ± 0.25	1.58 ± 0.37*	1.12 ± 0.28‡

Note: Healthy young adults and elderly of different ages and health status were selected according to the SENIEUR protocol (86) and added criteria (14,15). Mean values were significantly different from those for the young adults; *$p < 0.05$, **$p < 0.01$, ***$p < 0.001$. Mean values were significantly different from those for the young elderly: ‡$p < 0.05$, ‡‡$p < 0.05$.

Age is also associated with changes in the naive/memory T cell ratio (CD45RA/CD45R0), which reflects the antigenic exposure throughout life and the aging phenomenon on T cell maturation (19). In fact, the most important changes occur early in life, until age 30, during development of immune response to unknown antigens, changes that continue later on during the entire life but at lower speed (20). The occurrence of age-related naive/memory T cell disequilibrium is of great importance for immune reactivity, since memory T cells are poor secretors of IL-2 and poor proliferative T cells (21,22).

Is was also described that age leads to TH1/TH2 disequilibrium (14,23,24). In fact, aging is associated with decreased TH1 activities: decreased IL-2 (1,25,26) and IFN-γ (27) production, even if controversial results have been published for the latest (28). In addition, aging is associated with increased production of IL-4 (29), which reflects the increase in TH2 activity. TH1/TH2 dysequilibrium may be responsible for the often age-related decreased in CD8+ cytotoxic T cell subset (12,14,17) even if contradictory results have been published (16). The decrease in CD8+ cytotoxic T cell subset may be restored by exogenous IL-12, a TH1 cytokine (30). In contrast, the CD4+ subset seems to be more preserved in healthy elderly (12,14,17).

These changes in T cell subsets remain minor (<20%) in carefully selected healthy elderly (14,16,19; Table 10.2). In contrast, they are major in less carefully selected elderly. This shows the influence of the clinical and/or nutritional status on such modifications (12,14-16; Table 10.1).

B. Changes in T Lymphocyte Functions

Aging is associated with impairment of T cell functions, the most important being the decline in T cell proliferation (1,25,26,31). This is dependent to a great extent on the age-related changes in T cell subsets (11,12). Indeed, CD2+CD3– immature and CD45R0 memory T cells have lower capacity to replicate (11,22). In addition, memory T cells are poor IL-2 producers (21,22), both factors that may explain poor proliferative responses. In addition, decreased lymphocyte reactivity was also associated with increased membrane viscosity in lymphocytes from healthy elderly (32), showing that decreased lymphocyte reactivity is also due to other factors such as the membrane lipid composition, which partly reflects the lipid diet composition.

The age-related decrease in lymphocyte proliferation is probably less important than generally reported when the healthiness of the studied elderly is carefully analyzed. We have recently shown (15,18; Table 10.2) that such decrease is nonsignificant in the young olds at age 70 to 85 (18; Table 10.2) when the elderly are carefully selected for being fully healthy (15,16), using specific healthiness criteria (12,15), and is significant only in the old olds (>80 years). Furthermore, it was also reported that "healthy" nonagenarians have responses comparable to young adults (33), and this was related to natural selection of higher responders in this age population. Therefore, the decrease of lymphocyte reactivity with age is dependent on both extrinsic features, i.e. antigenic pressure throughout life and nutritional status, and intrinsic factors such as the genetic background.

Similar findings have been observed for the age-related decline in IL-2 (15,16), a TH1 function. Kubo and Cinader reported in 1990 that the age-related decline in IL-2 is not observed in all mice strains (34), and this was confirmed a few years later (35). The *in vivo* IL-2 secretion capacities have been reported to be comparable in healthy young adults and young olds (60–70 years) (36). We have reported similar findings for the *in vitro* Il-2 production from mononuclear cell cultures in young elderly (75–84 years) in carefully selected individuals (15,16). We observed a decrease in *in vitro* IL-2 productions only in the old olds (15).

If this is true, the decline in TH1 function is no longer obvious in the young elderly. Indeed, TH1 functions are quantified using IL-2, IFN-γ, or IL-12 productions. Contradictory results have been reported for IFN-γ, which was reported to decrease or to remain level in the elderly (27,28). In addition, IL-12 does not change with age (37). Therefore, it appears that TH1 function does not decline with age in young olds as long as they remain very healthy and declines only in the old olds.

C. Macrophage Functions

Macrophage functions are preserved during aging. Antigen processing does not change with age in mice (38,39). IL-1 is sustained in old mice (40) and in old olds (15,16; Table 10.3). IL-6 is even increased in the young olds (15, Table 10.3). Therefore, no major changes occur in macrophages during aging as long as the subject remains in very good health. In addition, peritoneal macrophages increased in mice in the last third of the life span (41), perhaps in relation to increased secretion with age of cytokines that act on monocyte-macrophage maturation (28,42) such as macrophage colony stimulating factor M-CSF (43).

On overall aging per se, there is little influence on CMI aging in young olds, as long as the subject remains in very good health. The age-related changes consist mainly in the occurrence of T cell subset disequilibrium, which leads to borderline changes in T cell functions in the young olds but becomes significant in the old olds.

D. Immune Responses in Frail Elderly

Frail elderly is the fastest growing elderly population. While aging, the very healthy elderly (Table 10.1) progressively lose some activities, and this leads to progressive decline either in physical or intellectual activities as well as to lower social connections. In some of them, frailty is only translated into decrease in food intake, which may be quantified by a slow decrease in nutritional status as observed in the Euronut/Seneca study (44). We have investigated immune responses in such "healthy frail elderly" selected with the same criteria of healthiness (15,16) but who have lower nutritional status (30 g/l < serum albumin < 39 g/l; 15,16). In such elderly all the age-related changes in T cell subsets are major (15,16) and the T cell functions, i.e., lymphocyte proliferation and IL-2 production, are always significantly decreased (Tables 10.2). In addition, even in the very healthy elderly, changes in nutritional status induce higher changes in T cell subsets and lower immune functions. We have shown that in comparing very healthy elderly with normal or low folate levels (seric folates more or less than 5 µg/l and hematic folates more or less than 400 µg/L) (12,14,17). Therefore, it appears obvious that undernutrition, even with no clinical consequences, may be responsible for lower immune responses even in apparently healthy elderly. Part of what has been described as immune aging may be related to undetected decreases in nutritional status, and this may explain why, in contrast to others who never checked their studied populations for nutritional status, we do not observe decreased immune functions in very healthy elderly. It is also possible that the normal immune functions we observed in the very healthy elderly we recruited may be due to selection bias. In fact, it was shown that age-related IL-2 decrease with age is not observed in all mouse strains (34), and this was related to differences in the major histocompatibility complex. In addition, it was shown that proliferative responses are not decreased in nonagenarians when compared with young adults and have responses higher than those of 70- to 80-year-old persons (33). In the studied nonagenarians, there was a higher proportion of high responders and a different major histocompatibility complex profile (33). Therefore, it seems obvious that the very healthy population selected on healthiness criteria may also be genetically selected for being immune high responders. If this is the case, aging influences in high immune responders could be detectable only at very old age, i.e., after 90 or 100 years. Those individuals who are high immune responders remain healthy for a longer period and may be a special group naturally selected for successful aging. Only long-term longitudinal study comparing the health evolution of individuals with different levels of immune responses and different genetic backgrounds will enable complete proof of such a hypothesis. Nevertheless, even in such a very healthy elderly group, lower nutritional status induces lower CMI and pushes them to accelerated aging, in increasing the age-related disequilibrium between macrophage and T cell functions.

In fact, with aging, the appearance of macrophage–T cell disequilibrium is of great importance. Indeed, any time one faces a disease, the macrophages release cytokines to activate the body defenses. Those cytokines have many nutritional activities, including body reserve liberation (proteolysis, osteolysis, etc.) and changes in metabolic functions (changes in protein synthesis within the liver, decrease in insulin, etc.), all modifications that characterize the classical hypercatabolic syndrome (45,46). At disease occurrence, the decreased T cell functions in the frail elderly push the macrophages to higher cytokine releases in order to stimulate depressed lymphocytes at a sufficient level of efficiency (47). It must be added that elevated serum IL-6 levels, a reflection of inflammation, are often observed in the elderly, even in the apparently healthy frail elderly (48). Therefore, any stress condition induces long-term cytokine releases in the elderly; this results in longer liberation of body nutritional reserves and therefore in higher body reserve depletion. As aging is characterized also by metabolic disequilibrium [calcium release from the bone, lower protein synthesis (49) while protein catabolism is preserved (50)], the used body reserves will not be fully reconstituted, and therefore, the aged person recovers from any stress with lower body reserves and in a frailer state (51). Disease after disease, the elderly become more and more frail. Nutritional deficiency or low intakes, in advancing the macrophage–T cell disequilibrium, may push the very healthy elderly to frailty and/or the frail elderly to a more frail state, and therefore, undernutrition is responsible for the occurrence of accelerated aging.

In addition, when undernutrition increases and reaches PEM state, all immune responses are decreased (1,51), including macrophage cytokine synthesis (1,52). The occurrence of any stress, in such PEM elderly, is associated with lower *in vivo* macrophage cytokine secretions (53), therefore with lower nutritional reserve liberation and, in consequence, with lower and inefficient lymphocyte activation. This leads to prolonged disease length, to further decreases in body nutritional reserves, and to a more profound PEM (53). When recovering, under a more profound PEM state, the elderly have far lower defense capacities. It was shown that prolonged secretion of macrophage cytokines is associated with increased mortality in the elderly (54). In PEM elderly, important nutritional support during disease permits a faster recovery (55), and this is associated with a quicker improvement of immune capacities of macrophages to synthesize cytokines (48). Such a finding points out the importance of nutritional supplements on immune responses of PEM elderly patients on recovery speed.

In summary, undernutrition in majoring the macrophage–T cell disequilibrium leads to progressive losses of nutritional body reserves after any stress or disease. This pushes the very healthy elderly to frailty, the frail elderly to a more frail state and then to PEM, the PEM elderly to a more profound PEM state and then to death. Undernutrition, which usually starts when intake declines, is an important factor of accelerated aging through the progressive occurrence of lower immune functions.

II. INFLUENCES OF NUTRITIONAL SUPPLEMENTATION IN THE SELF-SUFFICIENT ELDERLY

Many studies in the past 15 years have investigated the relation between nutrition and immunology in the elderly in placebo double-blind well-controlled intervention studies. Most of them were done in home-living, self-sufficient, apparently healthy elderly (56–60), but generally the health selection criteria are quite poor. In particular, the micronutrient status was generally measured only for the micronutrients included in the studied supplements. In addition, protein status, namely albumin and acute phase proteins, was not quantified in spite of the important influences of protein-energy malnutrition (PEM) and of acute phase responses on the immune responses, especially in aged persons (47). Therefore, those studies really concerned micronutrient interventions in frail elderly rather than in very healthy elderly and will be analyzed as so. Fewer intervention studies were done in institutionalized aged persons (62–66) and concerned diseased elderly in which immune responses are even lower (53). We will focus on those double-blind well-controlled studies, since they all show that such nutritional interventions may improve immune responses in the frail (and/or diseased) elderly. Therefore, they brought additional information on some mechanisms that are responsible for decreased immune responses in the aged, and further insight into the mechanisms that push the elderly into frailty.

A. Single Nutrient Supplementations

Some studies gave a single micronutrient as a supplement, using either zinc (60,62), vitamin B_6 (57,59) or vitamin E (58), the latest being given at very high doses (5 to 20 times the RDAs). Some others used few micronutrients as a supplement (61,63–66), generally a combination of antioxidants: vitamins (61,63–66), trace elements (63–66), or combinations of both micronutrient types (63–66). All of those studies have investigated the action of such supplements on the immune system of the frail elderly in analyzing different mechanisms that may depress immune responses of the aged persons.

Zinc and vitamin B_6 are important cofactors of several enzymes involved in cell division (67). Both zinc and vitamin B_6 deficits have been described to be associated with immunodeficiencies (68,69). Both deficits are quite common in aged persons, being always present in at least 5 to 10% of the home-living elderly, mostly in those with low meat consumption (8). Talbott et al. (57) reported a supplementation study using physiologic (RDAs) doses of vitamin B_6 and showed improvement of *in vitro* T cell proliferation in aged persons. Such effect was only significant in individuals with low PLP serum levels, showing the importance of vitamin B_6 status on immune responses of aged persons. In fact low PLP level, the best marker of vitamin B_6 low intakes (70) has been observed in 6 to 26% of the autonomous European elderly of the EURONUT/Seneca study (71) and in up to 40% in the U.S. (72). In addition, in a depletion-repletion study, S. Meydani showed that depletion of vitamin B_6 intakes induces cell-mediated immunodeficiency in elderly and that rapid recovery of this immunodeficiency may be obtained by vitamin B_6 supplementation using high doses (several times the RDAs) of vitamin B_6 (59). Therefore, it seems obvious that some of the immunodeficiencies observed in home-living self-sufficient elderly may be due to vitamin B_6 deficits. Zinc deficit has been long known to lead to cell-mediated immunodeficiency in children, the same being true in aged persons (60). Recently, several studies investigated the efficacy of zinc supplements on cell-mediated immunity in the elderly. Zinc supplementation increases immune responses in self-sufficient home-living (60) as well as in institutionalized (62) elderly. This effect was obtained using only zinc in the supplement. In contrast, when zinc was associated with other micronutrients in the supplement, an opposite effect was observed (73,63). Bogden showed that adding zinc at physiologic (15 mg/d) or therapeutic (100 mg/d) doses to a multimineral/vitamin supplement leads to lower effect on delayed type hypersensitivity responses in home-living elderly (73). This depressive effect due to additive zinc was observed as long as (1 year) the supplement was given. After stopping supplementation, the enhancing effect on immune responses remains, at least for few a months, and the suppressive effect of zinc disappears, so that the group who received 15 mg/d of zinc reached comparable immune responses that the group without zinc 4 months after the supplement was stopped (73). In contrast, elderly who received 100 mg/d of zinc had still lower immune responses at that time, showing that the immunosuppressive effect of zinc in aged individuals is dose dependent (73). In the Min.Vit.AOx study, we similarly observed that the enhancing effect linked to antioxidant vitamin supplementation on IL-1 synthesis is abolished in the group who also received trace elements, i.e., zinc and selenium, in the supplement (63,64). Those findings may lead to cautious uses of zinc supplement in the elderly: zinc supplement to restore immune responses may be useful in elderly with zinc deficit, but zinc must be used only as a single supplement in the elderly, only for short periods, and only at physiologic doses. In contrast, vitamin B_6 must be extensively used as a supplement in elderly with vitamin B_6 deficiencies.

Simin Meydani and her group have conducted several studies using a large range (50, 200, and 800 mg dl-α-tocopherol in soybean oil per day, 5 to 20 times the RDAs) of vitamin E supplements in humans for 4 to 5 months (58,74). They confirmed in home-living, self-sufficient "healthy" humans that vitamin E supplements induce *in vivo* (delayed type hypersensitivity) and *in vitro* (lymphocyte proliferation or IL-2 production) increased cell-mediated immune responses, an effect they previously reported in aged healthy rats (75). Furthermore, such effect was associated with simultaneous decreases in lipoperoxydation products (serum MDA) and in monocyte prostaglandin E_2 (PGE_2) production (76,77), both effects being strongly correlated with the immune-enhancing effect (77). Such studies strongly suggest that, even in the "healthy frail" elderly, decreased immune responses may be due to age-related "pathological" mechanisms, i.e., decreases in free radical scavenging.

Indeed, it has been shown that aging per se is associated both with increased free radical production (78) and increased monocyte PGE_2 production (79). Increased free radical production is associated with changes in monocyte functions: i.e., decreased cytokine releases and increased PGE_2 production (79), both phenomena that induce lower lymphocyte functions. In addition, lymphocytes from elderly are particularly sensitive to the immunosuppressive effect of PGE_2 (80). As vitamin E deficiency is uncommon in the aged population — less than 1% in the EURONUT/Seneca study (44,51) — the probability that an immunodeficiency may be due to vitamin E deficit in the aged population is quite low. Therefore, vitamin E supplementation raises immune responses of aged population upon "normal" level. The fact that very high doses of vitamin E reduces both monocyte PGE_2 secretion as well as level of lipoperoxidation products (and then induces higher immune responses) shows that even in the "healthy frail elderly," age-related mechanisms occur in relation to insufficient intakes of antioxidants, even in the absence of vitamin E deficit. In consequence, the need for free radical scavenging agents (antioxidants) is probably higher than previously thought in the elderly. Some nutritional supplements, given at doses that permit a reduction in age-related mechanisms (here a higher free-radical scavenging supplement, i.e., a higher antioxidant micronutrient level) may be a very useful tool to prevent aging and then to keep higher immune responses in the aged population. In other words, the antioxidant needs of the elderly may be far higher than presently recommended by RDAs. If it is so, food could not supply enough antioxidants for aging prevention, and therefore, there is a need in the elderly population for antioxidant-enriched food and/or antioxidant supplements.

B. FEW MICRONUTRIENT SUPPLEMENTATIONS

The antioxidant activity of micronutrient supplementation on immunity has been tested in several double blind studies using combinations of antioxidant micronutrients (61,63–66). Penn showed that an antioxidant vitamin supplement induces higher cell-mediated immunity in the self-sufficient elderly (61). Our group conducted a four-leg supplementation study using either trace elements (Se + Zn), vitamins (E + C + β-carotene), or the combination of both and a placebo as a supplement given in institutionalized elderly for 2 years (63–66). Such a supplement is able to restore selenium and vitamin micronutrient deficits within 6 months (63), but a longer period is needed for zinc deficit (64). Simultaneously, serum MDA, a lipoperoxidation product, decreases and monocyte functions (IL-1 release after *in vitro* LPS stimulation) are improved (63–65), showing the effect of vitamin antioxidant supplementation on immune functions and confirming the result from Meydani's group using vitamin E as an antioxidant supplement (74). In contrast, in the trace-element supplement group, no IL-1 enhancing effect was observed (63), but antibody responses (B lymphocyte functions) after influenza vaccine was higher (81). Furthermore, the IL-1 enhancing effect was also not observed in the vitamin–trace-element supplement group (63,81), showing opposite effect of the two types of supplements. Such opposite effect of different supplementation on different immune responses points out the problem of micronutrient equilibrium in the supplements in regards to the mechanism is that supposed to be improved by the supplement. Indeed, in this study, zinc and perhaps also selenium may have had detrimental effect on monocyte–macrophage functions, but may have improved antibody responses, while antioxidant vitamin supplements improved antioxidant defenses and monocyte functions but had little effect on lymphocyte functions. Later on, it was reported that the groups who received trace-element supplements had fewer respiratory tract infections over the 2-year study than the other groups (66,81). This points out again that both micronutrient supplements, i.e., vitamins and trace-elements, act on different mechanisms and have different, perhaps opposite, activities. This study provides an example of the future studies that must be conducted in this field of nutrition and immunity in the elderly: comparison of different types of supplements, at best different only for one micronutrient, on different activities by investigation of different possible activity mechanisms.

C. MULTI MICRONUTRIENT SUPPLEMENTATIONS

Other studies have investigated the efficacy of more complete multivitamin/multimineral supplements (64–67), using "cocktail" commercial supplements in which most of the major vitamins and trace-elements are present at 0.5 to 3 RDA levels. The rationale for those studies is to investigate the potential benefit of long-term (1 year) use of commercial supplements in frail self-sufficient, home-living elderly without focusing on a precise mechanism. It is intriguing that these studies focus on immune activity, as if immune system declining were considered the major change that pushes elderly to accelerate aging and as if micronutrient deficits were considered to be the major cause of age-related immune declines. Bogden and colleagues conducted an initial study to try to link micronutrient deficits to immunodeficiencies (82) and he was successful. Then he conducted a supplementation study with a multivitamin/multimineral "cocktail supplement," plus or minus zinc, and showed improvement of delayed type hypersensitivity in close connection to improvement in micronutrient status (73). In another study he confirms, a few years later, that increased immune responses are related to increased micronutrient status (83). Chandra and his group observed similar improvement using a different multivitamin/multimineral "cocktail" (56,84). Immune improvement includes increased mature CD3+ lymphocyte numbers in peripheral blood, as well as increased *in vitro* lymphoblastoid proliferation and IL-2 synthesis from mitogen stimulated mononuclear cell cultures (56,84), all parameters that had been reported to decline with aging and to decline even more in aged persons with nutritional deficits. In addition, Chandra found that such a cocktail reduces the length of infectious episodes over the year of supplementation, showing a clinical benefit of the improved immune responses. Nevertheless, no other study has reported such a clinical benefit since then. Furthermore, it was claimed that cocktails containing only vitamins have no activity on infectious episodes when given for shorter periods (85). Such a finding must be linked to our experience in institutionalized elderly (MIN.VIT.AOX. Study, 63–66) in which clinical benefit on infections was observed only in the trace-element supplemented group but not in the vitamin-supplemented group (66,81).

III. CONCLUSION

In the last days of the 20th century, it is obvious that aging induces changes on the immune system: mainly on cell-mediated immunity rather than on humoral or on nonspecific immunity. The main consistent age-related changes are noticed for T cell subset equilibriums, which are modified even at the beginning of old age (60–80 years), while T cell functions remain quite stably modified until very old age (> 90 years) in the healthy human population. Those age-related changes depend on intrinsic body changes, i.e., growth hormone decreases after puberty, and on extrinsic factors of which antigenic pressure throughout the life span and nutritional status are the most important. In the young olds (60–80 years) mild decreases in nutritional status, such as vitamin B_6, zinc, or folate serum low levels are associated with decreased cell-mediated immunity (CMI) responses, so that CMI responses are lower than those of the healthy old olds. CMI decreases are even greater in "healthy" frail elderly with more important decreases in nutritional status: low albumin levels. The fact that higher CMI responses are observed in old old (>90 years) healthy elderly than in young olds with low micronutrient status prompt some researchers to think that nutrition may be an important perhaps the major, factor responsible for decreased CMI responses in the "healthy" elderly. Very few studies have investigated this hypothesis in the past, and this needs strong investigation in the few next years. The fact that the influence of micronutrients on immune responses of healthy elderly is nowadays taken account of in RD definitions in different countries, such as the U.S. or France, will be responsible for developing research in this field in the near future.

In addition, it is important to notice that, in the "healthy" elderly, albumin levels are strongly linked on one hand to decreases in CMI responses (17,87) and on the other hand to life expectancy (88). The influence of undernutrition on the immune system may be one, and perhaps the major, explanation of the influence of undernutrition on life expectancy at old age. Furthermore, there is now true evidence that micronutrient needs are higher than previously thought: indeed, the studies from Meydani's group bring clear data showing that, in spite of no vitamin E deficit, the intake of higher doses of vitamin E induces increases in immune responses and decreases in other age-related factors such as MDA and/or PGE_2 production. The prevention of aging though higher doses of antioxidant (89) and of anti-homocysteine vitamins (90) may be one of the major fields of research in the 21st century. The immune system always takes a central place in the involved mechanisms.

Finally, in compounding the age-related mild immunodeficit and therefore in pushing the elderly into true immunodeficiency, undernutrition pushes the elderly to stress long-lasting acute phase responses and therefore to higher consumption of body nutritional reserves, mainly to higher muscle breakdown. As aged individuals are unable to fully rebuild destroyed body reserves; undernutrition pushes the elderly to a more undernourished state after any stress, and this phenomenon becomes more and more important stress after stress. In consequence, undernutrition, through its action on CMI responses, is a factor that pushes the elderly in a vicious circle from healthiness to frailty, from frailty to a more frail state and, later on, further. Even mild undernutrition from such as micronutrient deficit, is then a factor in accelerated aging, the intensity of this acceleration being related to the intensity of the undernutrition.

In summary, undernutrition, even at a mild stage such as micronutrient deficit and/or insufficient micronutrient intake (and this is probably not truly related to RDA levels), through its major action on immune responses , mainly on CMI responses, is a major factor of aging per se and of disease-related accelerated aging.

REFERENCES

1. Lesourd, B., Le vieillissement immunologique: influence de la dénutrition (immune aging: influence of nutrition), *Annal. Biol. Clin.,* 1990;48:309-318.
2. Miller, R.A., Aging and immune function, *Internat. Rev. Immunol.,* 1992;124:890-904.
3. Lesourd, B., Mazari, L., and Ferry, M., The role of nutrition in immunity in the aged, *Nutr. Review,* 1998;56:1:S113-S125
4. Chandra, R.K., Nutrition and immunology: Experience of an old traveller and recent observations. In *Nutrition and Immunology.* Chandra, R.K., Ed., ARTS Biomedical. St. John's, Newfoundland, Canada. 1992:9-43
5. Rudman, D. and Feller, A.G., Protein-calorie undernutrition in the nursing home, *J. Am. Geriatr. Soc.,* 1987;37:173-183.
6. Department of Health and Social Security. Nutrition and health in old age: report on health and social subjets. Her Majesty's Stationery Office, London, 1979;16:79-90.
7. Lesourd, B., La malnutrition protéino-énergétique chez les sujets âgés. (protein-energy malnutrition in old subjects). Semaine des Hôpitaux, 1994;31-32:957-963.
8. Lesourd, B., Vitamines et oligo-éléments chez la personne âgée. (vitamins and trace elements in old subjects), *Nutr. Clin. Métabol.,* 1994;8,4 (suppl.): 79-82.
9. Wahlqvist, M.L., Vitamins, nutrition and aging. In *Nutrition and Aging. Progress in Clinical and Biological Research.* Prinsley, D.M. and Sandstead H.H., Eds., Alan R. Liss, New York, 1990;326:175-202.
10. Boosalis, M.G., Stuart, M.A., McClain, C.J., Zinc metabolism in the elderly. In *Geriatric Nutrition.* Morley, J.E., Glick, Z., and Rubenstein, L.Z., Eds. Raven Press, New York, 1995:115-121.

11. Alés-Martinez, J.E., Alvarez-Mon, M., Merino, F., Bonilla, F., Martinez-Alés, G., Durantez, A., and De La Hera, A., Decreased TcR-CD3-T cell numbers in healthy aged humans. Evidence that T cell defects are masked by a reciprocal increase of TcR-CD3-CD2+ natural killer cells, *Eur. J. Immunol.*, 1988;18:1827-1830.

12. Lesourd, B., Laisney, C., Salvatore, R., Meaume, S., and Moulias, R., Decreased maturation of T cell population factors on the appearance of double negative CD4-, CD8-, CD2+ cells, *Arch. Gerontol. Geriatr.*, 1994;4 (suppl):139-154.

13. Weksler, M.E., Immune senescence: deficiency or dysregulation, *Nutr. Review*, 1995;53:S3-S7.

14. Lesourd, B. and Meaume, S., Cell-mediated immunity changes in aging: relative importance of cell subpopulation switches and of nutritional factors, *Immunol. Lett.*, 1994;40:235-242.

15. Lesourd, B. and Mazari, L., Nutrition and Immunity in the Elderly, *Proc. Nutr. Soc.*, 1999;58: 685-695.

16. Wick,, G. and Grubek-Loebenstein, Primary and secondary alterations of immune reactivity in the elderly: impact of dietary factors and disease. *Immunol. Rev.*, 1997;160:171-184.

17. Mazari, L. and Lesourd, B., Nutritional influences on immune response in healthy aged persons, *Mech. Aging Develop.*, 1998;104:25-40.

18. Abo, T., Extrathymic differentiation of T lymphocytes and its biological function, *Bio. Med. Res.*, 1992;13:1-39.

19. Thoman, M.L., Effects of the aged microenvironment on CD4+ T cell maturation, *Mech. Aging Dev.*, 1997;96:75-88.

20. Cossarizza, A., Ortolani, C., and Paganelli, R. et al. Age-related imbalance of virgin (CD45RA+) and memory (CD45RO+) cells between CD4+ and CD8+ T lymphocytes in humans: study from newborns to centenarians, *J. Immunol. Res.*, 1992;4:117-126.

21. Nagelkerken, L., Hertogh-Huijbregts, A., Dobber, R., and Dräger, A., Age-related changes in lymphokine production related to a decreased number of CD45Rbohi CD4+ T cells, *Eur. J. Immunol.*, 1991;21:273-281.

22. Hobbs, M.V. and Ernst, D.N., T cell differentiation and cytokine expression in late life, *Dev. Compar. Immunol.*, 1997;21:464-470.

23. Cakman, I., Rohwer, J., and Schûtz, R.M. et al., Dysregulation between TH1 and TH2 cell subpopulations in the elderly, *Mech. Aging. Dev.*, 1996;87:197-209.

24. Shearer, G.M., Th1/Th2 changes in aging, *Mech. Aging. Dev.*, 1997;94:1-5.

25. Rabinowich, H., Goses, Y., Reshef, T., and Klajman, A., Interleukin 2 production and activity in aged humans, *Mech. Aging. Dev.*, 1995;32:213-226.

26. Nagel, J.E., Chopra, R.K., Chrest, F.J., McCoy, M.T., Schneider, E.L., Holbrook, N.J., and Adler, W.H., Decreased proliferation interleukin 2 synthesis and interleukin 2 receptor expression are accompanied by decreased mRNA expression, in phytohemagglutinin-stimulated cells from elderly donors, *J. Clin. Invest.*, 1988;81:1096-1102.

27. Chen, W.F, Liu, S.L, and Gao, X.M. et al., The capacity of lymphokine production by peripheral blood lymphocytes from aged humans, *Immunol. Invest.*, 1987;15:575-583.

28. Sinderman, J., Kruse, A., and Frercks, H.J. et al., Investigations of the lymphokine system in elderly individuals, *Mech. Aging Dev.*, 1993;70:149-159.

29. Barrat, F., Lesourd, B., Boulouis, H.J., Thibault, D., Vincent-Naulleau, S., Gjata, B., Louise, A., Neway, T., and Pilet, C., Sex and parity modulate cytokine production during murine ageing, *Clin. Exp. Immunol.*, 1997;110:562-568.

30. Mbawuike, I.N., Acuna, C.L., Walz, K.C., Atmar R.L., Greenberg, S.B., and Couch, R.B., Cytokines and impaired CD8+ CTL activity among elderly persons and the enhancing effect of IL-12, *Mech. Aging Dev.*, 1997;94:25-39.

31. Murasko, D.M., Weiner, P., and Kaynes, D., Decline in mitogen induced proliferation of lymphocytes with increasing age, *Clin. Exp. Immunol.*, 1987;70:440-448.

32. Wick, G., Huber, L.A., Xu, Q., Jarosch, E., Schönitzer, D., and Jürgens G., The decline of the immune response during aging: the role of an altered lipid metabolism, *Ann. N.Y. Acad. Sci.*, 1991;621:277-290.

33. Proust, J., Moulias, R., Mumeron, F., Beckkhoucha, F., Bussone, M., Schmid, M., and Hors, J., HLA and longevity, *Tissue Antigens*, 1982;19:168-173.

34. Kubo, M. and Cinader, B., Polymorphism of age-related changes in interleukin (IL) production: differential changes of T helper subpopulation, synthesizing IL-2, IL-3, and IL-4, *Eur. J. Immunol.*, 1990:24:133-136.

35. Engwerda, C.R., Fix, B.S., and Handwerger, B.S., Cytokine production by T lymphocytes from young and old mice, *J. Immunol.*, 1996;156:3621-3630.
36. Myslinska, J., Bryl, E., Foerster, J., and Myslinski, A., Increase of interleukin 6 and decrease of interleukin 2 production during the aging process are influenced by the health status, *Mech. Aging Dev.*, 1998;100:313-328.
37. Castle, S., Uyemura, K., Wong, W., Modlin, R., and Effros, R., Evidence of enhanced type 2 immune response and impaired upregulation of a type 1 response in frail elderly nursing home residents, *Mech. Aging Develop.*, 1997;94:7-16.
38. Goidl, E.A., Aging and autoimmunity. In *Aging and the Immune Response*. Goidl, E.A., Ed. Raven Press, New York, 1987:345-358.
39. Doria, G., Immunoregulation in aging, *Int. J. Med.*, 1988;4:83-85.
40. Goldberg, T.H., Baker, D.G., and Shumacher, H.R., Interleukin-1 and the immunology of aging and disease, *Aging Immunol. Infect. Dis.*, 3, 81-86. Goodwin, J.S., Changes in lymphocyte sensitivity to prostaglandin E_2 histamine, hydrocortisone, and X irradiation with age: studies in a healthy elderly population, *Clin. Exp. Immunol. Immunopathol.*, 1991;25:243-251.
41. Barrat, F., Lesourd, B.M., Louise, A., Boulouis, H.J., Vincent-Naulleau, S., Thibault, D., Neway, T., Sanaa, M., Pilet, C., Surface antigens expression in spleen cells of C57 BL/6 mice during aging: influence of sex and breeding, *Clin. Exp. Immunol.*, 1997;107:593-600.
42. Lesourd, B., Barrat, F., and Pilet, C., Vieillissement et système immunitaire. Quelques aspects expérimentaux (Aging and immune system. Influence of sex and parity), *Bull. Acad. Natle Méd.*, Thoman, M.L., Effects of the aged microenvironment on CD4+ T cell maturation, *Mech. Aging Dev.*, 96:75-88. 1999;183:1137-1151.
43. Suehiro, A., Imagawa, T., Hosokawa, H., Suehiro, M., Ohe, Y., and Kakishita, E., Age related elevation of serum macrophage colony stimulating factor (M-CSF) level, *Arch. Gerontol. Geriatr.*, 1999;29:13-20.
44. Haller, J., Weggemans, R.M., Lammi-Keefe, C.J., and Ferry, M., Changes in the vitamin status of elderly Europeans: plasma vitamins A, E, B-6, B-12, folic acid and carotenoids, *Eur. J. Clin. Nutr.*, 1996;50 (suppl. 2):S32-S46.
45. Lesourd, B.M., Hypermetabolism: a frightening symptom that pushes elderly to enter a vicious circle. In *Vitality Mortality and Aging*. Viidik, A. and Hofecker, G., Eds. Wien. Vienna Ageing Series, 1996;5:363-376.
46. Lesourd, B., Le vieillissement du système immunitaire. Un facteur favorisant la survenue et la gravité des infections chez les sujets âgés. (Aging of the immune system. A factor that increases infection occurrence and severity in the elderly). In *Infection chez les sujets âgés*. Veyssier, P., Ed., Ellipses Paris, 1997:60-70.
47. Lesourd, B. and Mazari, L., Immune responses during recovery from protein-energy malnutrition, *Clin. Nutr.*, 1997;16 (suppl 1):37-46.
48. Ballou, S.P. and Kushner, I., Chronic inflammation in older people. Recognition, consequences, and potential intervention, *Clinics Geriatr. Med.*, 1997;13:653-669.
49. Yarasheski, K.E., Zachwieja, J.J., and Bier, D.M., Acute effects of resistance exercise on muscle protein synthesis rat in young and elderly men and women, *Am. J. Physiol.*, 1993;265:E210-E214.
50. Fereday, A., Gibson, N.R., Cox, M., Pacy, P.J., and Millward, D.J., Protein requirements and aging: metabolic demand and efficiency of utilization, *Brit. J. Nutr.*, 1997;77:685-702.
51. Lesourd, BM., Mazari, L., and Ferry, M., The role of nutrition in immunity in the aged, *Nutr. Review*, 1998;56:S113-S125.
52. Nafziger, J., Bessege, J.P., Guillosson, J.J., Damais, C., and Lesourd, B., Decreased capacity of IL1 production by monocytes of infected elderly patients, *Aging, Immunol. Infect. Dis.*, 1993;4, 1:425-34.
53. Lesourd, B., Immune response during disease and recovery in the elderly, *Proc. Nutr. Soc.*, 1999;58:85-98.
54. Harris, T.B., Ferrucci, L., Tracy, R.P., Corti, M.C., Wacholder, S., Ettinger, W.H., Heimovitz, H., Cohen, H.J., and Wallace, R., Associations of elevated interleukin-6 and C-reactive protein levels with mortality in the elderly, *Am. J. Med.*, 1999;106:506-512.
55. Lesourd, B., Salvatore, R., Guichardon, M., Raynaud-Simon, A., and Moulias, R.,Une unité de médecine nutritionnelle gériatrique pour la prise en charge des malnutritions protéino-énergétiques majeures, *Age Nutr.*, 1997;8:93-99.

56. Chandra, R.K., Effect of vitamin and trace-element supplementation on immune responses and infection in elderly subjects, *Lancet*, 1992;340:1124-1127.

57 . Talbott, M.C., Miller, L.T., and Kerkvliet, N.I. Pyridoxine supplementation: effect on lymphocyte responses in elderly person, *Am. J. Clin. Nutr.*, 1987, 46:659-664.

58. Meydani, S.N., Barklund, M.P., Lui, S., Meydani, N., and Miller, R.A. Vitamin E supplementation enhances cell-mediated immunity in healthy elderly, *Am. J. Clin. Nutr.*, 1990;52:557-563.

59. Meydani, S.N., Ribaya-Mercado, J.D., Russell, R.M., Sahyoun, N., Morrow, F.D., and Gershoff, S.N., Vitamin B_6 deficiency impairs interleukin 2 production and lymphocyte proliferation in elderly adults, *Am J. Clin. Nutr.*, 1991;53:1275-1280.

60. Prasad, A.S., Fitzgerald, J.T., Hess, J.W., Kaplan, J., Pelen, F., and Dardenne, M., Zinc deficiency in elderly patients, *Nutrition*, 1993;9:218-224.

61. Penn, N.D., Purkins, L., Kelleher, J., Heartley, R.V., Masie-Taylor, B.H., and Belfield, P.W., The effect of dietary supplementation with vitamins A, C, and E on cell-mediated immune function in elderly long-stay patients: a randomized, controlled trial, *Age Aging*, 1991;20:169-174.

62. Boukaïba, N., Flament, C., Acher, S., Chappuis, P., Pian, A., Fusselier, M., Dardenne, M., and Lemonnier, D., A physiological amount of zinc supplementation: effects on nutritional, lipid, and thymic status in an elderly population, *Am. J. Clin. Nutr.*, 1993;57:566-572.

63. Galan, P., Preziosi, P., Richard, M.J., Monget, A.L., Arnaud, J., Lesourd, B., Favier, A., Girodon, F., Laisney, C., Bourgeois, C.F., Keller, H., and Hercberg, S. et le réseau gériatrie/ MIN.VIT.AOX. Biological and immunological effects of trace element and/or vitamin supplementation in the elderly, Proc. 4th Int. Conference on Trace-Elements in Medicine and Biology. Paris, 1994:197-210.

64. Girodon, F., Blache, D., Monget, A.L., Lombart, M., Brunet-Lecompte, P., Arnaud, J., Richard, M.J., and Galan, P., Effect of a two-year supplementation with low doses of antioxidant vitamins and/or minerals in elderly subjects on levels of nutrients and antioxidant defense parameters, *J. Am. Coll. Nutr.*, 1997;4:357-365.

65. Galan, P., Preziosi, P., Monget, A.L., Richard, M.J., Amaud, J., Lesourd, B., Girodon, F., Munoz-Alferez, M.J., Bourgeois, C., Keller, H., Favier, A., Hercberg, G., and the Geriatric Network MIN. VIT. AOX. Effects of trace element and/or vitamin supplementation on vitamin and mineral status, free radical metabolism and immunological markers in elderly long term hospitalized subjects, *Int. J. Vit. Nutr. Res.*, 1997:67:450-460.

66. Girodon, F., Lombard, M., Galan, P., Brunet-Lecomte, P., Monget, A.L., Arnaud, J., Preziosi, P., and Hercberg, S., Effect of micronutrient supplementation on infection in institutionalized elderly subjects: a controlled trial, *Ann. Nutr. Metabol.*, 1997;41:98-107.

67. Cunningham-Rundles, S., Bockam, R.S., Lin, A., Giardana, P.V., Hilgartner, M.W., Caldwell-Brown, D., and Carter, R.M., Physiological and pharmacological effects of zinc on immune responses, *Ann. N.Y. Acad. Sci.*, 1991;613:113-122.

68. Keen, C.L. and Gerswhin, M.E., Zinc deficiency and immune function, *Ann. Rev. Nutr.*, 1991;10:415-431,

69. Rall, L.C. and Meydani, S.N., Vitamin B_6 and immune competence, *Nutr. Rev.*, 1993;51:217-225,

70. Gary, P.J., Goodwin, J.S., and Hunt, W. et al., Nutritional status in a healthy elderly population: dietary and supplementation intakes, *Am. J. Clin. Nutr.*, 1982;36:319-331.

71. Amorin-Cruz, J.A., Moreiras, O., and Brzozowska, A., Longitudinal changes in the intakes of vitamins and minerals of elderly Europeans, *Eur. J. Clin. Nutr.*, 1996;50 (suppl 2):S77-S85.

72. Manore, M.M., Vaughan, L.A., Carroll, S.S., and Leklem, J.E., Plasma pyridoxal 5′-phosphate concentration and dietary vitamin B_6 intake in free-living, low-income elderly people, *Am. J. Clin. Nutr.*, 1989;50:339-345.

73. Bogden, J.D., Oleske, J.M., Lavenhar, M.A., Munves, E.M., Kemp, F.W., Bruening, K.S., Holding, K.J., Denny, T.N., Guarino, M.A., and Holland, B.K., Effects of one year of supplementation with zinc and other micronutrients on cellular immunity in the elderly, *J. Am. Coll. Nutr.*, 1990;9:214-225.

74. Meydani, S.N., Meydani, M., and Blumberg, J.B., et al., Vitamin E supplementation and *in vivo* immune response in healthy elderly subjects, *JAMA*, 1997;277:117-120.

75. Meydani, S.N., Meydani, M., Verdon, C.P., Shapiro, A.C., Blumberg, J.B., and Hayes, K.C., Vitamin E supplementation suppresses prostaglandin E2 synthesis and enhances the immune response of aged mice, *Mec. Age. Dev.*, 1986;34:191-201.

76. Cannon, J.G., Meydani, S.N., Fielding, R.A., Meydani, M., Fiatarone, M.A., Farhangmehr, M., Orencole, S.F., Blumberg, J.B., and Ewans, W.J., Tha acute phase response in exercise. II. Associations between vitamin E, cytokines and muscle proteolysis, *Am. J. Physiol.*, 1991;260:R1235-R1240.

77. Meydani, S.N., Wu, D., and Santos, M.S. et al., Antioxidants and immune response in aged persons: overview of the present evidence, *Am. J. Clin. Nutr.*, 1995;62 (suppl):1462S-1476S.

78. Harman, D., Role of antioxidant nutrients in aging: overview, *Age*, 1995;18:51-62.

79. Hayek, G.M., Mura, C., Wu, D., Beharka, A.A., Han, S.N., Paulson, E., Hwang, D., and Meydani, S.N., Enhanced expression of inducible cyclooxygenase with age in murine macrophages, *J. Immunol.*, 1997;159:2445-2451.

80. Goodwin, J.S., Changes in lymphocyte sensitivity to prostaglandin E$_2$, histamine, hydrocortisone, and X irradiation with age: studies in a healthy elderly population, *Clin. Exp. Immunol. Immunopathol.*, 1992;25:243-251.

81. Girodon, F., Galan, P., Monget, A,-L., Boutron-Ruault, M,-C., Brunet-Lecomte, P., Preciozi, P., Arnaud, J., Manuguerra, J,-C,, Hercberg, S., and the MIN.VIT.AOX Geriatric Network. Impact of trace elements and vitamin supplementation on immunity and infections in institutionalized elderly patients, *Arch. Intern. Med.*, 1999;159:748-754.

82. Bogden, J.D., Oleske, J.M., Munves, E.M., Lavenhar, M.A., Bruening, K.S., Kemp, F.W., Holding, K.J., Denny, T.N., Louria, D.B., Zinc and immunocompetence in the elderly: baseline data on zinc nutriture and immunity in unsupplemented subjects, *Am. J. Clin. Nutr.*, 1987;45:101-109.

83. Bogden, J.D., Bendich, A., and Kemp, F.W., Daily micronutrient supplements enhance delayed-hypersensitivity skin test responses in older people, *Am. J. of Clin. Nutr.*, 1994;60:437-747.

84. Pike, J. and Chandra, R.K., Effect of vitamin and trace element supplementation on immune indices in healthy elderly, *Int. J. Vit. Nutr. Res.*, 1995;65:117-121.

85. Chavance, M., Herbeth, B., Lemoine, A., and Zhu, B.P., Does Multivitamin Supplementation Prevent Infections in Healthy Elderly Subjects? A Controlled trial, *Int. J. Vit. Nutr. Res.*, 1993;63:11-16.

86. Ligthart, G.J., Corberand, J.X., Fournier, C., Galanaud, P., Hijmans, W., Kennes, B., Muller-Hermelink, H.K., and Steinmann ,G.G., Admission criteria for immunogerontological studies in man: the Senieur protocol, *Mech. Aging. Dev.*, 1984, 28, 47-55.

87. Lesourd, B.M., Moulias, R., Favre-Berrone, M., and Rapin, C.H., Nutritional influences on immune responses in elderly. In *Nutrition and Immunology*, Chandra, R.K., Ed., ARTS Biomedical, St John's, Newfoundland, Canada, 1992;211-223.

88. Corti, M.C., Guralnik, J.M., Salive, M.E., and Sorkin, J.D., Serum albumin level and physical disability as predictors of mortality in older persons, *JAMA*, 1994;272:1036-1042.

89. Matsuo, M., Age-related alterations in antioxidant defence. In *Free Radicals and Aging*;Yu, B.P., Ed., CRC Press, Boca Raton, FL, 1993:143-181.

90. Selhub, J., Homocysteine metabolism, *Ann. Rev. Nutr.*, 1999:217-246.

Section III

Mechanistic Studies of Nutrition and Health in the Elderly

11 Nutrition in the Aged: Nursing Perspectives

M. Anne Woodtli

CONTENTS

I. INTRODUCTION

Nurses, as the single largest professional health care group in the U.S., provide care to elderly persons in all institutional health care settings, in their homes, and in various other community locations. Because a major focus of nursing practice is health promotion, nurses are involved in nutrition-related health education activities in diverse locations, such as churches, senior citizens centers, health fairs, and congregate meal sites, and they participate in adult education programs in schools, support groups, and volunteer organizations. The variety and demand for nursing activities that promote elder wellness, including those associated with improved nutrition, will continue to expand as the numbers of elderly rapidly increase and as persons of all ages continue to explore ways to promote healthy aging.

Nursing care of elders, however, encompasses professional health care activities well beyond those related to health promotion. Nurses are actively engaged in disease prevention, symptom management, illness care, rehabilitation, and health maintenance. They practice in a wide range of settings: acute care hospitals, clinics, nursing homes, assisted living facilities, physician offices, health maintenance organizations, and public and community health organizations. Because the care of elders has rapidly become a primary focus of nursing care, wherever the client is, nurses must address nutritional issues with every client at every level of care. A growing body of literature addresses the relationship between adequate nutrition in the elderly and their physical and mental well being.[1-5] Nurses, often the first health care provider elders encounter, are well positioned to identify nutritional needs and intervene in ways that improve and promote nutritional health.[6]

The purpose of this chapter is to provide a brief overview of nursing practice as it relates to elder nutrition across a heterogenous population of older people with varied needs in diverse settings. Nursing assessment, nursing interventions, selected special care needs, setting-specific implications, and general nursing education activities that target the elderly will be addressed.

II. NURSING SCREENING AND ASSESSMENT

Nurses routinely use nutritional screening procedures to identify elders who are malnourished or who are at risk for nutritional deficiencies, to prevent and treat malnutrition early and to change the plan of treatment as indicated.[7-9] Identifying elderly persons at risk at any point in the continuum of care is a first step in preventing disease or successfully managing existing disease processes. At an initial first level of prevention, nurses have the opportunity to screen elderly clients in a variety of locations outside of formal health facilities. For example, nurses, who are usually present at health fairs, wellness clinics, or other community health care events, screen older persons to identify the presence of risk factors for many health problems, including those related to nutrition. Nurses provide health and nutrition information and counseling and, in situations in which immediate care is indicated, they refer the client to physicians or dietitians for more in-depth examination, diagnosis, and follow up.[10]

The Nutrition Screening Initiative (NSI), a multidisciplinary project of the American Academy of Physicians, American Dietetic Association, and National Council on Aging, has provided valuable tools for nurses and other health care professionals to use in screening, assessing, and intervening at three different levels and in different health care settings to meet the nutritional needs of older persons.[11,12] The three levels of nutritional screening are classified as follows: initial identification of those who may have key risk factors for nutritional problems; a level-1 screen to identify those who may need medical or nutritional attention; and a level-2 screen that provides more in-depth nutritional assessment. The initial screening tool nurses and others can use in community settings, such as congregate meal sites or health fairs, is the "Determine Your Nutritional Health Checklist." One advantage of this checklist is that it can be administered and interpreted by nonprofessionals and can become a part of many community programs for older people. This is a particularly helpful feature for nurses, as they may be the only professional health care provider present at many health screening programs sponsored by the community or specialty volunteer organizations. The checklist consists of ten warning signs of poor nutritional health that clients check if the statement applies to them. It is quick, easy to read and administer, and provides a simple rating scale that ranges from good or little risk, to moderate risk, to high risk.[12] In using this initial checklist, nurses can provide general nutritional information and counseling and can also refer clients who checked six or more of the ten warning signs to other health care professionals for additional diagnosis and care.

At the second level of screening, nurses regularly use the level 1 screen in which height and weight measurements are used to compute body mass index (BMI). Nomograms are available for nurses to use in determining the body mass index, which enables them to rapidly identify older adults who are below or above the accepted BMI range of 24 to 27. A major warning sign nurses screen for is a client-reported unintended weight loss or gain of 5 pounds in the previous 3 months or 10 pounds within the past 6 months. Some sources indicate a better measure might be 10% of body weight. In either case, abnormal weight loss or gain and abnormal BMI, nurses refer the elder to a physician for additional assessment. In addition to determining the body mass index, nurses question clients about their eating habits, living arrangements, and functional status. The foci of this level of screening are to identify those at risk for poor nutritional status and to obtain the appropriate health care or social services. Nurses readily refer elders to health care professionals such as dentists, dietitians, and social workers as the client situation or symptoms indicate. Timely nurse referrals to social service professionals are especially important if elders are to obtain needed community services such as meals brought to the home, counseling for alcohol abuse, or transportation to congregate meal sites as soon as possible once the needs are recognized. These community outreach efforts by nurses provide an early link to the health care system and may prevent onset of more serious problems.

Because nurses recognize the need to identify nutritional problems and plan interventions, they also use the third level of screening instruments, the level 2 screen. The level 2 screen provides additional information about anthropometric measurements, laboratory data, drug use, mental/cognitive status, and the presence of specific clinical features. The focus at this third level of screening is to recognize nutritional problems, intervene, and refer for additional professional attention as indicated. With various assessment tools now available to nurses and as their knowledge of nutritional risks and problems of the elderly continues to increase, nurses need to continue to emphasize the importance of their role in risk identification through their participation in community screening programs. The need for an integrated approach to risk factor identification was one reason for the development of the Nutrition Screening Initiative. Nurses play a major role in this effort as they interact with elderly persons in multiple community environments and, as such, are often the first people to recognize elders at risk and initiate referrals.[13]

For nurses in health care settings other than the community, nutritional assessment is an essential component of all comprehensive nursing assessments at the time of admission to acute care hospitals and long-term care facilities. Nursing assessments incorporate both objective and subjective data and minimally include patent history; physical, mental, and social assessment; and review of medications and laboratory data. Nurses are particularly alert to an elder's history of medical, surgical, psychological, or social conditions, such as neurological impairment, gastrointestinal surgery, chemotherapy or radiation, alcoholism, depression or isolation, that place him or her at high nutritional risk. They carefully document the patient's pattern of weight change, identify current symptoms such as diarrhea or dysphagia that may limit oral intake, and compile a dietary history. In hospitals and long-term care facilities, nurses care for patients on a 24-hour basis and are particularly aware of the elderly patient's physical appearance. They remain alert for and are able to recognize early changes in eating patterns, nutritional intake, and signs of eating disorders.[10] They also monitor patients who initially are not at risk for signs of declining nutritional status. Due to medications, treatments, surgery, or stress, elderly hospitalized patients may develop symptoms that can cause rapid deterioration in nutritional status. Bankhead notes that patients with conditions that have obvious nutritional consequences are usually monitored closely and treated appropriately, but patients who gradually decline during their stay may be temporarily overlooked and their nutritional treatment delayed.[7] For those patients who are identified at risk for or are already diagnosed with nutritional problems, nurses collaborate in developing a multidisciplinary plan. They implement independent nursing interventions as well as carry out those prescribed by other disciplines, such as administering parenteral or enteral feedings, calculating intake, or using specific assistive devices at mealtimes.

The Subjective Global Assessment (SGA) and the Admission Nutrition Screening Tool are two examples of other nutritional assessment tools available to nurses in institutional settings that provide systematic assessment of the elder's nutritional status or nutritional risk.[10] Nurses use the SGA to assess nutritional status; it is based on clinical history and physical examination findings. It has been found to be valid and reliable when compared with a standard objective measure.[14] The Admission Nutrition Screening Tool is useful at the time of patient admission to a hospital, nursing home or other health care facility to identify patients at nutritional risk. The rating scale identifies persons as either "at low risk" or "at risk" based on subjective and objective information related to diagnosis, symptoms, and weight.[15] The authors report a high degree of sensitivity and high interobserver agreement between the nurse and the nutritionist.

Mezey and Fulmer developed an assessment tool and process to identify risk factors that contribute to poor outcomes for hospitalized older adults.[16,104] It was part of a national initiative to improve geriatric care in hospitals and focuses on a screening process using the acronym SPICES:

skin impairment, poor nutrition, incontinence, confusion, evidence of falls or functional decline, and sleep disturbance. When nurses identify the presence of any of these assessment criteria, they take immediate steps to minimize the risk factors and to prevent development of associated health problems, such as decubiti, malnutrition, falls, or increased confusion, which are often aggravated during acute care episodes. The nursing screening process and the proactive plan of care that resulted from the Nurses Improving Care to the Hospitalized Elderly (NICHE) project also incorporated nutritional screenings at the time of admission. Proactive investigation of unexplained weight loss prior to hospitalization with referral to a dietitian, assessment of prehospital food preferences, food intake patterns, and limitations to ingestion are components of the nutritional assessment that also includes team interventions as an ongoing part of care.[17] Nutritional assessment from various disciplinary perspectives is an essential component in the process in an attempt to keep hospitalized elderly functioning at optimal levels.

Many nutrition assessment tools are available for nurses to use with community-dwelling elderly persons and with patients or residents in health care institutional settings. Nutritional assessment of all clients is a recognized nursing care responsibility. However, the problem that often arises in this era of cost constraints and reduction in staff is the lack of time to conduct an optimal, comprehensive nutritional assessment. When confronted with fewer nursing staff and more high-acuity patients, comprehensive nutritional assessments may not be considered high-priority nursing activities. This is unfortunate, as accurate nursing nutritional assessments provide valuable information that serves as the basis for developing individualized and appropriate plans of care, not just for the nurse but for use by other health professionals as well. Nursing nutritional assessments, observations, and care plans provide reliable information and insights that members of other health care disciplines use as part of their discipline-specific assessments, evaluations, and interventions.

III. NURSING INTERVENTIONS

Nurses review and analyze the objective and subjective assessment data they have collected and make clinical judgments that direct their care. Often these clinical judgments take the form of a nursing diagnosis, or a conclusion, which provides the basis on which the patient's individual care plan is developed. The care plan is mutually developed between the nurse and the patient and outlines the desired patient outcomes and associated nursing interventions.

A simplistic example will be used to illustrate the planning process. A nursing diagnosis based on assessment data might be "feeding self-care deficit," which is an impaired ability of the elderly person to perform or complete feeding activities.[18] Nurses might make this nursing diagnosis based on one or more factors that contribute to the inability of the patient to feed himself, such as weakness, pain on movement of arm or hand, cognitive impairment, musculoskeletal impairment, or lack of motivation. In addition, the elderly person might demonstrate one or more of the following characteristics: inability to handle utensils, open containers, pick up a cup, or chew food. The elder's functional ability might range from requiring the use of an assistive device to requiring help from another person to needing both the device and personal assistance, or he may be completely dependent. Based on these data, optimally the nurse and patient and/or family develop an individual care plan. Included in the plan are the patient's individual goals and expected outcomes related to self-feeding and nursing actions that will be implemented to facilitate goal achievement. Both short-term and long-term goals/outcomes are identified as well as the expected date of achievement. Patient progress is continually monitored; the plan is reviewed on an ongoing basis and modified as necessary.

As part of the care planning process, the nurse identifies appropriate nursing interventions, often in collaboration with other team members such as the physical therapist, occupational therapist, or dietitian. Based on the elder's signs and symptoms and the individual factors contributing to the self-feeding deficit, nursing interventions might include providing adequate pain relief before meals, positioning the elder in a chair rather than bed during meals, flexing the head and neck slightly forward during feeding, or providing a drinking straw or finger foods, and providing nutritional supplements between meals. Depending on the elder's specific deficits, the nurse might instruct nonprofessional staff to cut meat, avoid placing food on the person's blind side, provide adaptive devices such as long or large-circumference handles, use weighted dishes, or provide frequent cueing.[19] Regardless of the elder's functional status, nurses recognize that those at nutritional risk must be identified early if nurses are to minimize poor nutritional intake, prevent onset of more serious nutritional complications or aggravation of already existing conditions, and promote optimal self-care.

In summary, nurses systematically assess the nutritional status of elderly clients; make informed clinical judgments based on their assessments, knowledge and experience; identify and implement nursing interventions; and evaluate achievement of expected outcomes. Meeting the nutritional needs of elderly clients is a nurse-intensive effort which, in acute and long-term care facilities, takes place not just at designated mealtimes, but over a 24-hour period every day. Often the success of the interventions of other health team members, including the physician, is dependent on the effectiveness and the quality of the interactions that occur between the nurse and the patient, not just at meals but throughout the patient's hospitalization. The expertise of the nurse at the bedside is more often than not related to the quality of nutritional care the patient ultimately receives. The nurse is the professional on whom physicians, dietitians, occupational therapists, and others depend to implement nutritional interventions, consistently monitor the elderly patient's progress, and evaluate the outcomes on a daily, and in some acute situations hourly, basis.

A. Selected Special Care Needs

Elderly persons frequently have conditions that require extensive nursing assessment and complex nursing interventions. Their increased nutritional nursing needs are often related to the higher incidence of neurological, musculoskeletal, and cognitive impairments in the aging population. Nutritional implications of stroke, Parkinson's disease, arthritis, fractures, and cognitive impairments have significant implications for patient nutrition and, in turn, for nursing.[20,97] Dysphagia, dementia, and undernutrition are primary examples. Related to the nutritional implications of these complex health problems is the additional and associated nursing intervention of medication administration. In this section, special care needs related to impaired swallowing, dementia, undernutrition, and medication administration are discussed.

1. Impaired Swallowing

Impaired swallowing has been reported in numerous studies as a significant problem in patients with stroke, Parkinson's disease, and multiple sclerosis.[21-24] Aspiration, a risk in patients with impaired swallowing, was found to have occurred in 34 to 48% of 70 stroke patients who underwent videofluoroscopic examinations[21] and has been associated with pneumonia, sepsis, and increased mortality and morbidity.[25] McHale et al. describe two significant themes in nursing care of the patients with impaired swallowing: assessment and feeding.[25] The assessment function of the nursing role includes nursing assessment of the mechanics of swallowing, oral and pharyngeal stages of swallowing, and the effects of mental status on swallowing ability. They identified five major components of assessment nurses can use to identify patients at risk, several of which are similar to those included in an assessment tool developed by Johnson et al. for use in intensive care units.[26] The major assessment components relate to cardiopulmonary, neurological, and motor factors, and specific signs unique to the oral and pharyngeal stages of swallowing. Nursing assessment is enhanced by consultation and close collaboration with and formal assessment by speech pathologists regarding diagnosis of specific swallowing dysfunctions, efficiency of swallow, and use of appropriate food textures.[27]

The feeding function of nursing care for patients with dysphagia, as described by McHale et al.,[25] includes clinical management, feeding techniques and, most importantly, knowing the patient. Nurses who know their patients are able to be more creative, intuitive, and effective in their approaches to assessment and feeding practices. Nurses in McHale et al.'s study identified two major clinical management outcomes in dysphagic patients: providing nutrition and preventing aspiration. They emphasized the need for skilled assessment of swallowing ability and strongly recommended professional nursing guidance and direction of nonprofessional staff who are often responsible for feeding patients who are at risk for or have impaired swallowing. Again, the need for multidisciplinary assessment to ensure appropriate nursing interventions is critical. Specific nursing interventions related to swallowing therapy are identified in several nursing texts.[28-32]

2. Dementia

Dementia is one of the most common mental health conditions affecting older persons living in the community as well as those residing in long-term care facilities.[33,34] The degree of cognitive impairment and the associated behavioral manifestations provide challenges in all areas of nursing care but are of special concern in assuring patients receive adequate nutrition. Nurses are responsible for assessing and monitoring patient nutrition as well as feeding, documenting intake, educating family caregivers in the home, and training and supervising nonprofessional staff in health care facilities. According to Cohen,[35] malnutrition is a widespread problem among older patients in mental hospitals and on psychiatric units; older persons with dementia are at the highest risk for malnutrition. In these facilities as well as dementia care units in nursing homes and hospital skilled care units, nurses are present at all meals and are creative in their attempts to ensure adequate food intake.

Enumerating the diverse strategies nurses use to encourage eating and ensure adequate food intake is beyond the scope of this chapter, but these include attention to assessing the patient's eating habits and patterns, assessing patient-specific difficulties with feeding, and identifying the appropriate level, time, and frequency of feeding assistance.[36] Patients with dementia present the nurse with numerous feeding challenges. They sometimes pace relentlessly, fail to recognize food or utensils, forget how to feed themselves, how to chew, or how to swallow. At mealtimes, they sometimes demonstrate hostile and aggressive behaviors toward staff and other residents. Watson and Dreay[37] investigated the different aspects of feeding difficulty of elderly persons with dementia and developed a questionnaire that identifies three different facets of difficulty in feeding elderly patients with dementia: patient obstinacy or passivity (lack of cooperation with feeding), nursing intervention, and indicators of feeding difficulty. In subsequent testings, the scale was clinically significant in that the level of feeding difficulty assessed by the scale was positively and significantly correlated with the level of nursing intervention. These nursing research findings should guide future research, as they provide a strong empirical base for rationalizing into three factors a multiplicity of components of problems in feeding demented patients.

As the severity of dementia increases, patients become increasingly dependent on nurses or family caregivers to maintain nutritional intake. Van Ort and Phillips,[38,39] in a study of feeding problems of demented residents in a nursing home, found environmental, organizational, and interactional patterns at mealtime that made an already chaotic care environment even noisier and characterized by more staff involvement, more interruptions, many distractions, frequent non-feeding related events, and great variation in the organization of the feeding experience. They reported few systematic attempts by staff to elicit normal resident eating behaviors and observed that few fluids were offered during the meals. They described both feeder and resident behaviors that elicited, sustained, and extinguished functional feeding of the demented residents. Van Ort and Phillips suggested nursing interventions aimed at modifying the feeding environment and altering the behavioral context of the feeding interactions and recommended developing and implementing specific protocols that could promote functional feeding for each resident. Cohen[35] lists practical interventions that can be used for eating-related behavioral problems such as pacing, attention deficit, and constant chewing in persons with dementia (p. 112). These interventions have been adapted from the American Dietetic Association and are helpful suggestions for all caregivers, including nursing personnel.

3. Undernutrition

Although research studies investigating nutritional intake in the elderly report evidence of over-, adequate, and undernutrition, Clarke et al.,[40] in their review of studies of the prevalence of under-nutrition in the elderly, found high degrees of elder undernutrition. They reported that subnutrition occurs in 10 to 20% of the elderly living at home and up to 60% of elderly patients in long-term care facilities and acute care hospitals. It is well established that undernutrition increases with age and dependence and is related to a host of social, psychological, economic, and physical factors. Its contribution to increased morbidity and mortality in older persons continues to be well documented.[2,3,41-43,100]

To a large extent, undernutrition may go unrecognized.[2,42] Although the role of nurses in promoting good nutrition in the elderly and in identifying those at risk has been described earlier, nurses also have a major role in implementing corrective interventions such as oral, parenteral, and enteral nutritional support. Nutritional support is critical in many acute situations, but its general use is often controversial.[44,99] In any case, nursing care is essential to the effective implementation of nutritional support therapy as well as to counseling elders about their use of non-prescribed dietary supplements. Research findings indicate that 33 to 72% of elderly take nonprescription supplements including single nutrients, multivitamin and mineral combinations, and liquid supple-ments.[46] Unfortunately these supplements are often used without consultation with a physician or dietitian and without dietary assessment or counseling. Nurses, in carrying out their various roles in the community, clinics, or physicians' offices, are often the first health care providers to identify their use and provide appropriate assessment, counseling, or referral. Nursing interventions are related to their concerns about elders' being at higher risks for toxicity, drug interactions, and susceptibility to quackery as well as their attention to financial constraints and unnecessary or unrealistic costs.[46]

In more acute situations, nurses are responsible for administering oral supplements, tube feedings, and parenteral nutrition. Specific recommendations for nursing procedures or protocols related to these interventions can be found in many nursing textbooks, but the concern here is to emphasize the essential role nursing plays in safely administering, continuously monitoring, accu-rately documenting, and knowledgeably evaluating the effectiveness and outcomes of nutritional supplements to patients in the home, acute care, and long-term care environments.[102] Transitional or permanent feeding using more aggressive methods of nutrition such as nasogastric tubes or percutaneous endoscopic gastrostomy or jejunostomy tube feedings are very nurse-sensitive inter-ventions. The interdisciplinary team efforts, in which nursing plays a role, are invaluable in this transition process. However, it is often nursing observations and assessments that provide the practical data on which the course for transitioning from tube or parenteral feeding to oral intake is determined. Guenter et al.[47] describe specific nursing responsibilities and interventions for initiating tube feeding, assessing subjective and objective parameters for monitoring tolerance during therapy, and identifying common gastrointestinal, metabolic, and mechanical complications. In implementing nutritional interventions, as with many other clinical nursing interventions, clinical pathways provide guidance in tracking patient outcomes and documenting variances.[48]

The increasing importance of the nurse case manager and the home health nurse in providing home nutritional support cannot be underestimated. The advances in nutritional support equipment and techniques have made it technically possible for patients to receive sophisticated and complex types of nutritional support in their homes. In large part, however, the reality of home nutritional support is made possible by nurses teaching, supervising, and assisting the patient, family, or friends in administering enteral feedings and parenteral infusions. The role of the nurse case manager is critical in arranging patient discharge with the patient, family, and home health agency; assuring compliance with Medicare, Medicaid, or other insurer regulations; ensuring no interruption in treatment; and confirming that patient and family education will continue during the transition. The home health nurse is responsible for continuing the teaching that was begun in the hospital, being present for initial infusions or feedings, providing subsequent home visits to teach and to ensure that techniques are being safely and confidently performed, and being available for any problems that arise.[49] In summary, nursing care is a principal factor in achieving successful outcomes with patients who are undernourished and who are receiving oral, enteral, or parenteral nutritional therapy whether in the hospital or at home.

4. Medication Administration

One important responsibility of nurses is to administer medications or, in settings such as home health or in roles such as case manager or nurse practitioner, to prescribe, review, or monitor patients' medications. These medication-related nursing activities are especially challenging in elderly patients because of their high potential for toxicity, counterindications, and interactions. Risk assessment becomes even more essential, and more complicated, by the polypharmacy that seems to be a part of many elders' lives.[50] Consideration of drug–nutrient interactions is just one component of nursing assessment and monitoring that is part of nurses' professional responsibilities when they administer medications.

A related concern nurses address is the form in which the medication is given. Some older patients are at higher risk for swallowing, choking, or chewing problems, while others are receiving nutrition and medications by other than the oral route. For example, nurses are aware that changing the form in which medications are administered, such as crushing, may change their therapeutic effectiveness. Some medications need to be diluted, others should never be diluted. Some medications are incompatible with enteral formulas, some are less effective when given with food, while others are less effective when given on an empty stomach. Some medications should not be given with milk, others with citrus juices, others with alcohol, and yet others with over-the-counter remedies.[51] However, sometimes — perhaps too often — this information is not given to, understood, or remembered by families, nonprofessional caregivers, or patients themselves. Perhaps it would be ideal if the physician or a pharmacist were always aware of all of the prescription and nonprescription medications and nutrient supplements elderly persons take, but this is not the case. Therefore, the role of the nurse becomes even more important in institutional, community, and home settings to review, monitor, and/or supervise medications of elderly people. The nurse's role includes being alert for nutrient–drug interactions and incompatibilities as well as the timing and the form in which medications are administered in relation to specific foods, altered routes, and sensory and physical deficits. Again, the success of multidisciplinary therapies related to medications often depends on the nurse's knowledge, skills, experience, and consistent interaction with elderly patients and their families.

IV NURSING CARE SETTINGS

Nurses are present in most settings where nursing care is provided to elderly persons, and therefore have multiple and ongoing responsibilities for ensuring adequate nutrition to their patients. Certainly some challenges are common to all care settings, for example, the dependent eater, elders with special dietary requirements, or potential medication–food interactions. However, individual care settings also present nurses with unique nutritional problems related to the special needs of the clients in specific health care environments with different institutional considerations such as acuity levels, staffing ratios, staffing mix, or cost constraints. Regardless of setting, the overriding concern for nurses is ensuring quality care, which includes close attention to nutritional aspects of patient care. This section includes descriptions of acute care, subacute care, nursing home and home care settings.

A. ACUTE CARE

Elders aged 85 years and older are the fastest growing segment of the American population. Their numbers increased 41% in the decade between 1981 and 1990 and they accounted for 60% of all acute care beds.[52] The percentage of hospitalized elders who may experience functional decline, reported to be as high as 75%, has significant impact on the potential for increase in adverse outcomes.[53-57] Nutritional decline is no exception. A recent study of geriatric patients in an acute care hospital found inadequate nutritional support for geriatric patients, which placed malnourished and dependent patients at higher risk for starvation and hospital mortality. The investigators reported inadequate caloric intake across surgical, medical, and geriatric wards and found functional dependency in elders to be a strong predictor of mortality independent of mental deterioration.[43] Findings also indicated patients with inadequate oral intake were not provided adequate supplementation. Watson[58] also addressed this issue of nutritional supplementation in his concern for the need for nursing clarity about whether nutritional supplements were being used as replacements for oral intake or as a supplement to oral intake.

Both of these findings have serious implications for nurses, as the numbers of elderly patients continue to make up a increasingly larger percentage of the patients in acute care settings.

The consequences of poor nutritional status were found to be the best predictor of readmission to hospitals in elderly rehabilitation patients.[4] Nurses and nursing staff need to be alert for nutritional deficiencies, especially inadequate caloric intake, and to be aware of predictors such as functional dependency. These findings may reflect other institutional factors related to quality of care issues. Staffing numbers, mix, availability, shortened lengths of stay, and often insufficient time for patient and family teaching and discharge planning continue to be of concern to nurses. If nurses are not present to supervise or assist with nutritional intake, they cannot make the observations necessary to ensure appropriate nutrition-related interventions are implemented. Kresevic et al.[52] describe a hospital unit designed especially for acute care of elderly patients with care planned and provided by interdisciplinary core teams. Nursing protocols are designed to prevent functional decline and encourage self-care in relation to common geriatric problems encountered with older hospitalized patients, including malnutrition. The malnutrition nursing protocol includes interventions to prevent decline, such as nursing attention to caloric and fluid intake, oral care, and progress toward a more liberal diet. The restorative care protocol includes attention to snacks and dietary referrals. Nurses who are accessible to elderly hospitalized patients and their families 24 hours a day every day are a critical resource in a patient-centered acute care setting.[52] Nevertheless, nurses cannot overlook other possible contributing factors to nutritional depletion in acutely ill patients, such as the effects of physical and emotional stress in surgical patients, history of preadmission weight loss, patient dissatisfaction with diet or the lack of institutional clarity related to development of nursing protocols and implementation of independent nursing interventions based on professional nursing assessment. In summary, nursing observations, assessment, and documentation of nutritional intake of elderly patients in acute care hospitals are vital links in recognizing patients at risk for nutritional decline and instituting nursing interventions and appropriate interdisciplinary referrals to prevent or correct nutritional depletion.

B. SUBACUTE CARE

Although variously known as transitional care, skilled care, or step-down care, subacute care units provide less intensive care and longer lengths of stay than acute care units but more intensive care than nursing homes. They are designed to provide care immediately following acute care or instead of acute care. Many types of subacute services can now be obtained, but the specific types of care available are defined by each individual provider. In all instances however, nutritional support is a basic consideration. According to Robertson,[27] two thirds of current subacute patients are over the age of 65. Nurses are responsible for providing nutritional repletion, facilitating transition from functionally dependent feeding to more independent or self-feeding, and assisting with transition from various types of tube feeding or parenteral infusion to oral intake. In a subacute setting, nurses actively monitor patients' nutritional status, intake, and progress; implement various independent and interdependent nutrition-related interventions, and collaborate with interdisciplinary teams in goal setting, care planning, and outcome evaluation. This emerging care setting will continue to be an area where nurses can provide the specialized care necessary to promote functional independence and improve nutritional status of the growing numbers of elderly who require longer times to achieve functional and nutritional goals necessary for transition to more independent living.

C. Nursing Home

In the long-term care setting, the very term "nursing" home indicates the major purpose of care and the degree to which nurses are involved in providing or supervising resident care. Unfortunately, malnutrition among nursing home residents is an ongoing, significant, and serious problem for both nursing staff and the elderly for whom they care. Kayser-Jones and Schell[59] reported that from 30 to 50% of nursing home residents had below-normal body weights, serum albumin levels, and mid-arm-muscle circumferences. In a recently published study, they reported findings related to their investigation of the social, cultural, environmental, and clinical factors that influenced eating behavior in two proprietary nursing homes. Data were gathered from participant observation and in-depth interviews with physicians, nursing staff, residents, and families over a 23-month period. Qualitative methods were used for data analysis in order to identify patterns that explained resident behavior. The authors found that the major factor influencing nutritional care was an inadequate number of qualified staff. This finding reflected observations of insufficient nursing staff to feed and assist residents at mealtime, nursing assistants' lack of knowledge of feeding residents safely, and inadequate supervision of nonprofessional staff.

Among other findings, the investigators reported inadequate staffing affected care before and after meals and influenced how and where meals were served. For example, oral hygiene was neglected, dentures were not put in, residents were served meals in bed and not positioned correctly, and meal trays were poorly placed. The mealtime experience was often unpleasant, with staff enhancing dependency, feeding residents quickly and forcefully, mixing solid foods with liquids, not recognizing dysphagia, using liquid supplements inappropriately, and not feeding or underfeeding the most impaired residents. Kayser-Jones and Schell[59] concluded that, for some residents, the quality of care at mealtime was adequate; for most it was poor. They described mealtime as an "often frightening, unpleasant ordeal for the residents and an arduous task for the staff" (p. 70). To improve the quality of care at mealtime, the authors suggested that knowledgeable, professional gerontological nurses, nurse practitioners, or clinical nurse specialists assume leadership, management, and supervisory positions in nursing homes to provide much-needed role models, education, and supervision. They strongly recommended higher staff-to-resident ratios at mealtime along with recruiting other facility staff, family members, and community volunteers to assist residents with meals.

Although Kayser-Jones and Schell[59] describe mealtime conditions in two nursing homes, unfortunately these findings are not unique to this study. Van Ort and Phillips[38,39] reported many of the same findings: staff mixing food and liquid together, not setting up trays appropriately, discontinuing feeding residents before they were finished eating, and not attending to resident visual or behavioral cues. However, they also found that by implementing several nursing actions that modified the meal time and feeding environments, they were able to promote resident self-feeding without increasing the length of meal time. They also found that by implementing behavioral interventions that included systematic prompting, cueing, and reinforcing behaviors, residents consumed greater amounts of food and fluid and initiated self-feeding more often. They concluded that by designing and implementing specific nursing protocols, functional feeding for demented elders in nursing homes can be enhanced.

Johnson et al.[60] noted discrepancies between nutrient values provided by menus and those consumed by residents. Their findings included low intakes of iron, zinc, vitamin D, and calcium among residents. They recommended greater attention to delivery of food to long-term care residents and to staff feeding practices. Groher and McKaig,[61] in a study of 740 residents in two nursing homes, concluded that many nursing home residents were prescribed and maintained on mechanically altered diets unnecessarily. They reported that 91% of residents were at dietary levels below the recommended amount; of that number, 87% were receiving either pureed or tube feedings. Only 5% of residents were considered at the appropriate diet level. These findings support those of earlier studies.[62,63] Nurses need to be alert to the necessity for regular reevaluation of residents' dietary levels to ensure residents are placed on diets as close to normal as they can safely tolerate. Nursing home staff confront additional nutritional and feeding challenges when one considers that, according to Burns et al.,[64] at least 80% of nursing home residents have diagnosed mental disorders. As the severity of the disorder progresses from mild memory loss to profound dementia, so do the demands for increased staff time and creativity necessary to meet the nutritional needs of these residents with widely varying symptoms, functional abilities, and cognitive capacities.[35]

In summary, the current health care system's concerns with cost may have had unfortunate consequences in decreasing quality of care in many nursing homes. The nutritional care of residents may be one casualty in the restructured system's attempt to reduce nursing home costs by decreasing the number of staff, replacing professional nurses with less prepared or nonprofessional staff, and eliminating or severely reducing orientation and staff education activities. Adequate attention to the nutritional components of nursing home care has been and continues to be a priority in meeting nutritional requirements and improving the nutritional status of elderly residents.

D. HOME

Nurses are the primary formal care providers in community settings.[65] The home as a setting for nursing care is one in which nurses increasingly provide or supervise and monitor nutritional care for elderly persons. The use of home health care services, measured in dollars generated, increased five-fold in the decade between 1985 and 1995.[51,66] The growth in the number of home health agencies reflects consumer demand for delivery of health services in the home setting. Several factors have influenced the recent growth of home care as a health care industry, including the current ability to provide more technologically advanced therapies in the home setting, earlier release of patients from hospitals, cost constraints that accompanied introduction of managed care and prospective payment systems, and elders' relentless pursuit of independent living arrangements in their desire to remain outside of institutional settings. As expected, persons 65 years of age and older make up a large percentage of home care clients.

The overwhelming focus of home care is provision of nursing services, not the least of which is attention to nutritional needs and dietary management. Because few home care agencies currently employ full-time dietitians, home health nurses are responsible for nutritional care as one component of the professional nursing services they provide to homebound clients.[67] Nutrition-related nursing care in the home includes assessing the elder's nutritional status with special attention to preventing malnutrition and, if that is not possible, to identifying early signs of under- or overnutrition. In addition to promoting good general nutrition and eating habits in home-dwelling clients and their families, nurses regularly engage in nutrition-related activities such as dietary counseling and recommending diet modifications, oral supplements, or other dietary therapies. They refer elders living at home to their physicians for further examination or treatment, to dietitians for more extensive and in-depth dietary counseling and management, and to social workers for referrals for home delivery of meals, congregate meal sites, day care centers, food stamps, or other federal, state, or local nutrition programs. In addition to their health promotion, prevention, and screening activities, home health nurses assist elders in managing the nutrition and dietary aspects of diseases such as diabetes, renal disease, Crohn's disease, or AIDS; modified diets related to health problems associated with hypertension, radiation or hypercholestemia; and dietary control of symptoms such as nausea, vomiting, diarrhea, or anorexia.

The nutritional factors in nursing care of elders at home are multiple, often complex and frequently family focused. Currently, the vast majority of persons over the age of 65 live, not in institutions, but at home or at other locations in the community. With the dramatic projected increase in the percentage of the population over age 65 in the next 10 years and their seemingly increasing desire to remain at home as they age, the role of nurses in home care will continue be a significant component of a community-focused health care system that provides nutritional services to elderly people.

V.   NURSING EDUCATION ACTIVITIES

Nurses have multiple opportunities to provide information to elderly persons and to participate in various educational activities related to nutrition. Frequently, nurses are present either as volunteers or as part of formal community programs for the aging at congregate meal sites, senior citizen centers, health fairs, and shelters for women or the homeless. The potential for nurses to participate in formal and informal nutrition educational programs is almost limitless. They are regularly sought out as speakers on various health-related topics, participants in health care forums, and as representatives of health care professionals at community educational programs and health-related events. Topics range from helping patients modify food-related practices to identifying and using community resources to educating families about feeding dependent adults to the combined benefits of nutrition and exercise.

To increase their educational effectiveness, it is important that nurses be familiar with the variety of nutrition-focused educational resources currently available. Using appropriate printed, pictorial, audiotape, videotape, or computer-assisted materials along with other teaching models and strategies is a necessary prerequisite to facilitating effective instruction. Information that can be presented in various formats, congruent with different levels of cognitive abilities and targeted to the individual or group needs and interests, helps to assure positive learning outcomes in older learners. Not surprisingly, it is fairly well accepted that years of formal education correlate highly with level of reading ability. Certainly, a segment of the today's older population did not have the opportunity for long years of formal schooling and, indeed, may not have attained the eighth-grade level. The National Adult Literacy Survey found a significant percentage of American adults were able to perform at only the most basic literacy levels.[68,69] The lack of adequate literacy skills limits many elders in reading or understanding nutritional information necessary for improving their nutritional status or reducing their risk of nutrition-related health problems. Assessment of literacy is an early step in the instructional process that nurses cannot overlook. Fortunately, several brief and easy to administer literacy assessment instruments are available.[70,71] Once elders with low literacy skills are identified, nurses must be knowledgeable about availability and use of alternate methods and formats that meet the literacy skill level of the elder client or group.[72-75] One example of the use of an easy-to-administer literacy screening instrument is described in a study of outpatient nutrition counseling for cardiovascular risk reduction in 339 urban African-American adults, nearly half of whom scored at or below the eighth-grade level.[68] In summary, the link between literacy and health is becoming widely acknowledged and, therefore, awareness of literacy skills will become increasingly important to nurses if their nutritional educational efforts with the elderly are to be effective.

Assessing the grade reading level of written materials is necessary before nurses provide pamphlets or other written information to elderly clients. Several formulas and methods, including computer programs, are available to assist nurses to assess the degree of reading difficulty. The

SMOG formula is a commonly used formula to predict grade level readability of reading materials. It consists of counting the number of words containing three or more syllables in a total of 30 sentences selected from the beginning, middle, and end of the written material. The total number of words containing three or more syllables is compared with a conversion table. For example, if there are between 21 and 30 words that have at least three syllables, the predicted reading grade level is eighth.[76] However, the ability to read the words does not necessarily mean the elder is able to understand or use the information.[77] Nurses, therefore, need to ensure that elders comprehend the material they read and are able to apply the concepts. Nurses recognize that elderly persons do have special learning needs and try to adapt educational programs accordingly.[78-82]. For example, Weinrich et al.[78,90] examined the effect of three educational interventions with 135 elderly subjects who were participating in a fecal occult blood cancer screening project conducted at congregate meal sites. A significantly greater percentage of participants (94%, $p = .02$) taught by the educational intervention that included a practice session of the collection procedure for fecal occult blood screening completed the actual screening protocol than did those who were taught by either of the other two methods. The investigators suggest that findings support that need for nurses to take more time, address the relevance of the task, provide practice sessions, and adapt the teaching methods to accommodate aging changes when educational activities are designed for elderly clients.[81,78,90] These findings may have implications for nutrition-related educational activities for older adults.

Johnston and Gueldner[83] used a mnemonics program to improve the efficiency of memory in a group of older adults. They found significant differences between the experimental and control groups in improvement in memory and self-esteem after participation in the memory skills classes. They recommended nurses and others use a mnemonics approach to assist the elderly to cope with the effects of aging related memory loss. They suggested mnemonics programs may have long-range benefits in extending the time elders are able to function independently. These teaching techniques may well have valuable implications for nutrition education of older persons.[82] Theiss and Merrit,[84] in a study of coronary artery disease patients, found that older subjects preferred a structured learning situation in which they could listen to the presentation supplemented with visual aids and one in which materials were presented in a detailed manner. Findings indicated that reading was not a highly preferred learning style with these older adults and that women preferred higher affiliation relationships with peers than did men. The investigators also reported that elders with lower educational levels preferred to engage in friendly relationships with the instructor and peers, liked to set their own goals, chose to learn from an expert, and preferred iconics to listening and reading.[84-86]

A second general consideration for nurses in their efforts to teach the elderly is awareness of clients' cultural differences in food preferences, food preparation, daily diets, and eating patterns. Recognition that ethnic, religious, and social eating habits are major influences on lifestyle of the elderly increases the likelihood of achieving positive behavioral changes related to nutrition. Nurses, because of their interactions with clients and families over time, are particularly responsive to foods and dietary customs unique to specific cultures, especially those that are prevalent in their practice.[87] Nurses' recognition of cultural needs and practices of their patients increases the likelihood that elders will adhere to dietary modifications. Cultural differences may affect patient's acceptance of educational interventions and their ultimate incorporation of dietary changes into their eating patterns.[101] General knowledge of cultural patterns provides a beginning background for nursing intervention but does not consider individual preferences or intracultural differences. Nurses who are able to maintain open and trusting relationships with patients from different cultures have the opportunity to problem-solve, negotiate, and adjust dietary regimens to facilitate individualized modifications of dietary recommendations. By providing information and other nutritional resources and using communication techniques, language, and behaviors that are culturally appropriate, nurses can enhance their ability to motivate elderly persons and their families to make the changes necessary to reduce their risk factors and improve or maintain their nutritional status.[88,89,103] As the numbers of elderly increase, the health care system will be faced with more culturally diverse elders suffering with various chronic illnesses that demand nutritional intervention. The role of nurses in providing early screening and assessment in ways that are culturally appropriate will result in improving the health of all elderly persons.

Similarly, nurses, especially those who provide care in the home, clinic, private practice, or case management environments, are more likely than other care providers to be aware of financial and budget constraints that impose limitations on an elder's ability to purchase food, afford transportation to grocery stores, or pay for assistance with food preparation. Physical functional deficits that limit shopping and meal preparation are obvious; lack of adequate facilities for keeping foods cold, heating food, and properly storing foods are less so. Nevertheless, their potential impact on elder nutrition is significant and is often first identified by the nurse in discussions with the elders and their families or during home visits.

A final consideration in nursing educational activities are those targeted at older women. It has been well documented that women in the U.S. live longer than men. Not only are there more women than men in the over-65 population, but after age 75, 70% of women are widows.[92] Many older women have chronic illnesses, low incomes, and live alone. They compose a sizeable portion of the population who receive care in various community health centers, clinics, and in the home and who visit congregate meal sites or senior citizen centers. Nurses interact frequently and over long periods of time with older women and have many opportunities for health promotion and risk reduction activities, including those related to general nutrition, special diets, meal planning, shopping, and food selection. For example, nurses regularly discuss, either with individual clients, groups, or in formal classes, topics such as calcium needs, recommended fat intake, high-fiber foods, vitamin use, balanced meals, and heart-healthy diets. They are available to answer questions, provide nutritional information, offer suggestions, provide reinforcement and encouragement, or give sensible advice.[93-96]

A common risk factor nurses regularly address with older aged women is inadequate fluid intake.[98] Older women are at somewhat greater risk for dehydration than their younger counterparts. Physiological changes related to reduced protein stores, decreased urine concentration, diminished sensation of thirst combined with increased use of diuretics, difficulty with mobility, and concern about incontinence can result in below recommended daily intake of fluids. Unfortunately, elderly women often use fluid restriction as a means to control or manage incontinent episodes, which identifies yet another area for nursing education and intervention.

In summary, the need and the opportunities for nurses to assist elderly women to maintain or achieve sound nutritional practices through planned and unplanned patient education activities are endless. Unfortunately, the contributions of nurses to identifying elderly women at nutritional risk and providing appropriate and timely educational interventions are not well documented, yet this is an integral part of daily nursing practice.

VI. CONCLUSION

Currently, there are 38 million Americans who are age 65 and older. Nurses are the single largest group of health care professionals who provide care to these aging members of our society. Nurses are present at the bedside in acute and long-term care facilities, in patient homes, and in community health care centers in overwhelming numbers. Not infrequently, they are either the only or the primary health care provider in rural areas, in underserved urban centers, or in clinics serving vulnerable populations. Nutrition screening, assessment, intervention, and education are an essential and daily part of their professional nursing care practice. This role will become even more important as the numbers of elderly increase and they are faced with predicted limitations in federal health care assistance, rising health care costs, and new measures of health care rationing. These constraints will inevitably have consequences for elder nutrition as elders and their families try to balance the increasing financial demands for obtaining health care. Heitkemper and Jarrett[91] described the roles nurse scientists have played in advancing knowledge that has contributed to improving nutritional care services to the elderly. They emphasize the continuing challenges facing nurse scientists in their efforts to document the effectiveness of nutritional interventions and to move forward the nursing research agenda that supports developments in technology, changing care environments, and emergence of advanced nursing roles in directing nutritional support therapies. Nurses need to join other health care providers to advocate for nutritional services, evaluate nutrition-focused programs, assess nutritional outcomes, and investigate patterns of nutritional care and costs. If the goal of multidisciplinary team efforts is to provide optimal nutrition to older persons, nurses have the professional knowledge, skills, and realistic appreciation of nutrition-related health care needs of elderly persons to make unique and meaningful contributions.

REFERENCES

1. NSI, A Consensus Conference, sponsored by the Nutrition Screening Initiative, *Report of Nutrition Screening 1: Toward a Common View*, Washington, D.C. The Nutrition Screening Initiative, April 8-10, 1991.
2. Mowe, M. and Bohmer, T., The prevalence of undiagnosed protein-calorie undernutrition in a population of hospitalized elderly patients, *J. Am. Geriatric. Soc.*, 39, 1089, 1994.
3. Mowe, M., Bohmer, T., and Kindt, E., Reduced nutritional status in an elderly population (>70y) is probable before disease and possibly contributes to the development of disease, *Am. J. Clin. Nutr.*, 59, 317, 1994.
4. Sullivan, D., Risk factors for early hospital readmission in a select population of geriatric rehabilitation patients: The significance of nutritional status, *J. Am. Geriatr. Soc.*, 40, 792, 1992.
5. Mason, J.B., The pervasive nature of nutritional issues: The need for increased awareness, *Gerontologist,* 37, 277, 1997.
6. Morrisson, S., Feeding the elderly population, *Nurs. Clin. North Am.*, 32(4), 791, 1997.
7. Bankhead, R.R., Integration of nutrition screening into case management practice, *Nursing Case Management,* 4(3), 1999.
8. McMahon, K., Decker, G., and Sottery, F.D., Integrating proactive nutritional assessment in clinical practice to prevent complications and cost, *Semin. Oncol.,* 25, 20, 1998.
9. American Dietetic Association. ADA's definitions for nutrition screening and assessment, *J. American Dietetic Association*, 94, 838, 1994.
10. Evans-Stoner, N., Nutrition assessment. A practical approach, *Nurs. Clin. North Am.*, 32(4), 637, 1997.
11. Nutrition Screening Initiative. *Nutrition Screening Manual for Professionals Caring for Elder Americans*, Nutrition Screening Initiative, Washington, DC., 1991
12. Dwyer, J.T., Screening Older Americans' Nutritional Health: Current Practices and Future Possibilities, Washington, D.C. The Nutrition Screening Initiative, 1991.
13. Quinn, M.E., Johnson, M.A., Poon, L.W., Martin, P., and Nickols-Richardson, S.M., Factors of nutritional health-seeking behaviors, *Aging Health*, 9(1), 90, 1997.
14. Detsky, A.S., McLaughlin, J.R., Baker, J.P., et al. What is subjective global assessment of nutritional status? *JPEN J. Parenter. Enteral. Nutr.*, 11, 8, 1987.
15. Kovacevich, D.S., Boney, A.R., Braunschweig, C.L., et al. Nutrition risk classification: A reproducible and valid tool for nurses, *Nutr. Clin. Prac.*, 12, 20, 1997.
16. Kresevic, D.M. and Mezey, M., Assessment of function: Critically important to acute care of elders, The NICHE Faculty, *Geriatr. Nurs.*, 18, 216, 1997.
17. Simon, L.J., and Russell, C., Impact of the physiologic changes associated with aging on nutrition assessment, *Support Line,* 20(3), 3, 1998.
18. North American Nursing Diagnoses Association, NANDA nursing diagnoses: definitions and classifications, 1997-1998, NANDA, 1996.
19. McCloskey, J. and Bulechek, G., *Nursing Interventions Classification (NIC)*, St. Louis, MO: Mosby, 1992.
20. Norberg, A. and Athlin, E., Eating problems in severely demented patients: Issues and ethical dilemmas. *Nurs. Clin. North Am.*, 24, 789, 1989.

21. Horner, J., Massey, E., and Brazer, S., Aspiration in bilateral stroke patients, *Neurology*, 40(11), 1686, 1990.
22. Johnson, B., Castell, J., and Castell, D., Swallowing and esophagal function in Parkinson's disease, *Am. J. Gastroenterol.*, 90(1), 1741, 1995.
23. Maat, M.T. and Tandy, L., Impaired swallowing. In M. Maas, K. Buckwalter, and M. Hardy, (Eds.), *Nursing Diagnoses and Interventions for the Elderly*, 106, 1991.
24. Wheeler, D., Communication and swallowing problems in the frail older person, *Topics in Geriatric Rehabilitation*, 11(2), 11, 1995.
25. McHale, J.M., Phipps, M.A., Horvath, K., and Schmelz J., Expert nursing knowledge in the care of patients at risk of impaired swallowing, *Image Nurs. Scholarship*, 30(2), 137, 1998.
26. Johnson, D., Anderson, C., and Kosek, S., A tool for screening patients for oral-pharyngeal dysphagia in a medical-surgical intensive care unit, presented at the 4th Multidisciplinary Symposium on Dysphagia, Johns Hopkins University Hospital, Baltimore, MD, 1992.
27. Roberton, B.J., Geriatric nutrition support in subacute-care facilities, *Support Line*, 20(3), 8, 1998.
28. McCloskey, J.C., and Bulechek, J.M., Teaching: Prescribed diet in *Nursing Interventions Classification (NIC)*: Iowa Intervention Project, Mosby, St. Louis, 2nd Ed., 1996.
29. Glick, O.J., Interventions related to activity and movement. In G.M. Bulechek and J.C. McCloskey (Eds.), Symposium on Nursing Interventions, *Nurs. Clin. North Am.*, 27(2), 541, 1992.
30. Baker, D., Assessment and management of impairments in swallowing, *Nurs. Clin. North Am.*, 28(4), 793, 1993.
31. Goodwin, R., Prevention of aspiration: A research-based protocol, *Dimensions Crit. Care Nurs.*, 15(2), 58, 1996.
32. Rankin, J., The nursing diagnosis: Swallowing, impaired and bedside assessment of swallowing in neurologically involved care, *J. Neurosci. Nurs.*, 24(2), 117, 1992.
33. Larson, E., Illness causing dementia in the very elderly, *New Engl. J. Med.*, 328, 203, 1993.
34. Alzheimer's Association. What Does the Future Hold? National Program to Conquer Alzheimer's Disease, Chicago, Alzheimer's Association, 1991.
35. Cohen, D., Dementia, depression, and nutritional status, *Primary Care*, 21(1), 107, 1994.
36. Sanders, H.N., Hoffman, S., and Lund, C.A., Feeding strategy for dependent eaters, *J. Am. Dietet. Assoc.*, 92(11), 1992.
37. Watson, R. and Deary, I.J., Measuring feeding difficult in patients with demential multivariate analysis of feeding problems, nursing intervention and indicators of feeding difficulty, *J. Adv. Nurs.*, 20, 283, 1994.
38. Van Ort, S. and Phillips, L.R., Feeding nursing home residents with Alzheimer's disease, *Geriatr. Nurs.*, 13(5), 249, 1992.
39. Van Ort, S. and Phillips, L.R., Nursing interventions to promote functional feeding, *J. Gerontol. Nurs.*, 21(10), 36, 1995.
40. Clarke, D.M., Wahlqvist, M.L., and Strauss, B.J.G., Undereating and undernutrition in old age: Integrating bio-psychosocial aspects, *Age Ageing*, 27, 527, 1998.
41. Unosson, M., Ek, A.C., Bjurulf, P., and Larsson, J., Demographical, sociomedical and physical characteristics in relation to malnutrition in geriatric patients, *J. Adv. Nurs.*, 16, 1406, 1991.
42. McWhirter, J.P. and Pennington, C.R., Incidence and recognition of malnutrition in hospital, *Br. Med. J.*, 308, 945, 1994.
43. Incalzi, R.A., Capparella, O., Gemma, A., Landi, F., Pagano, F., Cipriani, L., and Cardonin, P., Inadequate caloric intake: A risk factor for mortality of geriatric patients in the acute-care hospital, *Age Aging*, 27, 303, 1998.
44. Larsson, J., Unosson, M., Ek, A.-C., Nilsson, K., Thorslund, S., and Bjurulf, P., Effect of dietary supplement on nutritional status and clinical outcomes in 501 geriatric patients — a randomized study, *Clin. Nutr.*, 9, 179, 1990.
45. Schlenker, E.D., *Nutrition in Aging*, 2nd ed., St. Louis, MO, CV Mosby, 1993.
46. Tripp, F., The use of dietary supplements in the elderly: Current issues and recommendations, *J. Am. Diet. Assoc.*, 19(1), 1, 1997.
47. Guenter, P., Jones, S., and Ericson, M., Enteral nutrition therapy, *Nurs. Clin. North Am.*, 32(4), 651, 1997.
48. Lykins, T.C., Nutrition support clinical pathways, *Nutr. Clin. Prac.*, 11, 16, 1996.

49. Goff, K., Enteral and parenteral nutrition transitioning from hospital to home, *Nurs. Case Management*, 3(2), 67, 1998.
50. Roe, D.A., Medications and nutrition in the elderly, *Primary Care*, 21(1), 1994.
51. Hussey, L.C., Overcoming the clinical barriers of low literacy and medication non-compliance among the elderly, *J. Gerontol. Nurs.*, 17(3), 77, 1991.
52. Kresevic, D.M., Counsell, S.R., Covinsky, K., Palmer, R., Landefeld, C.S., Holder, C., and Beeler, J., A patient-centered model of acute care for elders, *Nurs. Clin. North Am.*, 33(3), 515, 1998.
53. Francis, D., Fletcher, K., and Simon, L.J., The geriatric resource nurse model of care. A vision for the future, *Nurs. Clin. North Am.,* 33(3), 481, 1998.
54. Sager, M.A., Franke, T., Inouye, S.K., et al., Functional outcomes of acute medical illness and hospitalization in older persons, *Arch. Intern. Med.*, 256, 645, 1996.
55. Hirsch, C.H., Sommers, L., Olsen, A., et al., The natural history of functional morbidity in hospitalized older patients, *J. Am. Geriatr. Soc.*, 38, 1296, 1990.
56. Winograd, C.H., Kindenberger, E.E., Chavez, C.M., et al., Identifying hospitalized older patients at varying risk for physical performance decline: A new approach, *J. Am. Geriatr. Soc.*, 45, 604, 1997.
57. Creditor, M.C., Hazards of hospitalization of the elderly, *Ann. Intern. Med.*, 118, 219, 1993.
58. Watson, R., Nutrition standards and the older adult, Guest editorial, *J. Adv. Nurs.*, 20, 205, 1994.
59. Kayser-Jones, J., and Schell, E., The effect of staffing on the quality of care at mealtime, *Nurs. Outlook*, 45(2), 64, 1997.
60. Johnson, R.M., Smiciklas-Wright, H., Soucy, I.M., and Rizzo, J.A., Nutrient intake of nursing-home residents receiving pureed foods or a regular diet, *J. Am. Geriatr. Soc.*, 43, 344, 1995.
61. Groher, M.E. and McKaig, T.N., Dysphagia and dietary levels in skilled nursing facilities, *J. Am. Geriatr. Soc.*, 43, 528, 1995.
62. Cluskey, M.M. The use of texture-modified diets among the institutionalized elderly, *J. Nutr. Eld.*, 9, 3, 1989.
63. Siebens, H., Trupe, E., Siebens, A., Cook, F., Anshen, S. Hanauer, R., et al. Correlates and consequences of eating dependency in institutionalized elderly, *J. Am. Geriatr. Soc.*, 34, 192, 1986.
64. Burns, B.J., Wagner, H.R., Taube, J.E., et al. Mental health service use by the elderly in nursing homes, *Am. J. Public Health*, 83, 331, 1993.
65. Buhler-Willkerson, K., Naylor, M.D., Holt, S.W., and Rinke, L.T. An alliance for academic home care: Integrating research, education, and practice, *Nurs. Outlook*, March/April, 77, 1998.
66. Freedman, V. Long-term admissions to home health agencies: A life table analysis, *Gerontologist*, 39, 1, 1999.
67. Shoaf, L.R. and Mitchell, M.C., Nutrition for the older adult, *Topics Clin. Nutr.*, June, 70, 1996.
68. TenHave, T.R., Van Horn, B., Kumanyika, S., Askov, E., Matthews, Y., and Adams-Campbell, L., Literacy assessment in a cardiovascular nutrition education setting, *Patient Educ. Counseling*, 31, 139, 1997.
69. Kirsh, I.S., Jungeblut, A., Jenkins, L., and Kolstad, A., *Adult Literacy in America: A first look at the Results of the National Adult Literacy Survey*, Washington, DC, U.S. Government Printing Office, 1993.
70. Davis, T.C., Long, S.W., Jackson, R.I., Mayeau, E.J., and Crouch, M.A., Rapid estimate of adult literacy in medicine. A shortened screening instrument, *Fam. Med.*, 25, 391, 1993.
71. Parker, R., Baker, D., Williams, M., and Nurss, J., The test of functional health literacy in adults (TOFHLA): A new instrument for measuring patients' literacy skills, *J. Gen. Intern. Med.*, 10, 537, 1995.
72. Doak, C.C., Doak, L.G., and Root, J.H., Teaching Patients with Low-Literacy Skills, 2nd ed., Philadelphia, PA, JB Lippincott, 1995.
73. Weiss, B.D., Reed, R.L., and Kligman, E.W., Literacy skills and communication methods of low-income older persons, *Patient Education and Counseling*, 25, 109, 1995.
74. AMC Cancer Research Center, Beyond the Brochure: Alternative Approaches to Effective Health Communication, Denver, CO, AMC Cancer Research Center, 1993.
75. Gagliano, M.E., A literature review on the efficacy of video in patient education, *J. Med. Ed.*, 63, 785, 1988.
76. McLaughlin, G.H., SMOG — Grading: New readability formula, *J. Reading*, 12, 639, 1969.

77. Davis, T.C., et al. The gap between patient reading comprehension and the readability of patient education materials, *J. Family Practice*, 31(5), 533, 1990.

78. Weinrich, S.P., Weinrich, M.C., Boyd, M.D., Atwood, J., and Cervenka, B., Teaching older adults by adapting for aging changes, *Cancer Nurs.*, 17(6), 494, 1994.

79. Welch-McCaffrey, D., To teach or not to teach? Overcoming barriers to patient education in geriatric oncology, *Oncol. Nurs. Forum.*, 13, 25, 1986.

80. Weinrich, S.P., Boyd, M., and Nussbaum, J., Teaching the elderly: Adaptations for aging changes, *J. Gerontol. Nurs.*, 15, 17, 1989.

81. Weinrich, S.P. and Boyd, M., Education in the elderly: Adapting and evaluating teaching tools, *J. Gerontol. Nurs.*, 18, 15, 1992.

82. Dellasega, C., Clark, D., McCreary, D., Helmuth, A., and Schan, P., Nursing process: Teaching elderly clients, *J. Gerontol. Nurs.*, 29, 31, 1994.

83. Johnston, L.J. and Gueldner, S.H., Remember when ...? Using mnemonics to boost memory in the elderly, *J. Gerontol. Nurs.*, 15(8), 22.

84. Theis, S.L. and Merritt, S.L., Learning style preferences of elderly coronary artery disease patients, *Educ. Gerontol.*, 18, 677, 1992.

85. Theis, S.L., Using previous knowledge to teaching elderly clients, *J. Gerontol. Nurs.*, 17(8), 34, 1991.

86. Theis, S.L. and Merritt, S.L., A learning model to guide research and practice for teaching of elder clients, *Nurs. Health Care*, 15(9), 464, 1994.

87. Moore, S.A., Educating the faculty and the patient about nutrition, *Primary Care,* 21(1), 69, 1994.

88. Sidenvall, B., Fjellstrom, C., and Ek, A.C., The meal situation in geriatric care — intentions and experiences, *J. Adv. Nurs.*, 20, 613, 1994.

89. Leininger, M., Transcultural care diversity and universality: A theory of nursing, *Nurs. Health Care*, 6, 209, 1985.

90. Weinrich, S.W., Weinrich, M.C. Stromborg, M., Boyd, M.D., and Weiss, H., Using elderly educator to increase colorectal cancer screening, *Gerontologist*, 33, 401, 1993.

91. Heitkemper, M. and Jarrett, M., Research issues in nutrition support, *Nurs. Clin. North Am.*, 32(4), 755, 1997.

92. Chernoff, R., Nutritional needs of elderly women, in Krummel, D., Dris-Etherton, P.M., *Nutrition in Women's Health*, Gaithersberg, MD, Aspen, 1996.

93. Yen, P., When food doesn't taste good anymore*, Geriatri. Nurs.*, 44, 1996.

94. Bonnel, Blaser, W., Meal management strategies of older adult women, *J. Gerontol. Nurs.*, 41, 1999.

95. Yen, P., Focus on women's nutrition, *Geriatr. Nurs.*, 15(4), 225, 1994.

96. Small, S.P., Best, D.G., and Hustins, K.A., Energy and nutrient intakes of independently living elderly women, *Can. J. Nurs. Res.*, 26(1), 71.

97. Norberg, A., Athlin, E., and Winbald, B., A model for the assessment of eating problems in patients with Parkinson's disease, *J. Adv. Nurs.*, 12, 473, 1987.

98. Gaspar, P.M., Water intake of nursing home residents, *J. Gerontol. Nurs.*, April, 23, 1999.

99. Larsson, J., Unosson, M., Ek, A.C., et al. Effect of dietary supplement on nutritional status and clinical outcome in 501 geriatric patients — a randomized study, *Clin. Nutr.*, 9, 179, 1990.

100. Lipschitz, D.A., Nutrition, in Cassel, C.K., Cohen, H.J., Larson, E.B., Meier, D.E., Resnick, N.M., Rubenstein, L.Z., and Sorensen, L.B., Eds., *Geriatric Medicine,* New York, Springer, 801, 1997.

101. Kayser-Jones, J., Mealtime in nursing homes: The importance of individualized care, *J. Gerontol. Nurs.*, 22(3), 26, 1996.

102. Evans-Stoner, N., Guidelines for care of the patient on home nutrition support, *Nurs. Clin. North Am.,* 32(4), 769, 1997.

103. Poss, J., Providing culturally competent care: Is there a role for health promoters? *Nurs. Outlook*, 47, 30, 1999.

104. Nurses Improving Care to the Hospitalized Elderly (NICHE) Project Faculty. Geriatric models of care: Which one's right for your institution? *Am. J. Nurs.*, 94, 21, 1994.

12 Overweight and Obesity in the Aged

Debashish Kumar Dey and Bertil Steen

CONTENTS

I. INTRODUCTION

Despite certain controversies regarding the relative epidemiological and clinical significance of obesity in relation to morbidity and mortality at different ages, the fact remains that obesity is a very common type of malnutrition among the elderly in developed countries. Most authors agree that the definition of obesity is "too much body fat in relation to body weight." The discrepancies concern the definition of "too much." Thus, practical cut-off limits of, e.g., body mass index (BMI), for a diagnosis of overweight and obesity are difficult to assess, and they may be different in different population and age groups. Furthermore, it should be borne in mind that body weight and BMI are not necessarily good estimates of body fat, since they comprise also body cell mass, intra- and extracellular body water, and fat-free extracellular solids, such as the calcium content of bone mass.

The problem and management of obesity in individuals are, in many respects, much the same whether the obese individuals are middle-aged or old. In this respect, the relevance of a special review on obesity at higher age groups can be questioned. However, there are differences that justify separate considerations in the elderly, such as the body composition and the different impact of body weight and BMI as risk indicators and risk factors in higher age groups. The group of elderly — defined as 65 years of age or older — is a very heterogenous one regarding such factors as prevalance of disease, socioeconomic conditions, and age *per se* with an age span of more than 40 years. Therefore, the grouping together of these heterogenous groups of people can also be questioned.

Recent longitudinal studies[1,2] have shown that many functional parameters remain rather constant through middle life until age 70 to 75, where a more pronounced decrease can be seen. To this might be added that there is an increasing variability in functional capacity among individuals during life up to at least age 75. From these points of view the classification of elderly people into "young elderly" (age 65 to 75) and "old elderly" (over 75) seems, therefore, to bear a physiological meaning. On the other hand, "young elderly" might not be classified as "elderly" at all.

The literature on overweight and obesity is abundant. Excellent up-to-date reviews on selected topics can be found in the proceedings from the international congresses on obesity and from other reviewers.[3-11] The aim of the present chapter is to review some aspects on overweight and obesity of special gerontological and geriatric interest.

II. EPIDEMIOLOGY

Obesity (BMI over 30 kg/m^2) is a major nutritional condition and a public health problem in many parts of the world, irrespective of developed and developing countries. This is true also regarding overweight (BMI between 25 and 30 kg/m^2) and morbidity, although to a lesser degree, but of lower significance regarding mortality. The prevalence of obesity and overweight varies considerably between countries and between regions within countries. For example, the overall prevalence of obesity varies from 7% in France to 33% in Brazil, and the trends in developed as well as developing countries suggest that the rates of obesity are increasing.[12] The prevalence of obesity among older persons is also growing, partly since the percentage of older individuals is increasing worldwide, but it has only recently become a recognized public health problem in this population.[13,14]

At least one third of North Americans are obese, and the prevalence of obesity as well as overweight has increased rapidly in the U.S. and other developed countries during the past decades.[13,15,16] A comparison between the National Health Examination Survey (NHES I: 1960–62) and the National Health and Nutrition Examination Surveys (NHANES I: 1971–74; NHANES II: 1976–80; NHANES III: 1988–94) in the U.S. show a large increase of obesity between NHANES II (14.5%) and NHANES III (22.5%).[17] Almost one third of adult Canadians are at increased risk of disability, disease, and premature death due to obesity.[18]

Obesity is relatively common in Europe, especially in southern and eastern countries, and recent studies from repeated surveys suggest that the prevalence of obesity has been increasing during the past 15 years.[19] The average prevalence of obesity among Europeans between 1983 and 1986 was about 15% in men with a range from 7% in Gothenburg, Sweden to 22% in Lithuania. In women, the prevalence figure was 22%, with a range from 9% to 45% in the same locations.[20] It is estimated that more than half of adults aged 35 to 65 living in Europe are either overweight or obese, overweight thereby being more common among men than women, but obesity being more common among women.[21] Numerical values for prevalence of obesity are highly dependent on the criteria used to identify the condition and its gradations of severity. Recently, the prevalance of body mass index of 30 kg/m^2 or more in U.S. adults was compared with findings in adults in the U.K., France, the Netherlands, and Italy, the differences of prevalence ratios ranging from approximately 1.5 (U.S. vs. U.K.) to 3.0 (U.S. vs. France).[22]

III. BODY WEIGHT

Some general trends in body weight along with aging have been found, including an increase of body weight in middle age[23] followed by a decrease at older ages.[24,25] In a 25-year longitudinal population study of individuals from age 70 to 95 in Gothenburg, Sweden, it was found that body weight decreased 3.2 and 5.1 kg in males and females, respectively, during this period of time.[25] This decreasing trend can be explained partly by the physiological changes in body composition with age that influences the loss of body weight due to decrease in cell mass through cell death, impaired function of surviving cells,[26] decrease of body fat and body water,[27] and partly by changes in internal organs, bone mass, skeletal muscles, and lean body mass in elderly subjects.[26,28] However, a distinct gender difference has also been observed in this pattern where weight loss corresponded more to a loss of body cell mass in males than in females, and more to a decrease of body fat in females.

When talking about body weight, one should also keep in mind the secular trend of body composition, i.e., earlier generations being physically smaller than recent ones.[29] In a cohort comparison study from the gerontological and geriatric population studies in Gothenburg, Sweden – the H 70 study[1,30] — with five representative samples of 70-, 75-, and 79-year-old individuals born within a time span of 21 years, it has been found that individuals in the later-born cohorts were 1 to 2 cm taller and 1.5 to 6.3 kg heavier than the earlier-born cohorts.[31] The reason for that may be, at least partly, childhood nutrition and living conditions, changed food habits, upward social mobility, and less physical activity in later-born cohorts.[31]

IV. BODY FAT

The measurement or estimation of body fat can be performed in several ways.[32-34] These include cadaver analyses[35] and methods using absorption of fat-soluble gases such as krypton.[36] Isotope dilution methods to calculate total body water [37] and whole body potassium counting[38] to estimate body cell mass[32] can be used to estimate body fat.[32,39] The measurement of subcutaneous fat thickness with roentgenography[40] and calipers[41] is frequently performed. Furthermore, sophisticated techniques such as neutron activation or dual-photon (or X-ray) absorptiometry, computed tomography or nuclear magnetic resonance imaging are available for the determination of specific body components and the assessment of regional fat distribution.[42-44] The bioelectric impedance analysis[45,46] has substantially improved the estimation of total body fat, and nowadays body density may be considered as a "gold standard," from which fat and fat-free body mass can be calculated.[47] For estimating regional adiposity and adipose tissue distribution, several anthropometric methods have also been found useful, i.e., waist circumference,[48] waist to hip circumference ratio,[10,47,49,50] waist circumference to height ratio,[51] and subscapular skinfold.[47]

The correlations between simple anthropometric parameters and body fat are usually rather high in the elderly. In a Swedish population study of 70-year-olds,[34] it was shown that such correlations to body fat estimated with a combined approach of total body water measurement using tritiated water and whole body potassium counting were higher in females than in males regarding body weight, waist girth, upper arm girth, thigh skinfold, and body cell mass. Regarding subscapular and suprailiac skinfolds, the correlations were of the same order of magnitude in both sexes. The correlation coefficients between body fat and body weight, waist girth, and subscapular and triceps skinfold, respectively, ranged from $r = 0.47$ (triceps skinfold in males) to $r = 0.83$ (body weight in females) in that study. The correlation coefficient between body fat and the difference between body weight and "ideal body weight"[52] was $r = 0.71$ in males and $r = 0.91$ in females. A multiple regression analysis with body fat as the dependent variable revealed body weight as the most important independent variable in both sexes.

Energy intake and expenditure vary markedly between different populations, which means that the average amount of body fat — in absolute as well as in relative terms — varies accordingly. In the above-mentioned Swedish study of body composition,[34] the average percentage of body fat relative to body weight at age 70 was 16.1 and 26.6 for males and females, respectively. As judged from comparisons of body weight/height measurements and skinfold measurements between Sweden on the one hand and the U.K. and U.S. on the other, Swedish people seem to have a lower amount of body fat than in the other countries mentioned.[53-55]

A longitudinal population study of the same subjects from age 70 to age 79 in Gothenburg, Sweden[56] showed that the absolute amount of body fat did not change in any noteworthy way between age 70 and 75, but decreased in an order of magnitude of 2 kg between age 75 and 79 in females. However, the percentage of body fat to body weight seems to increase to about age 70 to 75 as judged from cross-sectional studies.[34]

It is well known that very old people are thin. Many clinicians have interpreted this fact as caused by a selective mortality of obese people. However, at least to some degree, it seems that the explanation is a decreasing degree of fatness in the same individuals. This decrease seems to start somewhat earlier (age 75) in females than in males. This fact has an obvious bearing when discussing the diagnosis of overweight and obesity, and indications for the therapy of obesity in the elderly. Some age-dependent changes have been described concerning the distribution of body fat. Skerlj and collaborators[57] found that subcutaneous fat was deposited more on the trunk than on the extremities in old compared to young women. Furthermore, Durnin and Womersley[55] described an increase of deep adipose tissue compared with subcutaneous fat with age. A centralized distribution of adipose tissue, especially in the trunk, is more hazardous in young and middle-aged men than in the elderly.[58]

V.   DEFINITIONS OF OVERWEIGHT AND OBESITY

According to Keys and collaborators,[59] a common clinically and epidemiologically useful way to express the degree of overweight and obesity is the use of weight/height indices of different kinds. Bray[60] defined overweight and obesity according to BMI calculated as the ratio of body weight in kilograms divided by the square of the height in meters (Quetelet index), where individuals with a BMI value between 25 and 30 kg/m^2 were classified as overweight and those with 30 kg/m^2 and above were obese, irrespective of age and sex.

The World Health Organization (WHO) recommended an adult range of desirable weights for heights of BMI 22.0 kg/m^2 (20.1–25.0 kg/m^2) for men and 20.8 kg/m^2 (18.7–23.8 kg/m^2) for women.[61] It is well recognized that age modifies the risks associated with BMI and certain diseases, but whether different cut-offs are more appropriate for individuals aged 70 or more is uncertain.[62] Andres and collaborators[63] suggested a modification of the Metropolitan desirable weight tables so that age is also taken into account. The American Committee on Diet and Health in its 1989 report stated that BMIs of less than 24 kg/m^2 and more than 29 kg/m^2 are undesirable for individuals over 65 years of age.[64] In a recent review, Beck and Ovesen [65] indicated that the optimal range of BMI for elderly people is increasing from 20–25 kg/m^2 to 24–29 kg/m^2, and have suggested for a new cut-off points for the elderly to be used in clinical practice.[65]

However, there are certain limitations to using BMI values for classifying obesity and overweight, particularly in the elderly. For example, BMI cannot distinguish between the contribution to body weight of fat tissue and that of muscle, bone, and water.[4,27] This problem is more pronounced in elderly, who tend to experience a redistribution of body fat from subcutaneous to intra-abdominal and intramuscular sites.[29] The sensitivity of BMI cutpoints with respect to body fatness decreases with age, since the same values of BMI correspond to different amounts of fat and fat-free mass at different ages, and the use of a fixed cutpoint for all age groups results in a "differential misclassification bias."[10]

VI.   RISKS OF OVERWEIGHT AND OBESITY

A. Morbidity

The risks of overweight and obesity in the elderly are still under debate. It is generally, agreed that obesity is associated with a number of major conditions such as cardiovascular diseases, i.e., coronary heart disease[50,66-69] and hypertension[44,70,71]; cerebrovascular disease, i.e., stroke[44,70]; diabetes mellitus[44,72-75]; impaired glucose tolerance[76]; gallbladder disease[44]; colorectal and prostate cancer in men[77,78]; renal cell, cervix, endometrial, ovarian, and breast cancer in women.[77,79,80] Evidence has also been found regarding serious consequences of obesity on conditions like cardiac dysfunction, pulmonary problems, digestive diseases, endocrine disorders, obstetric, orthopedic, dermal and immunologic disorders.[81-84] However, considerable inconsistencies have been reported among different age, gender, and ethnic groups for the relationship between obesity and diseases, i.e., coronary heart disease, stroke, diabetes, cancer, etc.[3,5,10,50,80,85-87] Suggested reasons for that are, e.g., misclassification, confounders, unknown protective factors, surrogate risk factors, and the small, short-term studies from which, in most of the cases, conclusions have been drawn.[5,88]

Furthermore, studies on risks of overweight and obesity for developing diseases have been mostly performed in middle-aged or relatively young adults. There is little or no population-based reported data in this regards on subjects aged 70 years and older. An attempt was made to investigate the relationship between baseline BMI values at age 70 and the subsequent incidence of coronary heart disease, stroke, cancer, and diabetes during a 15-year follow-up from age 70 to 85 years [89] with longitudinal cohort data from the gerontological and geriatric population studies in Gothenburg — the H70 study.[1,30] Significant positive trends were found between the quintiles of BMI for the relative risk of coronary heart disease in males, and diabetes in both sexes, where the lowest quintile was used as a reference group. However, a positive but nonsignificant trend was found for the relative risk of stroke in males.[89]

B. Mortality

The relation of obesity to mortality is still somewhat unclear. The well-known Build and Blood pressure Study from 1959[90] describes an almost linear relation between overweight and excess mortality in both sexes starting from 10% overweight. Epidemiologic studies have found four major types of relation between body weight and mortality, namely — no relation,[91-93] direct association,[94-96] inverse association,[97] and a U-shaped or J-shaped realtion.[23,63,98-102]

However, these studies are mostly from middle-aged people[103] and substantial differences have been found between body weight and mortality relationship among the elderly compared with that in younger adults.[104] A significant linear relationship was found between body weight and mortality in males from age 70 to 95 years after adjustment for serum cholesterol level, smoking, and cancer, but such a trend was significant for females only from age 70 to 80 years[105] within our gerontological and geriatric population studies in Gothenburg, Sweden.[1,30]

It is thus necessary to clarify whether age modifies the relation between body weight and mortality.[106] A Norwegian study by Waaler[107] found that the U-shaped mortality curve for weight flattened out with advancing age, and from 80 years or older the curve was almost horizontal. An increase in mortality risk for low weight with age has been interpreted as suggesting that a modest weight gain with increasing age may be protective and desirable.[7]

However, results from crude relation analyses between overweight and mortality have to be interpreted with great caution. They can certainly not tell us about the impact of obesity on morbidity; also, the impact on mortality may be obscure because of possible confounding factors, which can also be different in different populations. Several reviewers have indicated some methodological limitations, including the failure to control smoking, inappropriate control of physiologic and metabolic effects of obesity, and the failure to eliminate early mortality from the analysis.[4,6]

VII.   ETIOLOGICAL FACTORS

As pointed out by several leading authors in the field such as Björntorp[108] and Bray,[109] the understanding of obesity requires knowledge of the many different etiological and pathophysiological aspects of this condition. Bray suggested an anatomical classification of the syndromes of obesity in generalized or diffuse accumulation of fat and localized fat accumulation. This has no special geriatric implication. He also suggested an etiological classification into hypothalamic, endocrine, nutritional, physical-inactivity-induced, predominantly genetic-, and drug-induced obesity, where some have an obvious geriatric importance (i.e., the high fat nutritional, the physical inactivity, and the drug-induced obesity types of Bray).

The nutrient density of the food is especially important in the elderly, who on the average constitute a low-energy consumer group. The major explanation for the reduction of energy expenditure with age is probably the decreasing number of cells in the organs, loss of metabolizing tissue, and reduced physical activity,[110] although some intracellular aged-induced changes on the enzyme level might also be responsible. In the Baltimore longitudinal study of males,[111] the average total energy expenditure amounted to 2811 kcal/11.8 MJ and 1924 kcal/8.2 MJ at age 30 and 80, respectively.

It was shown in a study of three cohorts of 70-year-olds in Gothenburg, Sweden in 1971, 1981, and 1993, respectively, that food choice changed markedly over a 22-year perspective.[112] For example, sugar and potato intake had decreased, and intake of rice, pasta, and fresh vegetables increased. Energy intake seemed, however, to be quite stable during the period. Thus, food choice seemed to have changed more than nutrient intake, and many of these changes were due to an obvious trend of increasing diversity.[112] There is no reason to believe that elderly people are more conservative regarding their food choices.[113] Ordinary food in most industrialized countries has a low nutrient density because of a high proportion of fat and refined sugar. Therefore, intake of the same type of food in old age as earlier in life might obviously give either too much energy, too few essential nutrients, or both.

The energy "recommendations" of the 10th Recommended Dietary Allowances[114] for the age group 51 years and over (2300 kcal/9.7 MJ and 1900 kcal/7.6 MJ for males and females, respectively) are obviously too difficult to apply to such a heterogeneous group of individuals as the elderly. Body weight, among many other things, varies widely among age groups above 50 and among different populations. Thus, as an example, average body weight at age 70, 75, and 79 in a Swedish population[56] were 73, 70, and 69 kg for males, and 67, 65, and 63 kg for females, which for females means much more than the reference woman aged 51 or over of the Recommended Dietary Allowances.[114]

In this context it is important to point out that malnutrition means undernutrition, overnutrition, or both at the same time, as undernutrition of essential nutrients can be combined with overnutrition of fat, refined sugar, and energy. Physical inactivity is a not uncommon cause of overweight and obesity, as shown in many studies such as the seven-country study of Keys and collaborators.[115] This is a general phenomenon and not related to age; however, obese subjects are significantly less active than non-obese people.[116] Physical inactivity in the elderly, however, may — more than in younger age groups — be the result of not only sedentary occupation but also of physical handicap.

Social factors are of importance to obesity in the aged for several reasons. Especially in females, the socioeconomic state is inversely related to the prevalence of obesity.[109,117] Furthermore, although many elderly suffering from loneliness have a bad appetite, there is also a tendency in the opposite direction with an overrepresentation of increasing appetite in lonely elderly as judged from a Swedish study.[118] This has also been found by others.[119]

VIII.   OTHER COMPLICATIONS OF OBESITY FOR HEALTH CARE AND NURSING OF THE ELDERLY

Some special problems of advanced obesity are diagnostic difficulties when examining neck, thorax, and abdomen. Jugular venous pressure has been reported to be difficult to assess because of cervical adiposity.[120] The apex beat is not easily felt in obese patients, and heart sounds and murmurs are muffled.[121] The amplitude of precordial T-waves in the electrocardiogram has been reported to be reduced to half the normal.[122] These diagnostic difficulties are common in all age groups, but add to already existing diagnostic difficulties in elderly patients (for review see Steen[123]).

The practical handling of obese elderly patients in, for instance, long-term care medicine is often a difficult task. Changing position from bed to chair and even walking may be difficult, and must be looked upon as potential hazards for falls, the result of which can be a fractured hip due to co-existing osteoporosis.

Intertrigo is commonly found on various parts of the body and is often difficult to treat effectively. Toileting is difficult especially together with co-existing urinary incontinence — a very common condition in geriatric medicine.[124] Pressure sores, hypostatic congestion of the lungs, and leg vein thrombosis are more likely to develop in obese patients if they have to stay in bed for some time.[121]

IX.   INDICATIONS FOR TREATMENT

Treatment of obesity in elderly patients does not require methods other than those that are used in other age groups. However, many existing methods are not applicable or feasible to elderly people, and only a few, therefore, remain to be discussed in this context.

As was mentioned earlier, the indications for treatment might be different in the higher age groups, the tendency being generally to have more rigorous indications before intervening. It has been found that thinner older people who lost weight and heavier people who gained weight showed increased risk of coronary heart disease compared with people with stable weight in old age.[69] This is especially true in the highest age groups — above age 75 or 80 — where there seems to be an ongoing decrease of body fat and body weight apparently related to normal aging.[56]

Surgical methods to treat obesity seem to be indicated in the elderly only in exceptional cases. Nonsurgical methods include jaw fixation, intragastric balloons, diets, exercise, behavior modification, drugs, and hypnosis.[125] The National Board of Health and Welfare withdrew anorectic drugs from Sweden in 1980. The reasons given were that the efficiency of the drugs was doubtful, that there were indications that overprescription occurred, and that the drugs were abused.[125] Therefore, of the methods mentioned, those of choice in geriatric medicine are obviously to try changes of diet, physical activity, and sometimes behavior. An attractive principle especially in elderly obese patients is the use of large amounts of dietary fiber as an adjunct in the treatment.[126] A rather slow, progressive weight loss is preferable, especially in the elderly.[127] A daily reduction of 500 kcal can be mentioned as an optimal example. Acute intermittent fasts should be avoided in these age groups. Most fat diets are unbalanced and therefore to be avoided in the elderly, because of the need for high-quality food in these low-energy consumers.

X.   PREVENTION

When dealing with prevention in the elderly it has to be borne in mind that the elderly population comprises a very heterogenous group, and several factors of importance for prevention are closely interrelated in this age group, such as psychosocial factors, physical activity, and dietary intake.[128] It has been shown from a study of 68-year-old Swedish men that overweight, obesity, low physical activity, and high alcohol consumption were more common among those men with inadequate diets.[129] Furthermore, low social anchorage, low physical activity, and high body mass index were independent risk indicators of inadequate dietary habits in that population. Thus, social network and social support have clear relationships to health and to the outcome of preventive measures.[128] Physical activity is of special importance in the treatment of overweight in the elderly, and dietary advice in old age should always include recommendations for increased physical activity.[128] Since elderly individuals are, on average, low-energy consumers and therefore at risk of having low intake of essential nutrients, an increase in physical activity, and thereby of energy needs, will improve food and nutrient intake.

Thus, a good "dietary" recommendation in the elderly is to increase physical activity. It is important that physical activity is maintained in the elderly.[130] Exercise should, however, be light to moderate. Every "exercise candidate" should have a thorough physical examination before any exercise program.[131] This is obviously especially true in the higher age groups.

REFERENCES

1. Rinder , L., Roupe, S., Steen, B., and Svanborg, A., 70-year-old people in Gothenburg. A population study in an industrialized Swedish city. I. General design of the study, *Acta Med. Scand.,* 198, 397, 1975.
2. Svanborg, A., Landahl, S., and Mellström, D., Basic issues of health care, in *New Perspectives on Old Age: A Message to Decision Makers.* Thomae, H. and Maddox, G. L., Eds., Springer-Verlag, New York, 1982, 31.
3. Larsson, B., Björntorp, P., and Tibblin, G., The health consequences of moderate obesity, *Int. J. Obes.,* 5, 97, 1981.
4. Manson, J. E., Stampfer, M. J., Hennekens, C. H., and Willett, W. C., Body weight and longevity, a reassessment, *JAMA,* 257, 353, 1987.
5. Sjöström, L. V., Morbidity of severely obese subjects, *Am. J. Clin. Nutr.,* suppl., 55, 508, 1992.
6. Sjöström, L. V., Mortality of severely obese subjects, *Am. J. Clin. Nutr.,* suppl., 55, 516, 1992.
7. Andres, R., Muller, D. C., and Sorkin, J. D., Long-term effects of change in body weight on all-cause mortality, a review, *Ann. Intern. Med.,* 119, 737, 1993.
8. Kushner, R. F., Body weight and mortality, *Nutr. Rev.,* 51, 127, 1993.
9. Williamson, D. F. and Pamuk, E. R., The association between weight loss and increased longevity, a review of the evidence, *Ann. Intern. Med.,* 119, 731, 1993.
10. Baumgartner, R. N., Heymsfield, S.B., and Roche, A. F., Human body composition and the epidemiology of chronic disease, *Obes. Res.,* 3, 73, 1995.
11. Troiano, R. P., Frongillo, E. A., Jr., and Levitsky, D. A., The relationship between body weight and mortality: a quantitative analysis of combined information from existing studies, *Int. J. Obes.,* 20, 63, 1996.
12. Saw, S. M. and Rajan, U., The epidemiology of obesity: a review, *Ann. Acad. Med. Singapore,* 26,489,1997.
13. Dvorak, R., Starling, R. D., Calles-Escandon, J., Sims, E. A., and Poehlman, E. T., Drug therapy for obesity in the elderly, *Drugs Aging,* 11, 338, 1997.
14. Jensen, G. L. and Rogers, J., Obesity in older persons, *J. Am. Diet. Assoc.,* 98, 1308, 1998.
15. Kuczmarski, R. J., Flegal, K. M., Campbell, S. M., and Johnson, C. L., Increasing prevalance of overweight among US adults. The National Health and Nutrition Examination Surveys, 1960 to 1991, *JAMA,* 272, 205, 1994.
16. Solomon, C. G. and Manson, J. E., Obesity and mortality: a review of the epidemiologic data, *Am. J. Clin. Nutr.,* suppl., 66, 1044, 1997.
17. Flegal, K. M., Carroll, M. D., Kuczmarski, R. J., and Johnson, C. L., Overweight and obesity in the United States: prevalence and trends, 1960-1994, *Int. J. Obes. Relat. Metab. Disord.,* 22, 39, 1998.
18. Birmingham, C. L., Muller, J. L., Palepu, A., Spinelli, J. J., and Anis, A. H., The cost of obesity in Canada, *CMAJ,* 160, 483, 1999.
19. Seidell, J. C., Obesity in Europe: scaling an epidemic, *Int. J. Obes. Relat. Metab. Disord.,* suppl., 19, 1, 1995.
20. Seidell, J. C., Time trends in obesity: an epidemiological perspective, *Horm. Metab. Res.,* 29, 155, 1997.
21. Seidell, J. C. and Flegal, K. M., Assessing obesity: classification and epidemiology, *Br. Med. Bull.,* 53, 238, 1997.
22. Van Itallie, T. B., Prevalence of obesity, *Endocrinol. Metab. Clin. North. Am.,* 25, 887, 1996.
23. Cornoni-Huntley, J. C., Harris, T. B., Everett, D. F., Albanes, D., Micozzi, M. S., Miles, T. P., and Feldman, J. J., An overview of body weight of older persons including the impact on mortality. The national health and nutrition examination survey I — epidemiologic follow-up study, *J. Clin. Epidemiol.,* 44, 743, 1991.
24. Going, S., Williams, D., and Lohman, T., Aging and body composition: biological changes and methodological issues, *Exerc. Sport. Sci. Rev.,* 23, 411, 1995.

25. Dey, D. K., Rothenberg, E., Sundh, V., Bosaeus, I., and Steen, B., Height and body weight in the elderly. I. A 25-year longitudinal population study from age 70 to 95, *Eur. J. Clin. Nutr.*, 53, 905, 1999.

26. Munro, H. N., Nutrition and ageing, *Br. Med. Bull.*, 37, 83, 1981.

27. Steen, B., Lundgren, B. K., and Isaksson, B., Body composition at age 70, 75, 79 and 81. A longitudinal population study, in *Nutrition, Immunity and Illness in the Elderly*, Chandra, R. K., Ed., Pergamon Press, New York, 1985, 49.

28. Kuczmarski, R. J., Need for body composition information in elderly subjects, *Am. J. Clin. Nutr.*, 50, 1150, 1989.

29. Borkan, G. A., Hults, D. E., Gerzof, S. G., Robbins, A. H., and Silbert, C. K., Age changes in body composition revealed by computed tomography, *J. Gerontol.*, 38, 673, 1983.

30. Steen, B. and Djurfeldt, H., The gerontological and geriatric population studies in Gothenburg, Sweden, *Z. Gerontol.*, 26, 163, 1993.

31. Dey, D. K., Height and body weight in the elderly. II. A 21-year cohort comparison study in 70-, 75- and 79-year-olds, submitted.

32. Moore, F. D., Olesen, K. M., McMurray, J. D., Parker, H. V., Ball, M. R., and Boyden, C. M., The Body Cell Mass and its Supporting Environment, W. B. Saunders, Philadelphia, 1963.

33. Steinkamp, R. C., Cohen, N. L., Siri, W. E., Sargent, T. W., and Walsh, H. E., Measures of body fat and related factors in normal adults. I. Introduction and methodology, *J. Chron. Dis.*, 18, 1279, 1965.

34. Steen, B., Nutrition in 70-year-olds. Dietary habits and body composition. A report from the population study "70-year-old people in Gothenburg, Sweden," *Näringsforskning,* 21, 201, 1977.

35. Forbes, R. M., Cooper, A. R., and Mitchell, H. H., The composition of the adult human body as determined by chemical analysis, *J. Biol. Chem.*, 203, 359, 1953.

36. Hytten, F. E., Taylor, K., and Taggart, N., Measurement of total body fat in men by absorption of 85 Kr, *Clin. Sci.*, 31, 111, 1966.

37. Lindholm, B., Changes in body composition during long-term treatment with cortisone and anabolic steroids in asthmatic subjects, *Acta Allerg.*, 22, 261, 1967.

38. Sköldborn, H., Arvidsson, B., and Andersson, M., A new whole body monitoring laboratory, *Acta Radiol.*, suppl., 313, 213, 1972.

39. Berg, K. and Isaksson, B., Body composition and nutrition of school children with cerebral palsy, *Acta Paediat. Scand.*, suppl., 204, 41, 1970.

40. Garn, S. M., Roentgenogrammetric determinations of body composition, *Human Biol.*, 29, 337, 1957.

41. Pascale, L. R., Grossman, M. J., Sloane, H. S., and Frankel, T., Correlations between thickness of skin folds and body density in Gothenburg, Sweden. A population study, *Acta Med. Scand.*, suppl., 611, 87, 1955.

42. Lukaski, H. D., Methods for the assessment of human body composition: traditional and new, *Am. J. Clin. Nutr.*, 46, 537, 1987.

43. Heymsfield, S. B., Lichtman, S., Baumgartner, R. N., Wang, J., Kamen, Y., Aliprantis, A., and Pierson, R. N., Jr., Human body composition: comparison of two improved four-compartment models that differ in expense, technical complexity, and radiation exposure, *Am. J. Clin. Nutr.*, 52, 52, 1990.

44. Bray, G. A. and Gray, P. G., Obesity. Part I — pathogenesis, *West. J. Med.*, 149, 429, 1988.

45. Lukaski, H. C., Johnsson, P. E., Bolonchuk, W. W., and Lykken, G. I., Assessment of fat-free mass using bioelectrical impedance measurements of the human body, *Am. J. Clin. Nutr.*, 41, 810, 1985.

46. Steen, B., Bosaeus, I., Elmståhl, S., Galvard, H., Isaksson, I., and Robertsson, E., Body composition in the elderly estimated with an electrical impedance method, *Compr. Gerontol. A.*, 1, 102, 1987.

47. Bray, G. A., Obesity: basic considerations and clinical approaches, *Dis. Mon.*, 35, 449, 1989.

48. Seidell, J. C., Cigolini, M., Charezewska, J., Ellsinger, B., Deslypere, J. P., and Cruz, A., Fat distribution in European men: a comparison of anthropometric measurements in relation to cardiovascular risk factors, *Int. J. Obes.*, 16, 17, 1991.

49. Björntorp, P., The association between obesity, adipose tissue distribution, and disease, *Acta Med. Scand.*, suppl., 723, 121, 1988.

50. Rimm, E. B., Stampfer, M. J., Giovannucci, E., Ascherio, A., Spiegelman, D., Colditz, G. A., and Willett, W. C., Body size and fat distribution as predictors of coronary heart disease among middle-aged and older US men, *Am. J. Epidemiol.*, 141, 1117, 1995.

51. Hsieh, S. D. and Yoshinaga, H., Abdominal fat distribution and coronary heart disease risk factors in men-waist/height ratio as a simple and useful predictor, *Int. J. Obes.*, 19, 585, 1995.

52. Lindberg, W., Natvig, H., Rygh, A., and Svendsen, K., Height and weight studies in adult men and women. Suggestion for new Norwegian height and weight norms (in Norwegian), *Tidsskr. Nor. Laegeforen.,* 76, 361, 1956.

53. Montoye, H. J., Epstein, F. H., and Kjelsberg, M. O., The measurement of body fatness. A study in a total community, *Am. J. Clin. Nutr.,* 16, 417, 1965.

54. Seltzer, C. C., Stoudt, H. W., Jr., Bell, B., and Mayer, J., Reliability of relative body weight as a criterion of obesity, *Am. J. Epidemiol.,* 92, 339, 1970.

55. Durnin, J. V. G. A. and Womersley, J., Body fat assessed from total body density and its estimation from skinfold thickness: measurements on 481 men and women aged from 16 to 72 years, *Br. J. Nutr.,* 32, 77, 1974.

56. Steen, B., Isaksson, B., and Svanborg, A., Body composition at age 70, 75, and 79 years of age. A longitudinal population study, *Proc. 12th Int. Congr. Nutr.,* San Diego, 1981, 102.

57. Skerlj, B., Brozek, J., and Hunt, E. E., Subcutaneous fat and age changes in body built and body form in women, *Am. J. Phys. Anthropol.,* 11, 577, 1953.

58. Lapidus, L., Bengtsson, C., and Larsson, B., Distribution of adipose tissue and risk of cardiovascular disease and death: a 12-year follow-up of participants in the population study of women in Gothenburg, Sweden, *BMJ,* 289, 1257, 1984.

59. Keys, A., Fidanza, F., Karvonen, M. J., Kimura, N., and Taylor, H. L., Indices of relative weight and obesity, *J. Chron. Dis.,* 25, 329, 1972.

60. Bray, G. A., Overweight is risking fate. Definition, classification, prevalence and risk, *Ann. N. Y. Acad. Sci.,* 499, 14, 1987.

61. WHO Technical Report Series 724, Energy and protein requirements: report of a FAO/WHO/UNU expert consultation, World Health Organization, 1985.

62. WHO Technical Report Series 854, Physical status: the use and interpretation of anthropometry; report of a WHO expert committee, World Health Organization, 1995.

63. Andres, R., Elahi, D., Tobin, J. D., Muller, D. C., and Brant, L., Impact of age on weight goals, *Ann. Intern. Med.,* 103, 1030, 1985.

64. Ham, R. J., Indicators of poor nutritional status in older Americans, *Am. Fam. Physician,* 45, 219, 1992.

65. Beck, A. M. and Ovesen, L., At which body mass index and degree of weight loss should hospitalized elderly patients be considered at nutritional risk? *Clin. Nutr.,* 17, 195, 1998.

66. Hubert, H. B., Feinleib, M., McNamara, P. M., and Castelli, W. P., Obesity as an independent risk factor for cardiovascular disease: a 26-year follow-up of participants in the Framingham Heart Study, *Circulation,* 67, 968, 1983.

67. Jooste, P. L., Steenkamp, H. J., Benadé, A. J. S., and Rossouw, J. E., Prevalence of overweight and obesity and its relation to coronary heart disease in the CORIS study, *S. Afr. Med. J.,* 74, 101, 1988.

68. Harris, T. B., Ballard-Barbasch, R., Madans, J., Makuc, D. M., and Feldman, J. J., Overweight, weight loss, and risk of coronary heart disease in older women. The NHANES I Epidemiologic Follow-up Study, *Am. J. Epidemiol.,* 137, 1318, 1993.

69. Harris, T. B., Launer, L. J., Madans, J., and Feldman, J. J., Cohort study of effect of being overweight and change in weight on risk of coronary heart disease in old age, *BMJ,* 314, 1791, 1997.

70. Barrett-Connor, E. L., Obesity, hypertension and stroke, *Clin. Exp. Hypertens.,* 12, 769, 1990.

71. Gryglewska, B., Grodzicki, T., and Kocemba, J., Obesity and blood pressure in the elderly free-living population, *J. Hum. Hypertens.,* 12, 645, 1998.

72. Lundgren, H., Bengtsson, C., Blohme, G., Lapidus, L., and Sjöström, L., Adiposity and adipose tissue distribution in relation to incidence of diabetes in women: results from a prospective population study in Gothenburg, Sweden, *Int. J. Obes.,* 13, 413, 1989.

73. Bray, G. A., Obesity and diabetes, *Acta Diabetol. Lat.,* 27, 81, 1990.

74. Chan, J. M., Rimm, E. B., Colditz, G. A., Stampfer, M. J., and Willett, W. C., Obesity, fat distribution, and weight gain as risk factors for clinical diabetes in men, *Diab. Care.,* 17, 961, 1994.

75. Colditz, G. A., Willett, W. C., Rotnitzky, A., and Manson, J. E., Weight gain as a risk factor for clinical diabetes mellitus in women, *Ann. Intern. Med.,* 122, 481, 1995.

76. Colman, E., Katzel, L. I., Sorkin, J., Coon, P. J., Engelhardt, S., Rogus, E., and Goldberg, A. P., The role of obesity and cardiovascular fitness in the impaired glucose tolerance of aging, *Exp. Gerontol.,* 30, 571, 1995.

77. Garfinkel, L., Overweight and cancer, *Ann. Intern. Med.,* 103, 1034, 1985.

78. Caan, B. J., Coates, A. O., Slattery, M. L., Potter, J. D., Quesenberry, C. P., Jr., and Edwards, S. M., Body size and the risk of colon cancer in a large case-control study, *Int. J. Obes.*, 22, 178, 1998.

79. Olson, S. H., Trevisan, M., Marshall, J. R., Graham, S., Zielezny, M., Vena, J. E., Hellmann, R., and Freudenheim, J. L., Body mass index, weight gain, and risk of endometrial cancer, *Nutr. Cancer*, 23, 141, 1995.

80. Chow, W., McLaughlin, J. K., Mandel, J. S., Wacholder, S., Niwa, S., and Fraumeni, J. F., Jr., Obesity and risk of renal cell cancer, *Cancer Epidemiol. Biomarkers Prev.*, 5, 17, 1996.

81. Bray, G. A., Complications of obesity, *Ann. Intern. Med.*, 103, 1052, 1985.

82. Kral, J., Morbid obesity and related health risks, *Ann. Intern. Med.*, 103, 1043, 1985.

83. Wadden, T. A. and Stunkard, A. J., Social and psychological consequences of obesity, *Ann. Intern. Med.*, 103, 1003, 1985.

84. Nieman, D.C., Henson, D. A., Nehlsen-Cannarella, S. L., Ekkens, M., Utter, A. C., Butterworth, D. E., and Fagoaga, O. R., Influence of obesity on immune function, *J. Am. Diet. Assoc.*, 99, 294, 1999.

85. Van Itallie, T. B., Health implications of overweight and obesity in the United States, *Ann. Intern. Med.*, 103, 983, 1985.

86. Curb, J. D. and Marcus, E. B., Body fat, coronary heart disease, and stroke in Japanese men, *Am. J. Clin. Nutr.*, 53, 1612S, 1991.

87. Stern, M., Epidemiology of obesity and its link to heart disease, *Metabolism*, suppl. 3, 44, 1, 1995.

88. Barrett-Connor, E. L., Obesity, atherosclerosis and coronary artery disease, *Ann. Intern. Med.*, 103, 1010, 1985.

89. Dey, D. K., Rothenberg, E., Sundh, V., Bosaeus, I., and Steen, B., Height and Body weight at age 70 as predictors of coronary heart disease, diabetes, stroke and cancer. A 15-year longitudinal study of a population aged 70 to 85 years, in preparation.

90. Society of Actuaries, *Build and Blood Pressure Study*, The Society of Actuaries, Chicago, 1960, 1:1.

91. Schroll, M., A longitudinal epidemiological survey of relative weight at age 25, 50, and 60 in the Glostrup population of men and women born in 1914, *Dan. Med. Bull.*, 28, 106, 1981.

92. Tumilehto, J., Salonen, J. T., Marti, B., Jalkanen, L., Puska, P., and Nissinen, A., Body weight and risk of myocardial infarction and death in the adult population of eastern Finland, *Br. Med. J.*, 295, 623, 1987.

93. Stevens, J., Keil, J. E., Rust, P. F., Verdugo, R. R., Davis, C. E., Tyroler, H. A., and Gazes, P. C., Body mass index and body girths as predictors of mortality in black and white men, *Am. J. Epidemiol.*, 135, 1137, 1992.

94. Garrison, R. J., Feinleib, M., Castelli, W. P., and McNamara, P. M., Cigarette smoking as a confounder of the relationship between relative weight and long-term mortality, *JAMA*, 249, 2199, 1983.

95. Lindsted, K., Tonstad, S., and Kuzma, J. W., Body mass index and patterns of mortality among Seventh-day Adventist men, *Int. J. Obes.*, 15, 397, 1991.

96. Lee, I. M., Manson, J. E., Hennekens, C. H., and Paffenbarger, R. S., Jr., Body weight and mortality: a 27-year follow-up of middle-aged men, *JAMA*, 270, 2823, 1993.

97. Wilcosky, T., Hyde, J., Anderson, J. J., Bangdiwala, S., and Duncan, B., Obesity and mortality in the Lipid Research Program Follow-up Study, *J. Clin. Epidemiol.*, 43, 743, 1990.

98. Lew, E. A. and Garfinkel, L., Variations in mortality by weight among 750,000 men and women, *J. Chron. Dis.*, 32, 563, 1979.

99. Harris, T., Cook, E. F., Garrison, R., Higgins, M., Kannel, W., and Goldman, L., Body mass index and mortality among nonsmoking older persons: the Framingham Heart Study, *JAMA*, 259, 1520, 1988.

100. Rissanen, A., Heliovaara, M., Knekt, P., Aromaa, A., Reunanen, A., and Maatela, J., Weight and mortality in Finnish men, *J. Clin. Epidemiol.*, 42, 781, 1989.

101. Rissanen, A., Knekt, P., Helivoara, M., Aromaa, A., Reunanen, A., and Maatela, J., Weight and mortality in Finnish women, *J. Clin. Epidemiol.*, 44, 787, 1991.

102. Manson, J. E., Willett, W. C., Stampfer, M. J., Colditz, G. A., Hunter, D. J., Hankinson, S. E., Hennekens, C. H., and Speizer, F. E., Body weight and mortality among women, *New Eng. J. Med.*, 333, 677, 1995.

103. Diehr, P., Bild, D. E., Harris, T. B., Duxbury, A., Siscovick, D., and Rossi, M., Body mass index and mortality in nonsmoking older adults: the Cardiovascular Health Study, *Am. J. Public Health.*, 88, 623, 1998.

104. Kinney, E. L. and Caldwell, J. W., Relationship between body weight and mortality in men aged 75 years and older, *South Med. J.,* 83, 1256, 1990.

105. Dey, D. K., Rothenberg, E., Sundh, V., Bosaeus, I., and Steen, B., Body weight, weight change and mortality in the elderly. A 25-year longitudinal population study from age 70 to 95, submitted.

106. Stevens, J., Cai, J., Pamuk, E. R., Williamson, D. F., Thun, M. J., and Wood, J. L., The effect of age on the association between body mass index and mortality, *New Eng. J. Med.,* 338, 1, 1998.

107. Waaler, H. T., Height, weight, and mortality: the Norwegian experience, *Acta Med. Scand.*, suppl., 679, 1, 1984.

108. Björntorp, P., Effects of age, sex, and clinical conditions on adipose tissue cellularity in man, *Metabolism,* 23, 1091, 1974.

109. Bray, G. A., Definition, measurement, and classification of the syndromes of obesity, *Int. J. Obesity,* 2, 99, 1978.

110. Shock, N. W., Energy metabolism, caloric intake and physical activity of the aging, in *Nutrition in Old Age,* Carlsson, L. A., Ed., 10th Symp. Swedish Nutr. Found., Almqvist & Wiksell, Uppsala, 1972, 12.

111. McGandy, R. B., Barrows, C. H., Jr., Spanias, A., Meredith, A., Stone, J. L., and Norris, A. H., Nutrient intakes and energy expenditure in men of different ages, *J. Gerontol.,* 21, 581, 1966.

112. Rothenberg, E., Bosaeus, I., and Steen, B., Food habits in three 70-year-old free-living populations in Gothenburg, Sweden. A 22-year cohort study, *Scand. J. Nutr.,* 40, 104, 1996.

113. Steen, B. and Rothenberg, E., Aspects of nutrition of the elderly at home — a review, *J. Nutr. Health Aging,* 2, 28, 1998.

114. National Research Council (U.S.) Food and Nutrition Board Subcommittee on the Tenth Edition of the Recommended Dietary Allowances, *Recommended Dietary Allowances*, 10th ed., National Academy Press, Washington, D.C., 1989, 3.

115. Keys, A. Ed., Coronary heart disease in seven countries, *Circulation, 41,* 1, 1970.

116. Chirico, A. M. and Stun kard, A. J., Physical activity and human obesity, *New Eng. J. Med.,* 263, 935, 1960.

117. Burnight, R. G. and Marden, P. G., Social correlates of weight in an aging population, *Milbank Mem. Fund Q.,* 45, 75, 1967.

118. Mellström, D. and Steen, B., Some examples of relations between social factors and dietary habits in 70-year-old people, in *Nordisk Gerontologi*, Beverfelt, E., Julsurd, A. C., Kjørstad, H., and Nygård, A. M., Eds., Hammerstad Boktrykkeri, Oslo, 1981, 176.

119. Price, J. H., Nutrition for the elderly, *J. Nurs. Care,* 12, 14, 1979.

120. Alexander, J. R., Chronic disease due to obesity, *J. Chron. Dis.,* 18, 895, 1965.

121. Haleem, M. A., The problem of obesity in the elderly, *Br. J. Clin. Prac.,* 32, 45, 1978.

122. Jaffe, H. L., Corday, E., and Master, A. M., Evaluation of the precordial leads of the electrocardiogram in obesity, *Am. Heart J.,* 39, 911, 1948.

123. Steen, B., The importance of diagnostic procedures to ensure quality of health care in geriatric medicine. Examples from recent studies, *Qual. Ass. Health Care.,* 2, 387, 1991.

124. Molander, U., Milsom, I., Ekelund, P., and Mellström, D., An epidemiological study of urinary incontinence and related urogenital symptoms in elderly women, *Maturitas,* 12, 51, 1990.

125. Rössner, S., Examples of non-surgical methods to treat overweight, *Näringsforskning*, 26, 125, 1982.

126. Van Itallie, T. B., Dietary fibers and obesity, *Am. J. Clin. Nutr.,* 31, 543, 1978.

127. Albanese, A. A., *Nutrition for the Elderly*, Alan R. Liss, New York, 1980.

128. Steen B., Preventive nutrition in later life, in *Medical Practice of Preventive Nutrition*, Wahlqvist, M.L. and Vodbecky, J. S., Eds., Smith-Gordon & Co., London, 1994, 277.

129. Hanson, B. S., Mattison, I., and Steen, B., Dietary intake and psychosocial factors in 68-year-old men. A population study, *Compr. Gerontol., B,* 1, 62, 1987.

130. Shepard, R. J., Physical activity and ageing, *Croom, Helm,* 136, 1987.

131. Stuart, R. B., Obesity, *Geriatric Med.,* 5, 84, 1976.

13 Immune Reactivity in the Elderly: Influence of Dietary Factors and Disease with Emphasis on Lipid Alterations

Thomas M. Stulnig

CONTENTS

I. INTRODUCTION

A. INHERENT PROBLEMS IN STUDYING AGING OF THE IMMUNE SYSTEM

Many publications report changes in the immune system of elderly subjects, but often with conflicting results. One of the major problems in studying age-associated changes of the immune system is the selection of an appropriate study population. Most working groups agree that age-related changes should be studied in a "healthy" population to avoid influences by underlying disease, but the applied definition of "health" varies widely. The Concerted Action Programme on Aging of the European Community (EURAGE) has established selection criteria for studying healthy aging. The exclusion criteria have been summarized in the so-called SENIEUR protocol, in which information on clinical history and living conditions, intake of medication, and a panel of laboratory values are evaluated in order to classify an apparently healthy volunteer as SENIEUR-compatible.[1] Both elderly individuals and young control subjects have to fulfill these criteria to be included in a gerontological study. However, the completeness of this exclusion protocol is an issue of debate, and several groups have suggested additional selection criteria, e.g., serum lipid values.[2] Nevertheless, studying aging of the immune system in a selected healthy population is highly recommended in order to obtain comparable results.

On the other hand, selection of "extraordinarily healthy" individuals may also bias the result of a gerontological study. This fact is particularly evident in studies with centenarians who obviously represent a privileged population with respect to health, and data with these very old subjects often do not correspond to those obtained in "normal" aged healthy subjects. The approach to study healthy aging of the immune system in a SENIEUR-selected population of 65 to 85 years of age appears to represent a good compromise to study aging of the immune system in a population of highest clinical relevance.

B. Primary, Pseudo-Secondary, and Secondary Alterations of the Immune System in the Elderly

Alterations of the immune system found in perfectly healthy older individuals have been classified as "primary" in contrast to "secondary" alterations of the immune system, which are due to underlying disease or influence of environmental factors.[3] According to Wick and Grubeck-Loebenstein,[3] secondary alterations of immune reactivity also include age-related changes in other systems with influence on immune reactivity, e.g., alterations in lymphocyte lipid metabolism.[4,5] However, age-related alterations in other systems with impact on immune reactivity can hardly be discriminated from direct effects, e.g., measured as disturbed lymphocyte signaling, since the underlying molecular cause for immunological alterations often remains obscure. For instance, altered lymphocyte transmembrane signaling in the elderly may be due to altered membrane lipid composition because of age-related changes in the regulation of cellular and systemic lipid metabolism. Due to these inherent problems, I would like to add to that highly useful concept, and summarize age-associated alterations in systems other than the immune system that indirectly affect immune responsiveness in perfectly healthy older individuals, as "pseudo-secondary" alterations of immune reactivity. This extended categorization is of particular importance in view of the fact that the major biological communication systems, i.e., nervous, immune, and endocrine systems, closely interact with each other.[6-8] Both primary and pseudo-secondary alterations are found in perfectly healthy elderly and well-nourished individuals, and are thus clearly discriminated from secondary alterations of the immune system, which should be confined to those influenced by underlying disease or by factors from an individual's environment including deficiencies in micro- or macronutrients.

In this review, I briefly summarize alterations of the immune system in the elderly and discuss possible interference from nutritional supplementations. In all issues, I concentrate on the immunomodulatory action of lipids that are supposed to substantially contribute to pseudo-secondary and secondary alterations of immune reactivity in the elderly. For the huge variety of other issues concerning the influence of nutritional deficits or supplementations on the immune system from the elderly, please refer to two recent series of excellent reviews.[9,10]

II. PRIMARY ALTERATIONS OF THE IMMUNE SYSTEM IN THE ELDERLY

Elderly people are particularly prone to infectious diseases, thus emphasizing the clinical importance of age-related changes of the immune system. Though many aspects of immune responsiveness are decreased in the elderly, recent advances point to a dysregulation rather than a global decrease in function of the immune system.[11] In general, cellular and humoral reactions against exogenous antigens are diminished in the elderly, whereas autoimmune phenomena occur more frequently in elderly compared with young individuals. The age-related dysregulation predominantly involves T lymphocyte function, but there are also alterations in the B cell and accessory cell system.

A. T CELL SYSTEM

The principal alteration in the T cell system from the elderly is the *involution of the thymic gland*,[12] which is responsible for positive selection of T cells directed against foreign antigens and negative selection of potential autoreactive T cells. Age-associated changes may exist in bone marrow-derived thymic progenitor cells,[13,14] but thymic atrophy seems to be primarily caused by a failure of thymic T cells to undergo the differentiation stage that is associated with rearrangement and expression of the T cell receptor (TCR) β-chain.[15] Normally, T cells are selected in the thymus so they can only react against antigens presented on accessory cells within syngeneic major histocompatibility complex (MHC) molecules. Interestingly, this MHC restriction of T cells is much less stringent in aged mice and humans,[16,17] emphasizing the importance of disturbed thymic T cell differentiation on the immune reactivity in the elderly. Thymic involution may be influenced not only by intrathymic but also by extrathymic factors, so that regrowth of the thymus could be induced by neuroendocrine and nutritional manipulations.[18] The direct association of age-associated thymic atrophy and immune dysfunction suggests that an efficient immune system may be restored by reversing thymic atrophy by endocrine and nutritional manipulations.

T lymphocyte subsets in peripheral blood change dramatically during aging. The overall number of T cells in peripheral blood decreases,[19-22] due to a decline in the number of CD4+ T helper/inducer cell subset particularly in subjects aged >75 yr.[19,21,23] Following contact with antigen, T cells are transformed from so-called naïve T cells, which express the high molecular isoform of CD45 (CD45RA) on their surface, to memory T cells expressing the low molecular isoform CD45RO. Most importantly, T cells with characteristics of memory cells are much more frequent in peripheral blood of elderly subjects, whereas the number of naïve T cells is markedly diminished.[22,24] The shift from naïve to memory T cells is apparent within both the CD4+ helper/inducer as well as for CD8+ (primarily cytotoxic) T cell subset.[22] Moreover, the number of T lymphocytes with an activated phenotype, i.e., those expressing major histocompatibility complex (MHC) class II molecules or the IL-2 receptor α-chain (CD25), within both the CD4+ as well as the CD8+ T cell subset is increased in peripheral blood from healthy aged individuals,[20,22,25] paralleling the higher frequency of autoimmune phenomena in the elderly population. Interestingly, according to thymic involution and the concomitant T cell differentiation defect, there is an increased number of immature double negative (CD2+ CD4- CD8-) and double positive (CD2+ CD4+ CD8+) T cells in peripheral blood in elderly subjects.[26]

In addition to age-associated alterations in number and phenotype, *functional capabilities of T cells* change considerably during the aging process. Proliferative responses upon antigenic or mitogenic stimulation are drastically decreased during aging in parallel with a marked impairment in the synthesis of interleukin (IL)-2, the major T cell growth factor.[27] The diminished IL-2 synthesis is due to impaired activation of the transcription factors AP-1 and NF-AT but not NF-κB,[28] pointing to defects in stimulating the IL-2 promoter. The decrease in IL-2 production may partly be due to the decrease in the proportion of naïve CD4+ T cells, which are more potent in the production of this cytokine. Addition of exogenous IL-2 only in part overcomes the proliferation defect in aged T cells,[29,30] suggesting additional changes in the generation of functional IL-2 receptors.[29-31]

The diminished secretion of IL-2 during immune responses in the elderly is part of a general shift in *cytokine production* of CD4+ T cells from cytokines typical for Th1 responses (e.g., IL-2) to those of Th2 responses (e.g., IL-4, IL-5, IL-10; reviewed in ref. 32). The shift in cytokine profiles emphasizes the presence of an age-related dysregulation of immune reactivity rather than a general decline.

The impaired T cell response to antigens or mitogens is reflected by inhibited *transmembrane signaling* in T cells from the elderly. Protein tyrosine phosphorylation of distinct T cell proteins are the first changes detectable within seconds or minutes following T cell stimulation and are indispensable for further T cell activation. Tyrosine phosphorylation of a number of proteins is reduced in cells from aged individuals. Protein tyrosine phosphorylation of CD3ζ chain, a component of the TCR/CD3 complex; ZAP-70, a protein tyrosine kinase that binds to phosphorylated CD3ζ chains; phospholipase C(PLC)γ1; and the adaptor protein Shc, an important link to p21ras activation, were all shown to be impaired in T cells from aged humans or mice.[33-36] Accordingly, the activation of mitogen activated protein kinases ERK1 and ERK2, which depends on functional ras signaling, was inhibited in cells from aged individuals.[37,38] According to the decrease in phosphorylation and hence activation of PLCγ1, which catalyzes the generation of inositol trisphosphate and diacylglycerol from phosphatidylinositol bisphosphate, the increase of these two second messengers was reduced, leading to a diminished calcium response and translocation of protein kinase C, respectively.[39-41] As detailed below, transmembrane signaling in T cells is particularly dependent on membrane lipid composition, emphasizing the close association of metabolic alterations and immune dysfunction in the elderly.[4,42-44]

B. B CELL SYSTEM

In parallel with the T cell system, the humoral immune response in the elderly is dysregulated by diminished antibody production against foreign antigens, but increased levels of autoantibodies.[45,46] Aged individuals also have higher titers of anti-idiotypic antibodies, which represent a particular type of autoantibodies with immunosuppressive function.[47,48] In addition, the kinetics of antibody production against foreign antigens is altered in the elderly, so that the primary antibody response is decreased with delayed peak responses as well as lower and rapidly declining antibody levels compared with the young.[49] Particularly, T cell-dependent antibody responses are diminished in the elderly, pointing to the predominant role of the T cell system for the decline in immune responsiveness in the elderly.

C. ACCESSORY CELLS

Accessory cells as monocytes/macrophages, dendritic cells, and B cells present antigens to T cells by binding of antigenic peptides to MHC molecules. Notably, the expression of MHC class II molecules, which are important for activating T helper cells, appears altered in monocytes from the elderly, with increased expression of HLA-DQ and decreased expression of HLA-DR/DP, though results on this issue are contradictory.[50,51] Beyond antigen presentation, these cells secrete a panel of important cytokines including IL-1, IL-6, tumor necrosis factor (TNF), and eicosanoids.[32] Though age-related alterations in cytokine secretion have not been unequivocally reported in accessory cells from the aged, the production of prostaglandin E_2 appears increased in the aged.[52] This finding may be of particular importance for age-associated T cell alterations since T cells from the elderly seem particular sensitive to the immunosuppressive action of PGE_2.[53]

III.   PSEUDO-SECONDARY ALTERATIONS OF THE IMMUNE SYSTEM

A. THE POSSIBLE INFLUENCE OF AN ALTERED LYMPHOCYTE LIPID METABOLISM

Lipids alter lymphocyte function particularly by interacting with various intra- and intercellular signal transduction pathways. As listed in Table 13.1, lipids and their modifications may not only

TABLE 13.1
Possible Impact of Lipids on T Lymphocyte Signaling

Lipids	Target Structures
Membrane Lipids/Membrane Domains	
Membrane fluidity	Transmembrane proteins (e.g., TCR/CD3 complex, CD28)
Cholesterol/sphingolipid-enriched membrane domains ("rafts")	GPI-anchored proteins (e.g., CD59)
	Non-receptor protein tyrosine kinases (e.g., Src family)
Polyunsaturated fatty acids	Enrichment leads to modification of rafts with inhibition of signal transduction, membrane microviscosity
Cholesterol	Depletion inhibits signaling via GPI-anchored proteins, membrane microviscosity
Protein Lipidation	
Myristoylation	Trimeric G-protein α-subunits
	Non-receptor protein tyrosine kinases
Palmitoylation	Trimeric G-protein α-subunits
	G-protein-coupled receptors
Prenylation	Trimeric G-protein γ-subunits
	Small G-proteins, ras
Glycosyl phosphatidylinositol (GPI)	Many cell surface proteins (e.g., CD59)
Lipid Second Messengers	
Phosphatidylinositol phosphates and products (IP3, DAG, etc.)	Calcium release
	Protein kinase C
Ceramide	Protein phosphatase 2A, etc.
Sphingosine-1-phosphate	Calcium release, etc.
Arachidonic acid	Protein kinase C?
Intercellular Lipid Messengers	
Platelet activating factor	Specific receptor
Lysophosphatidic acid	Specific receptor
Eicosanoids	Specific receptor
Lipid Peroxidation	
Vitamin E/tocopherol (antioxidant)	Inhibition of PGE_2 production
	Inhibition of membrane lipid peroxidation

affect plasma membrane composition and function as a whole but may also alter membrane domains, protein lipidation, and/or the generation of lipid-derived messenger substances.

1. Membrane Microviscosity

Over a couple of years, the influence of membrane microviscosity and its relation to lymphocyte response was extensively investigated, since early studies revealed that cells from elderly subjects exhibit higher membrane microviscosity (equaling lower membrane fluidity) than those from young controls. It was shown that membrane fluidity has to be maintained precisely within a narrow range for proper function of all cells including lymphocytes.[4,54,55] Moreover, higher membrane microviscosity markedly paralleled age-associated inhibition of T cell stimulation, emphasizing that a loss of homeostatic control of membrane microviscosity in resting lymphocytes is at least partially responsible for the age-related decline in immune function.[5,56,57] Lipid composition plays a major role for determining membrane microviscosity, and Huber and colleagues[57] have shown that the age-related increase in lymphocyte membrane microviscosity was reflected by an altered lymphocyte lipid content, suggesting an altered regulation of lipid homeostasis in cells from elderly subjects. A disturbed regulation of lipid metabolism in lymphocytes from healthy aged individuals could also be determined when analyzing the switch in lipid composition that occurs during blast transformation of lymphocytes, an essential step for initiating an effective immune response.[43] The exact nature of the influence of increased membrane microviscosity on cellular function is still under debate. Membrane microviscosity could alter T lymphocyte responsiveness in the elderly by directly interfering with membrane protein function, e.g., the constituents of the TCR/CD3 complex and several costimulatory molecules including CD28 are transmembrane proteins and hence prone to be functionally affected by alterations in membrane microviscosity. On the other hand, age-related molecular alterations in T cell lipids may, independently of each other, lead to increased membrane microviscosity and inhibition of lymphocyte activation.

2. Cholesterol Homeostasis

Cells from healthy elderly subjects have an elevated cholesterol content that appears to be a critical determinant of their increased membrane microviscosity.[57] Cells take up cholesterol mostly via receptor-mediated endocytosis of low-density lipoproteins (LDL).[58] On the other hand, every cell is capable of synthesizing cholesterol with the rate-limiting step being catalyzed by 3-hydroxy-3-methylglutaryl coenzyme A (HMG-CoA) reductase.[59] Both pathways have to be tightly controlled by feedback mechanisms to prevent cholesterol overaccumulation within cells. However, despite higher cholesterol concentrations in blood serum in contrast to young controls, lymphocytes from healthy elderly individuals express higher numbers of LDL-receptors leading to enhanced uptake of LDL cholesterol and increased cellular cholesterol content.[42,60] This enhanced expression of LDL receptors is due to a marked transcriptional dysregulation in lymphocytes from the elderly.[44] Consequently, lymphocytes from healthy aged subjects expressed higher amounts of LDL receptor mRNA at equal serum cholesterol levels, showing that the feedback mechanism of exogenous cholesterol on LDL receptor (and less on HMG-CoA reductase) expression is disturbed in the elderly.[44] Thus, dysregulated cellular cholesterol metabolism contributes to sterol overaccumulation in lymphocytes from healthy elderly subjects, leading to increased membrane microviscosity. Thus, the disturbed regulation of cholesterol homeostasis in lymphocytes from healthy elderly subjects could indirectly add to the age-associated alteration of the immune response.

3. Membrane Domains

Numerous other possibilities exist for lipid alterations to interfere with immune function (Table 13.1), but most of them have not yet been tested in detail with respect to their impact on age-related dysregulation of immune function. Recently, a huge body of evidence was accumulated for the existence of microdomains within the plane of the plasma membrane. These membrane domains have been termed "rafts"[61] or detergent-resistant microdomains (DRMs)[62] according to their insolubility in non-ionic detergents, which is due to their particular lipid composition rich in sphingolipids, cholesterol, and saturated fatty acids. Membrane rafts turned out to be essential for lymphocyte activation,[63] most probably by concentration of palmitoylated protein tyrosine kinases of the Src family and the important adapter protein LAT,[64] which are both indispensable for T cell activation. Notably, some proteins capable of providing costimulatory signals to T cells are attached to the plasma membrane via a glycosyl phosphatidylinositol (GPI) anchor causing selective localization within membrane rafts. Changes in cholesterol content or fatty acid unsaturation of lymphocytes have been shown to result in functional and/or structural alterations of rafts.[65,66] Interestingly, polyunsaturated fatty acids whose enrichment in membrane lipids alter raft composition and lymphocyte activation[66] have been found more prevalent in lymphocyte membranes from SENIEUR-compatible aged individuals than from young controls.[57] Moreover, during lymphoblast formation

T cells from elderly subjects retained higher amounts of PUFAs compared with cells from young donors.[43] Thus, molecular alterations in membrane rafts could be a possible mechanism for age-related lipid alterations to affect lymphocyte activation.

B. Lipid Oxidation

Though the causal role of lipid oxidation and radical formation on the aging process itself and its influence on immune function is still a matter of debate,[67,68] recent studies with antioxidants (discussed in Section V) may emphasize the influence of lipid oxidation on immune reactivity in the elderly. Previous studies found increased concentrations of lipid oxidation products in serum and particularly within the LDL fraction when measured as thiobarbituric acid reactive substances (TBARS).[69] Analysis of a specific modification of apolipoprotein B (apoB) induced by 4-hydroxy-nonenal (HNE), a natural derivative of oxidized polyunsaturated fatty acids,[70] revealed an increased proportion of HNE-modified apoB in healthy, i.e., SENIEUR-compatible, aged subjects compared with young controls.[71] Since the fractional catabolic rate of LDL is decreased in the elderly in parallel with the increased LDL serum concentration, the prolonged life-span of LDL particles in the circulation in aged individuals may facilitate accumulation of lipid peroxidation end-products. Intriguingly, the concentration of several lipophilic antioxidants, e.g., carotenes, is decreased in the elderly when related to serum lipids, which represents their site of action and whose concentration increased in sera from elderly subjects. Moreover, the amount of β-carotene per LDL particle is decreased in healthy elderly subjects.[71] However, other antioxidants, e.g., α-tocopherol, tended to be increased[71] in serum lipids from the elderly despite advanced oxidation of LDL, suggesting that lipid peroxidation occurs slowly in human serum permitting tocopherol replenishment during the process. However, only a minor part of serum LDL is oxidatively modified (less than 1%), and overall LDL binding to its receptor is not diminished with LDL from the aged proposing that altered receptor binding does not underlie the diminished downregulation of the LDL receptor on the transcriptional level.[44]

IV.   SECONDARY ALTERATIONS OF THE IMMUNE SYSTEM

Secondary alterations of the immune system have been defined as those resulting from underlying disease or environmental factors,[3] among those nutritional influences may play a major role.[72,73] These comprise, e.g., protein-energy malnutrition, deficiencies in various micronutrients (Zn, Se, Fe, Cu, vitamins A, C, E, B6, and folic acid), and oxidative changes, but also overnutrition. Also, advanced glycosylation end products (AGEs) of proteins and lipids which accumulate during aging can alter immune response by enhanced production of IFN-γ, which may result in immune responses leading to tissue injury.[74] In addition, oxidative stress may contribute to altered immunoregulation in the elderly.

A. Secondary Alterations Resulting from Disorders of Lipid Metabolism

Hypercholesterolemia, whose incidence increases with age, contributes to the overaccumulation of cholesterol in lymphocytes, which may indirectly affect immune response as discussed above.

Insulin resistance is tightly associated with the so-called metabolic syndrome describing the common or separate existence of diabetes mellitus type II, hyperlipidemia, hyperuricemia, and hypertension. This situation is typically associated by high serum concentrations of free, i.e., non-esterified fatty acids (FFA). FFA can considerably alter activation and cytolytic function of lymphocytes in the absence of FFA-binding proteins in vitro.[75-77] Since large concentrations of serum albumin tightly bind FFA in human serum, it was unknown whether high serum FFA values as they occur in states of insulin resistance may be able to inhibit lymphocyte activation. Recent data from our laboratory, however, revealed that high serum FFA concentrations inhibit calcium response of T cells and this inhibition involves both CD4+ and CD8+ subsets.[105] Thus, insulin resistance may not only be deleterious for glucose metabolism, hence promoting bacterial growth due to hyperglycemia and glucosuria, and alter cytokine production due to occurrence of AGEs, but also may inhibit immune response by serum FFA elevation.

V.   POSSIBLE INFLUENCE OF NUTRITIONAL INTERVENTIONS ON THE IMMUNE SYSTEM IN THE ELDERLY

When considering dietary interventions on the immune system in the elderly, a clear goal has to be defined first: In view of the fact that the immune system of the elderly is dysregulated rather than simply inhibited in function, it is important to achieve a normally regulated immune system rather than an augmentation of immune response. This aim is of particular importance when considering on the one hand the mortality by infection, e.g., pneumonia, and on the other hand, the wide variety of autoimmune phenomena occurring in healthy elderly subjects. However, a reversion of immune system dysregulation or "rejuvenation" is *a priori* difficult to achieve in otherwise healthy elderly individuals. Moreover, when attempting an "optimized" immune reactivity in already diseased individuals, augmentation or inhibition of an immune response is intended depending on the very clinical situation. Whereas vaccination response and infectious diseases will benefit from a diet augmenting immune responsiveness, autoimmune phenomena could be alleviated by adjuvant immunosuppression. These disorders include not only classical autoimmune diseases but perhaps also the development of atherosclerosis.[3,78]

A. LIPID-MODIFYING INTERVENTIONS

1. Cholesterol

In spite of experimental data on the influence of cholesterol accumulation on lymphocyte responsiveness, there has been, up to now, no study showing that diets poor in cholesterol may enhance immune response in the elderly. In contrast, the powerful cholesterol-lowering drugs of the "statin" group, which inhibit HMG-CoA reductase activity, may exert immunosuppressive effects,[79] which could contribute to their effect of preventing the progression of atherosclerosis. More refined analyses revealed that lowering of cellular cholesterol disturbs the function of membrane rafts, thus inhibiting T cell costimulation via glycosyl phosphatidylinositol (GPI)-anchored proteins.[65] Moreover, the inhibition of HMG-CoA reductase activity by statins also interferes with the provision of substrates needed for lipidation of signaling proteins, e.g., for prenylation of Ras proteins.[59] Thus, the mechanism of immunosuppression by statins is not yet clear, but the development of modern drugs to inhibit cholesterol biosynthesis on a more distal step, i.e., without inhibiting protein lipidation,[80] may contribute to our understanding of immunosuppression by cholesterol lowering.

2. Polyunsaturated Fatty Acids

Various aspects of immune function are inhibited in states of deficiency of overnutrition with polyunsaturated fatty acids (PUFA).[81] Fish oils include a high proportion of n-3 PUFA whose major constituents, eicosapentaenoic acid and docosahexaenoic acid, inhibit the generation of eicosanoids by interfering with the processing of arachidonic acid.[82] Moreover, eicosapentaenoic acid is a substrate for cyclooxygenase and 5-lipoxygenase leading to prostaglandins and thomboxans of the 3-series and 5-series leukotrienes, and many of these substances are biologically less active than those derived from arachidonic acid.[82]

   However, only part of the immunosuppressive effect of PUFA is due to altered eicosanoid synthesis. Notably, PUFA inhibit immune response by incorporation in membrane lipids and subsequent interference with lymphocyte function independent of their effect on prostaglandin synthesis.[83-85] Dietary lipid modifications generally revealed PUFA as potent modulators of various aspects of the immune response, with PUFA of the n-3 series being more effective than those of the n-6 series.[86] N-3 PUFA inhibit mitogen response of peripheral blood lymphocytes during and following PUFA supplementation.[87-89] PUFA also inhibit cytotoxic T cell responses as revealed by animal studies.[90] Human studies indicate that diets rich in n-3 PUFA may inhibit antigen presentation by MHC class II molecules, which is a prerequisite for stimulation of helper T cells.[91] In addition to decreased mitogen response, PUFA inhibit production of cytokines IL-1β, TNF, IL-6, and IL-2.[88,89,92,93] PUFA were also shown to inhibit cell-mediated immunity *in vivo*, e.g., endotoxin response[94] as well as delayed-type hypersensitivity (DTH) in animals[95,96] and humans.[89] Therefore, PUFA, particularly of the n-3 series, have found clinical application not only for the prevention of atherosclerosis[97] but also for the treatment of various inflammatory diseases[98,99] and as adjuvant immunosuppressive agents.[100] Unfortunately, little information is available investigating the role of PUFA with emphasis on the elderly. Negative correlations have been found between the PUFA content of habitual diets and basal as well as stimulated NK cell activity, but PUFA supplementation only increased NK cell number without affecting activity of NK cells.[101] Supplementation of n-3 PUFA resulted in a significant decrease in T cell mitogen response only in aged individuals and a more pronounced decrease in IL-2 production in elderly than in young women.[87] Moreover, synthesis of IL-1, IL-6, and TNF was more dramatically reduced in aged than in young subjects.[87] These data emphasize that elderly individuals are particularly sensitive to the immunosuppressive action of PUFA. Accordingly, elderly individuals with autoimmune diseases or progressive atherosclerosis may particularly benefit from PUFA supplementation. Though autoimmune and cardiovascular disorders are frequent problems in the elderly, only longitudinal studies will clarify whether dietary PUFA supplementation should be generally recommended in the elderly or whether adverse effects that as a increase the incidence of fatal infections may limit their application to particular groups of patients.

3. Antioxidants

Antioxidants such as vitamin E (tocopherol) may augment immune reactivity by inhibiting PGE_2 production, the immunosuppressive impact of which is particularly effective in the aged.[102] In addition, prevention of polyunsaturated fatty acid oxidation of membrane lipids may contribute to its beneficial effect on immune reactivity. A double-blind, placebo-controlled study supplemented 34 healthy aged (>60 yr) subjects with 800 mg α-tocopherol for 30 days.[103] This treatment augmented not only plasma vitamin E concentration but also DTH, T cell mitogen response, and IL-2 production. Recently, the effect of tocopherol substitution on indicators of T cell responsiveness was confirmed when evaluating not only DTH but also antibody production against hepatitis B with dose-dependent differences in these changes, suggesting 200 mg/day as an optimal substitution for the immune system.[104] Moreover, vitamin E may hinder the progression of atherosclerosis by prevention of serum lipoprotein oxidation. Thus, vitamin E and possibly also other antioxidants appear particularly useful dietary supplements for elderly individuals.

VI.   CONCLUSIONS

The immune system in healthy elderly subjects is characterized by a dysregulation of immune reactivity with diminished responses against foreign antigens and a high frequency of autoimmune disorders. This dysregulation is due to primary alterations, comprising direct effects of aging on the immune system, and pseudo-secondary alterations, which summarize age-related metabolic, endocrine, and neuropsychologic changes in healthy individuals that are indirectly able to affect immune function. This review focused on changes in lipid metabolism that occur during healthy aging and that can be, at least to some extent, modified by dietary factors. Since the regulation of the immune system is primarily altered in the elderly, dietary interventions should not simply "enhance" immune function. However, our primary goal should be a "rejuvenation" of the immune system with strengthened responses against foreign antigens and suppression of autoimmune phenomena. Therefore, large longitudinal studies have to be carried out to prove the efficacy of dietary interventions to increase expectancy and, particularly, quality of life.

ACKNOWLEDGMENTS

This work was supported by the Austrian Science Foundation (project no. P13507-MED), and the Austrian National Bank (project no. 7196).

REFERENCES

1. Ligthart, G. J., Corberand, J. X., Fournier, C., Galanaud, P., Hijmans, W., Kennes, B., Müller Hermelink, H. K., and Steinmann, G. G., Admission criteria for immunogerontological studies in man: the SENIEUR protocol, *Mech. Ageing Dev.*, 28, 47, 1984.
2. Stulnig, T., Mair, A., Jarosch, E., Schober, M., Schönitzer, D., Wick, G., and Huber, L. A., Estimation of reference intervals from a SENIEUR protocol compatible aged population for immunogerontological studies, *Mech. Ageing Dev.*, 68, 105, 1993.
3. Wick, G., and Grubeck-Loebenstein, B., Primary and secondary alterations of immune reactivity in the elderly: impact of dietary factors and disease, *Immunol. Rev.*, 160, 171, 1997.
4. Traill, K. N., and Wick, G., Lipids and lymphocyte function, *Immunol. Today*, 5, 70, 1984.
5. Traill, K. N., Huber, L. A., Böck, G., Jürgens, G., and Wick, G., Lipoproteins and immune function in the aged, in *Crossroads in Aging*, Bergener, M., Ermini, M., and Stähelin, H. B., Eds., Academic Press, London, 1988, 129.
6. Wick, G., Hu, Y., Schwarz, S., and Kroemer, G., Immunoendocrine communication via the hypothalamo-pituitary-adrenal axis in autoimmune diseases, *Endocr. Rev.*, 14, 539, 1993.
7. Spector, N. H., Neuroimmunomodulation: a brief review, *Regul. Toxicol. Pharmacol.*, 24, S32, 1996.
8. Tomaszewska, D., and Przekop, F., The immune-neuro-endocrine interactions, *J. Physiol. Pharmacol.*, 48, 139, 1997.
9. Nutrition, aging, and immune function, *Nutr. Rev.*, 53, S1, 1995.
10. Nutrition and immunity, *Nutr. Rev.*, 56, S1, 1998.
11. Weksler, M. E., Immune senescence: deficiency or dysregulation, *Nutr. Rev.*, 53, S3, 1995.
12. Steinmann, G. G., Changes in the human thymus during aging, *Curr. Top. Pathol.*, 75, 43, 1986.
13. Globerson, A., Thymocyte progenitors in aging, *Immunol. Lett.*, 40, 219, 1994.
14. Yu, S., Abel, L., and Globerson, A., Thymocyte progenitors and T cell development in aging, *Mech. Aging Dev.*, 94, 103, 1997.
15. Aspinall, R., Age-associated thymic atrophy in the mouse is due to a deficiency affecting rearrangement of the TCR during intrathymic T cell development, *J. Immunol.*, 158, 3037, 1997.
16. Schwab, R., Russo, C., and Weksler, M. E., Altered major histocompatibility complex-restricted antigen recognition by T cells from elderly humans, *Eur. J. Immunol.*, 22, 2989, 1992.
17. Russo, C., Cherniack, E. P., Wali, A., and Weksler, M. E., Age-dependent appearance of non-major histocompatibility complex-restricted helper T cells, *Proc. Natl. Acad. Sci. USA*, 90, 11718, 1993.
18. Fabris, N., Mocchegiani, E., Muzzioli, M., and Provinciali, M., Neuroendocrine-thymus interactions: perspectives for intervention in aging, *Ann. NY Acad. Sci.*, 521, 72, 1988.
19. Dworsky, R., Paganini Hill, A., Ducey, B., Hechinger, M., and Parker, J. W., Lymphocyte immunophenotyping in an elderly population: age, sex and medication effects — a flow cytometry study, *Mech. Ageing Dev.*, 48, 255, 1989.
20. Goto, M., and Nishioka, K., Age- and sex-related changes of the lymphocyte subsets in healthy individuals: An analysis by two-dimensional flow cytometry, *J. Gerontol.*, 44, M51, 1989.
21. Utsuyama, M., Hirokawa, K., Kurashima, C., Fukayama, M., Inamatsu, T., Suzuki, K., Hashimoto, W., and Sato, K., Differential age-change in the numbers of CD4+CD45RA+ and CD4+CD29+ T-cell subsets in human peripheral blood, *Mech. Ageing Dev.*, 63, 57, 1992.

22. Stulnig, T., Maczek, C., Böck, G., Majdic, O., and Wick, G., Reference intervals for human peripheral blood lymphocyte subpopulations from "healthy" young and aged subjects, *Int. Arch. Allerg. Immunol.*, 108, 205, 1995.

23. Traill, K. N., Schönitzer, D., Jürgens, G., Böck, G., Pfeilschifter, R., Hilchenbach, M., Holasek, A., Förster, O., and Wick, G., Age related changes in lymphocyte subset proportions, surface differentiation antigen density and plasma membrane fluidity: application of the EURAGE SENIEUR protocol admission criteria, *Mech. Ageing Dev.*, 33, 39, 1985.

24. Sanders, M. E., Makgoba, M. W., and Shaw, S., Human naive and memory cells, *Immunol. Today*, 9, 195, 1988.

25. Yamashiki, M., Nishimura, A., Kosaka, Y., and James, S. P., Two-color analysis of peripheral lymphocyte surface antigens in inherently healthy adults, *J. Clin. Lab. Anal.*, 8, 22, 1994.

26. Lesourd, B. M., and Meaume, S., Cell mediated immunity changes in ageing, relative importance of cell subpopulation switches and of nutritional factors, *Immunol. Lett.*, 40, 235, 1994.

27. Pahlavani, M. A., and Richardson, A., The effect of age on the expression of interleukin-2, *Mech. Ageing Dev.*, 89, 125, 1996.

28. Whisler, R. L., Beiqing, L., and Chen, M., Age-related decreases in IL-2 production by human T cells are associated with impaired activation of nuclear transcriptional factors AP-1 and NF-AT, *Cell. Immunol.*, 169, 185, 1996.

29. Ernst, D. N., Weigle, W. O., McQuitty, D. N., Rothermel, A. L., and Hobbs, M. V., Stimulation of murine T cell subsets with anti-CD3 antibody. Age-related defects in the expression of early activation molecules, *J. Immunol.*, 142, 1413, 1989.

30. Orson, F. M., Saadeh, C. K., Lewis, D. E., and Nelson, D. L., Interleukin 2 receptor expression by T cells in human aging, *Cell. Immunol.*, 124, 278, 1989.

31. Schwab, R., Pfeffer, L. M., Szabo, P., Gamble, D., Schnurr, C. M., and Weksler, M. E., Defective expression of high affinity IL-2 receptors on activated T cells from aged humans, *Int. Immunol.*, 2, 239, 1990.

32. Chakravarti, B., and Abraham, G. N., Aging and T-cell-mediated immunity, *Mech. Ageing Dev.*, 108, 183, 1999.

33. Ghosh, J., and Miller, R. A., Rapid tyrosine phosphorylation of Grb2 and Shc in T cells exposed to anti-CD3, anti-CD4, and anti-CD45 stimuli: differential effects of aging, *Mech. Ageing Dev.*, 80, 171, 1995.

34. Grossmann, A., Rabinovitch, P. S., Kavanagh, T. J., Jinneman, J. C., Gilliland, L. K., Ledbetter, J. A., and Kanner, S. B., Activation of murine T-cells via phospholipase-C gamma 1-associated protein tyrosine phosphorylation is reduced with aging, *J. Gerontol.*, 50, B205, 1995.

35. Garcia, G. G., and Miller, R. A., Differential tyrosine phosphorylation of zeta chain dimers in mouse CD4 T lymphocytes: effect of age, *Cell. Immunol.*, 175, 51, 1997.

36. Chakravarti, B., Chakravarti, D. N., Devecis, J., Seshi, B., and Abraham, G. N., Effect of age on mitogen induced protein tyrosine phosphorylation in human T cell and its subsets: down-regulation of tyrosine phosphorylation of ZAP-70, *Mech. Ageing Dev.*, 104, 41, 1998.

37. Whisler, R. L., Newhouse, Y. G., and Bagenstose, S. E., Age-related reductions in the activation of mitogen-activated protein kinases p44mapk/ERK1 and p42mapk/ERK2 in human T cells stimulated via ligation of the T cell receptor complex, *Cell. Immunol.*, 168, 201, 1996.

38. Gorgas, G., Butch, E. R., Guan, K. L., and Miller, R. A., Diminished activation of the MAP kinase pathway in CD3-stimulated T lymphocytes from old mice, *Mech. Ageing Dev.*, 94, 71, 1997.

39. Gupta, S., Membrane signal transduction in T cells in aging humans, *Ann. NY Acad. Sci.*, 568, 277, 1989.

40. Varga, Z., Bressani, N., Zaia, A. M., Bene, L., Fulop, T., Leovey, A., Fabris, N., Damjanovich, S., and Zaid, A. M., Cell surface markers, inositol phosphate levels and membrane potential of lymphocytes from young and old human patients, *Immunol. Lett.*, 23, 275, 1990.

41. Utsuyama, M., Varga, Z., Fukami, K., Homma, Y., Takenawa, T., and Hirokawa, K., Influence of age on the signal transduction of T cells in mice, *Int. Immunol.*, 5, 1177, 1993.

42. Traill, K. N., Huber, L. A., Wick, G., and Jürgens, G., Lipoprotein interactions with T cells: an update, *Immunol. Today*, 11, 411, 1990.

43. Stulnig, T. M., Bühler, E., Böck, G., Kirchebner, C., Schönitzer, D., and Wick, G., Altered switch in lipid composition during T-cell blast transformation in the healthy elderly, *J. Gerontol.*, B383, 1995.

44. Stulnig, T. M., Klocker, H., Harwood, H. J., Jr., Jürgens, G., Schönitzer, D., Jarosch, E., Huber, L. A., Amberger, A., and Wick, G., *In vivo* low-density lipoprotein receptor and 3-hydroxy-3-methylglutaryl coenzyme A reductase regulation in human lymphocytes and its alterations during aging, *Arterioscler. Thromb. Vasc. Biol.*, 15, 872, 1995.

45. Rowley, M. J., Buchanan, H., and Mackay, I. R., Reciprocal change with age in antibody to extrinsic and intrinsic antigens, *Lancet*, 2, 24, 1968.

46. Hallgren, H. M., Buckley, C. E. D., Gilbertsen, V. A., and Yunis, E. J., Lymphocyte phytohemagglutinin responsiveness, immunoglobulins and autoantibodies in aging humans, *J. Immunol.*, 111, 1101, 1973.

47. Goidl, E. A., Schrater, A. F., Thorbecke, G. H., and Siskind, G. W., Production of auto-anti-idiotypic antibody during the normal immune response. IV. Studies of the primary and secondary responses to thymus- dependent and -independent antigens, *Eur. J. Immunol.*, 10, 810, 1980.

48. Arreaza, E. E., Gibbons, J. J., Jr., Siskind, G. W., and Weksler, M. E., Lower antibody response to tetanus toxoid associated with higher auto-anti-idiotypic antibody in old compared with young humans, *Clin. Exp. Immunol.*, 92, 169, 1993.

49. Lesourd, B. M., Mazari, L., and Ferry, M., The role of nutrition in immunity in the aged, *Nutr. Rev.*, 56, S113, 1998.

50. Villanueva, J. L., Solana, R., Alonso, M. C., and Pena, J., Changes in the expression of HLA-class II antigens on peripheral blood monocytes from aged humans, *Dis. Markers*, 8, 85, 1990.

51. Rich, E. A., Mincek, M. A., Armitage, K. B., Duffy, E. G., Owen, D. C., Fayen, J. D., Hom, D. L., and Ellner, J. J., Accessory function and properties of monocytes from healthy elderly humans for T lymphocyte responses to mitogen and antigen, *Gerontology*, 39, 93, 1993.

52. Hayek, M. G., Meydani, S. N., Meydani, M., and Blumberg, J. B., Age differences in eicosanoid production of mouse splenocytes: effects on mitogen-induced T-cell proliferation, *J. Gerontol.*, 49, B197, 1994.

53. Goodwin, J. S., Changes in lymphocyte sensitivity to prostaglandin E, histamine, hydrocortisone, and X irradiation with age: studies in a healthy elderly population, *Clin. Immunol. Immunopathol.*, 25, 243, 1982.

54. Grunberger, D., Haimovitz, R., and Shinitzky, M., Resolution of plasma membrane lipid fluidity in intact cells labelled with diphenylhexatriene, *Biochim. Biophys. Acta*, 688, 764, 1982.

55. Shinitzky, M., The lipid fluidity of cell membranes, in *Physiology of Membrane Fluidity*, Shinitzky, M., CRC Press, Boca Raton, FL, 1984, 1.

56. Rivnay, B., Bergman, S., Shinitzky, M., and Globerson, A., Correlations between membrane viscosity, serum cholesterol, lymphocyte activation and aging in man, *Mech. Ageing Dev.*, 12, 119, 1980.

57. Huber, L. A., Xu, Q., Jürgens, G., Böck, G., Bühler, E., Gey, F., Schönitzer, D., Traill, K. N., and Wick, G., Correlation of lymphocyte lipid composition, membrane microviscosity and mitogen response in the aged, *Eur. J. Immunol.*, 21, 2761, 1991.

58. Brown, M. S., and Goldstein, J. L., A receptor-mediated pathway for cholesterol homeostasis, *Science*, 232, 34, 1986.

59. Goldstein, J. L., and Brown, M. S., Regulation of the mevalonate pathway, *Nature*, 343, 425, 1990.

60. Traill, K. N., Jürgens, G., Böck, G., Huber, L., Schönitzer, D., Widhalm, K., Winter, U., and Wick, G., Analysis of fluorescent low density lipoprotein uptake by lymphocytes. Paradoxical increase in the elderly, *Mech. Ageing Dev.*, 40, 261, 1987.

61. Simons, K., and Ikonen, E., Functional rafts in cell membranes, *Nature*, 387, 569, 1997.

62. Melkonian, K. A., Chu, T., Tortorella, L. B., and Brown, D. A., Characterization of proteins in detergent-resistant membrane complexes from Madin-Darby canine kidney epithelial cells, *Biochemistry*, 34, 16161, 1995.

63. Xavier, R., Brennan, T., Li, Q. Q., McCormack, C., and Seed, B., Membrane compartmentation is required for efficient T cell activation, *Immunity*, 8, 723, 1998.

64. Zhang, W. G., Sloan, Lancaster, J., Kitchen, J., Trible, R. P., and Samelson, L. E., LAT: The ZAP-70 tyrosine kinase substrate that links T cell receptor to cellular activation, *Cell*, 92, 83, 1998.

65. Stulnig, T. M., Berger, M., Sigmund, T., Stockinger, H., Hořejší, V., and Waldhäusl, W., Signal transduction via glycosyl phosphatidylinositol-anchored proteins in T cells is inhibited by lowering cellular cholesterol, *J. Biol. Chem.*, 272, 19242, 1997.

66. Stulnig, T. M., Berger, M., Sigmund, T., Raederstorff, D., Stockinger, H., and Waldhäusl, W., Polyunsaturated fatty acids inhibit T cell signal transduction by modification of detergent-insoluble membrane domains, *J. Cell Biol.*, 143, 637, 1998.

67. Cutler, R. G., Antioxidants and aging, *Am. J. Clin. Nutr.*, 53, 373s, 1991.

68. Gardner, E. M., Bernstein, E. D., Dorfman, M., Abrutyn, E., and Murasko, D. M., The age-associated decline in immune function of healthy individuals is not related to changes in plasma concentrations of beta-carotene, retinol, alpha-tocopherol or zinc, *Mech. Ageing Dev.*, 94, 55, 1997.

69. Hagihara, M., Nishigaki, I., Maseki, M., and Yagi, K., Age-dependent changes in lipid peroxide levels in the lipoprotein fractions of human serum, *J. Gerontol.*, 39, 269, 1984.

70. Jürgens, G., Ashy, A., and Esterbauer, H., Detection of new epitopes formed upon oxidation of low-density lipoprotein, lipoprotein (a) and very-low-density lipoprotein, *Biochem. J.*, 265, 605, 1990.

71. Stulnig, T. M., Jürgens, G., Chen, Q., Moll, D., Schönitzer, D., Jarosch, E., and Wick, G., Properties of low density lipoproteins relevant to oxidative modifications change paradoxically during aging, *Atherosclerosis*, 126, 85, 1996.

72. Chandra, R. K., 1990 McCollum Award lecture. Nutrition and immunity: lessons from the past and new insights into the future, *Am. J. Clin. Nutr.*, 53, 1087, 1991.

73. Chandra, R. K., Nutrition and the immune system: an introduction, *Am. J. Clin. Nutr.*, 66, 460s, 1997.

74. Imani, F., Horii, Y., Suthanthiran, M., Skolnik, E. Y., Makita, Z., Sharma, V., Sehajpal, P., and Vlassara, H., Advanced glycosylation endproduct-specific receptors on human and rat T-lymphocytes mediate synthesis of interferon gamma: role in tissue remodeling, *J. Exp. Med.*, 178, 2165, 1993.

75. Richieri, G. V., and Kleinfeld, A. M., Free fatty acids inhibit cytotoxic T lymphocyte-mediated lysis of allogeneic target cells, *J. Immunol.*, 145, 1074, 1990.

76. Richieri, G. V., Mescher, M. F., and Kleinfeld, A. M., Short term exposure to cis unsaturated free fatty acids inhibits degranulation of cytotoxic T lymphocytes, *J. Immunol.*, 144, 671, 1990.

77. Breittmayer, J. P., Pelassy, C., Cousin, J. L., Bernard, A., and Aussel, C., The inhibition by fatty acids of receptor-mediated calcium movements in Jurkat T-cells is due to increased calcium extrusion, *J. Biol. Chem.*, 268, 20812, 1993.

78. Wick, G., Kleindienst, R., Dietrich, H., and Xu, Q., Is atherosclerosis an autoimmune disease? *Trends Food Sci. Technol.*, 3, 114, 1992.

79. Wheeler, D. C., Are there potential non-lipid-lowering uses of statins? *Drugs*, 56, 517, 1998.

80. Thelin, A., Peterson, E., Hutson, J. L., McCarthy, A. D., Ericsson, J., and Dallner, G., Effect of squalestatin 1 on the biosynthesis of the mevalonate pathway lipids, *Biochim. Biophys. Acta*, 1215, 145, 1994.

81. Chandra, R. K., and Amorin, S. A. D., Lipids and immunoregulation, *Nutr. Res.*, 12, S137, 1992.

82. Calder, P. C., n-3 polyunsaturated fatty acids and cytokine production in health and disease, *Ann. Nutr. Metab.*, 41, 203, 1997.

83. Santoli, D., and Zurier, R. B., Prostaglandin E precursor fatty acids inhibit human IL-2 production by a prostaglandin E-independent mechanism, *J. Immunol.*, 143, 1303, 1989.

84. Valette, L., Croset, M., Prigent, A. F., Meskini, N., and Lagarde, M., Dietary polyunsaturated fatty acids modulate fatty acid composition and early activation steps of concanavalin A-stimulated rat thymocytes, *J. Nutr.*, 121, 1844, 1991.

85. Rossetti, R. G., Seiler, C. M., DeLuca, P., Laposata, M., and Zurier, R. B., Oral administration of unsaturated fatty acids: effects on human peripheral blood T lymphocyte proliferation, *J. Leuk. Biol.*, 62, 438, 1997.

86. Calder, P. C., Dietary fatty acids and the immune system, *Nutr. Rev.*, 56, S70, 1998.

87. Meydani, S. N., Endres, S., Woods, M. M., Goldin, B. R., Soo, C., Morrill Labrode, A., Dinarello, C. A., and Gorbach, S. L., Oral (n-3) fatty acid supplementation suppresses cytokine production and lymphocyte proliferation: comparison between young and older women, *J. Nutr.*, 121, 547, 1991.

88. Endres, S., Meydani, S. N., Ghorbani, R., Schindler, R., and Dinarello, C. A., Dietary supplementation with n-3 fatty acids suppresses interleukin-2 production and mononuclear cell proliferation, *J. Leukoc. Biol.*, 54, 599, 1993.

89. Meydani, S. N., Lichtenstein, A. H., Cornwall, S., Meydani, M., Goldin, B. R., Rasmussen, H., Dinarello, C. A., and Schaefer, E. J., Immunologic effects of national cholesterol education panel step-2 diets with and without fish-derived n-3 fatty acid enrichment, *J. Clin. Invest.*, 92, 105, 1993.

90. Olson, L. M., Clinton, S. K., Everitt, J. I., Johnston, P. V., and Visek, W. J., Lymphocyte activation, cell-mediated cytotoxicity and their relationship to dietary fat-enhanced mammary tumorigenesis in C3H/OUJ mice, *J. Nutr.*, 117, 955, 1987.

91. Hughes, D. A., Pinder, A. C., Piper, Z., Johnson, I. T., and Lund, E. K., Fish oil supplementation inhibits the expression of major histocompatibility complex class II molecules and adhesion molecules on human monocytes, *Am. J. Clin. Nutr.*, 63, 267, 1996.

92. Endres, S., Ghorbani, R., Kelley, V. E., Georgilis, K., Lonnemann, G., van der Meer, J. W., Cannon, J. G., Rogers, T. S., Klempner, M. S., Weber, P. C., and et al., The effect of dietary supplementation with n-3 polyunsaturated fatty acids on the synthesis of interleukin-1 and tumor necrosis factor by mononuclear cells, *New Eng. J. Med.*, 320, 265, 1989.

93. Virella, G., Fourspring, K., Hyman, B., Haskill Stroud, R., Long, L., Virella, I., La, V. M., Gross, A. J., and Lopes Virella, M., Immunosuppressive effects of fish oil in normal human volunteers: correlation with the *in vitro* effects of eicosapentanoic acid on human lymphocytes, *Clin. Immunol. Immunopathol.*, 61, 161, 1991.

94. Mascioli, E. A., Iwasa, Y., Trimbo, S., Leader, L., Bistrian, B. R., and Blackburn, G. L., Endotoxin challenge after menhaden oil diet: effects on survival of guinea pigs, *Am. J. Clin. Nutr.*, 49, 277, 1989.

95. Yoshino, S., and Ellis, E. F., Effect of a fish-oil-supplemented diet on inflammation and immunological processes in rats, *Int. Arch. Allergy Appl. Immunol.*, 84, 233, 1987.

96. Fowler, K. H., Chapkin, R. S., and McMurray, D. N., Effects of purified dietary n-3 ethyl esters on murine T lymphocyte function, *J. Immunol.*, 151, 5186, 1993.

97. Schmidt, E. B., and Dyerberg, J., Omega-3 fatty acids. Current status in cardiovascular medicine, *Drugs*, 47, 405, 1994.

98. Belluzzi, A., Brignola, C., Campieri, M., Pera, A., Boschi, S., and Miglioli, M., Effect of an enteric-coated fish-oil preparation on relapses in Crohn's disease, *New Eng. J. Med.*, 334, 1557, 1996.

99. Cappelli, P., DiLiberato, L., Stuard, S., Ballone, E., and Albertazzi, A., N-3 polyunsaturated fatty acid supplementation in chronic progressive renal disease, *J. Nephrol.*, 10, 157, 1997.

100. van der Heide, J. J., Bilo, H. J., Donker, J. M., Wilmink, J. M., and Tegzess, A. M., Effect of dietary fish oil on renal function and rejection in cyclosporine-treated recipients of renal transplants, *New Eng. J. Med.*, 329, 769, 1993.

101. Rasmussen, L. B., Kiens, B., Pedersen, B. K., and Richter, E. A., Effect of diet and plasma fatty acid composition on immune status in elderly men, *Am. J. Clin. Nutr.*, 59, 572, 1994.

102. Meydani, S. N., Vitamin E enhancement of T cell-mediated function in healthy elderly: mechanisms of action, *Nutr. Rev.*, 53, S52, 1995.

103. Meydani, S. N., Barklund, M. P., Liu, S., Meydani, M., Miller, R. A., Cannon, J. G., Morrow, F. D., Rocklin, R., and Blumberg, J. B., Vitamin E supplementation enhances cell-mediated immunity in healthy elderly subjects, *Am. J. Clin. Nutr.*, 52, 557, 1990.

104. Meydani, S. N., Meydani, M., Blumberg, J. B., Leka, L. S., Siber, G., Loszewski, R., Thompson, C., Pedrosa, M. C., Diamond, R. D., and Stollar, B. D., Vitamin E supplementation and *in vivo* immune response in healthy elderly subjects. A randomized controlled trial, *JAMA*, 277, 1380, 1997.

105. Stulnig, T. M., Berger, M., Roden, M., Stingl, H., Raederstorff, D., and Waldhäusl, W., Elevated serum free fatty acid concentrations inhibit T lymphocyte signaling, *FASEB J.*, 14, 939, 2000.

14 Carbohydrate Metabolism and Aging

Rodney C. Ruhe and Roger B. McDonald

CONTENTS

I.   INTRODUCTION

Aging in humans is associated with physiologic and metabolic changes that can have profound effects on the physical and psychological well being of the individual. Among these changes is the impaired ability to maintain glucose homeostasis. Proper control of blood glucose concentration is important at any age, but it is of particular concern in the elderly. Age-related alterations in the release and action of insulin are often exacerbated by modifiable factors that commonly occur as a function of age. The resulting dysregulation of glucose homeostasis can have serious consequences with respect to physical health and cognitive function. The purpose of this review is to present recent studies that examine how aging affects glucose homeostasis and insulin secretion. Investigations of the deleterious effects of altered glucose homeostasis, as well as possible measures aimed at mitigating these effects, will also be presented.

II.   CARBOHYDRATE METABOLISM AND GLUCOSE HOMEOSTASIS

Glucose is an essential nutrient, the major source of energy in the human body, and dietary carbohydrate is the most important source of glucose. Carbohydrate in the diet is normally in the form of disaccharides (sucrose and lactose) and polysaccharides (starch) that must be hydrolyzed to monosaccharides to be absorbed and used by the body. Specific hydrolytic enzymes called glycosidases, located in the saliva, pancreatic juice, and in the wall of the small intestine, break down disaccharides and polysaccharides into their constituent monosaccharides, including glucose, fructose, and galactose. The monosaccharides are transported across the intestinal wall and enter the portal circulation. In the liver, glucose is either delivered to the bloodstream to be distributed among the tissues or it is converted to glycogen for storage, depending on the body's need for energy. Fructose and galactose are rapidly converted to glucose, so blood concentrations of these monosaccharides are usually very low and largely unregulated. However, the most abundant and important monosaccharide, glucose, is subject to strict hormonal regulation that is critical to glucose homeostasis (138,155).

Glucose homeostasis is dependent almost entirely upon the normal synthesis and secretion of insulin. Although numerous other hormones are necessary to increase blood glucose concentrations during hypoglycemic episodes, only insulin is required to decrease blood glucose concentration by enhancing peripheral tissue glucose uptake and by reducing glycogenolysis by the liver (94,223,368). Variations in time and amount of food intake, as often occur in the human diet, require the presence of strict homeostatic controls to maintain blood glucose concentrations within a relatively narrow range (between 80 and 100 mg/100 ml in the postabsorptive state). This is particularly important to the central nervous system, which utilizes glucose as its primary substrate. The net effect of insulin's action is to promote conversion of metabolizable fuels into a form that can be stored. In the liver, insulin suppresses glycogenolysis and gluconeogenesis, and in adipose tissue, insulin accelerates glucose transport and suppresses lipolysis. Insulin accelerates the transport of glucose and amino acid into skeletal muscle and promotes protein synthesis (110). In summary, insulin acts to decrease hepatic glucose production and to accelerate the uptake of glucose into peripheral tissues, resulting in lowered blood glucose concentrations.

After the ingestion of carbohydrates, the β-cells within the islets of Langerhans respond rapidly and with high sensitivity to the increased blood glucose concentration by secreting insulin. The relatively short half-life of insulin in the blood (163) and the fact that the rate of insulin secretion alone regulates changes in plasma insulin concentration, as opposed to regulation by the uptake and catabolism of the hormone by peripheral tissues (41), make it essential that the secretion of insulin operates under an effective feedback control system. Any alterations in β-cell function that result in even minute delays or losses of sensitivity of the β-cell to changes in glucose concentration could disrupt the feedback loop sufficiently to cause metabolic disorders (49).

III. AGE-RELATED CHANGES IN GLUCOSE HOMEOSTASIS

A diminished ability to regulate blood glucose concentration is a common occurrence with advancing age. Many elderly individuals, in the absence of disease, experience changes in glucose homeostasis manifested as glucose intolerance, the inefficient uptake of glucose from the blood by the peripheral tissues. Glucose intolerance results in elevated blood glucose levels (hyperglycemia), which, over time, can lead to numerous pathological conditions and increased mortality (145). Although it has been the subject of intensive research for several decades, the exact cause of glucose intolerance is not known. However, glucose intolerance is known to be associated with insulin resistance, a state in which normal concentrations of insulin produce an attenuated biological response (113,200). Ongoing investigations are attempting to answer the question; Are glucose intolerance and insulin resistance normal consequences of aging, or are they the result of modifiable, environmental factors?

A. AGING AND THE DEVELOPMENT OF GLUCOSE INTOLERANCE

Glucose intolerance is characteristic of non-insulin-dependent diabetes mellitus (NIDDM) but may also occur in the absence of NIDDM (18,25,112,177,184,257,299,326). In the U.S., there is estimated to be approximately 15 million people with either diagnosed or undiagnosed NIDDM, and there are about 25 to 30 million people with impaired glucose tolerance (181). The prevalence of both NIDDM and glucose intolerance increases with age (108,150,159,244,317,327). For example, the average annual incidence of NIDDM per 100,000 persons triples between the ages of 50 and 70 compared with a less than 25% increase between the ages of 30 and 50 years (265). It is estimated that between 25 and 30% of the population aged 65 and older has NIDDM or impaired glucose tolerance (199). Older adults showing no clinical signs of diabetes often demonstrate decreased glucose tolerance, i.e., decreased glucose disposal rate as determined by the oral glucose tolerance test (8,9,65,70), even though resting levels of insulin secretion and fasting plasma glucose concentration remain stable with age (140).

Glucose intolerance in the elderly, when it does occur, can vary greatly among individuals due to genetic and environmental factors. Generally, however, the development of glucose intolerance follows a predictable course that may be described in the following manner. Over several decades there may occur a very gradual, genetically based diminution in the sensitivity of the pancreatic beta cells to glucose stimulation, resulting in decreased insulin secretion. Concomitantly, there may be an increased demand for insulin due to insulin resistance that is the result of age-related changes intrinsic to the insulin receptor and/or to environmental factors such as obesity and lack of physical activity. At some point the combination of increased insulin resistance and inadequate insulin secretion in response to a glucose challenge will result in hyperglycemia, a hallmark of glucose intolerance.

B. Endogenous Factors Affecting Glucose Intolerance

Several studies have revealed a general decline in carbohydrate and total energy intake with age (303). Carbohydrate hydrolysis and monosaccharide uptake by the intestine are well-maintained in aging humans and rodents (100,349). Taken together, these studies indicate that overnutrition, particularly with respect to carbohydrates, and carbohydrate digestion are not factors contributing to the development of glucose intolerance.

A gradual but significant rise in insulin resistance with age, independent of other variables (69,214,263,380), suggests the existence of an age-related alteration in the ability of insulin to mediate uptake of glucose in peripheral tissues. Binding of insulin to its receptor initiates a series of intracellular events that result in stimulation of the glucose transport system and an increase in intracellular glucose metabolism. Because the insulin receptor and glucose transport protein (325,363) are critical for insulin to exert its biological effect, any alterations of these mechanisms would have a serious effect on tissue insulin sensitivity. Although the results of several studies examining age-related changes in insulin binding are conflicting, the majority of evidence supports the conclusion that insulin receptor number and affinity are unaffected by age (85,103-105,218,250,264,307,340).

The observation that changes in glucose transporter expression occur during development in the rat (12) and in many physiological conditions such as NIDDM in the human (23,328) led Lin et al. (216) to hypothesize that quantitative changes of the expression of the adipose/muscle-type (GluT4) glucose transporter isoform may play a role in impaired glucose transport. These investigators found a decrease in GluT4 protein in the muscle and fat tissue of aged rats as compared with the younger animals. The authors emphasized, however, that although altered expression of GluT4 may contribute to glucose intolerance observed in some aging rats, differences in physical activity or tissue size between the young and the aged rats may have influenced the results. Nonetheless, Charron and Katz (50) found that in mouse models, genetic modification of the expression of GluT4 had a profound effect on whole body insulin action and on glucose metabolism. For example, mice that expressed no GluT4 exhibited insulin resistance and glucose intolerance. Restoration of GluT4 expression in the skeletal muscle of these mice resulted in increased insulin sensitivity and normal glucose metabolism. The results of this study appear to support the findings of Houmard et al. (152) that a decrement in GluT4 protein concentration in skeletal muscle may at least partially contribute to the insulin resistance of aging in humans.

Several previous studies of humans and of rats support the hypothesis that age-related glucose intolerance is due partially to a post-receptor alteration in insulin-mediated glucose uptake (103–105,218,264). Insulin stimulates the tyrosine kinase activity of its receptor, resulting in the phosphorylation of its cytosolic substrate, insulin receptor substrate-1 (IRS-1), which, in turn, associates with phosphatidylinositol 3-kinase (PI3-kinase), thereby activating the latter. It has been suggested that age-related changes in the regulation of the tyrosine kinase moiety may affect insulin sensitivity of the cell by altering insulin receptor function (195,249). However, Eiffert et al. (85), using the male Sprague-Dawley rat of ages 12 and 24 months, reported that insulin receptor function, as measured by insulin binding and tyrosine kinase activity, was influenced more by diet and/or exercise than by aging per se. Carvalho et al. (44) determined that phosphorylation of IRS-1 and insulin-stimulated IRS-1 association with PI3-kinase were decreased by 25 and 98%, respectively, in old vs. young rats, leading the authors to suggest that changes in the early steps of insulin signal transduction may have an important role in the insulin resistance observed in old animals. Donnelly and Qu (81) provide an excellent review of other possible post-receptor mechanisms of insulin resistance.

C. Modifiable Factors Effecting Glucose Intolerance

The findings reported above, together with several other studies of humans and of rodents (31,71,103,285,293,307,356) suggest that deteriorating glucose homeostasis may be an inevitable consequence of aging in some individuals. However, it must be emphasized that aging is not always associated with glucose intolerance (28,263,268). Ferrannini et al. (99) have suggested that in the absence of disease, aging per se is not a significant cause of insulin resistance. Numerous studies over the past 10 years have demonstrated the importance of modifiable environmental factors, such as obesity, diet, and physical inactivity, with respect to the development of glucose intolerance and insulin resistance (122,137).

Obesity is perhaps the most important factor contributing to the development of glucose intolerance in the aged. Some investigators have suggested that age-related glucose intolerance is independent of obesity (52,172,252,276). However, the vast majority of recent studies in humans and rodents have demonstrated a relationship between obesity and insulin resistance (62,291,294). Differences in conclusions regarding the effect of obesity on insulin resistance in the elderly may reflect the heterogeneity in the distribution of body fat. Upper body obesity, or visceral fat, is associated with a greater risk of decreased hepatic insulin extraction, impaired glucose tolerance, hyperinsulinemia, and NIDDM (196,255,271). The accumulation of visceral fat (fat in the intraabdominal cavity) is a common development of age. In a series of studies, Colman et al. (57–59) determined that an age-associated increase in total adiposity, particularly visceral fat, is the most important contributor to the development of insulin resistance and glucose intolerance in older men. It was also determined that weight loss resulted in reduced visceral fat and increased insulin action in older men suffering from impaired glucose tolerance. In agreement with the Colman studies, Cefalu et al. (46) concluded that accumulation of visceral fat is the most important determinant of the development of insulin resistance. These authors suggested that insulin resistance may be due more to changes in body composition, i.e., increased visceral fat, that often occur as a function of age rather than to aging itself. The results of subsequent studies by numerous investigators emphasize the importance of weight loss for the control or prevention of impaired glucose metabolism (20,75,347), insulin (46,91,93,225), and diabetes (15,21,111,350).

Aging is associated with a decrease in lean body mass, particularly muscle tissue, and with a concurrent relative increase in fat mass (30). Because muscle uses about 30% of total available glucose, it is reasonable to assume that a decrease in muscle mass would result in a reduction in glucose disposal. However, an extensive review of the literature by Kohrt and Holloszy (193) reveals that loss of muscle mass with age does not contribute to the development of glucose intolerance.

These findings suggest that, with regard to glucose intolerance and the age-related change in fat mass and muscle mass, the increase in fat mass is certainly the more important factor.

Another factor that may contribute to the impairment of glucose metabolism in the elderly is elevated plasma concentration of tissue necrosis factor-α(TNF-α). This cytokine has been implicated in the development of insulin resistance (97,151,179,344) and of NIDDM (11,147) and has been shown to increase with advancing age in rodents (54,133,243). Paolisso et al. (269) recently demonstrated that in healthy men and women, plasma TNF-α concentration was positively associated with advancing age and negatively correlated with insulin action. Although the mechanisms underlying these observations have yet to be determined, the authors provided evidence that plasma TNF-α concentration may parallel the age-related increase in body fatness. Therefore, while TNF-α may be associated with a general impairment of insulin-mediated glucose uptake with age, it may also be a factor that can be controlled by means of weight reduction.

Attenuated glucose tolerance and insulin sensitivity in the aged may be linked to physical activity. Decreased physical activity is common as people age and is a potentially reversible factor contributing to glucose intolerance (14). Exercise is known to increase insulin sensitivity and improve glucose tolerance (148,302,304), whereas physical inactivity has the opposite effect (141,319). Kahn et al. (171) evaluated the effect of exercise training on insulin resistance and insulin secretion of healthy older men. These authors demonstrated that 6 months of endurance training improved insulin sensitivity but not glucose tolerance. The lack of improvement in glucose tolerance was attributed to reduced insulin output by the β-cells. The results of this study concur with those of other studies suggesting that aging is not associated with decreased insulin sensitivity in non-obese individuals who exercise regularly (24,291,322,343). Exercise is an effective means of preventing and treating impaired glucose tolerance and non-insulin-dependent diabetes mellitus in aged men and women who already suffer from or are at risk for developing these conditions (76,89,121,162,267,314,339,347,353). The mechanism underlying the beneficial effects of exercise is unclear. Studies by Hughes et al. (154) and Cox et al. (61) have found that skeletal muscle in the elderly responds to exercise training by increasing GluT4 concentration, resulting in improved insulin action. This effect of exercise is apparently independent of diet (10) and the accumulation of visceral fat (79). It should be noted that the improved tissue insulin sensitivity occurring as a result of exercise is not always associated with increased glucose disposal (154,379). A study by Dengel et al. (76) suggests that exercise must be accompanied by weight loss to improve insulin sensitivity and glucose tolerance.

Changes in dietary composition are known to alter tissue insulin sensitivity and β-cell responsiveness (7,33,34,123,194,247). Chen et al. (53) examined the relationship between dietary carbohydrate- and age-related glucose intolerance. Elderly men eating an *ad libitum* diet were less tolerant to glucose than the younger participants, but after a 3- to 5-day regimen of very high (85%) carbohydrate intake, the results of insulin sensitivity and carbohydrate tolerance measurements of these same men were comparable to those of the younger men. The authors concluded that reduced glucose tolerance and insulin secretion, and increased insulin resistance, of aged non-obese men are related to diet, particularly decreased carbohydrate intake. These results were verified by Brunzell et al. (33,34), who observed that dietary carbohydrates in a physiological range (40–60%) did not seem to have a major impact on insulin sensitivity, while insulin sensitivity increased when carbohydrates composed more than 60% of the calories in the diet. However, the use of very high carbohydrate diets (>60% carbohydrate) as a means of improving insulin sensitivity has no major clinical significance, as these diets are not feasible in everyday life.

Barnard et al. (19) examined further the relationship between diet and the development of insulin resistance by comparing the effects of raising female Fischer rats on a low-fat, high complex carbohydrate (LFCC) diet versus a high-fat, sucrose (HFS) diet on serum glucose and insulin as well as skeletal muscle glucose transport. No significant differences were observed between 6- and 24-month-old rats raised on the LFCC diet. However, when the 24-month-old animals raised on the HFS diet were compared with age-matched rats raised on the LFCC diet, major differences were observed. Rats on the HFS diet had significantly higher fasting serum insulin and significantly reduced insulin-stimulated glucose transport than the rats on the LFCC diet. Taken together, these results led the authors to conclude that diet and not aging per se caused insulin resistance.

In summary, attenuated glucose tolerance in the aging human and rodent has been attributed to decreased secretion of insulin and to decreased peripheral tissue insulin sensitivity (51,55,82,241,286,287). Although much controversy has surrounded the question of which is the more important mechanism contributing to the apparent deterioration of glucose tolerance in the aged, the majority of recent studies point to insulin resistance (52,71,103,165,166,284,307) resulting from modifiable environmental factors and/or postreceptor modifications inherent to aging cells. However, changes in insulin secretion may also affect the ability of the aging animal to maintain proper glucose homeostasis.

IV. AGE-RELATED CHANGES IN THE ENDOCRINE PANCREAS AND IN INSULIN SECRETION

The effect of aging on insulin secretion and β-cell function is controversial. Studies of plasma insulin response to increased plasma glucose concentration in humans, and *in vivo* and *in vitro* studies of glucose-stimulated insulin secretion in rodents, have produced conflicting results. A review of the literature to 1979 by Davidson (66) revealed increased, decreased, and no change in insulin secretion with age in humans in response to a glucose load. Human studies using oral glucose tolerance as an index of insulin secretion indicate no age-related decline (65,71,83,172,228,284,323). The oral glucose tolerance test, considered an adequate index of glucose metabolism in general, has found limited application in defining β-cell function. Variability in plasma glucose levels due to gastrointestinal factors, e.g., differences in absorption rates, and neurohormonal effects, e.g., suppression of insulin secretion by epinephrine, cannot be controlled or quantified during this procedure. Plasma insulin concentrations of elderly subjects measured during the oral glucose tolerance test have been observed to be normal or even elevated (66,103). Conversely, Chen et al. (52) demonstrated that β-cell secretory capacity was 48% lower in older men (57–82 yr) than in younger men (18–36 yr). This apparent discrepancy has been attributed to an age-related reduction in the ability of the liver to metabolize insulin (101). Plasma insulin clearance in the elderly is reduced by about 40% as compared with younger individuals (238). Thus, plasma insulin concentration values obtained from the oral glucose tolerance test may reflect hepatic insulin extraction rate rather than β-cell secretory capacity.

Measurement of plasma insulin concentration in response to a glucose load, e.g., the oral glucose tolerance test, is an indirect and possibly inaccurate index of β-cell responsiveness to glucose. Thus, various techniques have been developed which provide a more accurate determination of glucose tolerance and of plasma insulin concentration. In the intravenous glucose tolerance test, a glucose load is administered intravenously, thereby avoiding possible variations associated with glucose absorption by the gastrointestinal tract. The euglycemic clamp technique (72) allows maintenance of blood glucose concentration at a steady state by continuous intravenous glucose infusion. The rate at which glucose is metabolized can then be determined by the rate of glucose infusion necessary to maintain the blood glucose level. Concurrent with the determination of glucose disposal rate, insulin release may be estimated from the measurement of plasma C-peptide concentration. Because C-peptide and insulin are stored and released by the β-cell in equimolar quantities, yet C-peptide is not metabolized by the liver, plasma C-peptide concentration may be a better indicator of prehepatic insulin concentration (278,279,308).

The intravenous glucose tolerance test and C-peptide measurement were utilized by Pacini et al. (262) in evaluating β-cell insulin release and the role of the liver in insulin disposal in healthy, oral glucose-tolerant young and old men. Results of the intravenous glucose tolerance test revealed no difference between the two groups with respect to plasma glucose and insulin concentration, although C-peptide secretion rate in the elderly subjects was much lower than in the young controls. These results led the authors to conclude that plasma insulin concentrations observed in the elderly subjects were similar to those seen in the younger men due to a net effect of reduced hepatic insulin extraction and a reduction in β-cell insulin secretion. However, this and other recent studies demonstrating diminished insulin secretion with age (52,171) have not attempted to control dietary intake or physical activity in the subjects. These environmental factors have a great impact on glucose metabolism at any age (52,53,342), and β-cell function is intimately linked to glucose metabolism. Therefore, it is critical that these factors be considered when examining the effects of age on glucose-stimulated insulin secretion.

If, as some studies suggest (52,171,262), attenuated insulin secretion is a true effect of age, then the question becomes, Is this attenuation of secretory capacity due to an age-related alteration(s) that is intrinsic to the β-cell, or is the β-cell merely responding to the affects of age-related changes in other tissues?

A. Aging and Physical Alterations in the Pancreas and Islets

Extensive vascularization of the islet enables the β-cells to react rapidly and with great sensitivity to even minor changes in blood glucose concentration. As such, any changes in islet or pancreatic vasculature that result in impeded blood flow will affect β-cell responsiveness to glucose stimulation. Pancreatic structural changes in the aged, including fibrosis of the exocrine tissue and pancreatic vascular degeneration, have been reported (37,364). These changes, however, were probably not a function of age but rather a consequence of diabetes, as they were observed in elderly subjects with NIDDM. In a study of the effects of aging on whole pancreatic blood flow and islet blood flow in the Sprague-Dawley rat, Jansson and Swenne (167) determined that although pancreatic blood flow decreased progressively with age, islet blood flow increased as the animal reached maturity (20 weeks) and remained constant into senescence (104 weeks). When islet blood flow was expressed as a fraction of pancreatic blood flow, the 20-week-old rats were found to have a fractional islet blood flow of about 10%, whereas a significantly larger fraction (20%) was diverted through the islets in the 104-week-old rats. Glucose administration increased significantly both pancreatic blood flow and islet blood flow, and this effect was most apparent in the older animals. These results indicate that in the healthy, aging animal, decreased blood flow to the islets is not a factor contributing to β-cell responsiveness. However, it is possible that an age-related increase in islet blood flow may have an adverse effect in individuals at risk for developing diabetes. Carlsson et al. (43) suggested that the increased islet blood flow observed in diabetes-prone NOD mice may augment homing to islets of inflammatory cells and soluble factors involved in β-cell destruction associated with the development of diabetes.

Amyloid polypeptide, a 37-amino acid polypeptide that has been linked to deleterious effects of aging, is produced by the β-cells of normal and NIDDM subjects (361) and may affect β-cell responsiveness. Although amyloid deposition occurs in the islets of non-diabetic subjects, it occurs to a much greater extent in the islets of those with NIDDM. Westermark et al. (362) found amyloid deposition in 20 to 99% of the islets in 12 of 13 NIDDM subjects as compared with 3 to 11% of the islets in 6 of 11 non-diabetic subjects. Extensive amyloidosis in islets correlates well with impaired insulin secretion and increased glucose intolerance in the diabetic macaque (153) and in genetically obese and diabetic mice (211,337). In human NIDDM, the extent of amyloid deposition increased along with disease severity (221). Ohsawa et al. (256) demonstrated that islet amyloid polypeptide inhibits glucose-stimulated insulin secretion in islets of Langerhans isolated from the rat. In a study involving lean, non-diabetic individuals, Edwards et al. (84) observed that after a 75-g glucose load, amylin secretion exhibited a U-shaped curve with greater secretion in young (20–40 yr) and old (61–90 yr) subjects than in middle-aged (41–60 yr) persons. A significant association was found between maximum amylin secretion and a glucose concentration greater than 120 mg/dl. The authors interpreted these results as indicative of a counterregulatory role for amylin. They also proposed that amylin may merely be acting as a marker of impaired glucose metabolism. Although the results reported by Edwards et al. (84) are suggestive, there have been no studies to date demonstrating an increase in islet amyloid deposition with age in non-diabetic persons, nor has an age-related increase in islet amyloid polypeptide secretion been demonstrated. Mitsukawa et al. (239) provided evidence that plasma islet amylyoid polypeptide concentrations at both basal and glucose-stimulated conditions were unaffected by age in the human. Nonetheless, the possibility that islet amyloid polypeptide plays a role in diminished β-cell responsiveness with age will no doubt remain an active area of investigation.

Studies concerned with the effects of aging on insulin secretion normally have focused on the secretory organ itself, with little consideration given as to how age-related changes in other tissues may influence the regulation of the β-cell. It has long been known that insulin secretion is enhanced by gastrointestinal hormones, e.g., gastric inhibitory peptide, enteroglucagon, gastrin, secretin, and cholecystokinin, which are stimulated by the presence of food within the lumen of the gut (227,229). The possibility exists that age-related changes occurring in the gut may compromise the enteroinsular axis, resulting in altered control input to the β-cell. Using gastric inhibitory peptide as a typical example of an enteric insulinotropic hormonal factor, Groop (124) examined the relationship between insulin secretion, gastric inhibitory peptide, and aging. Groop (124) observed in aged individuals an increased insulin/C-peptide response to a glucose load, while gastric inhibitory peptide response was comparable to that of the younger subjects. Elahi et al. (86) also showed that aging is associated with a normal gastric inhibitory peptide response to oral glucose, while β-cell sensitivity to gastric inhibitory peptide was decreased. Similarly, studies by Meneilly et al. (234) and Ranganath et al. (283) demonstrated that secretion of the major insulintropic hormones glucagon-like peptide and glucose-dependent insulintropic polypeptide was increased and β-cell sensitivity was decreased in old vs. younger subjects. Taken together, these results indicate that the enteric end of the enteroinsular axis is intact in the aged, suggesting that impaired insulin secretion with age must be intrinsic to the endocrine pancreas.

Certain pathological conditions associated with aging, e.g., NIDDM and chronic renal failure with secondary hyperparathyroidism (3,95,96,109,146,173,222,306), can contribute to diminished glucose-stimulated insulin secretion. However, normal age-related changes occurring in the healthy animal have little impact on β-cell responsiveness. It may thus be inferred that the presence of an age-related attenuation of insulin secretion is due to changes in stimulus-secretion coupling.

B. *In Vitro* Analysis of Insulin Secretion

Despite improved techniques for determining insulin secretion in response to glucose stimulation, *in vivo* assessment of β-cell function is indirect and is subject to the influences of neural and hormonal factors that cannot be controlled. As such, *in vivo* techniques for examining aging effects specific to the β-cells are inherently imprecise. Evaluation of age-related alterations intrinsic to the endocrine pancreas requires the use of a model for islet function that allows control over external influences. To this end, islet function has been studied *in vitro* using either the whole perfused pancreas, or isolated islets and β-cells. The whole perfused pancreas technique has the advantage of allowing the islets to remain in a relatively normal physiological environment in which anatomical relationships with other cells and tissues are intact, and the perfusion medium containing substrates and test substances arrive at the islet via blood vessels. The major disadvantage of this technique is that certain biochemical responses, such as islet glucose oxidation, cannot be studied directly and are thus difficult to evaluate.

The use of isolated islets of Langerhans is less physiological than the use of whole perfused pancreas. However, this technique provides the investigator the advantage of examining phenomena intrinsic to the islet, separate from neural effects and the influences of hormones from other endocrine organs. Because islets of Langerhans are normally isolated by collagenase digestion

(208), it is possible that islets may be damaged during the procedure, resulting in abnormal secretion (38,130). This is of particular concern during the isolation of islets from older rats whose collagen-rich pancreases require longer digestion time and/or a greater concentration of collagenase in the incubation solution (36). Techniques have been described in which collagenase-induced damage to islets during isolation is minimized (22,36,215,309). Regardless of method of isolation used, several studies have demonstrated that the pattern of glucose-induced insulin secretion are similar in isolated islets and in the whole perfused pancreas (157,161,215). These studies validate the use of isolated pancreatic islets of Langerhans for the study of insulin secretion at the cellular level.

Investigations using islets of Langerhans isolated from mice and rats have shown both decreased (51,52,55,63,185,241,285–289,318,354) and increased (36,214) insulin secretion with age. An investigation in our laboratory showed greater insulin secretion by islets isolated from young (6 mo.) vs. senescent (26 mo.) male Fischer 344 rats (309). The various results obtained from the studies cited above may reflect differences in strain and species of animal model used as well as varying definitions of senescence in rodents.

Islet size may also influence results of studies investigating the effect of age on insulin secretion. The proportion of large islets in the pancreas of the rat increases with age (118,131,142,186,297). Kitahara and Adelman (185) and Adelman (1) have shown that, regardless of the age of the rat, large islets secrete more insulin than do smaller islets. These authors suggested that the age-dependent decrease in insulin secretion of β-cells is observed only in small islets (50 to 80 μm diameter); larger islets are apparently less affected by aging. According to Adelman (1), the age-related differences in glucose sensitivity of large vs. small islets introduces a confounding factor that was rarely considered in past studies of islet responsiveness. As such, many previous investigations of islet insulin secretion may require reinterpretation.

Reaven et al. (287) observed that larger islets from older (18 mo.) Sprague-Dawley rats contained more β-cells, and more insulin per β-cell, than islets from younger (2 mo.) animals. A progressive, age-related decrease in glucose- and leucine-stimulated insulin secretion per islet was also observed (119,185), indicating that insulin release per β-cell declines significantly with age. Adelman (1) has suggested that this apparent alteration of insulin secretion during aging may be overcome *in vivo* by the capacity of older animals to compensate by expanding their pool of β-cells. The observation that the proportion of larger islets increases with age suggests that the insulin secretory function of the endocrine pancreas as a whole does not become impaired with age but rather adapts to the changing metabolic environment (1). The hypothesis of pancreatic adaptation is consistent with data that describe attenuated insulin secretion by isolated islets without a concomitant decrease during whole pancreatic perfusion (309).

In addition to islet size, the effects of aging on the relative proportions and sensitivity of all cell types that compose the islet must be considered. The normal islet consists of α-, β-, and δ-cells that secrete glucagon, insulin, and somatostatin, respectively. These cells are in proximity, which permits effective paracrine control of one cell type by another (260). Glucagon stimulates secretion of both insulin and somatostatin (4,191,270,321,357), while somatostatin inhibits insulin and glucagon release (4,191,220). Paracrine regulation of insulin secretion has been reported (174,275,346), so it is possible that any age-related change in relative proportions of the cell types, or even in the spatial relationships within the islet, may have a profound effect on β-cell responsiveness. Changes in paracrine regulation leading to altered insulin secretion is consistent with the observations of decreased density, mean area, and sensitivity of glucagon-containing α-cells (188,329). In addition, Casad et al. (45), using the whole perfused pancreas technique, observed that the inhibitory action of somatostatin on insulin secretion is increased with age. However, these findings are not supported by the work of Starnes et al. (332), who found no decrease in somatostatin or insulin secretion from the whole perfused pancreas of the aged rat. A possible explanation for the apparent discrepancy between Casad et al. (45) and Starnes et al. (332) may be found in the observations of Adelman and colleagues (1,51), who have proposed that the ability of smaller islets to secrete insulin is attenuated with age because of enhanced availability of somatostatin, while enhanced secretion of somatostatin with a subsequent decrease in insulin secretion was not seen in larger islets. It is thus possible that the greater proportion of larger islets in the pancreases of aged rats (118,131,142,186,297) is an adaptation that allows these animals to maintain insulin secretion.

Another possible adaptation that may help maintain the insulin secretory capacity of the whole endocrine pancreas was examined recently in our laboratory (310). Responsiveness and sensitivity to glucose stimulation, as determined by changes in cytoplasmic calcium concentration, were evaluated in individual β-cells isolated from senescent and young rats. A greater percentage of β-cells from the senescent rats (76%) responded to a stimulatory glucose concentration compared with the young animals (63%). Of the responsive β-cells, a greater percentage of those from the old rats (72%) responded to a low stimulatory glucose concentration as compared with the young rats (58%). These data indicate that in older rats, an increase in the percentage of β-cells that are responsive to stimuli, and/or an increase in the sensitivity of the responsive β-cells, contributes to the maintenance of islet function at a level comparable to that of younger animals.

C. AGING AND INSULIN BIOSYNTHESIS

There is little evidence to suggest that any age-related changes in β-cell function occur at the level of transcription. Microscopic analysis of 30-month-old rat β-cell nuclei reveals that with age, the relative volume of the condensed (nontranscribable) chromatin increases progressively at the expense of the dispersed (transcribable) form, suggesting that transcriptional activity could be reduced in these aged cells (67). It was noted in this study, however, that under nonphysiological *in vitro* conditons, old β-cell nuclei are able to react in the same way as young ones with respect to chromatin redistribution and nuclear size increase, suggesting that the machinery for transcription remains fully functional in the older cells. In a study of isolated islets from young and old Fischer rats (354), it was determined that the levels of preproinsulin mRNA, the direct product of transcription, did not change with age. These data strongly suggest that any alteration in the insulin synthesis/secretion pathway is post-transcriptional.

In studies using the isolated islet preparation (354), it was demonstrated that, although preproinsulin mRNA levels remained the same, glucose-stimulated proinsulin biosynthesis was decreased in islets of old animals, suggesting impaired translation. It was not determined if the impairment was due to a defect in the signaling mechanism or to degeneration of the biosynthetic apparatus. Evidence for the latter was provided by DeClercq et al. (67), who observed in freshly isolated islets a decrease with age in the volume density of rough endoplasmic reticulum and Golgi complex, changes that could affect proinsulin biosynthesis. It should be noted that DeClercq et al. observed few other structural changes occurring with age.

Despite an apparent decrease in proinsulin synthesis and degeneration of the insulin synthetic apparatus, the total insulin content of pancreases and of isolated islets is quite similar in both young and old rats (119,309,354). The fact that pancreatic insulin content is the same in young and old rats while insulin secretion is lessened with age implies that an age-related alteration may exist in the actual secretion of newly made and preformed insulin from the β-cell. Draznin et al. (82), working with islets isolated from 2- and 18-month-old Fischer 344 rats, concluded that the lower insulin secretory response to glucose in old islets was due to an age-related impairment of glucose-induced fusion of secretory vesicles with the plasma membrane. These investigators found that glyburide, a substance that can directly stimulate secretory vesicle fusion with the plasma membrane and subsequent vesicle lysis, will elicit insulin release from old islets that are unresponsive to glucose. This observation implies that the secretory pathway per se is likely to be intact but glucose signal recognition is impaired. Wang et al. (354) arrived at a similar conclusion, stating that decreased insulin secretion in old islets may be due to impaired transduction of the glucose stimulus into signals affecting steps in the insulin secretory pathway.

In summary, the studies discussed above demonstrated that biological aging does not result in significantly decreased insulin secretory capacity of the whole endocrine pancreas, and that insulin secretion is unaffected by age-related alterations in pancreatic structure. In addition, pancreatic islets of Langerhans undergo no significant physical changes with age that would impede insulin release, and the β-cells are unaltered with respect to structure and function of the insulin biosynthetic apparatus. Nonetheless, an age-related attenuation of β-cell responsiveness to secretagogues does occur (26,27,160,201,272,273), suggesting an alteration in the stimulus-secretion coupling mechanism, the complex, postreceptor series of events within the β-cell that links the increase in plasma glucose concentration to insulin secretion. The affects of aging on the stimulus-secretion coupling mechanism are discussed in detail in the previous edition of this book (311)

V. ADVERSE EFFECTS OF ALTERED GLUCOSE HOMEOSTASIS IN THE AGED

As discussed in the previous sections, aging is often associated with changes in glucose homeostasis resulting from insulin resistance and/or decreased insulin secretion. Although many of these changes can be prevented or controlled through lifestyle choices, the fact remains that perturbations in glucose homeostasis generally increase as a function of age. The end result is usually a large variation in blood glucose and/or insulin concentration. Hyperglycemia, hypoglycemia, and hyperinsulinemia are all related to pathological conditions. The deleterious effects of chronic dysregulation of blood glucose and insulin levels merit consideration, as they are prevalent among the elderly.

A. HYPERGLYCEMIA

Hyperglycemia is a chronic or acute increase in fasting or postprandial blood glucose concentration above those levels that are considered normal. In general, hyperglycemia occurs as a result of decreased transport and uptake of glucose into muscle and adipose tissue, and an increase in hepatic glucose output. Because blood glucose levels can vary widely depending on the influence of numerous factors, there is no precise definition of hyperglycemia. Recently, the Expert Committee on the Diagnosis and Classification of Diabetes Mellitus of the American Diabetes Association established new diagnostic criteria for impaired glucose tolerance and diabetes (231). The revised criteria were based on disease etiology, i.e., correlating blood glucose concentration with the development of various pathologies. According to the new criteria, a fasting plasma glucose level of 110 to 125 mg/dl indicates impaired fasting glucose and a value greater than 126 mg/dl indicates diabetes. A 2-hour postprandial (75 g glucose) value of 140 to 199 mg/dl indicates impaired glucose tolerance, while a value greater than 200 mg/dl is considered diagnostic of diabetes. Because of their demonstrated relationship to the development of specific disease states, these values may provide a quantitative and practical definition of hyperglycemia.

Glucose is an essential nutrient, but very high levels of glucose can produce adverse changes in glucose metabolism, an effect often referred to as *glucose toxicity* (178,242,376,377). Hyperglycemia can lead to a reduced number of glucose transporters and to insulin resistance (13,107). Hyperinsulinemia associated with hyperglycemia may also contribute to the development of insulin resistance by down-regulating the number of insulin receptors (42). Hyperglycemia can even have adverse effects on β-cell insulin secretion (158). Therefore, hyperglycemia resulting from insulin resistance and decreased insulin secretion can worsen glucose intolerance by promoting further insulin resistance and decreased insulin secretion, i.e., the effect contributes to its own cause. The effects of glucose toxicity are somewhat reversible, as a reduction in hyperglycemia by any means improves insulin sensitivity and insulin secretion in NIDDM (376).

It has been known for some time that acute and chronic hyperglycemia can accelerate aging and mortality (5,168,192,305,355). In addition to glucose toxicity, hyperglycemia is linked to numerous pathologic conditions that are usually associated with advancing age, including hearing loss (313), cataracts (290), impaired cognitive function (235,314), DNA damage and tumor growth

(64,280), osteoporosis (40,296), and impaired cellular immunity (280). In terms of prevalence, health care costs, and length and quality of life, cardiovascular disease (CVD) is perhaps the most important consequence of hyperglycemia. There is much evidence for an intimate association between hyperglycemia and the development of CVD, although epidemiological evidence is insufficient to verify causality (345,352). Nonetheless, its close relationship to CVD implicates hyperglycemia as a risk factor contributing to this condition (127,205). This is most apparent in cases of NIDDM. Persons with NIDDM have a twofold to fourfold increased risk of dying of heart disease as compared with non-diabetic individuals (330). Several studies have indicated a causal link between postprandial hyperglycemia and the development of CVD in persons with NIDDM (135,136,187,213,331), and it is well documented that all forms of CVD, including coronary heart disease, stroke, and peripheral vascular disease, are much more common in persons with NIDDM than in non-diabetic individuals (127,207,245,281,320). Based on an analysis of 12 long-term studies (> 5 years) of middle-aged to elderly subjects with NIDDM, Laakso (205) concluded that hyperglycemia and poor glycemic control are associated with an increased risk for cardiovascular disease. A meta-analysis of 20 different studies of 95,783 individuals followed for 12 years led Coutinho et al. (60) to suggest that glucose seems to be a risk factor for cardiovascular events even within a range that is below the diabetic threshold, and that glucose is likely to be a continuous cardiovascular risk factor, similar to total cholesterol and blood pressure.

As noted earlier, there are approximately 25 to 30 million people in the U.S. with impaired glucose tolerance (IGT). Persons with IGT exhibit elevated postprandial blood glucose concentrations, while fasting levels are usually within the normal range (126). Because the prevalence of IGT is known to increase with age, the deleterious effects of the poor glycemic control that usually accompanies IGT should be of particular concern to the elderly (176). This is especially important in light of growing evidence that IGT may be an independent risk factor for the development of CVD (139,175,180,189,366). The prevalence of CVD in individuals with IGT and in control populations with normal glucose tolerance has been investigated in numerous studies. In the majority of these studies, an increased prevalence of CVD in subjects with IGT has been reported (266,298). For example, in a study involving men aged 67 years, Ohlson et al. (254) observed an increased prevalence of CVD in the subjects with IGT. Rewers et al. (298) reported a twofold increase in coronary heart disease in non-Hispanic white individuals with IGT compared with those with normal glucose tolerance. In this same study, the prevalence of coronary heart disease in Hispanic individuals was similar for those with IGT and those with normal glucose tolerance, suggesting that ethnicity may influence the effect of IGT on coronary heart disease. Gender may also play a role in the relationship between IGT and CVD. The Tecumseh Community Health Study demonstrated that even after controlling for other coronary risk factors, higher glucose levels 1 hour after a 100 gm glucose load are associated with excess coronary heart disease mortality in non-diabetic men but not women (39). However, data from the Framingham Heart Study indicate that hyperglycemia is an independent risk factor for CVD in non-diabetic women, but not among men (366). The results of the Framingham study imply that, as they age, women may become more vulnerable than men to the deleterious effects of hyperglycemia.

Cardiovascular disease is the result of significant and adverse changes in the macrovasculature and in the microvasculature, changes due, in part, to an elevation of blood glucose either in the fasting state or postprandially. In cases of poorly controlled diabetes, hyperglycemia is a clear risk factor for microvascular complications, e.g., retinopathy, nephropathy, and, less directly, neuropathy (127,187,280). Yamada and Ohkubo (373) demonstrated that, in healthy mice, excessive glucose intake resulted in microvascular aging, indicating a direct effect of glucose. Macrovascular changes associated with hyperglycemia have received greater attention in recent years. The most significant finding has been that even a mild increase in chronic (fasting) or acute (postprandial) blood glucose concentration can contribute to macrovascular injury (180,205). Yamasaki et al. (374) investigated the effects of asymptomatic hyperglycemia on the thickness of the carotid artery wall, an indication of more extensive atherosclerosis. Using ultrasonography, these investigators measured the intima medial wall thickness of the carotid artery in healthy male subjects, subjects with IGT, subjects with moderately elevated postprandial glucose levels (non-IGT), and subjects with NIDDM. There were no significant differences observed between the NIDDM group and the IGT and non-IGT groups, and the values for intima medial wall thickness for all three of these groups were significantly greater than those of the age-matched controls. The results of this study, together with those of previous studies by others (106,251), suggest that atherosclerotic changes are an early consequence of even mild elevations in postprandial blood glucose levels.

The mechanisms by which glucose produces its deleterious effects are not completely understood. The harmful effects of acute hyperglycemia may occur rapidly through the generation of free radicals, which in turn may mediate some of the changes associated with the development of atherosclerosis, e.g., activation of coagulation, vasoconstriction (365), and the increased expression of adhesion molecules (246). Glucose can also have a rapid and direct effect on the activity of protein kinase C (198), which may result in increased endothelial permeability (132), increased macrophage migration (115), and increased secretion of endothelin, a cytokine believed to be involved in the development of atherosclerosis (367).

Another adverse effect of elevated glucose levels that has been described thoroughly in several previous reviews (47,48,212,372) is the nonenzymatic glycosylation of proteins. As a function of time and glucose concentration, protein amino groups react with aldehydes of sugars to form unstable Schiff bases that can undergo further transformation into more stable Amadori products. Through a complex series of dehydration and oxidation reactions, the Amadori products become advanced glycosylation endproducts (AGE) (351). AGEs can accumulate over time (73) and can induce excess cross-linking of collagen and other extracellular matrix proteins. The harmful effects of glycosylation occur in a wide variety of tissues, because virtually every protein in the body is subject to glycosylation. Among the tissues adversely affected by glycosylation are the eye (2,6,134,190), cartilage (16,74,277), skin (240,360), kidney (117), bone (338), and brain (182,183). Several age-related diseases and conditions are associated with glycosylation, including atherosclerosis (301,315), Alzheimer's disease (102,248), cataracts (282), neuropathy (56), and erectile dysfunction (316). Macrovascular and microvascular complications are the most common and the most significant consequences of glycosylation. The AGE-induced cross-linking of proteins in the vascular wall has been implicated in pathological changes associated with atherosclerosis (32,35). For example, extensive cross-linking can lead to the accumulation of LDL particles in the vascular wall. Modification of the LDL particles by AGE render them prone to oxidation (219), which in turn can hasten the uptake of LDL by macrophages and the conversion of these macrophages to foam cells, a component of atherosclerotic plaque (80,92). The thickening, loss of elasticity, and increased permeability of blood vessel walls that is associated with microvascular complications may be due, in part, to glycosylation of vascular proteins.

Because causality between hyperglycemia and CVD has not been proven, it cannot be stated with certainty that glycemic control will cause a significant reduction in cardiovascular events. However, intensive glycemic control has been shown to cause a significant delay in the development of microvascular complications in persons with type 1 diabetes (295). Similar results were observed in persons with type 2 diabetes (253). The development of diseases related to microvascular changes can be prevented with strict glycemic control (210). For example, Giansanti et al. (114) in a 10-year retrospective study of subjects with type 1 diabetes, reported that deterioration of glycemic control was related to a progression of retinopathy, while Matsumoto et al. (224) found that intensive glycemic control was essential to prevent distal polyneuropathy. The authors of both of these studies concluded that hyperglycemia is a major determinant for the development of these conditions independent of age and duration of diabetes. Several longitudinal studies have demonstrated an association between glycemic control and the presence of macrovascular disease. Kuusisto et al. (204), using glycated hemoglobin levels as a marker of glycemic control, observed a stepwise increase in coronary artery disease morbidity and mortality over 3.5 years in elderly Finnish men with type 2 diabetes as glycemic control deteriorated.

B. Hyperinsulinemia

Hyperinsulinemia is often considered a normal component of IGT, although it does not necessarily parallel the development of glucose intolerance. An age-related decrease in the biological effectiveness of insulin, i.e., insulin resistance, may be due to genetic predisposition or it may occur as a result of acquired factors, such as obesity, lack of physical activity, or glucose toxicity. Regardless of cause, the diminished responsiveness of insulin receptors requires an increased serum concentration of insulin to produce the appropriate biological response. Initially, the endocrine pancreas compensates for insulin resistance by increasing insulin secretion (203). Fasting and postprandial glucose levels can be maintained within the normal range by means of this compensatory hyperinsulinemia, but not indefinitely. Eventually, a combination of reduced insulin secretory capacity of the β-cells and further diminution of insulin receptor responsiveness leads to the development of IGT and hyperglycemia (370). Even with decreased insulin secretion, serum insulin levels usually remain high relative to a state of normal glucose tolerance. Thus, for a period of years, and possibly decades, hyperglycemia may occur in conjunction with hyperinsulinemia.

It is possible that hyperinsulinemia may play a role in the apparent association between CVD and hyperglycemia (143,206). Hyperinsulinemia is strongly associated with a constellation of risk factors that contribute to the development of CVD, including elevated triglyceride and LDL levels (87,129,209,292), hypertension (77,88,98,116,230,324), decreased levels of HDL (87,209), and increased plasminogen activator inhibitor-1 (169,170,348). Several investigators have proposed that hyperinsulinemia may contribute to the development of atherosclerosis (68,334), possibly through direct effects on the arterial wall. Insulin can stimulate smooth muscle cell proliferation and can potentiate the effects of vascular growth factors (17,274). For example, Niskanen et al. (251) suggested that greater carotid intima-media thickness observed in elderly subjects with NIDDM as compared with control subjects was due, in part, to high postprandial insulin levels, while Suzuki et al. (336) concluded from a study of non-diabetic subjects aged 50 to 59 years that insulin resistance is an independent risk factor for carotid wall thickening. Insulin has been shown to stimulate cholesterol synthesis and to promote the binding of LDL to smooth muscle cells (335), fibroblasts (378), and monocytes (202, 258), all of which can result in arterial wall lipid deposition. Insulin may also accelerate atherogenesis indirectly by promoting the development of hypertension, dyslipidemia, and impaired fibrinolysis.

Hyperinsulinemia has been identified as a risk factor for CVD (78,90,358), although epidemiological studies of non-diabetic persons have revealed that it is not a consistent risk factor (369) and may be restricted to Caucasians (312). Several investigators have shown that hyperinsulinemia is a risk factor for CVD only in populations with specific risk factor abnormalities, such as hypertriglyceridemia (375) or the apolipoprotein E 3/2 phenotype (259). Age may also affect the relation between hyperinsulinemia and CVD. Insulin levels have generally correlated with CVD risk in middle-aged (40 to 60 years) Caucasian men, but not in older populations (128). Welin et al. (359) concluded that hyperinsulinemia is not a major coronary risk factor in men over the age of 80 years, while Ferrara et al. (100) determined that high blood insulin levels do not increase the risk of fatal CVD in non-diabetic elderly men or women. It is thus possible that in general, hyperinsulinemia is not a threat to people beyond a certain age, as these individuals are apparently not genetically susceptible to any adverse effects of high insulin levels.

C. Hypoglycemia

Hypoglycemia is a syndrome characterized by symptoms of sympathetic nervous system stimulation or of central nervous system dysfunction that are provoked by an abnormally low plasma glucose concentration. Many factors can cause a decrease in blood glucose levels, including an inappropriately high blood concentration of insulin, either endogenous or exogenous, hypoglycemic drugs, e.g., sulfonylureas, and prolonged fasting. True hypoglycemia in older persons in the absence of disease is uncommon, and aging does not alter significantly the physiologic response to hypogly-cemia when it does occur. However, the glucose level at which the maximum physiologic response occurs is lower in the elderly. For example, at a glucose level of 60 mg/dl, young controls had a greater response than did their elderly counterparts in the release of counterregulatory hormones, i.e., epinephrine, glucagon, cortisol, and pancreatic polypeptide. At a glucose level of 50 mg/dl, the responses were comparable between young and old. Symptom responses, such as hunger, tremulousness, and palpitations, were similar in both groups (232,261).

Although the physiologic response to hypoglycemia is sufficient in healthy older individuals, occasional hypoglycemic episodes are not innocuous. There is considerable evidence that acute hypoglycemia causes cognitive dysfunction in diabetic (300) and nondiabetic (144,149,156,217,333) humans. Hypoglycemia can affect complex as well as simple cognitive skills such as visual reaction time (333) regardless of age. However, several recent studies suggest that the elderly are at an increased risk of impaired cognitive capability associated with hypoglycemia (164). Brierley et al. (29) reported that, despite an intact counterregulatory response, elderly subjects experienced a decreased awareness of hypoglycemia, an effect attributed to diminished end organ responsiveness to the counterregulatory hormones. Matyka et al. (226) determined that older men are more prone to profound cognitive impairment during hypoglycemia than are younger men and are less likely to experience prior warning symptoms when blood glucose levels fall. These investigators, and others (233), suggest that a decreased ability to sense the onset of hypoglycemia puts older diabetics, especially those who are treated with insulin or hypoglycemic agents, at greater risk for severe or even fatal hypoglycemia. To prevent such an outcome, Teo and Ee (341), based on a retrospective study of hypoglycemia in the elderly, have recommended regular meals, careful use of hypoglycemic agents, and regular monitoring of blood glucose levels. Numerous studies have demonstrated that, with regard to cognitive function, it is better to err on the side of higher blood glucose levels, as hyperglycemia does not cause impairment of cognitive function (125) and, in fact, appears to enhance memory and learning in elderly rodents and humans (120,197,236,237,371).

VI. SUMMARY AND CONCLUSIONS

In the human diet, carbohydrates are the primary source of glucose, an essential nutrient that is the major metabolic fuel of the body under most conditions. Glucose homeostasis, the maintenance of serum glucose concentration within a relatively narrow range, is dependent upon highly regulated neural and hormonal activity. A critical hormonal component of glucose homeostasis is insulin, which mediates the uptake of glucose in the peripheral tissues. Aging is associated with a decrease in tissue sensitivity to the action of insulin, an effect that can result in inappropriately high plasma glucose concentration, or glucose intolerance. The incidence of impaired glucose tolerance (IGT) and of non-insulin-dependent diabetes mellitus (NIDDM) is increasing as the population ages. However, aging is not always associated with IGT, and the development of glucose intolerance and NIDDM is not inevitable in the aged. Environmental factors over which the individual has some control, such as obesity, physical inactivity, and diet play a major role in the development of glucose intolerance, although a small but significant decline in tissue insulin sensitivity, possibly related to alterations in post-receptor events, appears inevitable with age.

Glucose-stimulated insulin secretion is generally well maintained in the healthy aging human and rodent. There is currently no evidence of age-related changes in the pancreas, the islets of Langerhans, or in the β-cell insulin biosynthetic apparatus that might hinder insulin release. However, responsiveness of the β-cells to glucose stimulation is attenuated in the aged animal, indicating that the stimulus-secretion coupling mechanism of insulin release is in some way altered with age. An age-related impairment within this coupling mechanism has yet to be defined. It now appears that any impairment of the β-cell coupling mechanism occurs in conjunction with an adaptive alteration of the β-cell population that allows the maintenance of insulin secretion, albeit insufficient at times, in the face of changing exogenous influences occurring with age.

In healthy individuals, there is no significant deterioration of insulin secretory capacity with age, and glucose intolerance can be prevented or at least delayed through lifestyle choices. Nonetheless, IGT and NIDDM are occurring in epidemic proportions among the aging populations of industrialized nations. IGT and NIDDM are associated with perturbations in glucose homeostasis manifested as hyperglycemia, hypoglycemia, and insulinemia. Hyperglycemia and insulinemia are strongly related to the development of cardiovascular disease and many other diseases and condition associated with aging. Hypoglycemia is known to cause deficits in cognitive function and can be especially dangerous in the elderly. However, because most of the age-related changes in glucose homeostasis are not caused by aging per se, the deleterious effects of these changes are largely preventable.

ACKNOWLEDGMENTS

This work was supported by NIH Grant AG06665, and a gift for the California Age Research Institute.

REFERENCES

1. Adelman, R. C. Secretion of insulin during aging. *J. Am. Geriatr. Soc.* 37: 983-990, 1989.
2. Ahmed, M. U., E. Brinkmann Frye, T. P. Degenhardt, S. R. Thorpe, and J. W. Baynes. N-epsilon-(carboxyethyl)lysine, a product of the chemical modification of proteins by methylglyoxal, increases with age in human lens proteins. *Biochem. J.* 324: 565-70, 1997.
3. Akmal, M., S. G. Massry, D. A. Goldstein, P. Fanti, A. Weisz, and R. A. DeFronzo. Role of parathyroid hormone in the glucose intolerance of chronic renal failure. *J. Clin. Invest.* 75: 1037-1044, 1985.
4. Alberti, K. G. M. M., N. J. Christensen, S. E. Christensen, A. P. Hansen, J. Iversen, K. Lundbaeck, K. Seyer-Hansen, and H. Orskov. Inhibition of insulin secretion by somatostatin. *Lancet* 2: 1299-1301, 1973.
5. Alberti, K. G. M. M., and T. D. R. Hockaday. The biochemistry of the complications of diabetes mellitus. In: *Complications of Diabetes*, edited by H. Keen and J. Jarrett. Chicago: Yearbook Medical, 1975, p. 221-64.
6. Albon, J., W. S. Karwatowski, N. Avery, D. L. Easty, and V. C. Duance. Changes in the collagenous matrix of the aging human lamina cribrosa. *Brit. J. Opthalmol.* 79: 368-75, 1995.
7. Anderson, J. W., R. H. Herman, and D. Zakim. Effect of high glucose and high sucrose diets on glucose tolerance of normal men. *Am. J. Clin. Nutr.* 26: 600-609, 1973.
8. Andres, R. Aging and diabetes. *Med. Clin. N. Am.* 55: 835-845, 1971.
9. Andres, R., and J. D. Tobin. Endocrine systems. In: *Handbook of the Biology of Aging*, edited by C. E. Finch and L. Hayflick. New York: Van Nostrand Reinhold, 1977.
10. Arciero, P. J., M. D. Vukovich, J. O. Holloszy, S. B. Racette, and W. M. Kohrt. Comparison of short-term diet and exercise on insulin action in individuals with abnormal glucose tolerance. *J. Appl. Physiol.* 86: 1930-5, 1999.
11. Argiles, J. M., J. Lopez-Soriano, and F. J. Lopez-Soriano. Cytokines and diabetes: the final step? Involvement of TNF-alpha in both type I and II diabetes mellitus. *Horm. Metab. Res.* 26: 447-449, 1994.
12. Asano, T., Y. Shibasaki, and M. Kasuga. Cloning of a rabbit brain glucose transporter cDNA and alteration of glucose transporter mRNA during tissue development. *Biochem. Biophys. Res. Commun.* 154: 1204-1211, 1988.
13. Azam, M., G. Gupta, and N. Z. Baquer. Effect of hyperglycemia and hyperinsulinemia on rat red blood cell insulin receptors and catecholamines: relationship with cellular ageing. *Biochem. Int.* 22: 21-30, 1990.

14. Baan, C. A., R. P. Stolk, D. E. Grobbee, J. C. Witteman, and E. J. Feskens. Physical activity in elderly subjects with impaired glucose tolerance and newly diagnosed diabetes mellitus. *Am. J. Epidemiol.* 149: 219-27, 1999.

15. Bak, J., N. Moller, O. Schmitz, A. Saaek, and O. Pedersen. *In vivo* action and muscle glycogen synthase activity in type II (noninsulin dependent) diabetes mellitus: effects of diet treatment. *Diabetologia* 35: 777-784, 1992.

16. Bank, R. A., M. T. Bayliss, F. P. Lafeber, A. Maroudas, and J. M. Tekoppele. Aging and zonal variation in post-translational modification of collagen in normal human articular cartilage. The age-related increase in non-enzymatic glycation affects biomechanical properties of cartilage. *Biochem. J.* 330: 345-51, 1998.

17. Banskota, N. K., R. Taub, K. Zellner, and G. L. King. Insulin, insulin-like growth factor I and platelet-derived growth factor interact additively in the induction of the protooncogene c-myc and cellular proliferation in cultured bovine aortic smooth muscle cells. *Mol. Endocrinol.* 3: 1183-1190, 1989.

18. Bantle, J. P., D. C. Laine, G. W. Castle, J. W. Thomas, B. J. Hoogwerf, and F. C. Goetz. Postprandial glucose and insulin responses to meals containing different carbohydrates in normal and diabetic subjects. *New Engl. J. Med.* 309: 7-12, 1983.

19. Barnard, R. J., J. F. Youngren, and D. A. Martin. Diet, not aging, causes skeletal muscle insulin resistance. *Gerontology* 41: 205-11, 1995.

20. Barzilai, N., S. Banerjee, M. Hawkins, W. Chen, and L. Rossetti. Caloric restriction reverses hepatic insulin resistance in aging rats by decreasing visceral fat. *J. Clin. Invest.* 101: 1353-61, 1998.

21. Beck-Nielsen, H., O. Pedersen, and H. Lindskov. Normalization of the insulin sensitivity and the cellular insulin binding during treatment of obese diabetics for one year. *Acta Endocrinol.* 90: 103-112, 1979.

22. Beigelman, P. M., M. J. Shu, and L. J. Thomas. Insulin from individual isolated mouse islets of Langerhans. *Biochem. Med.* 7: 91-97, 1973.

23. Berger, J., C. Biswas, P. P. Vicario, H. V. Strout, R. Saperstein, and P. Pilch. Decreased expression of the insulin-responsive glucose transporter in diabetes and fasting. *Nature* 340: 70-72, 1989.

24. Bjorntorp, P., M. Fahlen, G. Grimby, A. Gustafson, J. Holm, P. Renstrom, and T. Schersten. Carbohydrate and lipid metabolism in middle-aged, physically well-trained men. *Metabolism* 21: 1037-1044, 1972.

25. Bolli, G. B., E. Tsalikian, M. W. Haymond, P. E. Cryer, and J. E. Gerich. Defective glucose counter-regulation after subcutaneous insulin in non-insulin-dependent diabetes mellitus. Paradoxical suppression of glucose utilization and lack of compensatory increase in glucose production, roles of insulin resistance, abnormal neuroendocrine responses, and islet paracrine interactions. *J. Clin. Invest.* 73: 1532-1541, 1984.

26. Bombara, M., P. Masiello, M. Novelli, and E. Bergamini. Impairment of the priming effect of glucose on insulin secretion from isolated islets of aging rats. *Acta Diabetologica* 32: 69-73, 1995.

27. Borg, L. A., N. Dahl, and I. Swenne. Age-dependent differences in insulin secretion and intracellular handling of insulin in isolated pancreatic islets of the rat. *Diabete et Metabolisme* 21: 408-14, 1995.

28. Bourey, R. E., W. M. Kohrt, J. P. Kirwan, M. A. Staten, D. S. King, and J. O. Holloszy. Relationship between glucose tolerance and glucose-stimulated insulin response in 65-year-olds. *J. Gerontol.* 48, no.4: M122-M127, 1993.

29. Brierley, E. J., D. L. Broughton, O. F. James, and K. G. Alberti. Reduced awareness of hypoglycaemia in the elderly despite an intact counter-regulatory response. *QJM* 88: 439-45, 1995.

30. Broughton, D. L., K. G. M. M. Alberti, O. F. W. James, and R. Taylor. Peripheral tissue in insulin sensitivity in healthy elderly subjects. *Gerontology* 33: 357-362, 1987.

31. Broughton, D. L., and R. Taylor. Review. Deterioration of glucose tolerance with age: The role of insulin resistance. *Age Aging* 20: 221-225, 1977.

32. Brownlee, M. Glycation and diabetic complications. *Diabetes* 43: 836-841, 1994.

33. Brunzell, J. D., R. L. Lerner, W. R. Hazzard, D. Porte, and E. L. Bierman. Improved glucose tolerance with high carbohydrate feeding in mild diabetics. *New Engl. J. Med.* 284: 521-537, 1971.

34. Brunzell, J. D., R. L. Lerner, D. Porte, and E. L. Bierman. Effect of a fat free, high carbohydrate diet on diabetic subjects with fasting hyperglycemia. *Diabetes* 23: 138, 1974.

35. Bucala, R., K. J. Tracey, and A. Cerami. Advanced glycosylation products quench nitric oxide and mediate defective endothelium-dependent vasodilatation in experimental diabetes. *J. Clin. Invest.* 87: 432-438, 1991.

36. Burch, B., D. K. Berner, A. Leontire, A. Vogin, B. M. Matschinsky, and F. M. Matschinsky. Metabolic adaptation of pancreatic islet tissue in aging rats. *J. Gerontol.* 39: 2-6, 1984.

37. Burgess, J. A. Diabetes mellitus and aging. In: *Hypothalamus, Pituitary, and Aging*, A. V. Everitt and J. A. Burgess, Eds. Springfield, IL: Charles C. Thomas, 1976, p. 497-513.

38. Burr, I. M., E. B. Marliss, W. Stauffacher, and A. E. Renold. Differential effect of ouabain on glucose-induced biphasic insulin release *in vitro*. *Am. J. Physiol.* 221: 943-951, 1971.

39. Butler, W. J., L. D. Ostrander Jr., W. J. Carman, and D. E. Lamphiear. Mortality from coronary heart disease in the Tecumseh Study. Long-term effect of diabetes mellitus, glucose tolerance, and other risk factors. *Am. J. Epidemiol.* 121: 541-547, 1985.

40. Buysschaaert, M., F. Cauwe, and J. Jamaart. Proximal femur density in type 1 and 2 diabetic patients. *Diabetes Metab.* 18: 32-37, 1992.

41. Cahill, G. F. Insulin and glucagon. In: *Peptide Hormones*, J. A. Parsons, Ed. London: Macmillan, 1976, p. 85-100.

42. Carantoni, M., G. Zuliani, S. Volpato, E. Palmieri, A. Mezzetti, L. Vergnani, and R. Fellin. Relationships between fasting plasma insulin, anthropometrics, and metabolic parameters in a very old healthy population. Associazione Medica Sabin. *Metab: Clin. Exptl.* 47: 535-40, 1998.

43. Carlsson, P. O., S. Sandler, and L. Jansson. Pancreatic islet blood perfusion in the nonobese diabetic mouse: diabetes-prone female mice exhibit a higher blood flow compared with male mice in the prediabetic phase. *Endocrinology* 139: 3534-41, 1998.

44. Carvalho, C. R., S. L. Brenelli, A. C. Silva, A. L. Nunes, L. A. Velloso, and M. J. Saad. Effect of aging on insulin receptor, insulin receptor substrate-1, and phosphatidylinositol 3-kinase in liver and muscle of rats. *Endocrinology* 137: 151-9, 1996.

45. Casad, R. C., and R. C. Adelman. Aging enhances inhibitory action of somatostatin in rat pancreas. *Endocrinology* 130: 2420-2422, 1992.

46. Cefalu, W. T., Z. Q. Wang, S. Werbel, A. Bell-Farrow, J. R. Crouse, 3rd, W. H. Hinson, J. G. Terry, and R. Anderson. Contribution of visceral fat mass to the insulin resistance of aging. *Metab. Clin. Exp.* 44: 954-9, 1995.

47. Cerami, A. Hypothesis: glucose as a mediator of aging. *J. Am. Geriat. Soc.* 33: 626-634, 1985.

48. Cerami, A., H. Vlassare, and M. Brownlee. Glucose and aging. *Sci. Am.* 256: 90-96, 1987.

49. Cerasi, E. Mechanism of glucose stimulated insulin secretion in health and in diabetes: some re-evaluations and proposals. *Diabetologia* 11: 1-13, 1975.

50. Charron, M. J., and E. B. Katz. Metabolic and therapeutic lessons from genetic manipulation of GLUT4. *Mol. Cell. Biochem.* 182: 143-52, 1998.

51. Chaudhuri, M., J. L. Sartin, and R. C. Adelman. A role for somatostatin in the impaired insulin secretory response to glucose by islets from aging rats. *J. Geront.* 38: 431-435, 1983.

52. Chen, M., R. N. Bergman, G. Pacini, and D. Porte. Pathogenesis of age-related glucose intolerance in man: insulin resistance and decreased b-cell function. *J. Clin. Endocrinol. Metab.* 60: 13-20, 1985.

53. Chen, M., R. N. Bergman, and D. Porte. Insulin resistance and beta-cell dysfunction in aging: the importance of dietary carbohydrate. *J. Clin. Endocrinol. Metab.* 67: 951-957, 1988.

54. Chorinchath, B. B., L. Y. Kong, L. Mao, and R. E. McCallum. Age-associated differences in TNF-alpha and nitric oxide production in endotoxic mice. *J. Immunol.* 156: 1525-1530, 1996.

55. Coddling, J. A., A. Kalnins, and R. E. Haist. Effects of age and of fasting on the responsiveness of the insulin-secreting mechanism of the islets of Langerhans to glucose. *Can. J. Physiol. Pharmacol.* 53: 716-725, 1975.

56. Cohen, M. P., and F. N. Ziyadeh. Role of Amadori-modified nonenzymatically glycated serum proteins in the pathogenesis of diabetic nephropathy [editorial]. *J. Am. Soc. Nephrol.* 7: 183-90, 1996.

57. Colman, E., L. I. Katzel, E. Rogus, P. Coon, D. Muller, and A. P. Goldberg. Weight loss reduces abdominal fat and improves insulin action in middle-aged and older men with impaired glucose tolerance. *Metab. Clin. Exp.* 44: 1502-8, 1995.

58. Colman, E., L. I. Katzel, J. Sorkin, P. J. Coon, S. Engelhardt, E. Rogus, and A. P. Goldberg. The role of obesity and cardiovascular fitness in the impaired glucose tolerance of aging. *Exp. Gerontol.* 30: 571-80, 1995.

59. Colman, E., M. J. Toth, L. I. Katzel, T. Fonong, A. W. Gardner, and E. T. Poehlman. Body fatness and waist circumference are independent predictors of the age-associated increase in fasting insulin levels in healthy men and women. *Intl. J. Ob. Relate Metab. Disorders* 19: 798-803, 1995.

60. Coutinho, M., H. C. Gerstein, Y. Wang, and S. Yusuf. The relationship between glucose and incident cardiovascular events: a metaregression analysis of published data from 20 studies of 95,783 individuals followed for 12.4 years. *Diabetes Care* 22: 233-240, 1999.

61. Cox, J. H., R. N. Cortright, G. L. Dohm, and J. A. Houmard. Effect of aging on response to exercise training in humans: skeletal muscle GLUT-4 and insulin sensitivity. *J. Appl. Physiol.* 86: 2019-25, 1999.

62. Craig, B. W., S. M. Garthwaite, and J. O. Holloszy. Adipocyte insulin resistance: effects of aging, obesity, exercise, and food restriction. *J. Appl. Physiol.* 62: 95-100, 1987.

63. Curry, D. L., G. Reaven, and E. Reaven. Glucose-induced insulin secretion by perfused pancreas of 2- and 12-month-old Fischer 344 rats. *Am. J. Physiol.* 248: E375-E380, 1985.

64. Dandona, P., K. Thusu, S. Cook, B. Snyder, J. Makowski, D. Armstrong, and T. Nicotera. Oxidative damage to DNA in diabetes mellitus. *Lancet* 347: 444-5, 1996.

65. Davidson, M. B. The effect of aging on carbohydrate metabolism: a comprehensive review and a practical approach to the clinical problem. In: *Endocrine Aspects of Aging*, edited by S. G. Korenman. New York: Elsevier Biomedical, 1982.

66. Davidson, M. B. The effect of aging on carbohydrate metabolism: a review of the English literature and a practical approach to the diagnosis of diabetes mellitus in the elderly. *Metabolism* 28: 687-705, 1979.

67. DeClercq, L., P. Delaere, and C. Remacle. The aging of the endocrine pancreas of the rat. II. Cytoplasmic parameters of the B-cell, including insulin synthesis and secretion. *Mech. Ageing Dev.* 43: 11-29, 1988.

68. DeFronzo, R., and E. Ferrannini. Insulin resistance. A multifaceted syndrome responsible for NIDDM, obesity, hypertension, dyslipidemia, and atherosclerotic cardiovascular disease. *Diabetes Care* 14: 173-194, 1991.

69. DeFronzo, R. A. Glucose intolerance and aging. *Diabetes Care* 4: 493-501, 1981.

70. DeFronzo, R. A. Glucose intolerance and aging. In: *Biological Markers of Aging*, edited by M. E. Reff and E. L. Schneider, Bethesda, MD: NIH Publication , 1982, p. 98-119.

71. DeFronzo, R. A. Glucose intolerance and aging: evidence for tissue insensitivity to insulin. *Diabetes* 28: 1095-1101, 1979.

72. DeFronzo, R. A., J. D. Tobin, and R. A. Andres. Glucose clamp technique: a method for quantifying insulin secretion and resistance. *Am. J. Physiol.* 237: E214-E223, 1979.

73. Degenhardt, T. P., S. R. Thorpe, and J. W. Baynes. Chemical modification of proteins by methylglyoxal. *Cell. Mol. Biol.* 44: 1139-45, 1998.

74. DeGroot, J., N. Verzijl, R. A. Bank, F. P. Lafeber, J. W. Bijlsma, and J. M. TeKoppele. Age-related decrease in proteoglycan synthesis of human articular chondrocytes: the role of nonenzymatic glycation. *Arth. Rheum.* 42: 1003-9, 1999.

75. Dengel, D. R., J. M. Hagberg, R. E. Pratley, E. M. Rogus, and A. P. Goldberg. Improvements in blood pressure, glucose metabolism, and lipoprotein lipids after aerobic exercise plus weight loss in obese, hypertensive middle-aged men. *Metab. Clin. Exp.* 47: 1075-82, 1998.

76. Dengel, D. R., R. E. Pratley, J. M. Hagberg, E. M. Rogus, and A. P. Goldberg. Distinct effects of aerobic exercise training and weight loss on glucose homeostasis in obese sedentary men. *J. Appl. Physiol.* 81: 318-25, 1996.

77. Denker, P. S., and V. E. Pollock. Fasting serum insulin levels in essential hypertension. A meta-analysis. *Arch. Intern. Med.* 152: 1649-1651, 1992.

78. Depres, J. P., B. Lamarche, P. Mauriege, B. Cantin, G. R. Dagenais, S. Moorjani, and P. J. Lupien. Hyperinsulinemia as an independent risk factor for ischemic heart disease. *New Engl. J. Med.* 334: 952-957, 1996.

79. DiPietro, L., T. E. Seeman, N. S. Stachenfeld, L. D. Katz, and E. R. Nadel. Moderate-intensity aerobic training improves glucose tolerance in aging independent of abdominal adiposity. *J. Am. Geriatr. Soc.* 46: 875-9, 1998.

80. Diwadkar, V. A., J. W. Anderson, S. R. Bridges, M. S. Gowri, and P. R. Oelgten. Postprandial low-density lipoproteins in type 2 diabetes are oxidized more extensively than fasting diabetes and control samples. *Proc. Soc. Exp. Biol. Med.* 222: 178-184, 1999.

81. Donnelly, R., and X. Qu. Mechanisms of insulin resistance and new pharmacological approaches to metabolism and diabetic complications. *Clin. Exper. Pharm. Physiol.* 25: 79-87, 1998.

82. Draznin, B., J. P. Steinberg, J. W. Leitner, and K. E. Sussman. The nature of insulin secretory defect in aging rats. *Diabetes* 34: 1168-1173, 1985.

83. Dudl, R. J., and J. W. Ensinck. Insulin and glucagon relationships during aging in man. *Metabolism* 26: 33-41, 1977.

84. Edwards, B. J., H. M. Perry, F. E. Kaiser, J. E. Morley, D. Kraenzle, D. K. Kreutter, and R. W. Stevenson. Age-related changes in amylin secretion. *Mech. Ageing Dev.* 86: 39-51, 1996.

85. Eiffert, K. C., R. B. McDonald, and J. S. Stern. High sucrose diet and exercise: effects on insulin-receptor function of 12- and 24-mo-old Sprague-Dawley rats. *J. Nutr.* 121: 1081-1089, 1991.

86. Elahi, D., D. K. Andersen, D. C. Muller, J. D. Tobin, J. C. Brown, and R. Andres. The enteric enhancement of glucose-stimulated insulin release. The role of GIP in aging, obesity, and non-insulin-dependent diabetes mellitus. *Diabetes* 33: 950-957, 1984.

87. Elliott, T. G., and G. Viberti. Relationship between insulin resistance and coronary heart disease in diabetes mellitus and the general population: a critical appraisal. *Clin. Endocrin. Metab.* 7: 1079-1103, 1993.

88. Epstein, M. Diabetes and hypertension: the bad companions. *J. Hyperten. Suppl.* 15: S55-62, 1997.

89. Eriksson, J. G. Exercise and the treatment of type 2 diabetes mellitus. An update. *Sports Med.* 27: 381-91, 1999.

90. Eschwege, E., J. L. Richard, N. Thibult, P. Ducemetiere, J. M. Warnet, J. R. Claude, and G. E. Rosselin. Coronary heart disease mortality in relation to diabetes, blood glucose and plasma insulin levels. The Paris Prospective Study 10 years later. *Horm. Metab. Res.* 15: 41-46, 1985.

91. Escriva, F., M. Agote, E. Rubio, J. C. Molero, A. M. Pascual-Leone, A. Andres, J. Satrustegui, and J. M. Carrascosa. *In vivo* insulin-dependent glucose uptake of specific tissues is decreased during aging of mature Wistar rats. *Endocrinology* 138: 49-54, 1997.

92. Esterbauer, H., and P. Ramos. Chemistry and pathophysiology of oxidation of LDL. *Rev. Physiol. Biochem. Pharmacol.* 127: 31-64, 1995.

93. Everson, S. A., D. E. Goldberg, S. P. Helmrich, T. A. Lakka, J. W. Lynch, G. A. Kaplan, and J. T. Salonen. Weight gain and the risk of developing insulin resistance syndrome. *Diabetes Care* 21: 1637-43, 1998.

94. Exton, J. H., S. C. Harper, A. L. Tucker, and R. I. Ho. Effects of insulin on gluconeogenesis and cyclic AMP levels in perfused livers from diabetic rats. *Biochim. Biophys. Acta* 329: 23-40, 1973.

95. Fadda, G. Z., M. Akmal, F. H. Premdas, L. G. Lipson, and S. G. Massry. Insulin release from pancreatic islets: effects of CRF and excess PTH. *Kidney Intl.* 33: 1066-1072, 1988.

96. Fadda, G. Z., S. M. Hajjar, A. Perna, X. J. Zhou, L. G. Lipson, and S. G. Massry. On mechanism of impaired insulin secretion in chronic renal failure. *J. Clin. Invest.* 87: 255-216, 1991.

97. Feingold, K. R., and C. Grufeld. Role of cytokines in inducing hyperlipidemia. *Diabetes* 41: 97-101, 1992.

98. Ferrannini, E., G. Buzzigoli, R. Bonadonna, M. A. Giorico, M. Oleggini, L. Graziadei, R. Pedrinelli, L. Brandi, and S. Bevilacqua. Insulin resistance in essential hypertension. *New Engl. J. Med.* 317: 350-357, 1987.

99. Ferrannini, E., S. Vichi, H. Beck-Nielsen, M. Laakso, G. Paolisso, and U. Smith. Insulin action and age. European Group for the Study of Insulin Resistance (EGIR). *Diabetes* 45: 947-53, 1996.

100. Ferrara, A., E. L. Barrett-Connor, and S. L. Edelstein. Hyperinsulinemia does not increase the risk of fatal cardiovascular disease in elderly men or women without diabetes: the Rancho Bernardo Study, 1984-1991. *Am. J. Epidemiol.* 140: 857-869, 1994.

101. Field, J. B. Extraction of insulin by liver. *Annu. Rev. Med.* 24: 309-312, 1973.

102. Finch, C. E., and D. M. Cohen. Aging, metabolism, and Alzheimer disease: review and hypotheses. *Exp. Neurol.* 143: 82-102, 1997.

103. Fink, R. I., O. G. Kolterman, J. Griffin, and J. F. Olefsky. Mechanisms of insulin resistance in aging. *J. Clin. Invest.* 71: 1523-1531, 1983.

104. Fink, R. I., O. G. Kolterman, M. Kao, and M. J. Olefsky. The role of the glucose transport system in the postreceptor defect in insulin action associated with human aging. *J. Clin. Endocrinol. Metab.* 58: 721-725, 1984.

105. Fink, R. I., P. Wallace, and J. M. Olefsky. Effects of aging on glucose-mediated glucose disposal and glucose transport. *J. Clin. Invest.* 77: 2034-2041, 1986.

106. Folsom, A. R., J. H. Eckfeldt, S. Weitzman, J. Ma, L. E. Chambless, R. W. Barnes, K. B. Cram, and R. G. Hutchinson. Relation of carotid artery wall thickness to diabetes mellitus, fasting glucose and insulin, body size, and physical activity. Atherosclerosis Risk in Communities (ARIC) Study Investigators. *Stroke* 25: 66-73, 1994.

107. Fontbonne, A. Insulin-resistance syndrome and cardiovascular complications of non-insulin-dependent diabetes mellitus. *Diabetes Metab.* 22: 305-13, 1996.

108. Forbes, A., T. Elliott, H. Tildesley, D. Finegood, and G. S. Meneilly. Alterations in non-insulin-mediated glucose uptake in the elderly patient with diabetes. *Diabetes* 47: 1915-9, 1998.

109. Forero, M. S., R. F. Klein, R. A. Nissenson, K. Nelson, H. Heath, C. D. Arnaud, and B. L. Riggs. Effect of age on circulating immunoreactive and bioactive parathyroid hormone levels in women. *J. Bone Miner. Res.* 2: 363-366, 1987.

110. Foster, D. W., and J. D. McGarry. The metabolic derangements and treatments of diabetic ketoacidosis. *New Engl. J. Med.* 309: 159-169, 1983.

111. Freidenberg, G., D. Reichart, J. Olefsky, and R. Henry. Reversibility of defective adipocyte insulin receptor kinase activity in noninsulin-dependent diabetes mellitus. *J. Clin. Invest.* 82: 1398-1406, 1988.

112. Fujita, Y. A., A. L. Herron, and H. S. Seltzer. Confirmation of impaired early insulin response to glycemic stimulus in nonobese mild diabetes. *Diabetes* 24: 17-27, 1975.

113. Garcia, G. V., R. V. Freeman, M. A. Supiano, M. J. Smith, A. T. Galecki, and J. B. Halter. Glucose metabolism in older adults: a study including subjects more than 80 years of age. *J. Am. Geriatr. Soc.* 45: 813-7, 1997.

114. Giansanti, R., M. Boemi, L. Amodio, P. Fioravanti, R. A. Rabini, and P. Fumelli. Long-term metabolic control and retinopathy in type I diabetes: ten-year follow-up. *Diabetes Res.* 25: 77-84, 1994.

115. Gilcrease, M. Z., and R. L. Hoover. Examination of monocyte adherence to endothelium under hyperglycemic conditions. *Am. J. Pathol.* 139: 1089-1097, 1991.

116. Giugliano, D., T. Salvatore, G. Paolisso, R. Buoninconti, R. Torella, M. Varricchio, and F. D'Onofrio. Impaired glucose metabolism and reduced insulin clearance in elderly hypertensives. *Am. J. Hyperten.* 5: 345-53, 1992.

117. Goetz, F. C., D. R. Jacobs, Jr., B. Chavers, J. Roel, M. Yelle, and J. M. Sprafka. Risk factors for kidney damage in the adult population of Wadena, Minnesota. A prospective study. *Am. J. Epidemiol.* 145: 91-102, 1997.

118. Gold, G., E. Reaven, and G. Reaven. Changes in islets of Langerhans in aged rats. *Gerontol. Soc. Proc.* : 77, 1978.

119. Gold, G., G. M. Reaven, and E. P. Reaven. Effect of age on proinsulin and insulin secretory pattern in isolated rat islets. *Diabetes* 30: 77-87, 1981.

120. Gold, P. E. Role of glucose in regulating the brain and cognition. *Am. J. Clin. Nutr.* 61: 987S-995S, 1995.

121. Goodyear, L. J., and B. B. Kahn. Exercise, glucose transport, and insulin sensitivity. *Annu. Rev. Med.* 49: 235-61, 1998.

122. Granberry, M. C., and V. A. Fonseca. Insulin resistance syndrome: options for treatment. *Southern Med. J.* 92: 2-15, 1999.

123. Grey, N. G., and D. M. Kipnis. Effect of diet composition on the hyperinsulemia of obesity. *New Engl. J. Med.* 285: 827-842, 1971.

124. Groop, P.-H. The influence of body weight, age, and glucose tolerance on the relationship between GIP secretion and beta-cell function in man. *Scand. J. Clin. Lab. Invest.* 49: 367-379, 1989.

125. Gschwend, S., C. Ryan, J. Atchison, S. Arslanian, and D. Becker. Effects of acute hyperglycemia on mental efficiency and counterregulatory hormones in adolescents with insulin-dependent diabetes mellitus. *J. Pediatr.* 126: 178-84, 1995.

126. Haffner, S. M. The importance of hyperglycemia in the nonfasting state to the development of cardiovascular disease. *Endocr. Rev.* 19: 583-592, 1998.

127. Haffner, S. M., S. Lehto, T. Ronnemaa, K. Pyorala, and M. Laakso. Mortality from coronary heart disease in subjects with type 2 diabetes and in nondiabetic subjects with and without prior myocardial infarction. *New Engl. J. Med.* 339: 229-234, 1998.

128. Haffner, S. M., and H. Miettinen. Insulin resistance implications for type II diabetes mellitus and coronary heart disease. *Am. J. Med.* 103: 152-62, 1997.

129. Haffner, S. M., L. Mykkanen, M. Paidi, R. Valdez, B. V. Howard, and M. P. Stern. Small dense LDL is associated with the insulin resistance syndrome. *Diabetologia* 38: 1328-1336, 1995.

130. Hahn, H. J., M. Ziegler, H. Jahr, R. B. Butter, and K. D. Kohnert. Investigations on isolated islets of Langerhans *in vitro*. XIII. Experiments concerning the preparation conditions with collagenase. *Endokrinologie* 67: 67-75, 1976.

131. Hajdu, A., F. Herr, and G. Rona. Morphological observations on spontaneous pancreatic islet changes in rats. *Diabetes* 16: 198-110, 1967.

132. Haller, H., W. Ziegler, C. Lindschau, and F. C. Luft. Endothelial cell tyrosine kinase receptor and G protein-coupled receptor activation involves distinct protein kinase C isoforms. *Arteriol. Thromb. Vascul. Biol.* 16: 678-686, 1996.

133. Han, D., T. Hosokawa, A. Aoike, and K. Kawai. Age-related enhancement of tumor necrosis factor production in mice. *Mech. Ageing Dev.* 84: 39-54, 1995.

134. Handa, J. T., N. Verzijl, H. Matsunaga, A. Aotaki-Keen, G. A. Lutty, J. M. te Koppele, T. Miyata, and L. M. Hjelmeland. Increase in the advanced glycation end product pentosidine in Bruch's membrane with age. *Invest. Ophthal. Visual Sci.* 40: 775-9, 1999.

135. Hanefeld, M., S. Fischer, U. Julius, J. Schulze, U. Schwanebeck, H. Schmechel, H. J. Ziegelasch, J. Linder, and T. D. Group. Risk factors for myocardial infarction and death in newly detected NIDDM: the Diabetes Intervention Study, 11-year follow-up. *Diabetologia* 39: 1577-1583, 1996.

136. Hanefeld, M., S. Fischer, H. Schmechel, G. Rothe, J. Schulze, H. Dude, U. Schwanebeck, and U. Julius. Diabetes Intervention Study. Multi-intervention trial in newly diagnosed NIDDM. *Diabetes Care* 14: 308-317, 1991.

137. Hansen, B. C. Obesity, diabetes, and insulin resistance: implications from molecular biology, epidemiology, and experimental studies in humans and animals. Synopsis of the American Diabetes Association's 29th Research Symposium and Satellite Conference of the 7th International Congress on Obesity, Boston, Massachusetts. *Diabetes Care* 18: A2-9, 1995.

138. Harper, H. A., V. W. Rodwell, and P. A. Mayes. *Rev. Physiol. Chem.* Los Altos: Lange Medical Publications, 1977.

139. Harris, M. I. Impaired glucose tolerance in the U.S. population. *Diabetes Care* 12: 464-474, 1989.

140. Harris, M. I. Prevalence of noninsulin-dependent diabetes and impaired glucose tolerance. In: *Diabetes in America*. Washington, DC: NIH Publication, U. S. Department of Health and Human Services, 1985, p. VI-1 to VI-31.

141. Heath, G. W., J. R. Gavin, J. M. Hinderliter, J. M. Hagberg, S. A. Bloomfield, and J. O. Holloszy. Effects of exercise and lack of exercise on glucose tolerance and insulin sensitivity. *J. Appl. Physiol.* 55: 512-517, 1983.

142. Hellman, B. The total volume of the pancreatic islet tissue at different ages of the rat. *Act. Pathol. Jpn.* 47: 35-50, 1959.

143. Henry, R. R. Type 2 diabetes care: the role of insulin-sensitizing agents and practical implications for cardiovascular disease prevention. *Am. J. Med.* 105: 20S-26S, 1998.

144. Herold, K. C., K. S. Polonsky, and R. M. Cohen. Variable deterioration in cortical function during insulin-induced hypoglycemia. *Diabetes* 34: 677-685, 1985.

145. Hiltunen, L., E. Läärä, S. L. Kivelä, and S. Keinänen-Kiukaanniemi. Glucose tolerance and mortality in an elderly Finnish population. *Diab. Res. Clin. Pract.* 39: 75-81, 1998.

146. Hirokawa, K. Characterization of age-associated kidney disease in Wistar rats. *Mech. Aging Dev.* 4: 301-316, 1975.

147. Hofman, C., K. Lorenz, S. S. Braithwaite, J. R. Colca, B. J. Polaruk, G. S. Hotamisligil, and B. M. Spiegelman. Altered gene expression for tumor necrosis factor-alpha and its receptor during drug and dietary modulation of insulin resistance. *Endocrinology* 134: 264-270, 1994.

148. Holloszy, J. O., J. Schultz, J. Kusnierkiewicz, J. M. Hagberg, and A. A. Ehsani. Effects of exercise on glucose tolerance and insulin resistance. *Act Med. Scand. Suppl.* 711: 55-65, 1986.

149. Holmes, C. S., K. M. Koepke, and R. G. Thompson. Simple versus complex performance impairments at three blood glucose levels. *Psychoneuroendocrinology* 11: 353-357, 1986.

150. Horton, E. S. NIDDM — the devastating disease. *Diab. Res. Clin Pract.* 28 suppl: S3-11, 1995.

151. Hotamisligil, G. S., and B. M. Spiegelman. Tumor necrosis factor-alpha: a key component of the obesity-diabetes link. *Diabetes* 43: 1271-1278, 1994.

152. Houmard, J. A., M. D. Weidner, P. L. Dolan, N. Leggett-Frazier, K. E. Gavigan, M. S. Hickey, G. L. Tyndall, D. Zheng, A. Alshami, and G. L. Dohm. Skeletal muscle GLUT4 protein concentration and aging in humans. *Diabetes* 44: 555-60, 1995.

153. Howard, C. F. Longitudinal studies on the development of diabetes in individual *Macaca nigra.* *Diabetologia* 29: 301-306, 1986.

154. Hughes, V. A., M. A. Fiatarone, R. A. Fielding, B. B. Kahn, C. M. Ferrara, P. Shepherd, E. C. Fisher, R. R. Wolfe, D. Elahi, and W. J. Evans. Exercise increases muscle GLUT-4 levels and insulin action in subjects with impaired glucose tolerance. *Am. J. Physiol.* 264: E855-62, 1993.

155. Hunt, S. M., and J. L. Groff. *Adv. Nutr. Human Metab.* St. Paul: West Publishing Company, 1990.

156. Hvidberg, A., C. G. Fanelli, T. Hershey, C. Terkamp, S. Craft, and P. E. Cryer. Impact of recent antecedent hypoglycemia on hypoglycemic cognitive dysfunction in nondiabetic humans. *Diabetes* 45: 1030-6, 1996.

157. Idahl, L. A., A. Lernmark, J. Sehlin, and I. B. Taljedal. The dynamics of insulin release from mouse pancreatic islet cells in suspension. *Pfluegers Arch.* 366: 185-197, 1976.

158. Ihara, Y., S. Toyokuni, K. Uchida, H. Odaka, T. Tanaka, H. Ikeda, H. Hiai, Y. Seino, and Y. Yamada. Hyperglycemia causes oxidative stress in pancreatic beta-cells of GK rats, a model of type 2 diabetes. *Diabetes* 48: 927-32, 1999.

159. Ikegami, H., T. Fujisawa, H. Rakugi, Y. Kumahara, and T. Ogihara. Glucose tolerance and insulin resistance in the elderly. *Japanese J. Geriatr.* 34: 365-8, 1997.

160. Inoue, K., S. Norgren, H. Luthman, C. Möller , and V. Grill. B cells of aging rats: impaired stimulus-secretion coupling but normal susceptibility to adverse effects of a diabetic state. *Metab. Clin. Exp.* 46: 242-6, 1997.

161. Iversen, J., and D. W. Miles. Evidence for a feedback inhibition of insulin on insulin secretion in the isolated, perfused canine pancreas. *Diabetes* 20: 1-9, 1971.

162. Ivy, J. L. Role of exercise training in the prevention and treatment of insulin resistance and non-insulin-dependent diabetes mellitus. *Sports Med.* 24: 321-36, 1997.

163. Izzo, J. L. Pharmacokinetics of insulin. In: *Handbook of Experimental Pharmacology*, edited by A. Hasselblatt and F. von Bruchhausen. Berlin: Springer, 1975, p. 195-228.

164. Jaap, A. J., G. C. Jones, R. J. McCrimmon, I. J. Deary, and B. M. Frier. Perceived symptoms of hypoglycaemia in elderly type 2 diabetic patients treated with insulin. *Diab. Med.* 15: 398-401, 1998.

165. Jackson, R. A., P. M. Blix, and J. A. Matthews. Influence of aging on glucose homeostasis. *J. Clin. Invest.* 55: 840-848, 1982.

166. Jackson, R. A., M. I. Hawa, R. D. Roshania, B. M. Sim, L. Disilvo, and J. B. Jaspan. Influence of aging on hepatic and peripheral glucose metabolism in humans. *Diabetes* 37: 119-129, 1988.

167. Jansson, L., and I. Swenne. Age-dependent changes of pancreatic islet blood flow in the rat. *Int. J. Pancreatol.* 5: 157-163, 1989.

168. Jarrett, R. J. Diabetes, hyperglycemia, and arterial disease. In: *Blood Vessel Disease in Diabetes Mellitus*, edited by K. Lundbaek and H. Keen. Milano: Casa Editrice Il Ponte SRL, 1971, p. 7.

169. Juhan-Vague, I., M. C. Alessi, and P. Vague. Increased plasma plasminogen activator inhibitor-1 levels: a possible link between insulin resistance and atherothrombosis. *Diabetologia* 34: 457-462, 1991.

170. Juhan-Vague, I., S. G. Thompson, and J. Jespersen. Involvement of the hemostatic system in the insulin resistance syndrome. A study of 1500 patients with angina pectoris. The ECAT Angina Pectoris Study Group. *Arterioscl. Thromb.* 13: 1865-1873, 1993.

171. Kahn, S. E., V. G. Larson, J. C. Beard, K. C. Cain, and I. B. Abrass. Effect of exercise on insulin action, glucose tolerance, and insulin secretion in aging. *Am. J. Physiol.* 258: E937-E943, 1990.

172. Kalant, N., D. Leiborici, T. Leibovici, and N. Fukushima. Effect of age on glucose utilization and responsiveness to insulin in forearm muscle. *J. Am. Geriatr. Soc.* 28: 304-307, 1980.

173. Kalu, I. N., R. H. Hardin, R. Cockerham, and Y. G. Yu. Aging and dietary modulation of rat skeleton and parathyroid hormone. *Endocrinol.* 115: 1239-1247, 1984.

174. Kanatsuka, A., H. Makino, M. Osegawa, J. Kasanuki, T. Suzuki, S. Yoshida, and H. Horie. Is somatostatin a true local inhibitory regulator of insulin secretion? *Diabetes* 33: 510-515, 1984.

175. Kannel, W. B. Cardioprotection and antihypertensive therapy: the key importance of addressing the associated coronary risk factors (the Framingham experience). *Am. J. Cardiol.* 77: 6B-11B, 1996.

176. Kannel, W. B. Epidemiology of cardiovascular disease in the elderly: an assessment of risk factors. *Cardiovas. Clin.* 22: 9-22, 1992.

177. Kaplan, S. A., B. M. Lippe, C. R. Brinkman, M. B. Davidson, and M. E. Geffner. Diabetes mellitus. *Ann. Int. Med.* 96: 635-639, 1982.

178. Karam, J. H. Reversible insulin resistance in non-insulin-dependent diabetes mellitus. *Horm. Metab. Res.* 28: 440-4, 1996.

179. Kawadami, M., P. H. Pekala, M. D. Lone, and A. Cerami. Lipoprotein lipase suppression in 3T3-L1 cells by an endotoxin-induced mediator from exudate cells. *PNAS USA* 82: 912-916, 1982.

180. Kawamori, R. Asymptomatic hyperglycaemia and early atherosclerotic changes. *Diab. Res. Clin. Pract.* 40 suppl: S35-42, 1998.

181. Kenny, S. J., R. E. Aubert, and L. S. Geiss. Prevalence and incidence of non-insulin-dependent diabetes. In: *Diabetes in America* (2 nd ed.), edited by M. I. Harris. Washington, DC: National Institute of Diabetes and Digestive and Kidney Diseases NIH publication 95-1468, 1995, p. 47-67.

182. Kimura, T., J. Takamatsu, K. Ikeda, A. Kondo, T. Miyakawa, and S. Horiuchi. Accumulation of advanced glycation end products of the Maillard reaction with age in human hippocampal neurons [see comments]. *Neurosci. Lett.* 208: 53-6, 1996.

183. Kimura, T., J. Takamatsu, T. Miyata, T. Miyakawa, and S. Horiuchi. Localization of identified advanced glycation end-product structures, N epsilon(carboxymethyl)lysine and pentosidine, in age-related inclusions in human brains. *Pathol. Intl.* 48: 575-9, 1998.

184. Kipnis, D. M. Insulin secretion in diabetes mellitus. *Ann. Int. Med.* 69: 891-901, 1969.

185. Kitahara, A., and R. C. Adelman. Altered regulation of insulin secretion in isolated islets of different sizes in aging rats. *Biochem. Biophys. Res. Commun.* 87: 1207-1214, 1979.

186. Kitahara, A., M. Obenrader, A. Rosenfeld, T. Burch, and R. C. Adelman. Altered regulation of insulin production in aging rats. *Gerontol. Soc. Proc.* : 88, 1978.

187. Klein, R. Hyperglycemia and microvascular and macrovascular disease in diabetes. *Diab. Care* 18: 258-268, 1995.

188. Klug, T. L., C. Freeman, K. Karoly, and R. C. Adelman. Altered regulation of pancreatic glucagon in male rats during aging. *Biochem. Biophys. Res. Commun.* 89: 907-912, 1979.

189. Ko, G. T., J. C. Chan, J. Woo, E. Lau, V. T. Yeung, C. C. Chow, J. K. Li, W. Y. So, W. B. Chan, and C. S. Cockram. Glycated haemoglobin and cardiovascular risk factors in Chinese subjects with normal glucose tolerance. *Diab. Med.* 15: 573-8, 1998.

190. Koefoed Theil, P., T. Hansen, M. Larsen, O. Pedersen, and H. Lund-Andersen. Lens autofluorescence is increased in newly diagnosed patients with NIDDM. *Diabetologia* 39: 1524-7, 1996.

191. Koerker, D. J., W. Ruch, E. Chideckel, J. Palmer, C. J. Goodner, J. Ensinck, and C. C. Gale. Somatostatin: hypothalamic inhibitor of the endocrine pancreas. *Science* 184: 482-484, 1984.

192. Kohner, E. M. Abnormal physiological processes in the retina. In: *Handbook of Diabetes Mellitus*, edited by M. Brownlee. New York: Garland, 1981, p. 1-21.

193. Kohrt, W. M., and J. O. Holloszy. Loss of skeletal muscle mass with aging: effect on glucose tolerance. *J. Gerontol. Ser. A Biol. Sci. Med. Sci.* 50 spec. no.: 68-72, 1995.

194. Kolterman, O. G., M. Greenfield, G. M. Reaven, M. Saekow, and J. M. Olefsky. Effect of a high carbohydrate diet on insulin binding to adipocyte and on insulin action *in vivo* in man. *Diabetes* 28: 731-739, 1979.

195. Kono, S., H. Kuzuya, M. Okamoto, H. Nishimura, A. Kosaki, T. Kakehi, M. Okamoto, G. Inoue, I. Maeda, and H. Imura. Changes in insulin receptor kinase with aging in rat skeletal muscle and liver. *Am. J. Physiol.* 259: E27-E35, 1990.

196. Kopelman, P. G., T. R. E. Pilkington, N. White, and S. L. Jeffcoate. Evidence for the existence of two types of massive obesity. *Br. Med. J.* : 82-83, 1980.

197. Korol, D. L., and P. E. Gold. Glucose, memory, and aging. *Am. J. Nutr.* 67: 764S-771S, 1998.

198. Koya, D., and G. L. King. Protein kinase C and the development of diabetic complications. *Diabetes* 47: 859-866, 1998.

199. Kreisberg, R. A. Aging, glucose metabolism, and diabetes: current concepts. *Geriatrics* 42: 67-76, 1987.

200. Krentz, A. J., and M. Nattrass. Insulin resistance: a multifaceted metabolic syndrome. Insights gained using a low-dose insulin infusion technique. *Diab. Med.* 13: 30-9, 1996.

201. Krishnan, R. K., J. M. Hernandez, D. L. Williamson, D. J. O'Gorman, W. J. Evans, and J. P. Kirwan. Age-related differences in the pancreatic beta-cell response to hyperglycemia after eccentric exercise. *Am. J. Physiol.* 275: E463-70, 1998.

202. Krone, W., H. Naegele, B. Behnke, and H. Greten. Opposite effects of insulin and catecholamines on LDL-receptor activity in human mononuclear leukocytes. *Diabetes* 37: 1386-1391, 1988.

203. Kruszynska, Y. T., and J. M. Olefsky. Cellular and molecular mechanisms of non-insulin dependent diabetes mellitus. *J. Invest. Med.* 44: 413-428, 1996.

204. Kuusisto, J., L. Mykkanen, K. Pyorala, and M. Laakso. NIDDM and its metabolic control predict coronary heart disease in elderly subjects. *Diabetes* 43: 960-967, 1994.

205. Laakso, M. Hyperglycemia and cardiovascular disease in Type 2 diabetes. *Diabetes* 48: 937-942, 1999.

206. Laakso, M. Insulin resistance and coronary heart disease. *Curr. Op. Lipidol.* 7: 217-26, 1996.

207. Laakso, M., and S. Lehto. Epidemiology of macrovascular disease in diabetes. *Diab. Rev.* 5: 294-315, 1997.

208. Lacy, P. E., and M. Kostianovsky. Method for the isolation of intact islets of Langerhans from the rat pancreas. *Diabetes* 16: 35-39, 1967.

209. Laws, A., and G. M. Reaven. Insulin resistance and risk factors for coronary heart disease. *Clin. Endocrinol. Metab.* 7: 1063-1078, 1993.

210. Lebovitz, H. E. Effects of oral antihyperglycemic agents in modifying macrovascular risk factors in type 2 diabetes. *Diab. Care* 22 Suppl 3: C41-4, 1999.

211. Leckström, A., I. Lundquist, Z. Ma, and P. Westermark. Islet amyloid polypeptide and insulin relationship in a longitudinal study of the genetically obese (ob/ob) mouse. *Pancreas* 18: 266-73, 1999.

212. Lee, A. T., and A. Cerami. Role of glycation in aging. *Ann. N.Y. Acad. Sci.* 663: 63-72, 1992.

213. Lehto, S., T. Ronnemaa, S. M. Haffner, K. Pyorala, V. Kallio, and M. Laakso. Dyslipidemia and hyperglycemia predict coronary heart disease events in middle-aged patients with NIDDM. *Diabetes* 46: 1354-1359, 1997.

214. Leiter, E. H., F. Premdas, D. E. Harrison, and L. G. Lipson. Aging and glucose homeostasis in C57BL/6J male mice. *FASEB J.* 2: 2807-2811, 1988.

215. Lernmark, A. Isolated mouse islets as a model for studying insulin release. *Acta Diabetol. Lat.* 8: 649-655, 1971.

216. Lin, J.-L., T. Asano, Y. Shibasaki, K. Tsukuda, H. Katagiri, H. Ishihara, F. Takaku, and Y. Oka. Altered expression of glucose transporter isoforms with aging in rats — selective decrease in GluT4 in the fat tissue and skeletal muscle. *Diabetologia* 34: 477-482, 1991.

217. Lindgren, M., B. Eckert, G. Stenberg, and C. D. Agardh. Restitution of neurophysiological functions, performance, and subjective symptoms after moderate insulin-induced hypoglycaemia in non-diabetic men. *Diab. Med.* 13: 218-25, 1996.

218. Lonnroth, P., and U. Smith. Aging enhances the insulin resistance in obesity through both receptor and postreceptor alterations. *J. Clin Endocrinol. Metab.* 62: 433-437, 1986.

219. Lyons, T. J. Glycation and oxidation: a role in the pathogenesis of atherosclerosis. *Am. J. Cardiol.* 71: 26B-31B, 1993.

220. Magal, E., M. Chaudhuri, and R. C. Adelman. The capability for regulation of insulin secretion by somatostatin in purified pancreatic islet B cells during aging. *Mech. Ageing Dev.* 33: 139-146, 1986.

221. Maloy, A. L., D. S. Longnecker, and E. R. Greenberg. The relationship of islet amyloid to the clinical type of diabetes. *Hum. Pathol.* 12: 917-922, 1981.

222. Massry, S. G., G. Z. Fadda, X. Zhou, P. Chandrasoma, L. Cheng, and C. R. Filburn. Impaired insulin secretion of aging: role of renal failure and hyperparathyroidism. *Kidney Intl.* 40: 662-667, 1991.

223. Mathews, E. K. Insulin secretion. In: *Hormones and Cell Regulation.*, edited by A. W. Cuthbert. Amsterdam: North-Holland, 1977, p. 57-76.

224. Matsumoto, T., Y. Ohashi, N. Yamada, and M. Kikuchi. Hyperglycemia as a major determinant of distal polyneuropathy independent of age and diabetes duration in patients with recently diagnosed diabetes. *Diab. Res. Clin. Pract.* 26: 109-13, 1994.

225. Matsuzawa, Y., I. Shimomura, T. Nakamura, Y. Keno, K. Kotani, and K. Tokunaga. Pathophysiology and pathogenesis of visceral fat obesity. *Obesity Res.* 3 suppl 2: 187S-194S, 1995.

226. Matyka, K., M. Evans, J. Lomas, I. Cranston, I. Macdonald, and S. A. Amiel. Altered hierarchy of protective responses against severe hypoglycemia in normal aging in healthy men. *Diab. Care* 20: 135-41, 1997.

227. Mayhew, D. A., P. H. Wright, and J. Ashmore. Regulation of insulin secreton. *Pharmacol. Rev.* 21: 185-193, 1969.

228. McConnell, J. G., K. D. Buchanan, J. Ardill, and R. W. Stout. Glucose tolerance in the elderly: the role of insulin and its receptor. *Eur. J. Clin. Invest.* 12: 55-61, 1982.

229. McIntyre, N., C. D. Holdsworth, and D. S. Turner. Intestinal factors in the control of insulin secretion. *J. Clin. Endocrinol. Metab.* 25: 1317-1321, 1965.

230. Mediratta, S., A. Fozailoff, and W. H. Frishman. Insulin resistance in systemic hypertension: pharmacotherapeutic implications. *J. Clin. Pharmacol.* 35: 943-56, 1995.

231. Mellitus, T. E. C. o. t. D. a. C. o. D. Report on the Expert Committee on the Diagnosis and Classification of Diabetes Mellitus. *Diab. Care* 20: 1183-1197, 1997.

232. Meneilly, G. S., E. Cheung, and H. Tuokko. Altered responses to hypoglycemia of healthy older people. *J. Clin. Endocrinol. Met.* 78: 1341-1350, 1994.

233. Meneilly, G. S., W. P. Milberg, and H. Tuokko. Differential effects of human and animal insulin on the responses to hypoglycemia in elderly patients with NIDDM. *Diabetes* 44: 272-7, 1995.

234. Meneilly, G. S., A. S. Ryan, K. L. Minaker, and D. Elahi. The effect of age and glycemic level on the response of the beta-cell to glucose-dependent insulinotropic polypeptide and peripheral tissue sensitivity to endogenously released insulin. *J. Clin. Endocrinol. Met.* 83: 2925-32, 1998.

235. Messier, C., and M. Gagnon. Glucose regulation and cognitive functions: relation to Alzheimer's disease and diabetes. *Behav. Brain Res.* 75: 1-11, 1996.

236. Messier, C., M. Gagnon, and V. Knott. Effect of glucose and peripheral glucose regulation on memory in the elderly. *Neurobiol. Aging* 18: 297-304, 1997.

237. Messier, C., J. Pierre, A. Desrochers, and M. Gravel. Dose-dependent action of glucose on memory processes in women: effect on serial position and recall priority. *Cog. Brain Res.* 7: 221-33, 1998.

238. Minaker, K. L., J. W. Rowe, and R. Tonino. Influence of age on clearance of insulin in man. *Diab.* 31: 851-855, 1982.

239. Mitsukawa, T., J. Takemura, M. Nakazato, J. Asai, K. Kanagawa, H. Matsuo, and S. Matsu. Effects of aging on plasma islet amyloid polypeptide basal level and response to oral glucose load. *Diab. Res. Clin. Pract.* 15: 131-134, 1992.

240. Mizutari, K., T. Ono, K. Ikeda, K. Kayashima, and S. Horiuchi. Photo-enhanced modification of human skin elastin in actinic elastosis by N(epsilon)-(carboxymethyl)lysine, one of the glycoxidation products of the Maillard reaction. *J. Invest. Dermatol.* 108: 797-802, 1997.

241. Molina, J. M., F. H. Premdas, and L. G. Lipson. Insulin release in aging: dynamic response of isolated islets of Langerhans of the rat to D-glucose and D-glyceraldehyde. *Endocrinol.* 116: 821-826, 1985.

242. Mooradian, A. D., and J. E. Thurman. Glucotoxicity: potential mechanisms. *Clinics Geriatr. Med.* 15: 255, 1999.

243. Morin, C. L., M. J. Pagliassotti, D. Windmiller, and R. H. Eckel. Adipose tissue-derived tumor necrosis factor-alpha activity is elevated in older rats. *J. Gerontol. Series A, Biol. Sci. Med. Sci.* 52: B190-5, 1997.

244. Morley, J. E. The elderly Type 2 diabetic patient: special considerations. *Diab. Med.* 15 suppl 4: S41-6, 1998.

245. Muggeo, M., G. Verlato, E. Bonora, G. Zoppini, M. Corbellini, and R. de Marco. Long-term instability of fasting plasma glucose, a novel predictor of cardiovascular mortality in elderly patients with non-insulin-dependent diabetes mellitus: the Verona Diabetes Study. *Circulation* 96: 1750-4, 1997.

246. Mullarkey, C. J., D. Edelstein, and M. Brownlee. Free radical generation by early glycation products: a mechanism for accelerated atherogenesis in diabetes. *Biochem. Biophys. Res. Commun.* 173: 932-939, 1990.

247. Muller, W. A., G. R. Faloona, and R. H. Unger. The influence of the antecedent diet upon glucagon and insulin secretion. *New Engl. J. Med.* 285: 1450-1468, 1971.

248. Münch, G., R. Schinzel, C. Loske, A. Wong, N. Durany, J. J. Li, H. Vlassara, M. A. Smith, G. Perry, and P. Riederer. Alzheimer's disease — synergistic effects of glucose deficit, oxidative stress and advanced glycation endproducts. *J. Neur. Transmis.* 105: 439-61, 1998.

249. Nadiv, O., O. Cohen, and Y. Zick. Defects of insulin's signal transduction in old rat livers. *Endocrinology* 130: 1515-1524, 1992.

250. Nishimura, H., H. Kuzuya, and M. Okamoto. Change of insulin action with aging in conscious rats determined by euglycemic clamp. *Am. J. Physiol.* 254: E92-E98, 1988.

251. Niskanen, L., R. Rauramaa, H. Miettinen, S. M. Haffner, M. Mercuri, and M. Uusitupa. Carotid artery intima-media thickness in elderly patients with NIDDM and in nondiabetic subjects. *Stroke* 27: 1986-92, 1996.

252. O'Shaughnessy, I. M., G. M. Kasdorf, R. G. Hoffmann, and R. K. Kalkhoff. Does aging intensify the insulin resistance of human obesity? *J. Clin. Endocrinol. Metab.* 74: 1075-1081, 1992.

253. Ohkubo, Y., H. Kishikawa, and E. Araki. Intensive insulin therapy prevents the progression of diabetic microvascular complications in Japanese patients with non-insulin-dependent diabetes mellitus: a randomized prospective 6-year study. *Diab. Res. Clin. Pract.* 28: 103-117, 1995.

254. Ohlson, L. O., T. Bjuro, B. Larsson, H. Eriksson, K. Svardsudd, L. Welin, and L. Wilhelmsen. A cross-sectional analysis of glucose tolerance and cardiovascular disease in 67-year-old men. *Diab. Med.* 6: 112-120, 1989.

255. Ohlson, L. O., B. Larsson, and K. Svardsudd. The influence of body fat distribution on the incidence of diabetes mellitus. *Diabetes* 34: 1055-1058, 1985.

256. Ohsawa, H., A. Kanatsuka, T. Yamaguchi, H. Makino, and S. Yoshida. Islet amyloid polypeptide inhibits glucose-stimulated insulin secretion from isolated rat pancreatic islets. *Biochem. Biophys. Res. Comm.* 160: 961-967, 1989.

257. Olefsky, J. M. Insulin resistance and insulin action. An *in vitro* and *in vivo* perspective. *Diabetes* 30: 148-162, 1981.

258. Oppenheimer, M. J., K. Sundquist, and E. L. Bierman. Downregulation of high-density lipoprotein receptor in human fibroblasts by insulin and IGF-I. *Diabetes* 38: 117-122, 1989.

259. Orchard, T. J., J. Eichner, and L. H. Kuller. Insulin as a predictor of coronary heart disease: interaction with apolipoprotein E phenotype: a report from the Multiple Risk Factor Intervention Trial. *Ann. Epidemiol.* 4: 40-45, 1994.

260. Orci, I. The insulin factory: a tour of the plant surroundings and a visit to the assembly line. *Diabetologia* 28: 528-546, 1985.

261. Ortiz-Alonso, F. J., A. Galecki, W. H. Herman, M. J. Smith, J. A. Jacquez, and J. B. Halter. Hypoglycemia counterregulation in elderly humans: relationship to glucose levels. *Am. J. Physiol.* 267: E497-506, 1994.

262. Pacini, G., F. Beccaro, A. Valerio, R. Nosadini, and G. Crepaldi. Reduced beta-cell secretion and insulin hepatic extraction in healthy elderly subjects. *J. Am. Geriatr. Soc.* 38: 1283-1289, 1990.

263. Pacini, G., A. Valerio, R. Beccaro, C. Nosadini, C. Cobelli, and G. Crepaldi. Insulin sensitivity and beta-cell responsivity are not decreased in elderly subjects with normal OGTT. *J. Am. Geriatr. Soc.* 36: 317-323, 1988.

264. Pagano, G., M. Cassader, and P. Perin-Cavallo. Insulin resistance in the aged: a quantitative evaluation in *in vivo* insulin sensitivity and *in vitro* glucose transport. *Metabolism* 33: 976-981, 1984.

265. Palumbo, P. J., L. R. Elveback, C. P. Chu, D. C. Connolly, and L. T. Kurland. Diabetes mellitus: incidence, prevalence, survivorship, and causes of death in Rochester, Minnesota. *Diabetes* 25: 566-573, 1976.

266. Pan, X. R., Y. H. Hu, G. W. Li, P. A. Liu, P. H. Bennett, and B. V. Howard. Impaired glucose tolerance and its relationship to ECG-indicated coronary heart disease and risk factors among Chinese. Da Qing IGT and diabetes study. *Diab. Care* 16: 150-156, 1993.

267. Pan, X. R., G. W. Li, Y. H. Hu, J. X. Wang, W. Y. Yang, Z. X. An, Z. X. Hu, J. Lin, J. Z. Xiao, H. B. Cao, P. A. Liu, X. G. Jiang, Y. Y. Jiang, J. P. Wang, H. Zheng, H. Zhang, P. H. Bennett, and B. V. Howard. Effects of diet and exercise in preventing NIDDM in people with impaired glucose tolerance. The Da Qing IGT and Diabetes Study. *Diab. Care* 20: 537-44, 1997.

268. Paolisso, G., A. Gambardella, S. Ammendola, A. D'Amore, V. Balbi, M. Varricchio, and F. D'Onofrio. Glucose tolerance and insulin action in healty centenarians. *Am. J. Physiol.* 270: E890-4, 1996.

269. Paolisso, G., M. R. Rizzo, G. Mazziotti, M. R. Tagliamonte, A. Gambardella, M. Rotondi, C. Carella, D. Giugliano, M. Varricchio, and F. D'Onofrio. Advancing age and insulin resistance: role of plasma tumor necrosis factor-alpha. *Am. J. Physiol.* 275: E294-9, 1998.

270. Patton, G. S., E. Ipp, R. E. Dobbs, L. Orci, W. Vale, and R. H. Unger. Pancreatic immunoreactive somatostatin release. *Proc. Nat. Acad. Sci. USA* 74: 2140-2143, 1977.

271. Peiris, A. N., R. A. Mueller, G. A. Smith, M. F. Struve, and A. H. Kissebah. Splanchnic insulin metabolism in obesity: Influence of body fat distribution. *J. Clin. Invest.* 78: 1648-1657, 1986.

272. Perfetti, R., C. M. Rafizadeh, A. S. Liotta, and J. M. Egan. Age-dependent reduction in insulin secretion and insulin mRNA in isolated islets from rats. *Am. J. Physiol.* 269: E983-90, 1995.

273. Perfetti, R., Y. Wang, A. R. Shuldiner, and J. M. Egan. Molecular investigation of age-related changes in mouse endocrine pancreas. *J. Gerontol. Series A Biol. Sci. Med. Sci.* 51: B331-6, 1996.

274. Pfeifle, B., and H. Ditschuneit. Effect of insulin on growth of cultured human arterial smooth muscle cells. *Diabetologia* 20: 155-158, 1981.

275. Pipeleers, D. Islet cell interaction with pancreatic B-cells. *Experientia* 40: 1114-1125, 1984.

276. Poehlman, E. T., T. L. McAuliffe, D. R. Van Houten, and E. Danforth. Influence of age and endurance training on metabolic rate and hormones in healthy men. *Am. J. Physiol.* 259: E66-E72, 1990.

277. Pokharna, H. K., and L. A. Pottenger. Nonenzymatic glycation of cartilage proteoglycans: an in vivo and in vitro study. *Glycoconjugate J.* 14: 917-23, 1997.

278. Polonsky, K. S., J. B. Jaspan, and W. Pugh. Metabolism of C-peptide in the dog: in vivo demonstration of the absence of hepatic extraction. *J. Clin. Invest.* 72: 1114-1119, 1983.

279. Polonsky, K. S., and A. H. Rubenstein. C-peptide as a measure of the secretion and hepatic extraction of insulin: pitfalls and limitations. *Diabetes* 33: 486-489, 1984.

280. Preuss, H. G. Effects of glucose/insulin perturbations on aging and chronic disorders of aging: the evidence. *J. Am. Coll. Nutr.* 16: 397-403, 1997.

281. Pyorala, K., M. Laakso, and M. Uusitupa. Diabetes and atherosclerosis: an epidemiologic view. *Diab. Metab. Rev.* 3: 463-524, 1987.

282. Ramalho, J., C. Marques, P. Pereira, and M. C. Mota. Crystallin composition of human cataractous lens may be modulated by protein glycation. *Graefes Arch. Clin. Exp. Opthamol.* 234 suppl 1: S232-8, 1996.

283. Ranganath, L., I. Sedgwick, L. Morgan, J. Wright, and V. Marks. The ageing entero-insular axis. *Diabetologia* 41: 1309-13, 1998.

284. Ratzmann, K. P., S. Witt, P. Heinke, and B. Shulz. The effect of ageing on insulin sensitivity and insulin secretion in non-obese health subjects. *Acta Endocrinol.* 100: 543-549, 1982.

285. Reaven, E., D. Curry, J. Moore, and G. Reaven. Effect of age and environmental factors on insulin release from perifused pancreas of the rat. *J. Clin. Invest.* 71: 345-358, 1983.

286. Reaven, E., D. Wright, C. E. Mondon, R. Solomon, H. Ho, and G. M. Reaven. Effect of age and diet on insulin secretion and insulin action in the rat. *Diabetes* 32: 175-180, 1983.

287. Reaven, E. P., G. Gold, and G. Reaven. Effect of age on glucose-stimulated insulin release by the beta cell of the rat. *J. Clin. Invest.* 64: 591-597, 1979.

288. Reaven, E. P., and G. M. Reaven. Structure and function changes in the endocrine pancreas of aging rats with reference to the modulating effects of exercise and caloric restriction. *J. Clin. Invest.* 68: 75-84, 1981.

289. Reaven, G., and E. Reaven. Effect of age on glucose oxidation by isolated rat islets. 18: 69-71, 1980.

290. Reaven, G. M. Role of insulin resistance in human disease (Banting Lecture 1988). *Diabetes* 37: 1595-1607, 1988.

291. Reaven, G. M., N. Chen, C. Hollenbeck, and Y.-D. I. Chen. Effect of age on glucose tolerance and glucose uptake in healthy individuals. *J. Am. Geriatr. Soc.* 37: 735-740, 1989.

292. Reaven, G. M., Y. D. I. Chen, J. Jeppesen, P. Maheux, and R. M. Krauss. Insulin resistance and hyperinsulinemia in individuals with small dense, low density lipoprotein particles. *J. Clin. Invest.* 92: 141-146, 1993.

293. Reaven, G. M., M. S. Greenfield, C. E. Mondon, M. Rosenthal, D. Wright, and E. P. Reaven. Does insulin removal rate from plasma decline with age? *Diabetes* 31: 670-673, 1982.

294. Reaven, G. M., and E. P. Reaven. Age, glucose intolerance, and non-insulin-dependent diabetes mellitus. *J. Am. Geriatr. Soc.* 33: 286-290, 1985.

295. Reichard, P., B. Y. Nilsson, and U. Rosenqvist. The effect of long-term intensified insulin treatment on the development of microvascular complications of diabetes mellitus. *New Engl. J. Med.* 329: 304-309, 1993.

296. Reid, I. R., M. C. Evans, G. J. S. Cooper, R. W. Ames, and J. Stapleton. Circulating insulin levels are related to bone density in normal postmenopausal women. *Am. J. Physiol.* 265: E655-E659, 1993.

297. Remacle, C., N. Hauser, M. Jeanjean, and A. Gommers. Morphometric analysis of endocrine pancreas in old rats. *Exp. Gerontol.* 12: 207-214, 1977.

298. Rewers, M., S. M. Shetterly, J. Baxter, J. A. Marshall, and R. F. Hamman. Prevalence of coronary heart disease in subjects with normal and impaired glucose tolerance and non-insulin-dependent diabetes mellitus in a biethnic Colorado population. The San Luis Valley Diabetes Study. *Am. J. Epidemiol.* 135: 1321-1330, 1992.

299. Reynolds, C., D. L. Horwitz, G. D. Molnar, A. H. Rubenstein, and W. F. Taylor. Abnormalities of endogenous insulin and glucagon in insulin-treated unstable and stable diabetes. *Diabetes* 23: 343-347, 1974.

300. Richardson, J. T. E. Cognitive function in diabetes mellitus. *Neurosci. Biobehav. Rev.* 14: 385-388, 1990.

301. Ritthaler, U., Y. Deng, Y. Zhang, J. Greten, M. Abel, B. Sido, J. Allenberg, G. Otto, H. Roth, A. Bierhaus, et al. Expression of receptors for advanced glycation end products in peripheral occlusive vascular disease. *Am. J. Pathol.* 146: 688-94, 1995.

302. Rodnick, K. J., W. L. Haskell, A. L. M. Swislocki, J. E. Foley, and G. M. Reaven. Improved insulin action in muscle, liver, and adipose tissue in physically trained human subjects. *Am. J. Physiol.* 253: E489-E495, 1987.

303. Rolls, B. J., K. A. Dimeo, and D. J. Shide. Age-related impairments in the regulation of food intake. *Am. J. Clin. Nutr.* 62: 923-31, 1995.

304. Rosenthal, M., W. L. Haskell, and R. Solomon. Demonstration of a relationship between level of physical training and insulin-stimulated glucose utilization in normal humans. *Diabetes* 32: 408-416, 1983.

305. Ross, H., G. Bernstein, and H. Rifkin. Relationship of metabolic control of diabetes to long-term complications. In: *Diabetes Mellitus: Theory and Practice* (3rd ed.), edited by R. Ellenberg. New York: Med. Exam. Publ., 1983, p. 907-25.

306. Rowe, J. W., R. Andres, and J. D. Tobin. The effect of age on creatinine clearance in man: a cross sectional and longitudinal study. *J. Gerontol.* 31: 155-163, 1976.

307. Rowe, J. W., K. L. Minaker, J. A. Pallota, and J. S. Flier. Characterization of the insulin resistance of aging. *J. Clin. Invest.* 71: 1581-1589, 1983.

308. Rubenstein, A. H., J. L. Clark, F. Melani, and D. F. Steiner. Secretion of pro-insulin C-peptide by pancreatic beta cells and its circulation in blood. *Nature* 224: 697-704, 1969.

309. Ruhe, R. C., D. L. Curry, S. Herrmann, and R. B. McDonald. Age and gender effects on insulin secretion and glucose sensitivity of the endocrine pancreas. *Am. J. Physiol.* 262: R671-R676, 1992.

310. Ruhe, R. C., D. L. Curry, and R. B. McDonald. Altered cellular heterogeneity as a possible mechanism for the maintenance of organ function in senescent animals. *J. Gerontol. Series A Biol. Sci. Med. Sci.* 52: B53-8, 1997.

311. Ruhe, R. C., and R. B. McDonad. Aging, insulin secretion, and cellular senescence. In: *Handbook of Nutrition in the Aged* (2nd ed.), edited by R. R. Watson. Boca Raton, FL: CRC Press, 1994, p. 73-98.

312. Ruige, J. B., W. J. Assendelft, J. M. Dekker, P. J. Kostense, R. J. Heine, and L. M. Bouter. Insulin and risk of cardiovascular disease: a meta-analysis. *Circulation* 97: 996-1001, 1998.

313. Rust, K. R., J. Prazma, R. J. Triana, O. E. T. Michaelis, and H. C. Pillsbury. Inner ear damage secondary to diabetes mellitus. II. Changes in aging SHR/N-cp rats. *Arch. Otolaryn. Head Neck Surg.* 118: 397-400, 1992.

314. Ryan, A. S., R. E. Pratley, A. P. Goldberg, and D. Elahi. Resistive training increases insulin action in postmenopausal women. *J. Gerontol. Series A Biol. Sci. Med. Sci.* 51: M199-205, 1996.

315. Sakata, N., J. Meng, S. Jimi, and S. Takebayashi. Nonenzymatic glycation and extractability of collagen in human atherosclerotic plaques. *Atherosclerosis* 116: 63-75, 1995.

316. Salama, N., and S. Kagawa. Ultra-structural changes in collagen of penile tunica albuginea in aged and diabetic rats. *Int. J. Impot. Res.* 11: 99-105, 1999.

317. Samos, L. F., and B. A. Roos. Diabetes mellitus in older persons. *Med. Clin. N. Am.* 82: 791-803, 1998.

318. Sartin, J. L., M. Chaudhuri, M. Obenrader, and R. C. Adelman. The role of hormones in changing adaptive mechanisms during aging. *Fed. Proc.* 39: 3163-3167, 1980.

319. Sato, Y., K. Yamanouchi, H. Nakajima, T. Shinozaki, S. Fujii, N. Chikada, and Y. Suzuki. Effect of aging and physical inactivity on glucose tolerance and insulin sensitivity. *Jap. J. Geriatr.* 27: 564-569, 1990.

320. Savage, P. J. Treatment of diabetes mellitus to reduce its chronic cardiovascular complications. *Curr. Op. Cardiol.* 13: 131-8, 1998.

321. Schatz, H., and U. Kullek. Studies on the local (paracrine) actions of glucagon, somatostatin and insulin in isolated islets of rat pancreas. *FEBS Lett.* 122: 207-210, 1980.

322. Seals, D. R., J. M. Hagberg, B. F. Hurley, A. A. Ehsani, and J. G. Holloszy. Effects of endurance training on glucose tolerance and plasma lipid levels in older men and women. *JAMA* 252: 645-649, 1984.

323. Sherwin, R. S., P. A. Insel, J. D. Tobin, J. E. Liljenquist, R. Andres, and M. Berman. Computer modelings: an aid to understanding insulin action. *Diabetes* 21: 347-354, 1972.

324. Shimamoto, K., H. Takizawa, and N. Ura. Insulin resistance in elderly patients with hypertension. *Jap. J. Geriatr.* 34: 369-74, 1997.

325. Simpson, I. A., and S. W. Cushman. Hormonal regulation of mammalian glucose transport. *Ann. Rev. Biochem.* 55: 1059-1089, 1986.

326. Simpson, R. G., A. Benedetti, G. M. Grodsky, J. H. Karam, and P. H. Forsham. Early phase of insulin release. *Diabetes* 17: 684-692, 1968.

327. Singh, I., and M. C. Marshall, Jr. Diabetes mellitus in the elderly. *Endocrinol. Metab. Clin. N. Amer.* 24: 255-72, 1995.

328. Sivitz, W. I., S. L. DeSautel, T. Kayano, G. I. Bell, and J. E. Pessin. Regulation of glucose transporter messenger RNA in insulin deficient states. *Nature* 340: 72-74, 1989.

329. Slavin, B. G., and S. P. Lerner. Age-related immunohistochemical studies of A and D cells in pancreatic islets of C57BL/6J. *Anatom. Record* 228: 53-57, 1990.

330. Stamler, J., O. Vaccaro, and J. D. Neaton. Diabetes, other risk factors, and 12-yr cardiovascular mortality for men screened in the Multiple Risk Factor Intervention Trial. *Diab. Care* 16: 434-444, 1993.

331. Standl, E., B. Balletshofer, B. Dahl, B. Weichenhain, and H. Stiegler. Predictors of 10-year macrovascular and overall mortality in patients with NIDDM: the Munich General Practitioner Project. *Diabetologia* 39: 1540-1545, 1996.

332. Starnes, J. W., E. Cheong, and F. M. Matschinsky. Hormone secretion by isolated perfused pancreas of aging Fischer 344 rats. *Am. J. Physiol.* 260: E59-E66, 1991.

333. Stevens, A. B., W. R. McKane, P. M. Bell, P. Bell, D. J. King, and J. R. Hayes. Psychomotor performance and counterregulatory responses during mild hypoglycemia in healthy volunteers. *Diab. Care* 12: 12-17, 1989.

334. Stout, R. W. Insulin and atheroma: 20 year perspective. *Diab. Care* 13: 631-654, 1990.

335. Stout, R. W., E. L. Bierman, and R. Ross. Effect of insulin on the proliferation of cultured primate arterial smooth muscle cells. *Circul. Res.* 36: 319-327, 1975.

336. Suzuki, M., K. Shinozaki, A. Kanazawa, Y. Hara, Y. Hattori, M. Tsushima, and Y. Harano. Insulin resistance as an independent risk factor for carotid wall thickening. *Hypertension* 28: 593-8, 1996.

337. Takada, K., A. Kanatsuka, Y. Tokuyama, K. Yagui, M. Nishimura, Y. Saito, and H. Makino. Islet amyloid polypeptide/amylin contents in pancreas change with increasing age in genetically obese and diabetic mice. *Diab. Res. Clin. Pract.* 33: 153-8, 1996.

338. Takagi, M., S. Kasayama, T. Yamamoto, T. Motomura, K. Hashimoto, H. Yamamoto, B. Sato, S. Okada, and T. Kishimoto. Advanced glycation endproducts stimulate interleukin-6 production by human bone-derived cells. *J. Bone. Miner. Res.* 12: 439-46, 1997.

339. Takemura, Y., S. Kikuchi, Y. Inaba, H. Yasuda, and K. Nakagawa. The protective effect of good physical fitness when young on the risk of impaired glucose tolerance when old. *Preventive Med.* 28: 14-9, 1999.

340. Taylor, R., A. J. McCulloch, S. Zeuzem, P. Gray, F. Clark, and K. G. M. M. Alberti. Insulin secretion, adipocyte insulin binding, and insulin sensitivity in thyrotoxicosis. *Acta Endocrinol.* 109: 96-103, 1985.

341. Teo, S. K., and C. H. Ee. Hypoglycaemia in the elderly. *Singapore Med. J.* 38: 432-4, 1997.

342. Tonino, R. P. Effect of physical training on the insulin resistance of aging. *Am. J. Physiol.* 256: E352-E360, 1989.

343. Tonino, R. P., W. H. Nedde, and D. C. Robbins. Effect of physical training on the insulin resistance of aging. *Clin. Res.* 34: 557A-563A, 1986.

344. Torti, F. M., B. Dieckman, A. Beutler, A. Cerami, and G. M. Reingold. A macrophage factor inhibits adipocyte gene expression: an in vitro model of cachexia. *Science* 229: 867-869, 1985.

345. Tuomilehto, J., Q. Qiao, R. Salonen, A. Nissinen, and J. T. Salonen. Ultrasonographic manifestations of carotid atherosclerosis and glucose intolerance in elderly eastern Finnish men. *Diab. Care* 21: 1349-52, 1998.

346. Unger, R. H., and L. Orci. Possible role of the pancreatic D-cell in the normal and diabetic states. *Diabetes* 26: 241-244, 1977.

347. Uusitupa, M. I. Early lifestyle intervention in patients with non-insulin-dependent diabetes mellitus and impaired glucose tolerance. *Ann. Med.* 28: 445-9, 1996.

348. Vague, P., I. Juhan-Vague, M. F. Aillaud, C. Badier, R. Viard, M. C. Alessi, and D. Collen. Correlation between blood fibrinolytic activity, plasminogen activator inhibitor level, plasma insulin level, and relative body weight in normal and obese subjects. *Metabolism* 35: 250-253, 1996.

349. Valenkevich, L. N., and O. I. Iakhontova. [Carbohydrate hydrolysis and absorption in the human small intestine in aging]. *Fiziologicheskii Zhurnal Imeni I. M. Sechenova* 82: 111-6, 1996.

350. Viswanathan, M., C. Snehalatha, V. Viswanathan, P. Vidyavathi, J. Indu, and A. Ramachandran. Reduction in body weight helps to delay the onset of diabetes even in non-obese with strong family history of the disease. *Diab. Res. Clin. Pract.* 35: 107-12, 1997.

351. Vlassara, H. Recent progress in advanced glycation endproducts and diabetic complications. *Diabetes* 46: S19-S25, 1997.

352. Vokonas, P. S., and W. B. Kannel. Diabetes mellitus and coronary heart disease in the elderly. *Clin. Geriatr. Med.* 12: 69-78, 1996.

353. Wallberg-Henriksson, H., J. Rincon, and J. R. Zierath. Exercise in the management of non-insulin-dependent diabetes mellitus [published erratum appears in *Sports Med* 25(2):130, 1998]. *Sports Med.* 25: 25-35, 1998.

354. Wang, S. Y., P. A. Halban, and J. W. Rowe. Effects of aging on insulin synthesis and secretion: differential effects on preproinsulin messenger RNA levels, proinsulin biosynthesis, and secretion of newly made and preformed insulin in the rat. *J. Clin. Invest.* 81: 176-183, 1988.

355. Ward, J. D. Abnormal processes in the nerve. In: *Handbook of Diabetes Mellitus*, edited by M. Brownlee. New York: Garland, 1981, p. 87-113.

356. Weir, G. C. Non-insulin-dependent diabetes mellitus: interplay between b-cell inadequacy and insulin resistance. *Am. J. Med.* 73: 461-464, 1982.

357. Weir, G. C., E. Samols, R. Ramseur, J. A. Day, and Y. C. Patel. Influence of glucose and glucagon upon somatostatin secretion from the isolated perfused canine pancreas. *Clin. Res.* 25: 403A-409A, 1977.

358. Welborn, T. A., and K. Wearne. Coronary heart disease incidence and cardiovascular mortality in Busselton with reference to glucose and insulin concentrations. *Diab. Care* 2: 154-160, 1979.

359. Welin, L., H. Eriksson, B. Larsson, L. O. Ohlson, K. Svardsudd, and G. Tibblin. Hyperinsulinemia is not a major coronary risk factor in elderly men. The study of men born in 1913. *Diabetologia* 35: 766-770, 1992.

360. Wells-Knecht, M. C., T. J. Lyons, D. R. McCance, S. R. Thorpe, and J. W. Baynes. Age-dependent increase in ortho-tyrosine and methionine sulfoxide in human skin collagen is not accelerated in diabetes. Evidence against a generalized increase in oxidative stress in diabetes. *J. Clin. Invest.* 100: 839-46, 1997.

361. Westermark, P., C. Wernstedt, T. D. O'Brien, D. W. Hayden, and K. H. Johnson. Islet amyloid in type 2 human diabetes mellitus and adult diabetic cats contains novel putative polypeptide hormones. *Am. J. Pathol.* 127: 414-417, 1987.

362. Westermark, P., E. Wilander, G. T. Westermark, and K. H. Johnson. Islet amyloid polypeptide-like immunoreactivity in the islet B cells of type 2 (non-insulin-dependent) diabetic and non-diabetic individuals. *Diabetologia* 30: 887-892, 1987.

363. Wheeler, T. J., and P. C. Hinkle. The glucose transporter of mammalian cells. *Ann. Rev. Physiol.* 47: 503-517, 1985.

364. Williams, J. A., and I. A. Goldfine. The insulin-pancreatic acinar axis. *Diabetes* 34: 980-986, 1985.

365. Williams, S. B., J. A. Cusco, and M.-A. Roddy. Impaired nitric oxide-mediated vasodilation in non-insulin-dependent diabetes. *Circulation* 90: I-513, 1994.

366. Wilson, P. W. F., L. A. Cupples, and W. B. Kannel. Is hyperglycemia associated with cardiovascular disease — the Framingham Study. *Am. Heart J.* 121: 586-590, 1991.

367. Winegrad, A. I. Banting Lecture 1986. Does a common mechanism induce the diverse complications of diabetes? *Diabetes* 36: 396-406, 1987.

368. Winegrad, A. I., and A. E. Renold. Studies on rat adipose tissue in vitro. *J. Biol. Chem.* 233: 267-272, 1958.

369. Wingard, D. L., E. L. Barrett-Conner, and A. Ferrara. Is insulin really a heart disease risk factor? *Diab. Care* 18: 1299-1304, 1995.

370. Wingard, D. L., and E. Barrett-Connor. Heart disease and diabetes. In: *Diabetes in America* (2nd ed.), edited by M. I. Harris. Washington DC: National Institute of Diabetes and Digestive and Kidney Diseases, NIH publication 95-1468, 1995, p. 429-448.

371. Winocur, G., and S. Gagnon. Glucose treatment attenuates spatial learning and memory deficits of aged rats on tests of hippocampal function. *Neurobiol. Aging* 19: 233-41, 1998.

372. Wolff, S. P., Z. Y. Jiang, and J. V. Hunt. Protein glycation and oxidative stress in diabetes mellitus and ageing. *Free Radical Biol. Med.* 10: 339-52, 1991.

373. Yamada, S., and C. Ohkubo. The influence of frequent and excessive intake of glucose on microvascular aging in healthy mice. *Microcirculation* 6: 55-62, 1999.

374. Yamasaki, Y., R. Kawamori, H. Matsushima, H. Nishizawa, M. Kodan, M. Kubota, Y. Kajimoto, and T. Kamada. Asymptomatic hyperglycaemia is associated with increased intimal plus medial thickness of the carotid artery. *Diabetologia* 38: 585-591, 1995.

375. Yarnell, J. W. G., P. M. Sweetnam, and V. Marks. Insulin in ischaemic heart disease: are associations explained by triglyceride concentrations? The Caerphilly Prospective Study. *Brit. Heart J.* 71: 293-296, 1994.

376. Yki-Jarvinen, H. Glucose toxicity. *Endocr. Rev.* 13: 415-431, 1992.

377. Yki-Järvinen, H. Acute and chronic effects of hyperglycaemia on glucose metabolism: implications for the development of new therapies. *Diab. Med.* 14 suppl 3: S32-7, 1997.

378. Young, I. R., and R. W. Stout. Effects of insulin and glucose on the cells of the arterial wall: interaction of insulin with dibutyryl cyclic AMP and low density lipoprotein in arterial cells. *Diab. Metab.* 13: 301-306, 1987.

379. Youngren, J. F., and R. J. Barnard. Effects of acute and chronic exercise on skeletal muscle glucose transport in aged rats. *J. Appl. Physiol.* 78: 1750-6, 1995.

380. Zavaroni, I., E. Dall'Aglio, and F. Bruschi. Effect of age and environmental factors on glucose tolerance and insulin secretion in a worker population. *J. Am. Geriatr. Soc.* 34: 271-281, 1986.

15 Chemical Senses and Food Choices in Aging

Adam Drewnowski and Victoria Warren-Mears

CONTENTS

I. INTRODUCTION

The chemical senses, taste and smell, govern the perception of food flavors and help determine food preferences as well as eating habits.

Taste and smell deficits are thought to reduce the pleasure provided by food. Drug- or disease-induced disorders of taste and smell can lead to food aversions and to altered food intakes.[1-3] Patients typically complain of distorted or unpleasant tastes and reduced enjoyment of food.[2,4] While there is little evidence to link chemosensory deficits with overt malnutrition, clinicians have normally assumed that taste and smell disorders can lead to inadequate energy intakes and eventual weight loss.[5]

Taste and smell functioning also decline with advancing age.[6,7] Complaints regarding the taste of food have often been reported by the elderly.[8] While the most common complaint was that food tasted weak or flat, other age-related dysfunction has involved both olfaction and the oral perception of texture.[9,10] Clinical and survey studies of the elderly have variously reported a narrowing of food choices, a decline in food intakes, and an increased prevalence of malnutrition.[11-13]

Many investigators believe that these factors are causally linked. Some have stated that the irreversible age-related decline in taste and smell can lead to altered food preferences, inadequate food intake, and poor nutrition.[14-16] For example, impaired perception of sweet and salty tastes has been reported to enhance dietary intakes of sugar and salt, with potential implications for hypertension and diabetes among the aged.[17] Health, nutrition, and quality of life are all said to be compromised by chemosensory dysfunction.[18] Age-related deficits of taste and smell are very often listed as potential causes of anorexia and malnutrition among the elderly.[13,16,18]

The key assumption guiding most sensory studies in aging has been that age-related deficits in taste and smell have a causal impact on nutrition and health. However, no study has demonstrated a causal relationship between sensory deficits, altered food habits, and compromised health in the elderly. A critical appraisal of the available data is the chief purpose of this review.

A few points should be noted. First, not all sensory deficits observed among the elderly are age-related. Both taste and smell are influenced by acute and chronic disease and by a variety of pharmaceutical agents. Drug-induced disorders of taste and smell have been fully described elsewhere.[1,3,16] Since the elderly as a group suffer from a variety of chronic diseases and are more likely to be medicated than are younger people, some of the observed taste and smell dysfunctions may be illness- or drug-induced.

Second, sensory acuity in the elderly can vary across individuals. While some elderly subjects suffer from taste and smell deficits, others do not.[6,19] Both taste and smell functions are susceptible to age-related diseases.[20] Common causes of smell loss in the elderly include upper respiratory viral infection and head trauma. Alzheimer's disease and Parkinson's disease are among the neurological diseases also associated with smell losses.[20] Since, in many past studies, institutionalized elderly of uncertain health were compared with community-based samples of young people, some of the observed sensory deficits may have been secondary to the presence of acute or chronic disease.

Third, a wide range of psychological or sociocultural variables influences eating behaviors of the elderly. Studies citing the increased prevalence of frank malnutrition among the aged were often based on hospitalized patients and residents of nursing homes, as opposed to healthy elderly. Physical and mental health of the respondents was not always taken into account. Clinical depression, dementia and Alzheimer's disease, and memory losses may affect food habits and contribute to inadequate nutrition.[21] Marital status, education, income, and membership in diverse cultural or ethnic groups also influence food preferences and dietary choices. Food habits of the elderly are likely to be influenced by these and other factors.[22] Interestingly, a study of healthy, middle-class elderly subjects without medical or financial restrictions revealed no evidence of malnutrition.[23] There is always the possibility that anorexia and malnutrition among the elderly are due to age-associated economic, sociocultural, and psychological factors and not to physiological deficits in taste and smell.

Finally, the postulated causal relationship between altered chemical senses, eating habits, and malnutrition is itself open to question. This causal link is thought to be mediated through altered pleasure response to foods. Age-related sensory losses are said to be the main cause of altered food habits, diminished food consumption, and compromised nutritional status.

In reality, there are many intervening steps between the chemical senses and food consumption. Taste and smell sensitivity, hedonic preference profiles, and food choices are independent behavioral variables that need not be tightly linked.[24-26] It has even been questioned whether detection threshold for sweet, sour, salty and bitter tastes in water solutions has any relevance to food-related behaviors at any age.[26] For the most part, foods represent complex sensory stimuli, and even major shifts in detection thresholds for the four basic tastes may have no practical significance. In some studies, impaired detection thresholds of dilute taste stimuli were unrelated to perception of the same stimuli at above-threshold levels. Other studies have shown that intensity scaling of basic tastes in water solutions did not predict response to real-life foods.[24,26] While age-associated sensory changes may influence eating behaviors, their impact on food selection, nutritional status, and quality of life in the older person remains to be determined.

II. TASTE FUNCTIONING

A. ANATOMICAL STUDIES

The loss of taste sensitivity with age was for a long time attributed to the loss of taste buds.[27] Taste buds, found throughout the oral cavity, are most common on the papillae of the tongue. Fungiform papillae are found mainly at the tip and the front edges of the tongue; foliate papillae are on the folds along the outer edges of the tongue, while circumvallate papillae are found at the back of the tongue.

The density of taste buds varies widely among individuals, as does taste acuity.[18,28,29] Both the number of papillae and the number of taste buds per papilla have been reported to decline with age. Early studies have reported major atrophic disappearance of taste buds from the circumvallate papillae, especially after the age of 70.[27] However, it now appears that taste buds are replaced throughout life, and that taste function is in fact stable.[6] There were no age-related differences in number of taste buds in the fungiform papillae of humans, rhesus monkeys, and Wistar rats.[30-32] Arvidson found no difference in the number of taste buds per fungiform papillae between 2 days and 90 years of age.[30]

Taste losses in the elderly may thus be due to changes in cell membranes, or in receptor innervation.[33] However, electrophysiological responses from taste nerves were stable, and neural recordings showed that the peripheral taste system functions well in old age.[34] Redundancy in the neural mediation of taste may be one reason the sense of taste is so robust. Bortoshuk noted that a complete taste loss would require damage to multiple nerves, damage to all receptors, or damage to all taste areas in the central nervous system.[6] Although localized taste losses do occur in some elderly subjects, whole-mouth taste sensation is preserved and such losses often go unnoticed.[6]

Oral hygiene, the use of medications and a variety of acute and chronic diseases affect taste and smell functions.[3] For example, since taste nerves in the chorda tympani travel through the inner ear, ear infections and respiratory infections have sometimes been associated with taste loss.[10] Such taste losses as have been observed among the elderly may be the result of cumulative pathology, and not the result of normal aging.

B. PSYCHOPHYSICAL STUDIES

Taste sensitivity is reputed to decline with age. Early studies in this area have been reviewed by Cowart,[35] Murphy,[36,37] and Schiffman.[38,39] In general, taste sensitivity to water solutions of sweet, sour, salty, and bitter compounds was measured using detection and recognition thresholds. Detection threshold is the minimum concentration of a stimulus that is perceived as distinct from distilled water, while recognition threshold is the level at which it is perceived as salty or sweet. Responsiveness to more-concentrated solutions was measured using magnitude estimation procedures.[40,41]

C. DETECTION AND RECOGNITION THRESHOLDS

Early studies on taste thresholds pointed to a sharp decline of taste acuity with age, at least for some basic tastes. Sucrose detection and recognition thresholds in the elderly were higher that those of young adults.[42] Some studies showed that sensitivity to sweet, salty, and bitter (but not sour) tastes declined after the age of 60, while others found that older adults (ages 48 to 60 yr) were less sensitive to sweet, sour, and bitter (but not salty) tastes.[43,44]

Studies on bitter taste, conducted using phenylthiocarbamide (PTC) and propylthiouracil (PROP), reported a decline in sensitivity to PTC with age, corresponding to a mean 3% annual increase in threshold levels.[45,46] Subsequent research showed that only smokers showed an age-related decline in bitter taste sensitivity to quinine and PROP.[47]

However, threshold measures used in most early studies may have been subject to a variety of problems, such as lack of water rinse between stimuli, and may not have provided an accurate picture of taste sensitivity. In later studies, taste thresholds were determined using the method of limits.[37] In the ascending method, the concentration of the stimulus was increased until the subject detected its presence. In the descending method, the stimulus was progressively diluted until it was perceived as no different from water. Because studies on taste and aging were invariably cross-sectional as opposed to longitudinal, the concern was that older people may differ in their decision-making criteria, and may be more or less reluctant to say yes/no to ambiguous stimuli than are young people.[48] The forced-choice procedure, in which subjects are asked to choose between the stimulus and plain water, became the method of choice, since it minimized the response criterion bias.

Murphy examined detection thresholds for the four basic tastes among subjects aged from 17 to 83 yr. The oldest subject group was 65 to 83 years of age. The data showed a gradual decline in sensitivity, amounting to one log step over the age range studied.[36,37] Similar results were reported by Cowart,[35] while Dye and Koziatek[49] observed a significant drop in sensitivity to sweet taste, beginning in the eighth decade of life.

Detection thresholds for sweet and salty tastes appeared to be unaffected by either smoking or gender. In one study, salt taste detection thresholds were measured in 76 adults aged 23 to 92 yr, using a forced-choice staircase procedure, with water rinses between all stimuli.[48] Although an age-related drop in taste sensitivity was observed, it was smaller than reported in other studies.[36,43] Another study observed a twofold increase in thresholds for sucrose among subjects aged 60 to 88 yr as compared with subjects aged 20 to 45 yr.[49] However, individual sensitivities were highly variable and the average deficit was not large.[50]

Some basic tastes were affected more strongly than others. Weiffenbach et al.[51] showed that thresholds for salty and bitter tastes were typically more affected by age than thresholds for sweet and sour. Detection thresholds for the four basic tastes were obtained for 81 adults between 23 and 88 years of age. Sodium chloride thresholds showed a significant but small increase with age, amounting to 0.1 of a log step per age decade. Quinine sulfate thresholds showed a similar but weaker increase with age. No age-related effects were obtained for sucrose or citric acid. According to Schiffman, taste detection thresholds among the elderly were 2.7 times higher for sweeteners, 11.6 times higher for sodium salts, 4.3 times higher for acids, and 6.9 times higher for bitter compounds.[15]

Few studies have examined the sensitivity to other tastes. Schiffman and colleagues measured detection thresholds for 19 amino acids in subjects age 17 to 27 yr and 75 to 87 yr, using a three-cup forced choice procedure. Thresholds for older subjects were 2.5 times higher than for younger ones, and no gender differences were observed.[52]

Later studies of localized taste losses represent an important methodological innovation.[6] In this procedure, strong taste stimuli were "painted" on discrete areas of the tongue and the oral cavity. Localized taste deficits were obtained in patients with diagnosed bulimia, viral respiratory infection and a history of head trauma. The elderly were more likely to have localized taste losses than were young subjects.[10] However, whole-mouth taste sensation was relatively robust, and no profound decline in the sense of taste was observed. Whole-mouth sensory functioning, as assessed by the threshold method, seems to be quite resistant to the effects of age.

D. INTENSITY SCALING

The scaling of suprathreshold intensity may be more relevant to taste function in the elderly than are threshold measures. Early work in this area was previously reviewed by Cowart,[35] Murphy,[37] and Schiffman.[53] Observed taste losses in the elderly were largely limited to bitter taste.

In most studies, the perceived intensity of solutions was assessed using category scaling or magnitude estimation procedures. The decline in taste acuity was denoted by a change in slope of the intensity function with concentration, suggesting that the perceived sensation increased more slowly in the elderly than in the young. For example, the elderly had flatter slopes when rating taste intensities of serial dilutions of 23 amino acids.[53]

Studies of above-threshold stimuli, conducted using magnitude estimation and magnitude matching procedures, showed that sweetness perception was unaffected by age. Studies found no change in slope in sweetness intensity rating,[49] and no age or gender effects for intensity scaling of sucrose solutions.[54] The data were not always so consistent. One study found no difference in sweetness intensity slopes between the young and the elderly subjects.[55] However, the slopes for the two adult groups were flatter than for 12-year-olds. A study on the perceived intensity of citric acid among three groups of subjects also reported inconsistent results. Elderly subjects (ages 70 to 79 yr) showed flatter slopes than both young (age 20 to 29 yr) and very old subjects (ages 80 to 99 yr).[56]

Other studies reported major differences between taste qualities. Age-related effects were greatest for bitter, marginal for sour, and least for sweet and salty stimuli. Gender effects were obtained only for sour and bitter tastes.[54-56] Murphy and Gillmore also found age-related effects for bitter and sour, but not for salty and sweet tastes. In judging taste mixtures, the elderly (ages 56 to 83 yr) found bitter, but not the other three tastes, to be less intense than did young subjects (ages 18 to 31 yr).[57] Another study similarly observed an age-related decline in the sensitivity to bitter taste, but no decline in the perception of sweetness, saltiness, warmth or cold, or viscosity among men and women, ages 25 to 93 yr.[58] The only impairment was in the perception of local pressure on the dorsal tongue, which might be related to impaired perception of food texture, reported to be common among the elderly.[59]

E. STUDIES OF FOOD STIMULI

Intensity scaling of the four basic tastes in food media failed to show major effects of age. There were no age-related deficits in scaling of saltiness in tomato juice;[60] no decline in the perception of saltiness in potatoes or broth,[61] and no decline in the perception of citric acid in an apple drink.[56] Warwick and Schiffman found no age-related deficits in the intensity ratings for salt and sugar in salted or sweetened daily products.[59] Only Murphy and Withee[62] have reported an age-associated decline in the perception of protein taste (hydrolyzed casein) in soup.

In an early study on food recognition,[9] older subjects (ages 67 to 93 yr) were as accurate as young controls (ages 18 to 22 yr) in identifying a solution of salt thickened with cornstarch, and were only slightly worse in identifying sugar. A more recent study found that elderly subjects were not as good as middle-aged or the young in judging the presence or absence of salt in tomato soup.[63] Although detection thresholds for sodium chloride in tomato soup far exceeded those for salt in water, the age-related deficits still held. The authors suggested that higher sodium detection thresholds for salt in soup might impact on nutritional status, since the elderly may fail to detect excessive salt levels in their diet.[63]

Only one study addressed the oral sensory perception of fats. Warwick and Schiffman[59] reported that the elderly might show a reduced ability to detect the fat content of sweet and salty dairy products, ranging from milk to heavy cream. However, the perception of fat in foods is largely guided by stimulus consistency and texture and to a lesser degree by olfaction. The chief cues for perception of fat in dairy products are stimulus thickness, smoothness, and viscosity. While oral perception of food texture may be impaired in the elderly, it should be noted that sensory perception of dietary fats is problematic at any age. Even young subjects did not always discriminate among foods of low vs. high fat content.

III.   TASTE HEDONICS

For the most part, studies on aging and taste acuity did not examine taste or food preferences.[35] One study on preferences for sugar in pineapple juice showed that the elderly preferred less sweet stimuli. While not always consistent, later studies showed that the elderly preferred sweeter and saltier stimuli that did younger subjects. In most studies, the stimuli were aqueous solutions of sugar and salt, while some of the later studies also made use of beverages and soups.

Liking or disliking, often measured using magnitude estimates, or the perceived pleasantness of a stimulus were the typical measures of the hedonic response. An alternative measure of preference was the peak-preferred concentration of either sugar or salt in a food stimulus. Some studies assessed it directly, by measuring the amount of sugar added to lemonade or salt added to tomato juice or soup. For example, Pangborn, Braddock, and Stone[64] found that older people added more salt to chicken broth than did younger ones.

However, hedonic response profiles can be highly idiosyncratic. One study[55] reported that hedonic preferences for sweet taste did not differ between children, young adults, and the oldest adults. Chauhan and Hawrysh[65] examined pleasantness ratings for different levels of citric acid in water and in apple juice drink in three groups of subjects. The oldest group (ages 80 to 99 yr) disliked high levels of citric acid and showed a lower hedonic optimum for sour taste. The old group (ages 70 to 79 yr) showed a higher optimum than the younger group (20 to 29 yr), but only for the solutions and not for the lemon-based drink. The same experiment showed an increase of the salt "breakpoint" with age, but only for water solutions and not for chicken soup.[66] Again, age-related deficits in salt taste perception were offered as the most likely explanation for the observed preferences for higher levels of salt.

Only one study reported that hedonic rating for sodium chloride, sucrose, and citric acid increased with age.[62] Four concentrations of each stimulus were presented in both water and in appropriate beverage bases, such as vegetable juice and lemonade. In general, beverages were judged to be more pleasant than were aqueous stimuli. Older subjects preferred higher concentrations of sugar and salt in both water and beverages than did younger subjects. This shift in hedonic preferences toward higher levels of sugar and salt was again thought to be caused by age-related sensory deficits.[62] The suggestion made was that reduced perception of sweet and salty tastes among the elderly might be one reason for increased intakes of sweet and salty foods, with consequences for obesity, diabetes, and hypertension.[17]

The question whether chemosensory preferences are driven by nutritional status has important implications for nutrition and aging. At least one study suggests that it might be so. Murphy and Withee examined the impact of taste preferences and age on selected biochemical indices of nutritional status, including total protein, albumin, and blood urea nitrogen (BUN).[67] Young and elderly subjects rated the pleasantness of five concentrations of casein hydrolyzate prepared in an amino-acid deficient soup base. Elderly subjects preferred 3.0% casein, as opposed of 0.5% casein for younger people. Elevated preferences for casein were also reported for persons of lower biochemical status.[67]

IV. IDENTIFICATION OF FOODS

Classic studies of food identification by the elderly, conducted by Schiffman and colleagues, made use of the multidimensional scaling (MDS) procedure. MDS is a mathematical method that allows stimuli, including sensory stimuli, to be represented in points in space. Stimuli judged as similar to one another are position close in space, while those judged as dissimilar are located further apart. Proximity matrices can be obtained either by direct similarity scaling, or by calculating the inter-item similarities on the basis of multiple additive scales.[68]

Identifying real-life foods involves oral perception of taste, flavor, and texture. Studies on sensory identification of foods by the elderly minimized visual cues by the use of blindfolds or dim red light, while textural cues were minimized by the use of steamed and blended foods.[9,69] In a pioneering MDS study, Schiffman presented 27 young college students (ages 18 to 22 yr) and 29 elderly residents of a retirement home (ages 67 to 93 yr) with 21 different foods to taste and smell.[9] The foods included fresh unseasoned blended fruits, vegetables, meats, fish, nuts, grains, and dairy products. The foods were steamed, blended and strained, or pureed. Water was added to minimize texture differences. The four taste standards, representing sweet, salty, sour and bitter — sucrose, NaCl, lemon, and coffee — were presented in a cornstarch base. Blindfolded subjects were first presented with a container of food to smell. Later, they tasted a teaspoon of the food, spitting out the food into an opaque paper bag. The subjects were asked to identify the foods, and rate them along 51 attribute scales.

Elderly subjects were sometimes unable to identify blended foods by taste and smell. Out of 24 foods, 21 were more frequently identified by young people than by the elderly. More elderly subjects than younger ones commented on the weakness of taste and smell for the unseasoned blended foods.[9] MDS analysis of proximity data showed that elderly subjects used only a single dimension that was related to pleasure, while younger subjects used two dimensions, suggesting better discrimination.

A similar study by Stevens and Lawless compared the ability to identify pureed vegetables and fruits by subjects, ages 18 to 65 yr.[70] The foods were cantaloupe, peach, strawberry, broccoli, carrot, corn, green pepper, lima bean, onion, pea, spinach, and turnip. The foods were cooked, drained and pureed, and the experiment was conducted under dim red light. To minimize cognitive demands, the subjects rated the similarity of pairs of stimuli, using direct scaling, and rated the purees on 10 attribute scales. The optimal MDS solution obtained using the ALSCAL program was a four-dimensional one. In this study, no striking differences in food perception were obtained as a function of age. The principal MDS dimension distinguished peach and strawberry from broccoli and spinach. For older people, the intensity of flavor (flat vs. sharp) appears to be the single most important dimension.

Impaired food identification by the elderly may involve the olfactory/trigeminal as opposed to taste input. In a study by Murphy,[69] 40 young (ages 18 to 26) and 40 older people (ages 65 and over) attempted to identify pureed foods while blindfolded, using only taste and odor cues. The freshly prepared, steamed and blended foods were potato, tomato, carrot, broccoli, celery, lemon, pear, banana, beef, coffee, sugar, and salt.

Younger people identified more foods on the first attempt than did older subjects. While performance improved with feedback, the effect of age still held. Older women had higher scores than older men. In the second study, 20 younger and 17 older women repeated the task with their nostrils pinched to eliminate olfactory input. The rate of correct scores on the first attempt was now the same for the two groups, suggesting that smell rather than taste plays a major role in the identification of foods. This notion was confirmed by a later study showing that detection of the spice marjoram in soup was largely based on olfactory input.[71] In contrast, taste played a minor role.

The age-related drop in the ability to identify foods may also involve cognition. In Murphy's study,[69] younger women performed better than older women during repeated attempts at identifying foods, suggesting that learning and memory, and semantic retrieval may also be involved. Younger subjects were more likely to place incorrectly identified food into the correct semantic categories; for example, 37 of 40 young people assigned pureed pears to the fruit category. In contrast, more elderly subjects gave it a non-fruit label, mostly vegetable. Similar results were obtained with other fruits, such as bananas. Younger subjects were more likely to operate within the appropriate cognitive categories in assigning labels to foods, while the elderly showed greater variability and more frequent inappropriate judgments. Reduced ability to identify foods by elderly adults may result from a decline in olfactory sensitivity and in cognitive skills.

V. FOOD PREFERENCES

Food preferences are determined not only by taste and smell, but also by other sensory cues including food texture, temperature, color, and appearance.[72,73] The elderly rate the taste of foods as the main determinant of food selection,[74] and the chief reason for the enjoyment and appreciation of foods.[75] Food "taste" typically includes both taste and olfaction. Olfactory deficits are said to reduce food acceptability and result in diminished food intakes.[16] Amplifying foods by adding additional odor has been reported to increase hedonic tone and reverse age-related anorexia.[76]

In one early study on flavor amplification,[38] 14 elderly people (ages 77 to 84 yr) and 11 college students (ages 17 to 25 yr), tasted five blended foods that were fortified with artificial flavors at two levels of strength. The flavors included apple, beef, egg, pork, and walnut. The subjects tasted the foods, and rated them along visual analog scales. Flavor amplification reduced complaints of sourness and bitterness, and increased hedonic rating among the elderly, while reducing them for the young.

In a later study,[76] 75% of elderly subjects (ages 70 to 79 yr) were found to prefer those foods that had been amplified or enhanced with added flavors. The non-caloric flavors, added to cooked and drained foods, were carrot, pea, potato, tomato, apple, chicken, beef, and bacon. In some samples, carrots were amplified with carrot flavor, in other samples, peas were enhanced with bacon. The most frequently used enhancer was bacon, which was used 11 times in 22 samples.

Continuing this line of research, Schiffman and Warwick[77] reported that the elderly preferred 19 out of 20 enhanced foods. The flavors used were apple, bacon, beef, carrot, cheese, chicken, pea, peach, pear, potato, and tomato. About half of the manipulations involved flavor amplification and half involved flavor enhancement. In the amplification condition, carrots were amplified with carrot flavor, apple juice with apple flavor, and tuna salad with tuna flavor. Although the subjects did prefer the flavor-amplified foods, some of the observed increments were not large. More-dramatic results were obtained in the flavor enhancement condition, where broccoli and cauliflower were enhanced with cheese flavor, peas, beans, and turnip greens with bacon flavor, and spaghetti with both bacon and cheese. In most cases, the added non-caloric flavors (bacon or cheese) provided sensations commonly associated with dietary fats.

Although amplification and enhancement are distinct conditions, the two terms have sometimes been used interchangeably. While flavor amplification might compensate for perceptual losses, food enhancement with fat flavors adds a new sensory dimension. One study used fat-related flavors to enhance institutional foods, mostly vegetables ($n = 15$); sauces and gravies ($n = 8$); breakfast foods such as eggs, grits, maple syrup, and oatmeal, and main dishes such as beef barley soup, macaroni and cheese, and veal paprika stew.[77] The six flavors used were roast beef, ham, bacon, prime beef, maple, and cheese. One or two foods were enhanced at each meal, and food intakes and nutritional status of 39 elderly residents of a retirement home (average age 85 yr) were examined over a 3-week period. The study used a crossover within-subject design, with subjects serving as their own controls. Out of 30 enhanced foods, only peas and carrots, mushroom gravy, and maple syrup showed significant increases in intake. The most effective enhancers of food intake were meat flavors: roast beef, bacon, and ham. Flavor enhancement did not increase energy intakes and appeared to have no clinically significant effects on nutritional status.

VI. AGING AND FOOD SELECTION

Consumption of a varied diet is an effective way of assuring adequate nutrient intake.[74] The reported narrowing of food choices with age is thought to be a potential cause of inadequate nutrition among the elderly.

Data obtained from the 1977–78 Nationwide Food Consumption Survey (NFCS) are sometimes cited as evidence that dietary variety declines with age.[78] These data were based on a sample of adults more than 54 years old ($n = 4,983$) drawn from among more than 30,000 people interviewed in the NFCS study. Food consumption data were based on one 24-hour food recall and 2-day food records.[78] Approximately 2,500 different foods were reported over the 3-day period.

Consumption patterns of the elderly were analyzed using two separate measures of dietary variety. The first measure, the variety index, was calculated by counting the number of different foods in each of 18 previously defined food groups that were eaten by each individual over 3 days. The elderly respondents ate approximately 35 different foods over three days, with men reporting more different foods than did women. The variety index declined slightly from the youngest (age 55 to 64) to the oldest group (>75 yr). The age-related decline for men was from 37.0 to 33.5 foods, while the decline for women was from 35.2 to 32.7. Categories in which the decline occurred included meat, vegetables, and fruit. In contrast, other food categories showed no age-related decline in variety. No changes were observed for milk products, whole and refined grain products, sweets, soups, or desserts.[78]

The second measure of "core" foods was based on a straight frequency tally of foods consumed over the 3-day period, and a more complex calculation of a food frequency score over the three days. The first 20 items were the same by either score, and did not vary markedly with either age or gender. As shown in Table 15.1, items consumed on at least 1 of the 3 days by approximately 50% of the elderly respondents were whole milk, coffee, white bread, potatoes (other than fried), margarine, and sugar.[78] These items were relatively inexpensive, simple to chew, and easy to prepare. A higher proportion of the sample population 75 years and above lived alone, and had lower income and educational levels than did younger adults.

TABLE 15.1
The Most Frequently Consumed Foods in the U.S. Diet

	All Adults Ages 19–74	Adults Ages 75 and Over			
			Men		Women
1.	Coffee, tea	1.	White bread, rolls, crackers	1.	White bread, rolls, crackers
2.	White bread, rolls, crackers	2.	Whole milk	2.	Whole milk
3.	Margarine	3.	Sugar	3.	Coffee, tea
4.	Whole milk, whole milk beverages	4.	Coffee, tea	4.	Margarine
5.	Doughnuts, cookies, cake	5.	Margarine	5.	Sugar
6.	Sugar	6.	Potatoes, excluding fried	6.	Potatoes, excluding fried
7.	Green salad	7.	Bacon	7.	Orange juice
8.	Regular soft drinks	8.	Eggs	8.	Eggs
9.	Cheeses, excl. cottage cheese	9.	Butter	9.	Lettuce
10.	Eggs	10.	Orange juice	10.	Butter
11.	Mayonnaise, salad dressings	11.	Jam, jelly	11.	Low-fat milk
12.	Hot dogs, ham, lunch meats	12.	Lettuce	12.	Jam, jelly
13.	Alcoholic beverages	13.	Bananas	13.	Bananas
14.	Potatoes, excluding fried	14.	Whole-wheat, rye bread	14.	Ready-to-eat cereal
15.	Tomatoes, tomato juice	15.	Ready-to-eat cereal	15.	Whole-wheat, rye bread
16.	Whole-wheat, rye bread	16.	Tomatoes	16.	Bacon
17.	Beef steaks, roasts	17.	Low-fat milk	17.	Tomatoes
18.	Orange juice	18.	Gravy	18.	Ice cream
19.	Butter	19.	Ice cream	19.	Salad dressing
20.	French fries, fried potatoes	20.	Soup	20.	Soup

Note: Data from NHANES II (1976–80) and 1977 CSFII. Table based on data from Block et al.[79] and Fanelli and Stevenhagen.[78]

The foods listed in Table 15.1 are not so different from the "core" foods of the American diet. Block and colleagues published a similar analysis of the most frequently consumed foods in the 1976–80 NHANES II sample.[79] These data were based on 11, 658 adults, between 19 and 74 years of age, and a single 24-hour food recall. The food frequency score was the number of persons estimated to consume that food on any given day per 10,000 population.

Only three foods — coffee, white bread, and margarine — were consumed by more than 50% of the respondents on any given day. The most frequently consumed foods were coffee and tea, white bread, margarine, whole milk, doughnuts, cookies and cakes, and sugar.[79] The "core" foods, which appeared in the NHANES II data but not in the NFCS data, were doughnuts, regular (non-diet) soft drinks, cheese, hot dogs, alcohol, steaks, and french fries. In their place, the NFCS data reported bacon, jam/jelly, cereal, low-fat milk, ice cream, and soup.

Dietary trends among the elderly have followed those of the American public. A comparison of 1977–78 NFCS data with the 1985 CSFII study[80] showed that American women ages 19 to 50 reduced the consumption of meat and full-fat milk, but consumed more low-fat milk, and low-calorie soft drinks. A similar analysis of intake trends for the elderly[81] showed that they too reduced the consumption of meat, and increased the consumption of low-fat milk, low-calorie beverages, and take-out foods.

VII.   PSYCHOSOCIAL ISSUES IN AGING

A variety of factors other than taste and smell influence food intakes among the elderly. Studies in social nutrition have addressed cohort effects, social support networks, and alterations in family structure and gender roles.[22] Such studies place food selection in a broader sociocultural context, describing it as an integral part of food habits. Food habits have been defined as including actual food consumption, food purchasing, meal patterns, the frequency of consumption of specific foods, preferences for particular foods, and underlying nutrition-related attitudes and beliefs.

Aging is associated with a number of inevitable life changes, such as decreased income, altered social and family roles, death of spouse and friends, and declining health status. Chronic diseases and the use of medications, more prevalent with increasing age, may also require a change in food habits.[21,82] Medical nutrition therapy for obesity, diabetes, hypertension, and cardiovascular disease may be associated with restricted energy intakes and reduced consumption of fats, sugar, and salt. Any of those factors can have an influence on eating habits, as indicated in Table 15.2.

Social factors may play the dominant role in determining eating behaviors among the elderly. Fujita reported that the food habits of Japanese elderly depended for the most part on the socio-economic environment and the activities of daily living, and not on age-associated changes in sensory function.[83] Appropriate integration into social networks is another factor influencing food habits among the elderly. Beyond its positive influence on life satisfaction, social activity may indirectly influence the patterns of obtaining, preparing and consuming foods.[22] Income, gender, marital status, living alone, and the lack of socialization at meals have been found in some studies to affect food habits and have an impact on nutritional status.[84] Institutionalization in hospitals and nursing homes was also found to affect food habits and nutrition, although these effects could not be separated from those of poor health and sharply reduced physical activity.[85] Dentition and oral health also affect food acceptance.[86]

Food habits are also influenced by psychiatric and psychological factors.[13,21] The prevalence of clinical depression is high among the elderly.[13] However, the effects of depression on food habits are not always consistent. While some depressed patients complain of a diminished ability to taste and enjoy food, others reported a craving for sweets. Up to 15% of depressed patients showed increased appetite and consequent weight gain.

VIII.   CONCLUSIONS

While sensory losses in both taste and smell do occur in the elderly, there is little evidence that such losses are causally tied to altered eating habits, malnutrition, and ill health. Only a few studies have examined the impact of sensory dysfunction on eating habits and quality of life, and it remains a vital area for further research. There is also a need for more-extensive studies in social nutrition to investigate the mechanisms of food selection that lead to dietary variety or to a narrowing of food choices. In particular, such factors as poverty, education and occupation, marital status, living

TABLE 15.2
Potential Causes of Altered Eating Habits and Food Choices in the Elderly

Social Factors

Poverty
Institutional setting
Living arrangements
Marital status
Lack of socialization at meals

Psychiatric and Behavioral Factors

Depression
Loneliness
Dementia

Health Status and Physical Functioning

Decreased energy needs
Reduced energy expenditure
Acute and chronic disease
Immobility
Poor oral hygiene
Inability to chew

Metabolic Factors

Neurotransmitters
Hormones
Drug–nutrient interactions

Chemosensory Factors

Taste and smell deficits
Diminished perception of bitter taste
Reduced pleasure response to foods
Absence of sensory specific satiety

arrangements, physical activity, and social support networks are likely to be among the major determinants of physical and mental health and good nutrition among elderly adults.[87]

REFERENCES

1. Griffin JP. Drug-induced disorders of taste. *Adverse Drug React Toxicol Rev* 1992; 11: 229-239.
2. Mattes RD, Cowart BJ, Schiavo MA, Arnold C, Garrison B, Kane MR, Lowry LD. Dietary evaluation of patients with smell and/or taste disorders. *Am J Clin Nutr* 1990; 51: 233.
3. Schiffman SS. Taste and smell in disease. *New Engl J Med* 1983; 308: 1275-1279, 1337-1343
4. Ferris AM, Schlitzer JL, Schierberl, MJ. Nutrition and taste and smell deficits: A risk factor or an adjustment? In *Clinical Measurement of Taste and Smell*, HL Meiselman, RS Rivlin (Eds.), New York, Macmillan, 1986; 264-278.
5. Ferris AM, Duffy VB. Effect of olfactory deficits on nutritional status: Does age predict persons at risk? *Ann NY Acad Sci* 1989; 561: 113-123.
6. Bartoshuk LM. Taste: Robust across the age span? *Ann NY Acad Sci* 1989; 561: 65-75.
7. Cain WS, Stevens JC. Uniformity of olfactory loss in aging. *Ann NY Acad Sci* 1989; 561: 29-38.
8. Cohen T, Gitman L. Oral complaints and taste perception in the aged. *J Gerontol* 1959; 14: 294-298.
9. Schiffman SS. Food recognition by the elderly. *J Gerontol* 1977; 32: 586-592.

10. Weiffenbach JM, Bartoshuk LM. Taste and smell. *Clin Geriatric Med* 1992; 8: 543-555.
11. Fanelli MT, Woteki, CE. Nutrient intakes and health status of older Americans: Data from the NHANES II. *Ann NY Acad Sci* 1989; 561: 94-112.
12. Lowenstein FW. Nutritional status of the elderly in the United States of America. *J Am Coll Nutr* 1982; 1: 165.
13. Morley JE, Silver AJ. Anorexia in the elderly (Review) *Neurobiol. Aging* 1988; 9: 9-16.
14. Schiffman SS. Taste. In *Encyclopedia of Aging*, GL Maddox (Ed.), Springer, New York, 1987; 655-658.
15. Schiffman SS. Perception of taste and smell in elderly persons. In *Critical Reviews in Food Science Nutrition*, Vol. 33, FM Clydesdale (Ed.), CRC Press, Boca Raton, FL, 1993; 17-26.
16. Schiffman SS, Warwick ZS. Changes in taste and smell over the life span: effects on appetite and nutrition in the elderly. In *Chemical Senses: Appetite and Nutrition*, MI Friedman, MG Tordoff, MR Kare (Eds.), Marcel Dekker, New York, 1988; 367-382.
17. Murphy C. Aging and chemosensory perception of and preference for nutritionally significant stimuli. *Ann NY Acad Sci* 1989; 561: 251-266.
18. Murphy C. Nutrition and chemosensory perception in the elderly. In *Critical Reviews in Food Science and Nutrition*, Vol. 33, FM Clydesdale (ed), CRC Press, Boca Raton, FL, 1993, 3-15.
19. Doty RL, Shaman P, Applebaum SL, Giberson R, Siksorski L, Rosenberg L. Smell identification ability: changes with age. *Science* 1984; 226: 1441-1443.
20. Doty RL. Influence of age and age-related diseases on olfactory function. *Ann NY Acad Sci* 1989; 561: 76-86.
21. Fischer J, Johnson MA. Low body weight and weight loss in the aged. *J Am Diet Assoc* 1990; 90: 1697.
22. Davis MA, Randall E. Social change and food habits of the elderly. In *Aging in Society: Selected Reviews of Recent Research*, MW Riley, BB Hess, K Boud, (Eds.), Lawrence Erlbaum, NJ, 1983,199-217.
23. Garry PJ, Rhyne RL, Haliqua L, Nicholson C. Changes in dietary patterns over a 6-year period in an elderly population. *Ann NY Acad Sci* 1989.
24. Mattes RD. Gustation as a determinant of ingestion: Methodological uses. *Am J Clin Nutr* 1985; 41: 672-683.
25. Mattes RD, Mela DJ. Relationship between and among selected measures of sweet taste preference and dietary intake. *Chem Senses* 1986, 11: 523-539.
26. Pangborn RM, Pecore SD. The taste of sodium chloride in relation to dietary intake of salt. *Am J Clin Nutr* 1982; 35: 510-520.
27. Arey LE, Tremaine MJ, Monzingo FL. The numerical and topographical relations of taste buds to human circumvallate papillae throughout the life span. *Anat Rec* 1935; 64: 9-25.
28. Miller IJ. Human taste bud density across adult age groups. *J Gerontol*, 1988 Jan; 43: B26-30.
29. Miller IJ, Reedy FE. Variations in human taste bud density and taste intensity perception. *Physiol Behav* 1990; 47: 1213-1219.
30. Arvidson K. Location and variation in number of taste buds in human fungiform papillae. *Scand J Dent Res*, 1979; 87: 435-442.
31. Bradley RM, Stedman HM, Mistretta CM. Age does not affect numbers of taste buds and papillae in adult rhesus monkeys. *Anat Rec* 1985; 212: 246-249.
32. Mistretta CM, Oakley IA. Quantitative anatomical study of taste buds in fungiform papillae of young and old Fischer rats. *J Gerontol* 1986; 41: 315-318.
33. Mistretta CM. Aging effects of anatomy and neurophysiology of taste and smell. *Gerodontol* 1984; 3: 131-136.
34. McBride MR, Mistretta CM. Taste responses from the chorda tympani nerve in young and old Fischer rats. *J Gerontol* 1986; 41: 306-314.
35. Cowart BJ. Development of taste perception in humans: Sensitivity and preference throughout the life span. *Psychol Bull* 1981; 90: 43-73.
36. Murphy C. The effects of age on taste sensitivity. In *Special Senses in Aging*, SS Han, DH Coons (Eds.), University of Michigan Institute of Gerontology, Ann Arbor, MI, 1979.
37. Murphy C. Taste and smell in the elderly. In *Clinical Measurement of Taste and Smell*, HL Meiselman, RS Rivlin (Eds.), Macmillan, New York, 1986.
38. Schiffman SS. Changes in taste and smell with age: Psychophysical aspects. In *Sensory Systems and Communications in the Elderly*, JM Ordy, K Brizzee (Eds.), Raven Press, New York, 1979.

39. Schiffman SS. Recent developments in taste enhancement. *Food Technol* 1987;41:72-73.

40. Weiffenbach JM. Taste and smell perception in aging. *J Gerontol* 1984; 3: 137-146.

41. Weiffenbach JM. Assessment of chemosensory functioning in aging: Subjective and objective procedures. *Ann NY Acad Sci* 1989; 561: 56-64.

42. Richter C, Campbell K. Sucrose taste thresholds of rats and humans. *Am J Physiol* 1940; 28: 291-297.

43. Cooper RM, Bilash I, Zubek JP. The effect of age on taste sensitivity. *J Gerontol* 1959; 14:56-58.

44. Hermel J, Schonwetter S, Samueloff S. Taste sensations and age in man. *J Oral Med* 1970; 25: 39.

45. Harris H, Kalmus H. The measurement of taste sensitivity to phenylthiourea (PTC). *Ann Hum Genet* 1949; 15: 24-31.

46. Kalmus H, Trotter WR. Direct assessment of the effect of age on PTC sensitivity. *Ann Hum Genet* 1962; 26: 145-149.

47. Glanville EV, Kaplan AR, Fischer R. Age, sex and taste sensitivity. *J Gerontol* 1964; 19: 474-478.

48. Grzegorczyk PB, Jones SW, Mistretta CM. Age-related differences in salt-taste acuity. *J Gerontol* 1979; 34: 834-840.

49. Dye CJ, Koziatek DA. Age and diabetes effects on threshold and hedonic perception of sucrose solutions. *J Gerontol* 1981; 36: 310-315.

50. Moore LM, Nielsen CR, Mistretta CM. Sucrose taste thresholds: age-related differences. *J Gerontol* 1982; 37: 64-69.

51. Weiffenbach JM, Baum BJ, Burghauser R. Taste thresholds: quality specific variation with human aging. *J Gerontol* 1982; 37: 372-377.

52. Schiffman SS, Hornak K, Reilly D. Increased taste thresholds of amino acids with age. *Am J Clin Nutr* 1979; 32: 1622-1627.

53. Schiffman SS. Age-related changes in taste and smell and their possible causes. In *Clinical Measurement of Taste and Smell*, HL Meiselman, RS Rivlin (Eds.), Macmillan, New York, 1986.

53. Schiffman SS, Clark TB. Magnitude estimates of amino acids for young and elderly subjects. *Neurobiol Aging* 1980; 1: 81-91.

54. Hyde RJ, Feller RP. Age and sex effects on taste of sucrose, NaCl, citric acid and caffeine. *Neurobiol Aging* 1981; 2: 315-318.

55. Enns MP, Van Itallie TB, Grinker JA. Contributions of age, sex, and degree of fatness on preferences and magnitude estimations for sucrose in humans. *Physiol Behav* 1979; 22: 999-1003.

56. Chauhan J, Hawrysh ZJ. Suprathreshold sour taste intensity and pleasantness perception with age. *Physiol Behav* 1988; 43: 601-607.

57. Murphy C, Gilmore MM. Quality-specific effects of aging on the human taste system. *Percept Psychophys* 1989; 45: 121-128.

58. Weiffenbach JM, Tylenda CA, Baum BJ. Oral sensory changes in aging. *J Gerontol* 1990; 45: M121-125.

59. Warwick ZS, Schiffman SS. Sensory evaluations of fat-sucrose and fat-salt mixtures: relationship to age and weight status. *Physiol Behav* 1990; 48: 633-636.

60. Little AC, Brinner L. Taste responses to saltiness of experimentally prepared tomato juice samples. *J Am Diet Assoc* 1984; 21: 1022-1027.

61. Zallen E, Hooks LB, O'Brien K. Salt taste preferences and perceptions of elderly and young adults. *J Am Diet Assoc* 1990 Jul; 90:947-950.

62. Murphy C, Withee J. Age-related differences in the pleasantness of chemosensory stimuli. *Psychol Aging* 1986; 1: 312-318.

63. Stevens JC, Cain WS. Changes in taste and flavor in aging. In *Critical Reviews in Food Science and Nutrition*, vol. 33, FM Clydesdale (Ed.), CRC Press, Boca Raton, FL, 1993, 27-38.

64. Pangborn RN, Braddock KS, Stone LJ. *Ad libitum* mixing to preference versus hedonic scaling: salts in broth and sucrose in lemonade. *A Chems* abstract, 1983.

65. Chauhan J, Hawrysch ZJ. Salt and sour taste intensity and pleasantness perception with age. In *Food Acceptability*, DMM Thomson (Ed.), Elsevier, New York, 1988; 207-218.

66. Chauhan J. Pleasantness perception of salt in young vs. elderly adults. *J Am Diet Assoc* Jun 1989; 89: 834-5.

67. Murphy C, Withee J. Age and biochemical status predict preference for casein hydrolysate. *J Gerontol* 1987; 42: 73-77.

68. Drewnowski A. Food perceptions and preferences of obese adults: a multidimensional approach. *Int J Obesity* 1985; 9: 201-212.
69. Murphy C. Cognitive and chemosensory influences on age-related changes in the ability to identify blended foods. *J Gerontol* 1985; 40: 47-52.
70. Stevens DA, Lawless HT. Age-related changes in flavor perception. *Appetite* 1981; 2: 127-136.
71. Cain WS. Odor identification by males and females: Predictions vs. performance. *Chem Senses* 1982; 7: 129-142.
72. Christensen C. Effect of color on judgment of food aroma and flavor intensity in young and elderly adults. *Perception* 1985; 14: 755.
73. Clydesdale, FM. Color as a factor in food choice. In *Critical Reviews in Food Science and Nutrition*, vol. 33, FM Clydesdale (Ed.), CRC Press, Boca Raton, FL, 1993, 83-101.
74. Krondl M, Lau D, Yurkiw MA, Coleman PH. Food use and perceived food meanings of the elderly. *J Am Diet Assoc*, 1982; 80: 253.
75. Stevens JC, Bartoshuk LM, Cain WS. Chemical senses and aging: taste versus smell. *Chem Senses* 1984; 9: 167-179.
76. Schiffman SS, Warwick ZS. Flavor enhancement of foods for the elderly can reverse anorexia. *Neurobiol Aging* 1988; 9: 24-26.
77. Schiffman SS, Warwick ZS. Use of flavor-amplified foods to improve nutritional status in elderly patients. *Ann N Y Acad Sci* 1989; 561: 267-76.
78. Fanelli MT, Stevenhagen KJ. Characterizing consumption patterns by food frequency methodologies: Core foods and variety of foods in diets of older Americans. *J Am Diet Assoc* 1985; 85: 1570.
79. Block G, Dresser CM, Hartman AM, Carroll MD. Nutrient sources in the American diet: quantitative data from the NHANES II survey. *Am J Epidemiol* 1985; 122:13-40
80. Popkin BM, Haines PS, Reidy KC. Food consumption trends of US women: patterns and determinants between 1977 and 1985. *Am J Clin Nutr* 1989; 49: 1307-1319.
81. Popkin BM, Haines PS, Patterson RE. Dietary changes in older Americans, 1977-1985. *Am J Clin Nutr* 1992: 55: 823-830.
82. Darnton-Hill I. Psychological aspects of nutrition and aging. *Nutr Rev* 1992; 50: 476-479.
83. Fujita Y. Nutritional requirements of the elderly: A Japanese view. *Nutr Rev* 1992; 50: 449-453.
84. Walker D, Beauchene RE. The relationship of loneliness, social isolation, and physical health to dietary adequacy of independently living elderly. *J Am Diet Assoc* 1991; 91: 300.
85. Lowik MRH, van den Berg H, Schrijver J, Odink J, Wedel M, van Houten P. Marginal nutritional status among institutionalized elderly women as compared with those living more independently (Dutch nutrition surveillance system). *J Am Coll Nutr* 1992; 11: 673-81.
86. Wayler AH, Kapur KK, Feldman RS, Chauncey, HH. Effects of age and dentition status on measures of food acceptability. *J Gerontol* 1982; 37: 294-299.
87. Vailas LI, Nitzke SA, Becker M, Gast J. Risk indicators for malnutrition are associated inversely with quality of life for participants in meal programs for older adults. *J Am Diet Assoc* 1998;98:548-553.

16   Changes in Protein Turnover as a Function of Age and Nutritional Status

Walter F. Ward and Arlan Richardson

CONTENTS

I.   INTRODUCTION

Proteins are crucial to cellular function because of the roles they play as biological catalysts and as essential components of cell structure. Furthermore, proteins are in a state of constant turnover, i.e., proteins are continuously synthesized and degraded. It is therefore not surprising that there is strong interest in the effects of aging on protein turnover. Since our previous review of this field for this series,[1] there have been several reviews published.[2-5] The comprehensive review by Van Remmen et al.[3] is particularily noteworthy because of its focus on transcriptional processes in addition to translational processes. When these reviews are considered in total, the general conclusion that can be drawn is that protein synthesis and protein degradation decline with age.[2-5] In this review, we will discuss the more recent studies in this area in relationship to the previous studies in this area, which have been described in detail in previous reviews.

II.   EFFECT OF AGE ON PROTEIN SYNTHESIS

The view that protein synthesis declines with age is based primarily on measurement of general or total protein turnover.[1-6] When the effect of age on the synthesis of individual proteins is examined, it is found that synthetic rates of individual proteins may increase, decrease or not change.[7] Furthermore, within an individual organism there may be heterogenity both between and within tissues. For example, the rates of skeletal muscle protein synthesis in male Fischer 344/BN F1 rat soleus muscle declines with age, while there is no change in synthetic rates in gastrocnemius or extensor digitorus longus muscles.[8] In human liver, the fractional synthesis rate (FSR) of albumin is not affected by age while the FSR for fibrinogen decreases ~37%.[9] An examination of the synthesis of human myosin heavy-chain and sarcoplasmic reticulum protein turnover found that myosin heavy-chain synthesis decreased with age, which would correlate to an age-related decrease in whole body protein and mixed muscle protein synthesis.[10] In contrast, sarcoplasmic protein synthesis was not affected by aging.[10] Utilizing the double labeling technique for measuring protein turnover (synthesis + degradation), Ferrington et al.[11] observed that calcium regulatory proteins of the sarcoplasmic reticulum in hind limb muscles of Fischer 344 rats exhibit divergent turnover rates. They reported that Ca^{++}-ATPase and ryanodine receptor turnover rates decreased 27% and 25%, respectively, with age while the 53-kDa glycoprotein exhibited a 25% increase in rate of turnover and calsequestrin turnover was unchanged.[11] Changes in protein synthesis with age are not limited to the cytosol. For example, there is a roughly equivalent decrease in the rate of mitochondrial protein synthesis in human skeletal muscle (35% decrease) and rat heart (42% decrease).[12,13].

While it is still accepted that total protein synthesis declines with age, it has become obvious that a great deal of heterogenity exists in the effect of age on individual protein synthetic rates between as well as within tissues. This suggests that further studies on general/total protein synthesis will not make a significant contribution to our understanding of the role of alterations in protein synthetic rates in the aging process. While there is a general decrease in protein synthesis with age in liver, Butler et al.,[7] utilizing 2-D gel electrophoresis, observed that only 11 of ~500 hepatic proteins exhibited major age-related alterations, i.e., either appearing or disappearing with age. Thus, while the search for proteins whose turnover is age sensitive may be considered a fishing expedition, only when enough of the pieces of the puzzle are available will we be able to start putting the puzzle together and to then begin gaining an understanding of the interrelationships between protein synthesis and the aging process.

Over the past 3 decades, a large number of studies have focused on the effect of age on specific steps of protein synthesis (e.g., aminoacylation of tRNAs and the initiation and elongation steps of protein synthesis), and these studies have been described in detail in previous reviews.[1-6] While the actual steps of protein synthesis that are affected by age haven't been conclusively identified, it appears likely that ribosome aggregation to mRNA declines with age and that peptide chain elongation is reduced because of a decline in the activities of the elongation factors EF-1 and EF-2.[3-6,14] The potential role of oxidative stress in the age-related decline in protein synthesis was suggested by a study of Ayala et al.[15] They showed that oxidative stress (treatment with cumene hydroperoxide) significantly reduced protein synthesis in rats. It was found that the elongation step of protein synthesis was most sensitive to cumene hydroperoxide treatment and that EF-2 exhibited both oxidative modification and reduced activity. Thus, oxidation modification of elongation factors could provide an explanation for the reduced protein synthesis with age. This is of particular interest because of the popular concept that oxidative stress plays a role in the aging process, i.e., aging is associated with increasing levels of oxidative stress. In 1989, a great deal of interest in the role of elongation factors in aging was generated when transgenic *Drosophila melanogaster* were produced using a P-element vector containing a cDNA copy of the EF-1α gene under the control of the inducible hsp70 (70-kDa heat shock protein) promoter. Previous studies by Webster and Webster[16] showed that EF-1α decreased dramatically (over 90%) with age in *Drosophila*. Therefore, Shepard et al.[17] produced transgenic flies that would overexpress EF-1α. They reported that the life span of the transgenic flies was greater than non-transgenic flies. This was the first report of a transgenic manipulation extending the life span of an organism and suggested that the age-related decline in protein elongation was important in aging. Unfortunately, later studies showed that these transgenic flies were not expressing more EF-1α mRNA, EF-1α protein or exhibiting greater EF-1α activity.[18] It was concluded that the longer life span of the transgenic fly was not due to the overexpression of EF-1α but was due to a positional effect of where the transgene inserted into the genome.[18,19]

III. THE EFFECTS OF AGE ON PROTEIN DEGRADATION

The effects of age on protein degradation have received much less attention than has the effects of age on protein synthetic activity. There are three likely reason for this lack of attention. First, it has been generally accepted that protein degradation must decline with age since the total protein content of cells and tissues remains relatively constant in the face of significant declines in the rates of protein synthesis.[20,21] Second, it is difficult to accurately measure protein degradation. Third, there are multiple pathways of protein degradation and the mechanisms of action are not as well understood as the mechanisms of the protein synthetic pathway. Age-related decreases in protein degradation have been reported in nematodes (*Turbatrix aceti*), in a variey of rat tissues, and in senescent fibroblasts.[20,22-24] Taking into consideration all of the reviews of this topic leads to the general conclusion that protein degradation does indeed decline with age.[2,3,5,24,25]

There are two primary pathways of protein degradation, the lysosomal pathway and the extra-lysosomal, or cytosolic, pathway.[3] The degradation of intracellular proteins through the lysosomal pathway incorporates both macroautophagic and microautophagic sequestration of these proteins prior to degradation.[26] Dice's laboratory has discovered an additional pathway in which proteins are transferred directly across the lysosomal membrane through an hsc73-mediated transport process.[25,27] This direct transport pathway is inhibited by the aging process.[25] It has also been suggested that macroautophagic uptake of proteins is reduced with age.[24] There have been no studies of the effect of age on microautophagic activity.

The major proteolytic activity of the cytosolic fraction is contributed by the proteasome, which plays an important role in the turnover of oxidatively modified proteins.[28,29] Over the past decade, our knowledge of this pathway of protein degradation has increased enormously, and it is generally believed that the proteasome plays a major role in cellular protein degradation. The proteasome is a multisubunit complex that exists in two molecular forms, one having a molecular weight of ~750 kDa (20S) and the second of ~2,000 kDa (26S).[28] The 20S proteasome is a barrel-shaped structure composed of 28 subunits, representing 14 different gene products, arranged in four rings of seven subunits each.[28] The subunits are labeled α and β based on their homologies to the subunits of the archebacterial 20S proteasome, which has the same 28 subunit structure but is composed of only two gene products, α and β.[28] The subunit arrangement of the mammalian 20S proteasome is thus $\alpha_7\beta_7\beta_7\alpha_7$. Within the central cavity of this structure are found the active sites for three different peptidase activities, i.e., chymotrypsin-like, trypsin-like and caspase-like (PGPH) activities. The chymotrypsin-like activity appears to be the rate-limiting peptidase for proteasome-mediated protein degradation.[28,30] The 20S proteasome normally associates with a multisubunit regulatory protein, the 19S cap, forming the 26S proteasome.[28] The primary function of the 26S proteasome is to bind and degrade proteins that have been coupled with ubiquitin, ubiquintination being the major pathway for targeting proteins for degradation.[28]

Because of the importance of the proteasome in protein degradation, investigators have begun studying the effect of aging on the proteasome and its activity. These studies are listed in Table 16.1. Only the caspase-like activity was observed to decrease (~50–60%) with age in all four studies. Very little, if any, change in trypsin-like or chymotrypsin-like activity was observed with age in the proteasome by most studies. The decline in caspase-like activity does not affect the rate at which the proteasome degrades casein, a commonly used protein substrate for measurement of proteasomal proteolysis.[31] Therefore, Shibatani et al.[31] have concluded that it is unlikely that the age-related alterations of proteasomal peptidase activity are sufficient to account for the decline in protein degradation exhibited with aging, a conclusion with which Cuervo and Dice[25] concur.

If it is accepted that protein synthesis and degradation decline with age it can then be asked what the potential ramifications of decreased protein turnover would be for the cell. It is well established that cellular responsiveness to environmental and metabolic challenges is directly related to the rate of protein turnover. These responses are tied to the induction of critical enzymes, and a decrease in the rate of turnover would be predicted to lead to a decrease in the rate of enzyme induction.[21,35] In other words, the cellular levels of enzymes with short half-lives can be altered more rapidly than enzymes with long half-lives. Another consequence of slowed turnover would be an increased cellular dwell time for a protein. The greater the dwell time of a protein, the greater the probability that the protein will sustain damage.[36] There are, in fact, a significant number of studies that have demonstrated increases in the appearance of altered proteins with age.[36,37] These

TABLE 16.1
Effect of Age on Chymotrypsin-Like (ChT-L), Trypsin-Like (T-L) and Caspase-Like (C-L) Activities of the 20S Proteasome

Sex/Strain	Ages Studied (Months)	Change with Age			Reference
		Cht-L	T-L	C-L	
Male/Fischer 344	7 vs. 26	+30%	+15%	–40%	31
Male/Fischer 344	8–10 vs. 25–28	–30%	–17%	–60%	32
Male/Fischer 344	8 vs. 24	nc	nc	–50%	34
Female/Lou	18 vs. 33	nc	nc	–55%	33

Note: nc = no significant change.

alterations are largely post-translational in nature. For example, it has been reported that 40% of the inactive FDP-aldolase molecules found in the livers of old mice can be accounted for by the age-related decrease in degradation of these altered molecules.[38] At one time, it was thought that the production of altered proteins was due to errors in translation, but more-recent studies have shown that the accuracy of translation is not significantly affected by age.[3,6,20] A recent study by Heydari et al.[39] indicates that the transcription factor, HSF1 (heat shock transcription factor 1) becomes altered with age. This transcription factor plays a key role in the transcriptional regulation of the expression of heat shock proteins, especially hsp70.[40] Heydari et al.[39] showed that the degradation of HSF1 declined with age and that this decline was correlated with the appearance of altered HSF1. For example, the thermostability of HSF1 was reduced and the binding activity of the HSF to DNA was decreased. Because an age-related decline in the ability of organisms to respond to stress and to express heat shock proteins appears to be a universal phenomenon,[40,41] the age-related decrease in HSF1 activity could be a major factor in the reduced ability of senescent organisms to withstand stress. Marked decreases in the degradation rate of abnormal proteins in mouse liver and in cultured fibroblasts during cell senescence *in vitro* have also been reported.[42,43] Finally, one of the most important post-translational modifications is oxidative modification, or damage. Consistent with the Free Radical Theory of Aging, currently the most widely accepted theory of aging, it has been shown that oxidatively modified proteins accumulate with age, and it is proposed that this accumulation is due to an age-related decline in the rate of protein degradation.[44,45] The accumulation of post-translationally modified (damaged) proteins, in response to an age-related decline in the rate of protein degradation, would clearly be detrimental to an aging organism and is surely an important component of the aging process.

IV.   THE EFFECTS OF DIETARY RESTRICTION ON PROTEIN SYNTHESIS AND PROTEIN DEGRADATION

Dietary restriction is the only currently available experimental perturbation capable of altering the life span of mammals that directly affects the aging process.[46] Dietary restriction has been shown to modulate protein turnover in that it ameliorates the age-related declines in both protein synthesis and protein degradation.[3] These studies have thus far been restricted to rodents, i.e., rats and mice, with the effects of dietary restriction on protein synthetic activity being observed in most tissues and organs of these animals.[3] As was noted above, aging appears to have the greatest effect on the elongation phase of protein synthesis and this effect has been associated with an age-related decline in the activities of elongation factors EF-1 and EF-2.[4-6] It was thus a surprise, and a disappointment, when it was found that dietary restriction had no effect on elongation factor activity.[47] Therefore, at the present time, it is safe to say that dietary restriction maintains higher rates of protein synthesis throughout the life-span of an animal, but the mechanism of action for this effect remains unknown.

Dietary restriction has also been shown to maintain higher rates of protein degradation throughout the life-span.[1-3] Whether dietary restriction modulates the hsc73 degradation pathway has not yet been determined; however, it has been suggested that dietary restriction can modulate the age-related decline of the macroautophagic pathway.[24] Dietary restriction also modulates the age-related alterations in proteasomal peptidase activity. While not preventing the decline of caspase-like activity, at any age examined, the activity was significantly increased such that activity in the livers of 26-month-old caloric restricted rats was equivalent to that of 7-month-old rats fed *ad libitum*.[31]

V. CONCLUSION

The currently available data strongly support the hypothesis that, in general, the rates of total protein synthesis and total protein degradation decline with age. These data also demonstrate that the effects of aging are not homogeneous, i.e., the turnover rates of some proteins are unaffected by aging while the turnover rates of other proteins actually increase with age. Dietary restriction, while it doesn't prevent the age-related decline in the rates of either protein synthesis or protein degradation, maintains higher rates of both processes throughout the life span of an organism. In addition, there appears to be equivalent effects of dietary restriction on both processes because the total protein content of the cell does not appear to be significantly altered with age.[48,49] It appears that the higher rates of protein turnover exhibited by the rodents fed caloric restricted diets enhances the ability of the animals to respond to environmental and physiological challenges, whether it be induction of enzymes in response to exposure to xenobiotics or the removal of abnormal or damaged proteins. This ability to respond to stressful challenges may play a role in the increased survival and decreased pathology observed with dietary restriction.[50,51]

REFERENCES

1. Richardson, A. and Ward, W.F. Changes in protein turnover as a function of age and nutritional status, in *CRC Handbook of Nutrition in the Aged*, Watson, R.R., Ed., CRC Press, Boca Raton, FL, 1994, 309.
2. Ward, W.F. and Shibatani, T. Dietary modulation of protein turnover, in *CRC Handbook of Modulation of Aging Processes by Dietary Restriction*, Yu, B.P., Ed., CRC Press, Boca Raton, FL, 1994, 121.
3. Van Remmen, H., Ward, W.F., Sabia, R.V. and Richardson, A. Gene expression and protein degradation, in *Handbook of Physiology-Aging,* Masoro, E.J., Ed., Oxford University Press, New York, 1995, 171.
4. Rattan, S.I.S. and Clark, B.F.C. Intracellular protein synthesis, modifications and aging, *Biochem. Soc. Trans.* 24, 1043, 1996.
5. Rattan, S.I.S. Synthesis, modifications, and turnover of proteins during aging, *Exp. Gerontol.*, 31, 33, 1996.
6. Richardson, A. and Semsei, I. Effect of aging on translation and transcription, in *Biological Research in Aging*, Rothstein, M., Ed., Alan R. Liss, New York, 1987, 467.
7. Butler, J.S., Heydari, A.R. and Richardson, A. Analysis of the effect of age on synthesis of specific protein by hepatocytes, *J. Cell Physiol.*, 141, 400, 1989.
8. Fluckey, J.D., Vary, T.C., Jefferson, L.S., Evans, W.J. and Farrell, P.A. Insulin stimulation of protein synthesis in rat skeletal muscle following resistance exercise is maintained with advancing age, *J. Gerontol. Biol. Sci.*, 51A, B323, 1996.
9. Fu, A. and Nair, K.S. Age effect on fibrinogen and albumin synthesis in humans, *Am. J. Physiol.*, 275, E1023, 1998.
10. Balagopal, P., Rooyackers, O.E., Adey, D.B., Ades, P.A. and Nair, K.S., Effects of aging on *in vivo* synthesis of skeletal muscle myosin heavy-chain and sarcoplasmic protein in humans, *Am. J. Physiol.*, 273, 790, 1997.

11. Ferrington, D.A., Krainev, A.G. and Bigelow, D.J. Altered turnover of calcium regulatory proteins of the sarcoplasmic reticulum in aged skeletal muscle, *J. Biol. Chem.*, 273, 5885, 1998.

12. Rooyachers, O.E., Adey, D.B., Ades, P.A. and Nair, K.S., Effect of age on *in vivo* rates of mitochondrial protein synthesis in human skeletal muscle, *Proc. Natl. Acad. Sci. USA*, 93, 15364, 1996.

13. Hudson, E.K., Tsuchiya, N. and Hansford, R.G. Age-associated changes in mitochondrial mRNA expression and translation in the Wistar rat heart, *Mech. Aging Dev.*, 103, 1998.

14. Parrado, J., Bougria, B., Ayala, A., Castano, A. and Machado, A., Effects of aging on the various steps of protein synthesis: fragmentation of elongation factor 2, *Free Radical Biol. Med.*, 26, 362, 1999.

15. Ayala, A., Parrado, J., Bougria, M. and Machado, A. Effect of oxidative stress, produced by cumene hydroperoxide, on the various steps of protein synthesis, *J. Biol. Chem.*, 271, 23105, 1996.

16. Webster, G.C. and Webster, S.L., Decline in synthesis of elongation factor one (EF-1) precedes the decreased synthesis of total protein in aging *Drosophila melanogaster*, *Mech. Aging Dev.*, 22, 121, 1983.

17. Shepherd, J.C., Walldorf, U., Hug, P. and Gehring, W.J. Fruit flies with additional expression of the elongation factor EF-1α live longer, *Proc. Natl. Acad. Sci. USA*, 86, 7520, 1989.

18. Shikama, N., Ackermann, R. and Brack, C. Protein synthesis elongation factor EF-1α expression and longevity in *Drosophila melanogaster*, *Proc. Natl. Acad. Sci. USA*, 91, 4199, 1994.

19. Kaiser, M., Gasser, M., Ackermann, R. and Stearns, S.C. P-element inserts in transgenic flies: a cautionary tale, *Heredity*, 78, 1, 1996.

20. Ward, W. and Richardson, A. Effect of age on liver protein synthesis and degradation, *Hepatology*, 14, 935, 1991.

21. Richardson, A. and Cheung, H.T. The relationship between age-related changes in gene expression, protein turnover, and the responsiveness of an organism to stimuli, *Life Sci.*, 31, 605, 1982.

22. Makrides, S.C. Protein synthesis and degradation during aging and senescence, *Biol. Rev.*, 58, 343, 1983.

23. Dice, J.F. Altered intracellular protein degradaion in aging: a possible cause of proliferative arrest, *Exp. Gerontol.*, 24, 451, 1989.

24. Vittorini, S., Paradiso, C., Donati, A., Cavallini, G., Masini, M., Gori, Z., Pollera, M. and Bergamini, E. The age-related accumulation of protein carbonyl in rat liver correlates with the age-related decline in liver proteolytic activities, *J. Gerontol. Biol Sci.*, 54A, B318, 1999.

25. Cuervo, A.M. and Dice, J.F. How do intracellular proteolytic systems change with age? *Frontiers Biosci.*, 3, 25, 1998.

26. Blommaart, E.F.C., Luiken, J.J.F.P. and Meijer, A.J. Autophagic proteolysis: control and specificity, *Histochem. J.*, 29, 365, 1997.

27. Cuervo, A.M., Hayes, S.A. and Dice, J.F., Molecular chaperones and intracellular protein degradation with emphasis on a selective lysosomal pathway of proteolysis, in *Molecular Chaperones in the Life Cycle of Proteins*, Fink, A.L. and Goto, Y., Eds., Marcel Dekker, New York, 1997, 491.

28. Coux, O., Tanaka, K. and Goldberg, A.L., Structure and functions of the 20S and 26S proteasomes, *Annu. Rev. Biochem.*, 65, 801, 1996.

29. Pacifici, R.E., Salo, D.C. and Davies, K.J.A., Macroxyproteinase (M.O.P.): a 670 kDa proteinase complex that degrades oxidatively denatured proteins in red blood cells, *Free Radical Biol. Med.*, 7, 521, 1989.

30. Kisselev, A.F., Akopian, T.N., Castillo, V. and Goldberg, A.L., Proteasome activae sites allosterically regulate each other, suggesting a cyclical bite-chew mechanism for protein breakdown, *Mol. Cell*, 4, 395, 1999.

31. Shibatani, T., Nazir, M. and Ward, W.F., Alteration of rat liver 20S proteasome activities by age and food restriction, *J. Gerontol. Biol. Sci.*, 51A, B316, 1996.

32. Hayashi, T. and Goto, S., Age-related changes in the 20S and 26S proteasome activities in the liver of male F344 rats, *Mech. Aging Dev.*, 102, 55, 1998.

33. Anselmi, B., Conconi, M., Veyrat-Durebex, C., Turlin, E., Biville, F., Alliot, J. and Friguet, B., Dietary self-selection can compensate an age-related decrease of rat liver 20S proteasome activity observed with standard diet, *J. Gerontol. Biol. Sci.*, 53A, B173, 1998.

34. Conconi, M., Szweda, L.I., Levine, R.L., Stadtman, E.R. and Friguet, B., Age-related decline of rat liver multicatalytic proteinase activity and protection from oxidative damage by heat-shock protein 90, *Arch. Biochem. Biophys.*, 331, 232, 1996.

35. Schimke, R.T., Regulation of protein degradation in mammalian tissues, in *Mammalian Protein Metabolism*, vol. 4, Munro, H.N., Ed., Academic Press, New York, 1981, 178.

36. Rothstein, M. The formation of altered enzymes in aging animals, *Mech. Aging Dev.*, 9, 197, 1979.

37. Rothstein, M. Altered proteins, errors and aging, in *Protein Metabolism in Aging*, Segal, H.L., Rothstein, M. and Bergamini, E., Eds., Wiley-Liss, New York, 1990, 3.

38. Reznick, A.Z., Lavie, L., Gershon, H.E. and Gershon, D. Age associated accumulation of altered FPD aldolase B in mice, *FEBS Lett.*, 128, 221, 1981.

39. Heydari, A.R., You, S., Takahashi, R., Gutsman-Conrad, A., Sarge, K.D. and Richardson, A. Age-related alterations in the activation of heat shock transcription factor 1 in rat hepatocytes, *Exp. Cell Res.*, in press.

40. Heydari, A.R., Takahashi, R., Gutsman, A., You, S. and Richardson, A. HSP70 and aging, *Experientia*, 50, 1092, 1994.

41. Richardson, A. and Holbrook, N.J. Aging and the cellular response to stress: reduction in the heat shock response, in *Cellular Aging and Cell Death*, Holbrook, N.J., Martin, G.R. and Lockshin, R.A., Eds., John Wiley, New York, 1996, 67.

42. Lavie, L., Reznick, A.Z. and Gershon, D. Decreased protein and puromycinyl-peptide degradation in livers of senescent mice, *Biochem. J.*, 202, 47, 1982.

43. Dice, J.F. Altered degradation of proteins microinjected into senescent human fibroblasts, *J. Biol. Chem.*, 257, 14624, 1982.

44. Stadtman, E.R. Protein oxidation and aging, Science, 257, 1220, 1992.

45. Berlett, B.S. and Stadtman, E.R. Protein oxidation in aging, disease, and oxidative stress, *J. Biol. Chem.*, 272, 20313, 1997.

46. Masoro, E.J. Nutrition and aging: a current assessment, *J. Nutr.*, 115, 842, 1985.

47. Rattan, S.I.S., Ward, W.F., Glenting, M., Svendsen, L., Riis, B. and Clark, B.F.C. Dietary calorie restriction does not affect the levels of protein elongation factors in rat livers during aging, *Mech. Aging Dev.*, 58, 85, 1991.

48. Yu, B.P., Wong, G., Lee, H.C., Bertrand, H.B. and Masoro, E.J. Age changes in hepatic metabolic characteristics and their modulation by dietary restriction, *Mech. Aging Dev.*, 24, 67, 1984.

49. Iwasaki, K., Maeda, H., Shimokawa, I., Hayahida, M., Yu, B.P., Masoro, E.J. and Ikeda, T. An electron microscopic examination of age-related changes in the rat liver, *Acta Pathol. Jpn.*, 38, 1119, 1988.

50. Kapahi, P., Boulton, M.E. and Kirkwood, T.B. Positive correlation between mammalian lifespan and cellular resistance to stress, *Free Radical Biol. Med.*, 26, 495, 1999.

51. Masoro, E.J. Influence of caloric intake on aging on the response to stressors, *J. Toxicol. Environ. Health*, 1, 243, 1998.

17 Multifarious Health Benefits of Exercise and Nutrition

Mark D. Haub and Wayne W. Campbell

CONTENTS

I. INTRODUCTION

The greatest cause of all-cause mortality in the aged is cardiovascular disease (CVD) (1), which accounts for 70% of the deaths of older adults (2). Additionally, the risks of acquiring CVD and other disorders, including diabetes and obesity, are strongly related to lifestyle behaviors (e.g., nutrition, being sedentary, smoking) (3). Studies of diet and physical fitness focus primarily on younger adults. While many of the concepts developed in those investigations apply to elderly people, it is still important to acknowledge the substantial heterogeneity in age and fitness that characterizes this group. The population of older adults is continually growing in the U.S. It is estimated that older adults will compose 14.8% of the population of the U.S. by 2015; with the current older population being responsible for nearly a third (29%) of the national healthcare costs (2).

As people age they become less physically active (4), and there is a concomitant increase in the onset of disease and/or disability. For example, there are an estimated 20 to 25 million Americans stricken with non-insulin-dependent diabetes mellitus (NIDDM), with mortality resulting from circulatory disorders (stroke, infarction, renal dysfunction, atherosclerosis, etc.). It has been demonstrated that being physically inactive, participating in nonvigorous activity, and consuming foods high in total and saturated fat are risk factors for all-cause mortality (5). Therefore, since older adults tend to be less active and the population of older people is expected to increase, there will likely be an exponential increase in the number of persons attaining age-associated diseases and/or disabilities in the subsequent decades. This potential increase in the number of diseases and disorders will place more unnecessary costs on the already unstable healthcare system in the U.S. Therefore, a concerted effort must be made to prevent or effectively manage as much debilitation as possible, not only to keep healthcare costs minimal, but more importantly to heighten the quality of life of as many people as possible.

This review will focus on the beneficial role of physical activity in preventing or managing disease, and will include nutritional information with reference to specific disorders and issues related to active older adults. The sections were selected due to the established relationship between physical activity (or lack thereof) and the selected topic, given the topic's clinical relevancy and/or impact on quality of life.

II. CARDIOVASCULAR DISEASE

With the population of older persons increasing rapidly, there is an ever increasing need to prevent the onset of CVD to prolong the quality of life of those individuals and to reduce the financial costs that accrue from this prevalent disease. The majority of available data focuses on factors that, in theory, reduce the risk of acquiring CVD. Unfortunately, this approach only provides relationships and is, therefore, speculative; but the alternative of assessing the direct comparison with morbidity and mortality is impractical due to the inherent difficulties of long-term labor-intensive studies. The commonly used approach assumes that if the risks for acquiring CVD are reduced then the concomitant morbidity and mortality rates due to CVD will be reduced, as well. This section will focus on the risk factors most influenced by the incorporation of physical exercise into daily activities. These risk factors include physical inactivity, atherosclerosis, abnormal lipid-lipoprotein levels, lipid peroxidation (free radical "damage") and insulin resistance, and visceral obesity, which will be discussed in a subsequent section.

A. Physical Inactivity

It has been established that one's cardiovascular fitness and level of physical activity, or lack thereof, is not only related to CVD but also to all-cause mortality and other diseases such as diabetes (6,7), osteoporosis-related fractures (8,9), cancer (10), and cognitive dysfunction (8,11). It should be noted that sedentary individuals, even if they are in good cardiovascular condition, tend to be at greater risk for CVD-related mortality relative to those who are habitually active.

Increasing physical activity appears to reduce the risk of CVD by both direct and indirect effects. The available data indicate that both endurance training (e.g., prolonged aerobic exercises) and resistance training are beneficial means of increasing levels of physical activity in older adults, and thereby help to prevent the onset of CVD and minimize its effects on those already afflicted (12). As for the direct influence of exercise on the cardiovascular system, it has been observed that performing regular exercise reduces arrhythmias and lessens myocardial oxygen requirements (13). Additionally, endurance training has been shown to increase both blood flow capacity and capillary exchange through structural changes to the vessels and enhanced control of vascular resistance (14).

With respect to cardiovascular fitness, older men undergoing endurance training experience improved cardiovascular fitness by an enhanced left ventricular systolic function and diastolic filling, increased left ventricular hypertrophy, and increased arterial-venous O_2 content difference (a-vO_2) (15,16). Contrarily, older women do not experience left ventricular changes, their cardiovascular improvements are dependent on greatly enhancing the a-vO_2 (17). These gender differences have been related to the estrogen and/or progesterone levels of the elderly women due to the vascular influences of those gender-specific hormones (18,19).

Indirectly, exercise exerts its beneficial effects by reducing the risk for thrombosis due to alterations in the blood clotting process (20), and by influencing key metabolic enzymes of lipolysis and lipoprotein metabolism, thereby improving the lipid profile and possibly adipose distribution. Stefanick et al. (21), investigated the effects of the National Cholesterol Education Program diet and exercise on cholesterol and lipoprotein levels. They found that only the diet and exercise group

---

TABLE 17.1

Potential Means through which Exercise* Improves Health and Lessens Risks for Cardiovascular Disease

Maintain or Increase Myocardial Oxygen Supply

Improve HDL:LDL ratio

$\downarrow$ platelet aggregation

$\uparrow$ fibrinolysis

$\downarrow$ *chances for atherosclerosis, thrombosis*

Decrease Myocardial Oxygen Demand

$\downarrow$ heart at rest and submaximal exertion

$\downarrow$ cardiac output at submaximal exertion

$\downarrow$ catecholamine response to submaximal and maximal exertion (improved lipid metabolism)

$\downarrow$ afterload

$\downarrow$ *the work the heart must perform to function normally*

Improved Cardiovascular Fitness (VO$_{2max}$)

Improved functioning of cardiorespiratory system

$\downarrow$ hypertension

$\downarrow$ *physiological stress at an absolute workload*

Increase Insulin Sensitivity/Glucose Disposal

$\uparrow$ skeletal muscle GLUT4 content

$\uparrow$ insulin receptor sensitivity

$\downarrow$ *risk for developing insulin resistance and NIDDM*

Increase Lipid Metabolism

$\downarrow$ circulating catecholamines during exercise

$\uparrow$ lipoprotein lipase activity (increase triglyceride breakdown)

$\uparrow$ intramuscular lipolysis

$\uparrow$ lipid oxidation during exercise

$\downarrow$ *dyslipidemia and increase lipolysis*

Increase Bone Mineral Density (Weight Bearing or Strength Training Exercises)

$\downarrow$(*risk for osteoporosis and hip fractures*

Improved Body Composition

$\downarrow$ in fat mass (decrease risk for insulin resistance, hypertension, CVD)

Preservation of fat-free mass, especially with strength training

$\downarrow$ *Body Mass Index and obesity (enhanced day to day functioning)*

Note: In order to achieve the best benefits, exercise is defined as expending at least 2000 kcal(wk^{-1}), with at least 200 minutes expending at least 5 kcal(min^{-1}.

(compared with the control, diet only, and exercise only groups) lowered LDL cholesterol, thereby substantiating the importance of both diet and exercise in preventing CVD.

Most investigations have utilized estimates of energy expenditure (kcal(day^{-1}) or monitored endurance training as the mode of exercise for correlating physical activity with risk of developing CVD or all-cause mortality. As stated previously, endurance training directly and indirectly affects the cardiovascular system. These physiological adaptations appear to be dose dependent. That is, the more exercise that is performed or energy expended the lower the risk for CVD and premature mortality. This point is well illustrated by data from Paffenbarger et al. (22) that demonstrates the more energy that was expended by Harvard alumni, the lower the risk for all-cause mortality. They also determined that expending more than 2000 kcal(wk^{-1}, second only to avoiding cigarette smoking, provided the greatest reduction in all-cause mortality.

For the sedentary individual, a realistic initial goal would be to work up to expending 1000 kcal(wk^{-1}. Based on the Surgeon General's 1991 *Healthy People 2000* report, an attempt must be made to increase the physical activity of sedentary individuals, even if their activity is minimal (23). To put this level of energy expenditure in perspective, it is estimated that most adults expend 80 kcal·km^{-1} ($\approx$120 kcal·mile^{-1}) while walking. Therefore, in order to expend 1000 kcal each week, one must walk approximately 2 km·d^{-1}, or 12.5 km each week. For an average adult, this is may equate to walking 30 min·d^{-1}, 4 d·wk^{-1}. If the average adult walks at a rate of 10 min·km^{-1}, or 16 min·mile^{-1}, this would amount to about 960 kcal·wk^{-1}. As long as the individual has been given medical clearance to perform physical exercise, this would be an advisable initial goal. However, it must be stressed that the greatest health benefits seem to occur while expending 2,000 kcal·wk^{-1}, which would equate to walking about 24 km·wk^{-1} (15 miles). For specific guidelines to initiate an exercise program please refer to the position stand by the American College of Sports Medicine (24).

With regard to strength training, Ades et al. found that 12 weeks of strength training increased treadmill-walking endurance at 80% of VO$_{2max}$ by 38% in 65- to 79-yr-old women, although their VO$_{2max}$ did not change (25). Furthermore, the change in treadmill endurance time was significantly related to change in leg strength. Parker et al. (26) reported that 16 weeks of strength training in 60- to 77-yr-old women decreased heart rate, blood pressure, and rate pressure product (an index of myocardial VO$_2$) significantly during a weight-loaded submaximal treadmill-walking test). McCartney et al. (27) also found that heart rate, blood pressure, and rate pressure product during an acute resistive exercise are also lower after performing resistance training. Congruently, Frontera et al. (28) found that older men who performed high-intensity resistance training (80% of one-repetition maximum) not only experienced the expected strength gains, but increased cardiovascular fitness (1.9 ml·kg FFM^{-1}·min^{-1}), muscle fiber area, capillary distribution per fiber, and citrate synthase activity. Their results support the incorporation of resistance training in the exercise programs of adults to improve strength *and* cardiovascular health.

It is clear from studies comparing endurance training and strength training, and those assessing the effects of both training modes independently, that endurance training is the most effective intervention to improve cardiovascular fitness in older persons. Most results indicate that endurance training elicits greater improvements in cardiovascular fitness, as determined by measurements of VO$_{2max}$, than can be achieved following resistance training. Nonetheless, it is apparent that resistance training elicits other beneficial adaptations that might improve the cardiovascular systems of older persons in addition to the benefits of increased muscular strength. More importantly, given the substantial health risks associated with being sedentary, it is imperative that older individuals be encouraged to start and/or continue a vigorous and active lifestyle regardless of the type of exercise.

B. ATHEROSCLEROSIS AND LIPOPROTEINS

Similar to physical inactivity, abnormal serum cholesterol, lipoprotein, and lipid levels are strong risk factors for the onset of CVD by hastening the progression of atherosclerosis (29). Chronically elevated levels of total cholesterol and lipids tend to increase the accumulation of atherosclerotic plaque within the arteries; of special importance are the coronary arteries. This accumulation has a strong potential for progressing toward hypoxic and ischemic myocardial tissues due to the decreased vessel radius and subsequent occlusion of blood flow, after which a myocardial infarction or stroke will likely occur.

Initially, atherosclerosis develops with fatty streaks developing on the endothelium of arteries. These fatty streaks may develop as early as childhood and progress to life-threatening stages as years advance. Injury to the inner lining of arteries due to hypertensive trauma, inflammation, lipid impaction, or toxic chemicals may also lead to atherosclerosis. The progression of atherosclerosis results from the accumulation of monocytes (white blood cells), macrophages, and blood platelets on endothelial cells of the artery. The aggregation of these compounds in combination with the subsequent production of polypeptide and platelet-derived growth factors typically lead to the formation of fibrous plaque. A preventable factor that influences the pathogenesis of atherosclerosis is low-density lipoprotein (LDL) oxidation, particularly the small dense LDL phenotype. Free radicals oxidize LDLs, which enhances the likelihood of forming fibrous plaques (30). As the condition progresses, the location of the plaque may ulcerate, with the end result being thrombosis and subsequent necrosis of the affected region. The amount of tissue affected depends on the location of the thrombosis.

Prevention of atherosclerosis is suggested to focus on the lowering of circulating lipids (triglycerides, very low-density lipoproteins, VLDL, and low-density lipoproteins, LDL). The lowering of lipids decreases the availability of plaque components (fatty acids and cholesterol), as well as limits the availability of oxidizable LDL. Additionally, high-density lipoproteins (HDL) actually act to remove cholesterol via cholesterol ester transfer protein and lecithin cholesterol acyltransferase, which transfers cholesteryl esters to the liver to be incorporated into bile or bile salts (31). Therefore, incorporating a means through which VLDL, LDL, and triglycerides can be lowered with a concomitant increase in HDL and cholesterol transferring components would prove beneficial in reducing the chances for developing atherosclerosis.

Pharmacological and nonpharmacological means exist to reduce total cholesterol. However, the nonpharmacological approaches (e.g., diet and exercise) provide protection by altering cholesterol levels, and additional benefits that are unachievable using a pharmaceutical approach. The pharmaceutical method typically yields adverse or unwanted side effects, while the side effects of the nonpharmacological methods are typically beneficial (i.e., improved cognitive function, cardiovascular fitness, muscular strength, etc.).

With regard to improving one's cholesterol levels, the available data seem to indicate that exercise influences total cholesterol, LDL, and HDL levels when the exercise stimulus is within the guidelines established by the American College of Sports Medicine (24). Dengel et al. (7) demonstrated that 6 months of endurance training and weight loss led to significant changes in circulating cholesterol and lipid levels. They observed decreases of 14 and 34% in total cholesterol and triglyceride, respectively, in middle-aged hypertensive obese men. Following the intervention, there was also a twofold increase in HDL cholesterol. Halle et al. (32) observed reductions in serum total cholesterol, VLDL, and small dense LDL in obese men with NIDDM following 4 weeks of weight loss and endurance training intervention (exercise energy expenditure of 2,200 kcal·wk^{-1}).

The beneficial effects of exercise on decreasing atherogenic compounds have also been observed without inducing weight loss. Lehmann et al. (33) observed that HDL and HDL-subtype 3 significantly increased by 23 and 26%, respectively, following 3 months of endurance training (50–70% maximal effort, 3 d·wk^{-1}) in NIDDM men. In a long-term study by Ornish et al. (34), it was observed that aggressive coronary heart disease therapy (low-fat vegetarian diet, regular aerobic exercise, group counseling, smoking cessation, and stress management) led to a reduction in atherosclerotic development, whereas the nonintervention group experienced a continued progression of atherosclerosis. Granted, it is difficult to determine how much influence aerobic exercise had on the regression of atherosclerosis, but given the established data, exercise alone or in concert with other therapies seems to play a significant role in the prevention and/or reversal of atherosclerosis.

C. ANTIOXIDANTS

Exercise with all of its benefits may have some minor side effects. With regard to performing endurance training, high levels of oxidative metabolism have been shown to increase the excess oxygen free radicals, or reactive oxygen species (ROS) (35). At rest, the body has sufficient reserves of antioxidants to deal with normal (sedentary) free radical formation. However, if the production of free radicals exceeds the endogenous antioxidant pathways then oxidative stress occurs, which damages surrounding tissues if severe. Therefore, even though endurance training provides excellent protection against CVD, nutritional support focusing on antioxidants may further protect against disease beyond what can be achieved through the exercise alone.

The biochemical defenses consist of antioxidant vitamins and enzymes, glutathione (GSH), and sulfhydryls. Each component is complementary to the others when an oxidative stress is imposed. The antioxidant vitamins (e.g., α-tocopherol and β-carotene) generally are responsible for trapping ROS. Antioxidant enzymes (e.g., superoxide dismutase and GSH peroxidase) catalyze the reduction of the trapped ROS. Glutathione aids by maintaining the intracellular redox status.

Free radicals impose damage by oxidizing low-density lipoproteins (LDL), primarily the small dense LDL particles undergo lipid peroxidation. This oxidative process greatly increases the atherogenicity of LDLs, which in turn increases the degree of atherosclerosis (36). Generally, the total peroxyl radical trapping antioxidant capacity (TRAP), the body's circulating defense against free radical oxidation, is substantial enough to protect against normal daily free radical damage. However, if the amount of free radicals exceeds what TRAP can handle, then the chance for atherosclerosis increases.

With respect to aging and exercise, Bejma and Ji (35) observed in female Fisher rats that not only does endurance exercise increase free radical formation, but also, older rats have greater oxygen free radicals than their younger counterparts even at rest. To determine the intracellular oxdation rate, they measured the levels of malondialdehyde for the determination of peroxidation following exercise, and the oxidation rate of dichlorofluorescin, a synthetic probe for analyzing intracellular oxidants. Malondialdehyde, and therefore presumably peroxidation, increased significantly following vigorous and exhaustive exercise in both the young and old. However, the level of peroxidation was not different between the young and old, although this indifference may have been due to fiber type (35,37).

It appears that although the body experiences increased production of free radicals in response to both aging and exercise, the body is able to adapt and potentially tolerate the increased free radical oxidation. Vasankari et al. (38) observed that TRAP levels increase following acute oxidative stress (e.g., exercise). This acute adaptation effect was further substantiated by Liu et al. (39), who observed that serum TRAP increased significantly immediately after the completion of a marathon, and remained elevated for at least 4 days after the race. Bejma and Ji (35) also suggest that adaptations occur in the mitochondria to increase the transport of the free radicals to minimize mitochondrial damage.

There is strong evidence illustrating that the potential for increased oxidative stress increases not only with advancing age but with physical activity as well. However, the human body is fully capable of providing a line of defense against ROS. This protective system fluctuates as the body experiences oxidative stress, both acutely and chronically. Therefore, older adults may place emphasis on incorporating antioxidants into their diets for added protection against potential ROS-induced tissue damage, but it may not be necessary.

D. INSULIN RESISTANCE

A decrease in insulin's ability to stimulate glucose disposal, or insulin resistance, is strongly associated with several prevalent diseases such as hypertension, diabetes, obesity, and cardiovascular disease (40). It has been suggested that insulin resistance has a pathogenic role in the development of these abnormalities (40). However, the mechanisms responsible for the onset of insulin resistance are relatively unknown. Since skeletal muscle is the major site of insulin-stimulated glucose disposal (41), it is an essential tissue in which to examine issues relevant to insulin resistance. Insulin aids in lowering blood glucose levels by binding to its specific receptors on the sarcolemmal membrane, which elicits a cascade of intracellular responses that leads to glucose transport into the cell (42).

Critical components involved with insulin sensitivity are glucose transport proteins (GLUT). Specifically, for the person at risk for NIDDM it is critical to increase the number of GLUT proteins that are in the area where the majority of glucose is disposed. Skeletal muscle is the major depository for glucose, and the skeletal muscle isoforms of the GLUT proteins are GLUT-1 and GLUT-4 (43). During basal and postabsorptive periods GLUT-1 is responsible for transporting glucose into the muscle cell. However, following a meal or during exercise the GLUT-4 proteins transport the majority of glucose. The content of GLUT-4 proteins is greatly affected by the amount of physical activity. It has been routinely observed that individuals with insulin resistance have a decreased ability to translocate GLUT-4 proteins (44) and, therefore, when the cell is exposed to insulin are less able to dispose of the elevated glucose levels following a glucose load.

The most common outcome once insulin resistance is established is the onset of NIDDM (Type 2 diabetes), which accounts for at least 90% of the cases of diabetes, and afflicts millions of Americans (45). Also, NIDDM tends to develop in older individuals, as they have higher plasma glucose and insulin levels than younger people (46). However, the major factors that are involved in the pathogenesis of NIDDM are obesity and fat distribution, insulin resistance, insulin secretion, hepatic glucose production, and physical inactivity, regardless of chronological age. A major cause of morbidity, mortality, and disability in diabetics results from macrovascular complications. Howard et al. (47) found that individuals with NIDDM had a greater incidence of both fatal and nonfatal coronary heart disease. Therefore, the macrovascular complications of diabetes and the atherosclerotic predisposition of hyperglycemia place the NIDDM individual at a much greater risk of premature mortality.

It has been observed that those people who routinely engage in physical activity, vs. those who are sedentary, are less likely to acquire NIDDM. A potential mechanism for this decreased likelihood may be due to the morphological changes that exercise induces in skeletal muscle. One of the most beneficial changes is the increase in GLUT-4 protein content (48). Additionally, vigorous exercise tends to increase the size of fast-oxidative glycolytic fibers (Type IIa) and slow oxidative (Type I) as well as increase oxidative enzyme capacity (49). These morphologic alterations allow for greater carbohydrate metabolism via oxidative phosphorylation. Also following chronic exercise training, the muscle cells tend to increase glycogen synthase capacity, and thus their ability to form and store glycogen (50). Overall, this increase in glucose transport, oxidation, and storage permits the cell to dispose of more glucose, thereby lessening the hyperglycemia evident in individuals with NIDDM (assuming glucose intake and hepatic glucose production are under control).

Another factor that has been associated with affecting insulin action is the fatty acid composition of the sarcolemmal membrane. The sarcolemmal phospholipid composition has been observed to strongly affect the physicochemical attributes of the membrane (51). Altering the sarcolemmal composition by increasing the polyunsaturated fatty acid content of cultured cells has been shown to increase both membrane fluidity and the number of insulin receptors, thereby increasing insulin's ability to stimulate glucose transport (52). Additionally, it has been demonstrated that both omega-6 (n-6) and omega-3 (n-3) fatty acids play opposing roles in affecting insulin sensitivity, with decreased n-6 (53) and increased n-3 both enhancing insulin action (54).

A high amount of fat in the diet is known to actually induce insulin resistance (55,56). This metabolic conversion is well established in rodents, but data from human studies is ambiguous concerning the consistency of this association (57,58). The results illustrating a relationship in humans suggest that diets higher in fat lead to an increased saturation of the lipids in the membrane and decreasing membrane fluidity (59), thereby interfering with insulin binding (60) and/or insulin-stimulated glucose transport (61). However, the exact mechanism for any purposed associations between diet, membrane composition, and insulin resistance in humans is unclear (57). Of the available investigations, only Andersson et al. (53) have examined the role of exercise on decreasing the saturation of membrane phospholipids in humans. It was observed that chronic endurance training decreased the composition of n-6 fatty acids and insulin sensitivity increased.

Generally speaking, metabolic studies have demonstrated that physical activity enhances carbohydrate metabolism and glucose tolerance (62–64). Furthermore, training studies investigating the effect of physical activity on insulin sensitivity have suggested that incorporating exercise into activities of daily living will play a positive role in preventing NIDDM (6,65), thereby lessening premature mortality and health care costs brought about by diabetes.

As for the type of exercise to perform to prevent or manage NIDDM, both endurance and strength training exercises have been observed to be of benefit (66–68). It must be noted that, regardless of type of exercise, the program typically must result in weight loss for those with NIDDM or insulin resistance to conclusively increase insulin sensitivity (69).

III.   BODY COMPOSITION AND MUSCULOSKELETAL CHANGES

It is understood that as people age there is a decrease in energy expenditure (70,71) and alterations in skeletal muscle morphology (72,3). These alterations have been suggested as being related (74), but regardless, these changes may influence adiposity (75), resting metabolic rate, levels of circulating substrates and hormones (76), and functional capacity (71,77). Collectively, the typical loss of muscle mass and increases in fat mass and body weight have the potential to disrupt patterns of daily living in the older adult by increasing the risk for falls and decreasing functional ability due to loss of physical strength. These health risks are compounded by the higher risks for aquiring CVD that are associated with obesity.

A. OBESITY

As previously mentioned, fat mass tends to increase as we age. The level of excess body fat, or obesity, may lead to an increased health risk (78–80). It must be noted that obesity is a heterogeneous condition, in that some individuals with obesity do not exhibit the high risk pathologic conditions associated with CVD, NIDDM, or other deleterious health condition (81). In other words, overall excess body fat is not a definitive risk factor.

To better delineate how obesity influences health, the issue of body fat distribution must be addressed. Since excess body fat alone does not provide enough information as to the level of any potential health risks, researchers began investigating where the excess body fat tended to be distributed in those at greater risk for health complications. To examine this issue, studies have been conducted using computed tomography and magnetic resonance imaging to determine which region(s) tend to influence health the most (82,83). The results from Cefalu et al. (82) seem to indicate that those with greater amounts of body fat distributed in the visceral region also tend to be less insulin-sensitive. Specifically, visceral adiposity dyslipidemia and hyperinsulinemia tend to be positively correlated with atherogenesis (84), which heightens the risk for premature mortality.

Although there are limited data to support the use of a low-fat hypocaloric diet and/or exercise training, it is reasonable to expect that both of these lifestyle changes would prove beneficial in reducing the visceral adipose deposition (81). One such study examined the influence of a hypocaloric diet alone, a hypocaloric diet and endurance training, and a hypocaloric diet and resistance training on abdominal adipocity in obese men (85). It was observed that, regardless of treatment, each group experienced similar decreases in abdominal adipocity. Both exercise groups experienced greater preservation of skeletal muscle relative to the diet alone group.

As for visceral adipocity, Rice et al. (86) observed that obese men (BMI = 32–34 kg/m^2) who underwent a weight reduction program utilizing both a hypocaloric diet and exercise training (either endurance or resistance) had similar reductions in visceral adipocity (40 ± 14% and 40 ± 20%, respectively for endurance and resistance training groups) to the diet alone group (32 ± 9%). All subjects experienced increased insulin sensitivity as determined by reductions in fasting insulin and insulin area under the curve, but the two exercise groups experienced an even greater decrease in insulin area under the curve relative to diet alone (–208 ± 161 pmol·L^{-1}·2h^{-1}; –582 ± 244 pmol·L^{-1}·2h^{-1}; –594 ± 370 pmol·L^{-1}·2h^{-1} for diet alone, diet with endurance training, and diet with resistance training, respectively). Additionally, the diet only group experienced a significant reduction in muscle mass (–2.5 ± 1.0%) compared with the maintenance of muscle mass observed in the combined endurance training group (0.3 ± 1.0%) and combined resistance training group (0.2 ± 2.2%).

Based on these data, it is apparent that decreasing caloric consumption is critical to improving health risks associated with CVD, but the addition of exercise seems to provide further protection against insulin resistance and prevents losses in muscle mass. These data support the suggestion to both change one's nutritional habits and increase levels of physical to optimally reduce the risks for acquiring lifestyle-related diseases.

B. Sarcopenia and Protein Requirements

Sarcopenia develops as adults get older (87). This syndrome describes the age-associated loss of skeletal muscle mass. Older people also typically have excess body weight and fat mass, reduced fat-free mass, decreased total energy expenditure, lowered resting metabolic rate, altered protein metabolism and diminished physical activity. These factors contribute to an increased risk for many age-related disorders, including hypertension, diabetes, heart disease, obesity, and osteoporosis. Reduced muscle strength and muscle mass also contribute to a diminished muscle function, the onset of physical frailty, and the loss of an independent lifestyle for many older people (4,24). Effective therapies must be found to promote the maintenance of fat-free mass and muscle mass in older people.

One consequence of sarcopenia is a reduction in muscle strength. Frontera et al. (88) examined more than 200 men and women between the ages of 45 and 78 years old. Isokinetic and isometric strength of the upper and lower body were significantly lower for women than men and were decreased with advancing age for both groups. However, when corrected for FFM (estimated from body density using hydrostatic weighing) and total body muscle mass (estimated from 24-hour urinary creatinine excretion), age-related differences disappeared. These data suggest that loss of strength is mainly due to sarcopenia. Therefore, strategies to increase or preserve muscle mass may be used to cause long-term improvements in muscle function.

By far the best means of preventing and reversing sarcopenia is by incorporating an intense resistance training into one's lifestyle. Research has established that resistance training is an effective way to increase muscle strength and mass of older people (89). As previously discussed, Frontera et al. (28) observed increases in strength, muscle fiber cross-sectional area, capillarization of the fibers, and oxidative enzyme activity. Each of these alterations is beneficial in prolonging the ability to perform daily activities without undue stress.

Limited data also suggest that what an older person eats during the resistance training period can influence how much muscle mass is gained. For example, older men who consumed a nutritional supplement drink containing 560 calories of energy (17% energy from protein, 43% from carbohydrate, and 40% from fat) daily during a 12-week resistance training program gained more muscle mass (as determined by mid-thigh computed tomography) than age-matched men who did not consume the nutritional supplement drink (90). Further research has shown (91) that the level of dietary protein intake influences the relative uptake and efficiency of utilization of nitrogen in older people during resistance training. However, contrary to previous research (90), muscle hypertrophy did not occur with resistance training in these older people (91). It was questioned whether the lack of muscle hypertrophy was influenced by controlled lacto-ovo vegetarian (meat-free) menus the older subjects consumed (91), compared with self-selected habitual diets that presumably included meat (90) in those subjects who experienced skeletal muscle hypertrophy. If true, this would further establish the premise that nutrition and exercise interact synergistically to maintain and/or enhance skeletal muscle mass and function in older people.

Research has established several important findings with regard to the potential body composition benefits of resistance training. First, resistance training is an effective way for the frail elderly to improve indices of physical functional capacity, such as walking speed, stair-climbing power, and spontaneous physical activity (92). Second, resistance training increases FFM, total body energy expenditure, and dietary energy requirements in older men and women (93). Third, resistance training significantly improves whole-body nitrogen retention (91), thus providing a possible mechanism by which FFM and muscle mass are maintained or increased in older people. Collectively, these data suggest that resistance training is an effective tool in modifying body composition of older adults, even those considered frail.

With regard to nutritional status, age-related changes in body composition, physical functional capacity, physical activity, food intake, and the frequency of disease may all contribute to altered protein metabolism. There is an apparent redistribution of whole body protein metabolism in older people, with higher rates of protein turnover of the non-muscle tissues. Older men and women also have lower rates of muscle protein synthesis, compared with young adults (94), and this change may provide a mechanism of age-related muscle atrophy (95). The fact that the protein requirement appears to be higher in the older adult, despite generally decreased muscle mass, suggests that older people may have a lower efficiency of dietary protein utilization (91). The potential impact on protein metabolism of diet-induced weight loss is largely unknown in older people.

With regard to alterations in FFM as it occurs throughout the life span, muscle atrophy and hypertrophy are both associated with significant, and mostly opposite, changes in whole-body and muscle protein metabolism. Muscle atrophy occurs when there is a larger reduction in the rate of muscle protein synthesis relative to the rate of muscle proteolysis, contributing therefore to a reduction in net muscle protein synthesis. Furthermore, myofibrillar protein synthesis in both the fasting (94) and fed state (95) (assessed by the *in vivo* rate of infused ^{13}C-leucine incorporation into muscle protein) are reduced in older men and women, compared with young adults. After adjusting for age-related differences in FFM, the rates of muscle protein breakdown and synthesis were similar in young and older persons. Alternatively, resistance exercise significantly increases the fractional rate of muscle protein synthesis in older adults (94). The older adults studied by Yarasheski et al. (94) had a lower rate of muscle protein synthesis than the young adults before resistance exercise (0.030 ± 0.003 vs. $0.049 \pm 0.004\%$/h, respectively), but increased to a comparable rate (0.076 ± 0.011 vs. $0.075 \pm 0.009\%$/h, respectively) after 2 weeks of resistance exercise. Myofibrillar protein breakdown (assessed by urinary 3-methylhistidine excretion) was not changed during this short-term resistance exercise period, and may suggest that the balance between protein synthesis and protein breakdown was changed toward favoring net protein accretion. Therefore, it appears that older adults may need greater amounts of protein in their diets to account for the alterations in protein synthesis and degradation associated with aging (96). If this aspect of their nutrition is neglected, they may not benefit from the hypertrophic response associated with such activities.

IV. CONCLUDING REMARKS

It is evident from all available data that exercise provides a means of enhancing health through many systems. Therefore, exercise and physical activity should be prescribed to prevent or manage many diseases that plague the U.S. and other countries experiencing an increase of lifestyle-related diseases. Furthermore, the combination of healthy dietary habits with exercise provides a strong prevention strategy to prolong health and the ability to perform daily activities with vitality. The potential for exercise to prolong health extends beyond the diseases and conditions we discussed. However, CVD, insulin resistance, and sarcopenia are conditions that afflict older adults primarily.

With the increasing population of persons over 65 years of age, there will likely be a concomitant increase in the onset of these conditions. If these conditions can be prevented by even months, our families and respective nations would greatly benefit emotionally and financially. Exercise has been proven to improve these and other health-related conditions, but we must increase the number of persons who choose to become physically active. It is disparaging that given the available information regarding the risk prevention benefits of adequate exercise and nutritional consumption and the focus from the Surgeon General of the United States (23), people remain inactive while their health is deteriorating (97).

Given the available research and the increasing occurrences of disorders related to lifestyle choices, it is becoming apparent that merely providing information to the public is not the best means of altering unhealthy behaviors. Therefore, efforts should now be placed on finding the most effective means of incorporating these healthy behaviors into the lifestyles of the majority of the population.

ACKNOWLEDGMENTS

This effort was supported by funding from the National Cattlemen's Beef Association, National Institutes of Health (R01-AG15750 and R29-AG13409), and the U.S. Department of Agriculture (project 98-35200-6151).

REFERENCES

1. Blair, S.N., Horton, E., Leon, A.S., Lee, I.M., Drinkwater, B.L., Dishman, R.K., Mackey, M. and Kienholz, M.L., Physical activity, nutrition, and chronic disease, *Med Sci Sports Exerc*, 28(3), 335, 1996.
2. Kannel, W.B., The demographics of claudication and the aging of the American population, *Vasc Med*, 1(1), 60, 1996.
3. Winslow, E., Bohannon, N., Brunton, S.A. and Mayhew, H.E., Lifestyle modification: weight control, exercise, and smoking cessation, *Am J Med*, 101(4A), 25S, 1996.
4. Monthly estimates of leisure-time physical inactivity — United States, 1994, *MMWR Morb Mortal Wkly Rep*, 46(18), 393, 1997.
5. Lee, I.M., Hsieh, C.C. and Paffenbarger, R.S., Jr., Exercise intensity and longevity in men. The Harvard Alumni Health Study, *JAMA*, 273(15), 1179, 1995.
6. Goodyear, L.J. and Kahn, B.B., Exercise, glucose transport, and insulin sensitivity, *Annu Rev Med*, 49, 235, 1998.
7. Dengel, D.R., Hagberg, J.M., Pratley, R.E., Rogus, E.M. and Goldberg, A.P., Improvements in blood pressure, glucose metabolism, and lipoprotein lipids after aerobic exercise plus weight loss in obese, hypertensive middle-aged men, *Metabolism*, 47(9), 1075, 1998.
8. American College of Sports Medicine Position Stand. The recommended quantity and quality of exercise for developing and maintaining cardiorespiratory and muscular fitness, and flexibility in healthy adults, *Med Sci Sports Exerc*, 30(6), 975, 1998.
9. Kohrt, W.M., Ehsani, A.A. and Birge, S.J., Jr., HRT preserves increases in bone mineral density and reductions in body fat after a supervised exercise program, *J Appl Physiol*, 84(5), 1506, 1998.
10. Lee, I.M., Manson, J.E., Ajani, U., Paffenbarger, R.S., Jr., Hennekens, C.H. and Buring, J.E., Physical activity and risk of colon cancer: the Physicians' Health Study, *Cancer Causes Control*, 8(4), 568, 1997.
11. Perrig-Chiello, P., Perrig, W.J., Ehrsam, R., Staehelin, H.B. and Krings, F., The effects of resistance training on well-being and memory in elderly volunteers, *Age Ageing*, 27(4), 469, 1998.
12. Hurley, B.F. and Hagberg, J.M., Optimizing health in older persons: aerobic or strength training?, *Exerc Sport Sci Rev*, 26, 61, 1998.
13. Leon, A.S., Physiological interactions between diet and exercise in the etiology and prevention of ischaemic heart disease, *Ann Clin Res*, 20(1-2), 114, 1988.
14. Laughlin, M.H. and McAllister, R.M., Exercise training-induced coronary vascular adaptation, *J Appl Physiol*, 73(6), 2209, 1992.
15. Spina, R.J., Ogawa, T., Kohrt, W.M., Martin, W.H.D., Holloszy, J.O. and Ehsani, A.A., Differences in cardiovascular adaptations to endurance exercise training between older men and women, *J Appl Physiol*, 75(2), 849, 1993.
16. Spina, R.J., Turner, M.J. and Ehsani, A.A., Exercise training enhances cardiac function in response to an afterload stress in older men, *Am J Physiol*, 272(2 Pt 2), H995, 1997.

17. Spina, R.J., Miller, T.R., Bogenhagen, W.H., Schechtman, K.B. and Ehsani, A.A., Gender-related differences in left ventricular filling dynamics in older subjects after endurance exercise training, *J Gerontol A Biol Sci Med Sci*, 51(3), B232, 1996.

18. Spina, R.J., Cardiovascular adaptations to endurance exercise training in older men and women, *Exerc Sport Sci Rev*, 27, 317, 1999.

19. Gilligan, D., Badar, D., Panza, J., Quyyumi, A. and Cannon, R., Acute vascular effects of estrogen in postmenopausal women, *Circulation*, 90(2), 786, 1994.

20. Elwood, P.C., Yarnell, J.W., Pickering, J., Fehily, A.M. and JR, O.B., Exercise, fibrinogen, and other risk factors for ischaemic heart disease. Caerphilly Prospective Heart Disease Study, *Br Heart J*, 69(2), 183, 1993.

21. Stefanick, M.L., Mackey, S., Sheehan, M., Ellsworth, N., Haskell, W.L. and Wood, P.D., Effects of diet and exercise in men and postmenopausal women with low levels of HDL cholesterol and high levels of LDL cholesterol, *New Engl J Med*, 339(1), 12, 1998.

22. Paffenbarger, R.S., Jr., Hyde, R.T., Wing, A.L., Lee, I.M., Jung, D.L. and Kampert, J.B., The association of changes in physical-activity level and other lifestyle characteristics with mortality among men, *New Engl J Med*, 328(8), 538, 1993.

23. *Healthy People 2000, National Health Promotion and Disease Prevention Objectives*, vol. 91-50212, U.S. Government Printing Office, Washington DC, 1991.

24. American College of Sports Medicine Position Stand. Exercise and physical activity for older adults, *Med Sci Sports Exerc*, 30(6), 992, 1998.

25. Ades, P.A., Ballor, D.L., Ashikaga, T., Utton, J.L. and Nair, K.S., Weight training improves walking endurance in healthy elderly persons, *Ann Intern Med*, 124(6), 568, 1996.

26. Parker, N.D., Hunter, G.R., Treuth, M.S., Kekes-Szabo, T., Kell, S.H., Weinsier, R. and White, M., Effects of strength training on cardiovascular responses during a submaximal walk and a weight-loaded walking test in older females, *J Cardiopulm Rehabil*, 16(1), 56, 1996.

27. McCartney, N., McKelvie, R.S., Martin, J., Sale, D.G. and MacDougall, J.D., Weight-training-induced attenuation of the circulatory response of older males to weight lifting, *J Appl Physiol*, 74(3), 1056, 1993.

28. Frontera, W.R., Meredith, C.N., O'Reilly, K.P. and Evans, W.J., Strength training and determinants of VO_{2max} in older men, *J Appl Physiol*, 68(1), 329, 1990.

29. Kashyap, M.L., Cholesterol and atherosclerosis: a contemporary perspective, *Ann Acad Med Singapore*, 26(4), 517, 1997.

30. Holvoet, P. and Collen, D., Oxidation of low density lipoproteins in the pathogenesis of atherosclerosis, *Atherosclerosis*, 137 suppl, S33, 1998.

31. Dullaart, R.P., Sluiter, W.J., Dikkeschei, L.D., Hoogenberg, K. and Van Tol, A., Effect of adiposity on plasma lipid transfer protein activities: a possible link between insulin resistance and high density lipoprotein metabolism, *Eur J Clin Invest*, 24(3), 188, 1994.

32. Halle, M., Berg, A., Garwers, U., Baumstark, M.W., Knisel, W., Grathwohl, D., Konig, D. and Keul, J., Influence of 4 weeks' intervention by exercise and diet on low-density lipoprotein subfractions in obese men with type 2 diabetes, *Metabolism*, 48(5), 641, 1999.

33. Lehmann, R., Vokac, A., Niedermann, K., Agosti, K. and Spinas, G.A., Loss of abdominal fat and improvement of the cardiovascular risk profile by regular moderate exercise training in patients with NIDDM, *Diabetologia*, 38(11), 1313, 1995.

34. Ornish, D., Scherwitz, L.W., Billings, J.H., Brown, S.E., Gould, K.L., Merritt, T.A., Sparler, S., Armstrong, W.T., Ports, T.A., Kirkeeide, R.L., Hogeboom, C. and Brand, R.J., Intensive lifestyle changes for reversal of coronary heart disease, *JAMA*, 280(23), 2001, 1998.

35. Bejma, J. and Ji, L.L., Aging and acute exercise enhance free radical generation in rat skeletal muscle, *J Appl Physiol*, 87(1), 465, 1999.

36. Witztum, J.L., The oxidation hypothesis of atherosclerosis, *Lancet*, 344(8925), 793, 1994.

37. Leeuwenburgh, C., Fiebig, R., Chandwaney, R. and Ji, L.L., Aging and exercise training in skeletal muscle: responses of glutathione and antioxidant enzyme systems, *Am J Physiol*, 267(2 Pt 2), R439, 1994.

38. Vasankari, T.J., Kujala, U.M., Vasankari, T.M., Vuorimaa, T. and A., M., Effects of acute prolonged exercise on-serum and LDL oxidation and antioxidant defences, *Free Radical Biol Med*, 22(3), 509, 1997.

39. Liu, M.L., Bergholm, R., Makimatila, S., Lahdenpera, S., Valkonen, M., Hilden, H., Yki-Jarvinen, H. and Taskinen, M.-R., A marathon run increases the susceptibility of LDL to oxidation *in vitro* and modifies plasma antioxidants, *Am J Physiol*, 276(6 Pt 1), E1083, 1999.

40. Reaven, G.M., Role of insulin resistance in human disease (syndrome X): an expanded definition, *Annu Rev Med*, 44, 121, 1993.

41. DeFronzo, R.A., Jacot, E., Jequier, E., Maeder, E., Wahren, J. and Felber, J.P., The effect of insulin on the disposal of intravenous glucose. Results from indirect calorimetry and hepatic and femoral venous catheterization, *Diabetes*, 30(12), 1000, 1981.

42. Moller, D.E. and Flier, J.S., Insulin resistance — mechanisms, syndromes, and implications, *New Engl J Med*, 325(13), 938, 1991.

43. Pedersen, O., Bak, J.F., Andersen, P.H., Lund, S., Moller, D.E., Flier, J.S. and Kahn, B.B., Evidence against altered expression of GLUT1 or GLUT4 in skeletal muscle of patients with obesity or NIDDM, *Diabetes*, 39(7), 865, 1990.

44. Dohm, G.L., Elton, C.W., Friedman, J.E., Pilch, P.F., Pories, W.J., Atkinson, S.M., Jr. and Caro, J.F., Decreased expression of glucose transporter in muscle from insulin-resistant patients, *Am J Physiol*, 260(3 Pt 1), E459, 1991.

45. Kriska, A.M., Blair, S.N. and Pereira, M.A., The potential role of physical activity in the prevention of non-insulin-dependent diabetes mellitus: the epidemiological evidence, *Exerc Sport Sci Rev*, 22, 121, 1994.

46. Fink, R.I., Kolterman, O.G., Griffin, J. and Olefsky, J.M., Mechanisms of insulin resistance in aging, *J Clin Invest*, 71(6), 1523, 1983.

47. Howard, B.V., Cowan, L.D., Go, O., Welty, T.K., Robbins, D.C. and Lee, E.T., Adverse effects of diabetes on multiple cardiovascular disease risk factors in women. The Strong Heart Study, *Diabetes Care*, 21(8), 1258, 1998.

48. Hughes, V.A., Fiatarone, M.A., Fielding, R.A., Kahn, B.B., Ferrara, C.M., Shepherd, P., Fisher, E.C., Wolfe, R.R., Elahi, D. and Evans, W.J., Exercise increases muscle GLUT-4 levels and insulin action in subjects with impaired glucose tolerance, *Am J Physiol*, 264(6 Pt 1), E855, 1993.

49. Coggan, A.R., Spina, R.J., King, D.S., Rogers, M.A., Brown, M., Nemeth, P.M. and Holloszy, J.O., Skeletal muscle adaptations to endurance training in 60- to 70-yr-old men and women, *J Appl Physiol*, 72(5), 1780, 1992.

50. Allenberg, K., Johansen, K. and Saltin, B., Skeletal muscle adaptations to physical training in type II (non-insulin-dependent) diabetes mellitus, *Acta Med Scand*, 223(4), 365, 1988.

51. Hagve, T.A., Effects of unsaturated fatty acids on cell membrane functions, *Scand J Clin Lab Invest.*, 48(5), 381, 1988.

52. Ginsberg, B.H., Jabour, J. and Spector, A.A., Effect of alterations in membrane lipid unsaturation on the properties of the insulin receptor of Ehrlich ascites cells, *Biochim Biophys Acta*, 690(2), 157, 1982.

53. Andersson, A., Sjodin, A., Olsson, R. and Vessby, B., Effects of physical exercise on phospholipid fatty acid composition in skeletal muscle, *Am J Physiol*, 274(3 Pt 1), E432, 1998.

54. Storlien, L.H., Kraegen, E.W., Chisholm, D.J., Ford, G.L., Bruce, D.G. and Pascoe, W.S., Fish oil prevents insulin resistance induced by high-fat feeding in rats, *Science*, 237(4817), 885, 1987.

55. Storlien, L.H., Jenkins, A.B., Chisholm, D.J., Pascoe, W.S., Khouri, S. and Kraegen, E.W., Influence of dietary fat composition on development of insulin resistance in rats. Relationship to muscle triglyceride and omega-3 fatty acids in muscle phospholipid, *Diabetes*, 40(2), 280, 1991.

56. Kraegen, E.W., James, D.E., Storlien, L.H., Burleigh, K.M. and Chisholm, D.J., *In vivo* insulin resistance in individual peripheral tissues of the high fat fed rat: assessment by euglycaemic clamp plus deoxyglucose administration, *Diabetologia*, 29(3), 192, 1986.

57. Vessby, B., Andersson, A. and Sjodin, A., Training induced changes in the fatty acid composition of skeletal muscle lipids. Functional aspects, *Adv Exp Med Biol*, 441, 139, 1998.

58. Storlien, L.H., Pan, D.A., Kriketos, A.D., J, O.C., Caterson, I.D., Cooney, G.J., Jenkins, A.B. and Baur, L.A., Skeletal muscle membrane lipids and insulin resistance, *Lipids*, 31 Suppl, S261, 1996.

59. Borkman, M., Storlien, L.H., Pan, D.A., Jenkins, A.B., Chisholm, D.J. and Campbell, L.V., The relation between insulin sensitivity and the fatty-acid composition of skeletal-muscle phospholipids, *New Engl J Med*, 328(4), 238, 1993.

60. Grunfeld, C., Baird, K.L. and Kahn, C.R., Maintenance of 3T3-L1 cells in culture media containing saturated fatty acids decreases insulin binding and insulin action, *Biochem Biophys Res Commun*, 103(1), 219, 1981.

61. Storlien, L.H., Kriketos, A.D., Calvert, G.D., Baur, L.A. and Jenkins, A.B., Fatty acids, triglycerides and syndromes of insulin resistance, *Prostaglandins Leukot Essent Fatty Acids*, 57(4-5), 379, 1997.

62. Dela, F., Ploug, T., Handberg, A., Petersen, L.N., Larsen, J.J., Mikines, K.J. and Galbo, H., Physical training increases muscle GLUT4 protein and mRNA in patients with NIDDM, *Diabetes*, 43(7), 862, 1994.

63. Horton, E.S., Exercise and decreased risk of NIDDM, *New Engl J Med*, 325(3), 196, 1991.

64. Wallberg-Henriksson, H., Rincon, J. and Zierath, J.R., Exercise in the management of non-insulin-dependent diabetes mellitus, *Sports Med*, 25(1), 25, 1998.

65. Perseghin, G., Price, T.B., Petersen, K.F., Roden, M., Cline, G.W., Gerow, K., Rothman, D.L. and Shulman, G.I., Increased glucose transport-phosphorylation and muscle glycogen synthesis after exercise training in insulin-resistant subjects, *New Engl J Med*, 335(18), 1357, 1996.

66. Evans, W.J., Exercise training guidelines for the elderly, *Med Sci Sports Exerc*, 31(1), 12, 1999.

67. Ryan, A.S., Pratley, R.E., Goldberg, A.P. and Elahi, D., Resistive training increases insulin action in postmenopausal women, *J Gerontol A Biol Sci Med Sci*, 51(5), M199, 1996.

68. Smutok, M.A., Reece, C., Kokkinos, P.F., Farmer, C.M., Dawson, P.K., DeVane, J., Patterson, J., Goldberg, A.P. and Hurley, B.F., Effects of exercise training modality on glucose tolerance in men with abnormal glucose regulation, *Int J Sports Med*, 15(6), 283, 1994.

69. Hughes, V.A., Fiatarone, M.A., Fielding, R.A., Ferrara, C.M., Elahi, D. and Evans, W.J., Long-term effects of a high-carbohydrate diet and exercise on insulin action in older subjects with impaired glucose tolerance, *Am J Clin Nutr*, 62(2), 426, 1995.

70. Poehlman, E.T. and Tchernof, A., Traversing the menopause: changes in energy expenditure and body composition, *Coron Artery Dis*, 9(12), 799, 1998.

71. Evans, W.J. and Cyr-Campbell, D., Nutrition, exercise, and healthy aging, *J Am Diet Assoc*, 97(6), 632, 1997.

72. Houmard, J.A., Weidner, M.L., Gavigan, K.E., Tyndall, G.L., Hickey, M.S. and Alshami, A., Fiber type and citrate synthase activity in the human gastrocnemius and vastus lateralis with aging, *J Appl Physiol*, 85(4), 1337, 1998.

73. Proctor, D.N., Sinning, W.E., Walro, J.M., Sieck, G.C. and Lemon, P.W., Oxidative capacity of human muscle fiber types: effects of age and training status, *J Appl Physiol*, 78(6), 2033, 1995.

74. Evans, W.J., Exercise, nutrition and aging, *J Nutr*, 122(3 suppl), 796, 1992.

75. Calles-Escandon, J. and Poehlman, E.T., Aging, fat oxidation and exercise, *Aging (Milano)*, 9(1-2), 57, 1997.

76. Cefalu, W.T., Werbel, S., Bell-Farrow, A.D., Terry, J.G., Wang, Z.Q., Opara, E.C., Morgan, T., Hinson, W.H. and Crouse, J.R., 3rd, Insulin resistance and fat patterning with aging: relationship to metabolic risk factors for cardiovascular disease, *Metabolism*, 47(4), 401, 1998.

77. Bemben, M.G., Age-related alterations in muscular endurance, *Sports Med*, 25(4), 259, 1998.

78. Fox, A.A., Thompson, J.L., Butterfield, G.E., Gylfadottir, U., Moynihan, S. and Spiller, G., Effects of diet and exercise on common cardiovascular disease risk factors in moderately obese older women, *Am J Clin Nutr*, 63(2), 225, 1996.

79. Gurwitz, J.H., Field, T.S., Glynn, R.J., Manson, J.E., Avorn, J., Taylor, J.O. and Hennekens, C.H., Risk factors for non-insulin-dependent diabetes mellitus requiring treatment in the elderly, *J Am Geriatr Soc*, 42(12), 1235, 1994.

80. Lee, C.D., Blair, S.N. and Jackson, A.S., Cardiorespiratory fitness, body composition, and all-cause and cardiovascular disease mortality in men, *Am J Clin Nutr*, 69(3), 373, 1999.

81. Despres, J.P., Visceral obesity, insulin resistance, and dyslipidemia: contribution of endurance exercise training to the treatment of the plurimetabolic syndrome, *Exerc Sport Sci Rev*, 25, 271, 1997.

82. Cefalu, W.T., Wang, Z.Q., Werbel, S., Bell-Farrow, A., Crouse, J.R., 3rd, Hinson, W.H., Terry, J.G. and Anderson, R., Contribution of visceral fat mass to the insulin resistance of aging, *Metabolism*, 44(7), 954, 1995.

83. Matsuzawa, Y., Shimomura, I., Nakamura, T., Keno, Y., Kotani, K. and Tokunaga, K., Pathophysiology and pathogenesis of visceral fat obesity, *Obes Res*, 3 suppl 2, 187S, 1995.

84. Shantaram, V., Pathogenesis of atherosclerosis in diabetes and hypertension, *Clin Exp Hypertens*, 21(1-2), 69, 1999.
85. Ross, R., Rissanen, J., Pedwell, H., Clifford, J. and Shragge, P., Influence of diet and exercise on skeletal muscle and visceral adipose tissue in men, *J Appl Physiol*, 81(6), 2445, 1996.
86. Rice, B., Janssen, I., Hudson, R. and Ross, R., Effects of aerobic or resistance exercise and/or diet on glucose tolerance and plasma insulin levels in obese men, *Diabetes Care*, 22(5), 684, 1999.
87. Evans, W.J. and Campbell, W.W., Sarcopenia and age-related changes in body composition and functional capacity, *J Nutr*, 123(2 suppl), 465, 1993.
88. Frontera, W.R., Hughes, V.A., Lutz, K.J. and Evans, W.J., A cross-sectional study of muscle strength and mass in 45- to 78-yr-old men and women, *J Appl Physiol*, 71(2), 644, 1991.
89. Hurley, B.F., Redmond, R.A., Pratley, R.E., Treuth, M.S., Rogers, M.A. and Goldberg, A.P., Effects of strength training on muscle hypertrophy and muscle cell disruption in older men, *Int J Sports Med*, 16(6), 378, 1995.
90. Meredith, C.N., Frontera, W.R., O'Reilly, K.P. and Evans, W.J., Body composition in elderly men: effect of dietary modification during strength training, *J Am Geriatr Soc*, 40(2), 155, 1992.
91. Campbell, W.W., Crim, M.C., Young, V.R., Joseph, L.J. and Evans, W.J., Effects of resistance training and dietary protein intake on protein metabolism in older adults, *Am J Physiol*, 268(6 Pt 1), E1143, 1995.
92. Fiatarone, M.A., O'Neill, E.F., Ryan, N.D., Clements, K.M., Solares, G.R., Nelson, M.E., Roberts, S.B., Kehayias, J.J., Lipsitz, L.A. and Evans, W.J., Exercise training and nutritional supplementation for physical frailty in very elderly people, *New Engl J Med*, 330(25), 1769, 1994.
93. Campbell, W.W., Crim, M.C., Young, V.R. and Evans, W.J., Increased energy requirements and changes in body composition with resistance training in older adults, *Am J Clin Nutr*, 60(2), 167, 1994.
94. Yarasheski, K.E., Zachwieja, J.J. and Bier, D.M., Acute effects of resistance exercise on muscle protein synthesis rate in young and elderly men and women, *Am J Physiol*, 265(2 Pt 1), E210, 1993.
95. Welle, S., Thornton, C. and Statt, M., Myofibrillar protein synthesis in young and old human subjects after 3 months of resistance training, *Am J Physiol*, 268(3 Pt 1), E422, 1995.
96. Young, V.R., Protein and amino acid metabolism with reference to aging and the elderly, *Prog Clin Biol Res*, 326, 279, 1990.
97. Francis, K.T., Status of the year 2000 health goals for physical activity and fitness, *Phys Ther*, 79(4), 405, 1999.

18 Effect of Aging on Intestinal Lipid Absorption

M. Keelan and A.B.R. Thomson

CONTENTS

I. INTRODUCTION

Advances in technology and medicine have allowed the average life expectancy to increase. Awareness of the importance of exercise and nutrition also contributes to improved health and longevity. An emphasis to reduce the fat content and control the composition of fat in diet is beneficial in preventing the development of cardiovascular disease and several types of cancer. A healthy intestine is essential to maintaining good nutritional status, yet relatively little is known about changes in intestinal function with aging. Understanding age-associated alterations in intestinal function is necessary to prevent disease and maintain health.

How do we define aging? We begin to "age" from the moment we are born. The first year of life is a time of rapid development, followed by a period of steady continued growth. Another burst of development occurs with puberty. After achieving adult maturity, a type of steady state appears for a time, and then many physiological processes begin to slow down. Hosoda (1992) refers to these periods as infancy, growth, maturation, and senescence. The period of senescence can be described as the "regression of physiological function accompanied by the advancement of age" (Imahori, 1992).

Since intestinal lipid absorption is very complex, it is thought to be affected by the aging process more than other nutrients (Hosoda et al., 1992, 1976). Intestinal adaptation is the ability of the intestine to change functionally in response to differences in environmental conditions; aging is a type of adaptive response. The patterns, mechanisms, signals, and time course of intestinal adaptation have been reviewed (Karasov and Diamond, 1983; Diamond and Karasov, 1987; Thomson et al., 1990). The gut responds to differences in diet, metabolic requirements, and reproductive status concurrently with the process of aging. The mechanisms of the adaptive response describe

0-8493-2228-6/01/$0.00+$.50
© 2001 by CRC Press LLC

the manner in which function may be altered, such as changes in intestinal transport kinetics, membrane permeability, or cell maturity. Alterations in hormone levels, ATP levels or changes in solute concentration are all signals in this adaptive response. An acute adaptive response occurs in cells situated along the villus, while a longer-term adaptive response occurs in cells in the crypt. Adaptive responses may differ in the jejunum and ileum, where function may also differ. The reserve capacity of the small intestine may mask age-related impairment of digestion and absorption (Hosoda, 1992; Hosoda et al., 1992). Studies of animal and human tissue permit the examination of the adaptive aging response in the various phases of lipid absorption.

II. INTRALUMINAL DIGESTION AND SOLUBILIZATION OF LIPIDS

Several reviews describe the digestion and absorption of lipids (Shiau, 1987; Thomson et al., 1989a; Davidson, 1994; Tso and Fujimoto, 1991; Tso, 1994). The majority of dietary fat is triacylglycerol, which is hydrolyzed by gastric and pancreatic lipases to form monoacylglycerols and free fatty acids. Less than 5% of dietary fat is phospholipid, which is hydrolyzed in the presence of pancreatic phospholipase to lysophosphatidylcholine and free fatty acids. Dietary cholesterol may be in the free or esterifed form. Esterifed cholesterol is hydrolyzed by cholesterol ester hydrolase to free cholesterol and free fatty acid. The products of lipid digestion (free fatty acids, monoacylglycerols, lysophosphatidylcholine, and free cholesterol) are solubilized in mixed micelles composed of bile acids, cholesterol, and phospholipids, which dissociate prior to absorption.

Digestive enzyme activity may be reduced with aging. Gastric lipase activity is decreased in human gastric biopsies obtained from subjects over the age of 70 (Gargouri et al., 1989). Although early reports suggested that pancreatic enzyme excretion is decreased with age, later studies report no change in pancreatic enzyme secretion with age in rats (Miyasaka and Kitani, 1987, 1989; Miyasaka et al., 1989) and humans (Gullo et al., 1976, 1983, 1986; Tiscornia et al., 1986; Vellas et al., 1988). Other studies report a decrease in pancreatic secretions with age in rats following the acute stress of surgery (Pelot et al., 1987; Khalil et al., 1984, 1985). The relevance of any reported decreases in pancreatic secretion is likely small, since triglyceride hydrolysis is not affected until pancreatic secretions fall by greater than 90% (Holt and Balint, 1993). Reduced plasma chylomicron levels observed in older subjects are at least partially reversed with concurrent administration of pancreatic enzymes with the meal, suggesting that fat malabsorption occurs with age (Becker et al., 1950; Webster et al., 1977). Fat absorption is observed to be unaffected with increasing age in most persons (Simko and Michael, 1989, Arora et al., 1989). In those subjects with impaired lipid absorption, steatorrhea was present due to pancreatic insufficiency (Simko and Michael, 1989).

Bile acid secretion may be altered with aging (Holt and Balint, 1993). Bile acid excretion falls in older rats when expressed per 100 g body weight, but not per animal (Uchida et al., 1978). In human subjects, bile acid synthesis and excretion is reported to decrease with age (Einarsson et al., 1985). Bile acid metabolism may also increase with aging, while ileal reabsorption of bile acid may decrease (Van der Werf et al., 1981). Another study does not support any alterations in bile acid secretion with age (Valdivieso et al., 1978). A decline in bile acid concentration in the intestinal lumen with age would impair lipid solubilzation and subsequent absorption. To date, the data does not conclusively point to alterations in bile acid secretion.

Alterations in response to cholecystokinin (CCK) with age may influence intraluminal digestion. CCK is released by mucosal cells in the duodenum to stimulate the release of pancreatic juices to the small intestine, as well as to relax the sphincter of Oddi and cause gallbladder contraction to release bile into the duodenal lumen. CCK levels in the plasma increase with age in human subjects without any effect on gallbladder contraction (Khalil et al., 1985), although one study suggested that gallbladder contractility may decrease with age (Boyden and Grantham, 1926). A study in guinea pigs reports a decreased sensitivity to CCK with age (Poston et al., 1988a), which may be related to a decline in gallbladder CCK receptor density (Poston et al., 1988b). Reductions in bile release into the intestinal lumen with age could potentially impair the digestion and solubilization of lipids.

III. INTESTINAL MORPHOLOGY

In order to understand lipid absorption, it is important to consider the morphology of the small intestine. The intestinal mucosa consists of a layer of epithelial cells (enterocytes) supported by the lamina propria, which are seen as finger-like projections called villi. The crypts of Lieberkühn are located at the base of the villi, and serve as the origin of immature, undifferentiated cells. These immature cells leave the crypt and migrate to the villus tip over a period of approximately 2 to 3 days, over which time they develop into fully functional absorptive cells. Villus height may be altered with differences in the number of enterocytes, cell dimensions or the crypt cell production rate.

Aging does not significantly alter villus height, cell number, or cell dimensions in rats (Holt et al., 1984), but does increase the villus cell production rate (Holt et al., 1988). Human small bowel enterocyte morphology or cell number are not altered with aging (Corazza et al., 1986). It is important to consider the aging response under normal conditions as well as under conditions of stress (Holt and Balint, 1993). This response is important as it may address this issue of the functional reserve capacity of the intestine. For example, the villus cell proliferation rate is not controlled as tightly in older rats as compared with younger rats in response to starvation and refeeding (Holt et al., 1988).

The mucosal surface area of the jejunum declines with age in rabbits (Keelan et al., 1985), yet remains unchanged with aging in rats (Meshkinpour et al., 1981). *In vivo* perfusion studies in rats report an increase with age in the intestinal unstirred water layer surface area per unit length of gut, thereby increasing the effective surface area available for lipid absorption (Hollander and Dadufalza, 1983a, Hollander, 1984; Hollander and Tarnawski, 1984). An increase in fecal fat following a high fat meal, a potential indicator of lipid malabsorption, has been observed in elderly patients in conjunction with impaired xylose absorption, suggesting a decline in effective absorbing area with age (Pelz et al., 1968; Montgomery et al., 1978). Another study confirmed a decline in xylose absorption with age (Weiner et al., 1984). A recent pharmacokinetic study reports no change in the absorption rate constant of xylose with age in rats, but does show an increase in the fraction of xylose absorbed (Yuasa et al., 1995). Although a decline in the effective absorptive area may occur with aging, this change in intestinal morphology does not fully explain the magnitude of changes observed in lipid absorption (Thomson et al., 1980).

IV. INTESTINAL MUCOSAL SURFACE

The plasma membrane of the enterocytes is polarized in composition and function. Tight junctions divide the plasma membrane into two domains: the apical brush border membrane (BBM) and the basolateral membrane (BLM). At the luminal surface of each enterocyte is the BBM, which lies in direct contact with the luminal contents. The surface area of the BBM increases the surface area of the villus up to 40-fold (Brown, 1962; Kapadia and Baker, 1976; Penzes and Skala, 1977; Hardin et al., 1993), and is subject to direct or indirect regulation by food (Johnston and McCormack, 1994). Direct regulation of mucosal surface area occurs via polyamines (spermine, spermidine, putrescine), which bind nucleic acids, modify growth-regulating genes (c-myc, c-fos, H_2A), regulate membrane-bound proteins, and second messengers, and stabilize membranes (Seidel et al., 1985; Schuber, 1989; Wang and Johnson, 1992). Indirect modulation of mucosal surface area is achieved by the release of intestinal peptides (i.e., gastrin, enteroglucogon, neurotensin), increased pancreato-biliary secretions, and motor stimulation (Schuber, 1989).

The BBM serves as a permeability barrier which separates the enterocyte from the intestinal lumen. Nutrients are transported from the lumen across the BBM into the enterocyte by endocytosis, carrier-proteins, and permeability properties of the membrane. Absorbed nutrients exit the entero-cyte across the BLM into the portal blood and into the lymph. The BLM is also the entry site of nutrients, hormones, and ions from the blood.

The uptake of lipids occurs predominantly at the upper third of the villus (Haglund et al., 1973; Thomson et al., 1994). Nutrients must cross two barriers in series in order to be taken up by the enterocyte: the intestinal unstirred water layer (UWL) and the BBM. The rate of nutrient uptake is determined by the dimensions and properties of these two barriers, as well as by the activity of protein-mediated components of transport (Dietschy et al., 1971; Thomson and Dietschy, 1977; Westergaard and Dietschy, 1974; Wilson and Dietschy, 1975; Winne, 1976).

A. THE UNSTIRRED WATER LAYER

The UWL is formed by "a hydrated mucus and a series of water lamellae extending outward from the BBM, each progressively more stirred, until the layers blend imperceptibly with the bulk phase" (Thomson, 1979a). The thickness of the UWL is at least 500 Å in humans (Read et al., 1977), although lower values have been reported (Levitt et al., 1996). The effective resistance of this layer must be taken into consideration when describing nutrient absorption. The rate of solute diffusion across the UWL is determined by the thickness of the UWL, the surface area of the UWL, the aqueous diffusion constant of the solute, and the concentration of the solute from the bulk phase of the lumen to the BBM (Wilson et al., 1971). Failure to correct for the effective resistance of the unstirred water layer will lead to an underestimation of the permeability of the BBM, and may also lead to errors in the interpretation of the qualitative aspects of nutrient absorption and its adaptive potential.

The pH of the UWL is below 6, which is lower than in the bulk phase of the lumen, and is lowest in the mucus layer immediately adjacent to the BBM (Matsueda et al., 1989). The low pH of this acidic microclimate is maintained by the activity of the Na^+/H^+ exchanger in the BBM, and the physical properties of the mucus that retard the diffusion of H^+ to the bulk phase of the lumen (Shiau et al., 1985). The acidic microclimate may alter the proportion of ionized and non-ionized solutes, which may influence the ability of the solutes to be taken up by the BBM (Shiau et al., 1985; Small et al., 1984). This is particularly important for fatty acids (pKa ~4.2), since the majority would exist in the non-ionized form in the acidic microclimate, and thereby allow these protonated fatty acids to permeate the BBM more readily (Perkins and Cafiso, 1987). Mucus may also play a role in the absorption of cholesterol, since a component of mucus has been reported to have a high affinity for cholesterol and the ability to bind it in a stoichiometric manner (Mayer et al., 1985).

Aging is associated with a decrease in the thickness of the UWL in rabbits and rats with a concomitant decline in the resistance of the UWL (Thomson, 1979b, 1980, 1981; Hollander et al., 1984; Hollander and Tarnawski, 1984). Only one study reports no change in UWL resistance with age (Hollander and Dadufalza, 1983a). A decline in UWL resistance would tend to increase the net absorption of nutrients, or partially compensate for a change in the transport properties of the BBM.

B. BRUSH BORDER MEMBRANE (BBM)

Alterations in intestinal membrane lipid composition may alter the physical properties of the membrane, which may result in alterations in the activity of membrane-bound proteins. These changes in membrane composition may produce alterations in cell function, including nutrient transport. Alterations in BBM lipid composition with aging have been reported for rat intestine (Brasitus et al., 1984; Meddings and Thiessen, 1989;) and rabbit intestine (Keelan et al., 1985; Meddings et al., 1990). The ratio of total phospholipid to cholesterol in the brush border membrane increases with aging, primarily due to an increase in the phospholipid content of the membrane.

Fluidity is a property of membranes that describes the motional freedom of lipid molecules in the membrane. Alterations in fluidity are associated with changes in membrane lipid composition and function (Schachter et al., 1984; Stubbs and Smith, 1984; Meddings et al., 1990). The passive and carrier-mediated nutrient transport processes depend on the nature of the fluidity of the BBM and its lipid composition (fatty acids, phospholipid head group charge, interaction between phospholipid and cholesterol, protein–lipid interactions).

The low fluidity of the BBM reflects a low phospholipid-to-cholesterol ratio, and may be functionally important for efficient nutrient transport (Schachter and Shinitzky, 1977). Enterocyte BBM fluidity is greater in proximal, compared with distal small intestine, and decreases as cells migrate from the crypt to the villus (Brasitus and Dudeja, 1985; Meddings, 1988; Meddings et al., 1990). BBM fluidity decreases with age (Brasitus et al., 1989; Omodeo-Sale et al., 1991) and is associated with changes in lipid composition (Meddings and Thiesen, 1989). Passive lipid permeability and carrier-mediated glucose uptake are influenced by changes in BBM fluidity (Brasitus et al., 1989; Meddings, 1988, 1990; Meddings and Thiesen, 1989; Meddings et al., 1990). Weaning young animals from the high-fat breast milk diet to a high carbohydrate diet is associated with a decline in membrane lipid permeability. Alterations in BBM fluidity and membrane lipid composition may reduce lipid absorption with aging.

V.   INTESTINAL LIPID ABSORPTION

Lipid absorption involves the uptake of lipids across the BBM into the enterocyte where the lipids must be transferred intracellularly to sites of metabolism, or directly exit the cell across the BLM into the lymph or blood.

A. Lipid Uptake across the BBM

Lipid uptake across the BBM is the rate-limiting step for the uptake of short- and medium-chain fatty acids, while the passive uptake of long-chain fatty acids is rate-limited by the passage through the UWL (Proulx et al., 1984; Westergaard and Dietschy, 1974). The most likely model of fatty uptake involves the dissociation of fatty acids from the mixed micelles in the intestinal lumen mediated by the low pH of the acidic microclimate adjacent to the BBM (Shiau and Levine, 1980; Shiau, 1990). Fatty acids then become protonated and passively partition across the BBM. As mentioned previously, the lipid composition and fluidity influence the permeability properties of the BBM. Alternatively, fatty acids may cross the BBM using a protein-mediated process involving the plasma membrane fatty acid binding protein (FABP$_{pm}$) (Stremmel, 1988) or the fatty acid transporter (FAT) (Poirier et al., 1996). FABP$_{pm}$ has a high affinity for long-chain fatty acids, but can also transport monoacylglycerol, lysophosphatidylcholine, and cholesterol, but not bile acids. Cholesterol and phosphatidylcholine uptake may also be passive or protein-mediated (Thurnhofer and Hauser, 1990a, 1990b). The major site of bile acid absorption is in the terminal ileum (Lewis and Root, 1990). Bile acids are taken up by passive or protein-mediated processes, and this topic has been reviewed recently (Aldini et al., 1995; Montagnani et al., 1998). The apical Na$^+$/bile acid cotransporter (ASBT) has been cloned from rat, hamster, and human ileum (Schneider et al., 1995; Wong et al., 1994, 1995), and is subject to both translational and post-translational regulation (Minami et al., 1993). When this ileal bile acid transporter is chemically inhibited in rabbits, the development of hypercholesterolemia is also inhibited (Higaki et al., 1998).

Lipid absorption is reported to decrease with aging (Bowman and Rosenberg, 1983). Although *in vivo* perfusion studies in rats demonstrate an increase in the uptake of fatty acids and cholesterol with age (Hollander and Morgan, 1979; Hollander and Dadufalza, 1983a, 1983b, Hollander et al., 1984; Hollander and Tarnawski, 1984, 1985), *in vitro* uptake studies done on jejunal discs report a decline in the uptake of fatty acids and cholesterol with age, possibly due to a more permeable membrane in younger rabbits (Thomson, 1979b, 1980, 1981). Methodology differences may explain the contradictory results observed with *in vivo* vs. *in vitro* studies of lipid uptake. Radiolabeled fat breath tests have confirmed that lipid absorption is reduced in adult as compared with suckling rats

(Flores et al., 1989). Whether the age-associated alteration in lipid absorption is due to alterations in passive or protein-mediated permeability has not been resolved.

B. Intracellular Transport of Absorbed Lipids

In the cytosol of the enterocyte, fatty acids are bound and transported by two cytosolic fatty acid binding proteins ($FABP_c$) to their sites of metabolism: the intestinal type (I-$FABP_c$), which is present exclusively in the intestine, and the liver type (L-$FABP_c$), which is present in both liver and intestine. I-$FABP_c$ is localized to mature villus tip cells and is not usually present in the crypt cells, while L-$FABP_c$ is confined to the crypt–villus junction and is not present in villus tip cells (Iseki and Kondo, 1990a, 1990b; Iseki et al., 1990; Sweetser et al., 1988a, 1988b). L-$FABP_c$ appears in the crypt cells only under the conditions of fasting, likely in order to obtain fatty acids from the blood (Iseki and Kondo, 1990a, 1990b). I-$FABP_c$ binds palmitic, oleic, and arachidonic acid, while L-$FABP_c$ binds both saturated and unsaturated fatty acids, monoacylglycerols, lysophospholipids and bile salts, but not cholesterol (Cistola et al., 1989, 1990; Kaikaus et al., 1990; Peeters and Veerkamp, 1989). I-$FABP_c$ is thought to be important for binding luminally derived fatty acids absorbed across the BBM, while L-$FABP_c$ binds fatty acids from the bloodstream (Gangl and Ockner, 1975). I-$FABP_c$ is pH-insensitive, which suggests that it binds protonated fatty acids, while L-$FABP_c$ binds only the unprotonated fatty acids (Cistola, et al., 1989, 1990). L-$FABP_c$ also binds growth factors, prostaglandins and leukotrienes, which suggests that L-$FABP_c$ plays a role in enterocyte growth and differentiation (Ockner, 1990). These differences in binding specificities and properties may aid in the targeting of lipids to their sites of metabolism. Low molecular weight cytosolic bile acid binding proteins (I-BABP) are also involved in the intracellular transport of bile acids (Lin et al., 1990), and may be subject to transcriptional regulation (Kanda et al., 1998). Bile acids may provide positive feedback regulation for active bile acid uptake by binding the ileal lipid-binding protein (ILBP) (Kramer et al., 1998).

The rat intestinal I-$FABP_c$ and L-$FABP_c$ genes and the human I-$FABP_c$ have been cloned (Gordon and Lowe, 1985; Gordon et al., 1985; Lowe et al., 1987; Sweetser et al., 1986, 1987). Starvation, diet and peroximsomal proliferators influence the quantity of $FABP_c$ in rat intestine and suggest a differential nutritional regulation of I-$FABP_c$ and L-$FABP_c$ gene expression. The effect of aging on these functions of the intracellular lipid transport proteins is unknown.

C. Re-esterification, Packaging, and Exit of Lipids from Enterocytes

Absorbed free fatty acids and monoacylglycerols are re-esterified to monoacylglycerols, diacylglycerols, and triacylglycerols; lysophosphatidylcholine and cholesterol are esterified to phosphatidylcholine and cholesterol ester. Monoacylglycerol esterification is not influenced by age in mice or rats (Poirier et al., 1997), but this esterification is reduced in human intestinal mucosa (Nakajo, 1979; Hosoda et al., 1992). In contrast, less glycerophospholipid esterification of oleic and linoleic acid occurs with age in rats (Poirier et al., 1997).

Intestinal lipoprotein synthesis, secretion, and transport have been reviewed extensively (Thomson et al., 1989a, 1993; Vance and Vance, 1990; Davidson, 1994; Shepherd, 1994; Levy et al., 1995). The intestine synthesizes triacylglycerol-rich very low density lipoproteins (VLDL) and chylomicrons (CM), and some cholesterol-rich high density lipoproteins (HDL). VLDL are the major lipoproteins secreted by the intestine during fasting, while CM become the major lipoproteins secreted by the intestine following fat feeding. CM and VLDL are synthesized as pre-CM and pre-VLDL in the smooth endoplasmic reticulum. Triacylglycerols resynthesized at the outer membrane of the endoplasmic reticulum (Lehner and Kuksis, 1995) must flip to the inner membrane where they are transported to growing CM by the microsomal transport protein (Wetterau, et al., 1992). Lipid droplets bud off from the smooth endoplasmic reticulum to merge with the Golgi. An active transport mechanism has been proposed to transport triacylglycerols from the endoplasmic reticulum to the Golgi, which may be the regulatory step in triglyceride transport from the enterocyte (Kumar and Mansbach, 1997). Vesicles containing pre-CM and pre-VLDL pinch off from the Golgi to become secretory vesicles containing coated pits that later incorporate into the BLM (Pearse 1978). In the *trans* Golgi, the apoproteins of the pre-CM and pre-VLDL are glycosylated before release as CM and VLDL across the BLM into the lymphatic circulation (Swift et al., 1984).

Triacylglycerols make up the core of the CM, with cholesterol, phospholipids (phosphatidylcholine), several apolipoproteins (apoB$_{48}$, A-I, A-IV and C) at the surface (Green and Glickman, 1981). A number of apoproteins are synthesized by the intestine and incorporated into lipoproteins. ApoA-IV is a major apoprotein synthesized in the fed or fasting state. ApoB$_{48}$ is synthesized exclusively by the small intestine, while apoB$_{100}$ is synthesized by both liver and intestine. The molecular biology of the human apolipoprotein genes has been reviewed (Zannis et al., 1992), including knowledge of the transcription of the human apoB gene (Kardassis et al., 1990a, 1990b, 1992). Lipid transport from the intestine may be regulated by a process that edits apoB mRNA (Scott et al., 1989; Funahashi et al., 1995). Post-translational editing has been described in baboon enterocytes (Driscoll and Casanova, 1990) and in differentiating human enterocytes (Teng et al., 1990).

Availability of any of the components of CM formation influences the export of triacylglycerols from the enterocyte. Dietary lipids and fiber affect transcriptional and post-transcriptional mechanisms of apoprotein production (Srivastava et al., 1992; Mazur et al., 1991; Felgines et al., 1993, 1994; Sonoyama et al., 1995). Triolein perfusion in rats suggests that impaired exit of lipid from the mucosa occurs with age, possibly due to a defect in lipoprotein assembly (Holt and Dominguez, 1981). To date, no studies have examined the effect of age on lipoprotein assembly.

VI. DIET

Approximately 34% of the North American diet is composed of fat, which translates to approximately 83 g of triacylglycerol, 4 to 8 g phospholipid, and 0.5 g cholesterol per day per average adult. The addition of fiber to the diet increases the thickness of the UWL and alters the absorption of nutrients (Fuse et al., 1989). In Japan, dietary eating habits have become more like that of North America, with fiber intake dropping to 16 g from 23 g per day and fat intake increasing to 56 g from 18 g per day (Hosoda, 1992). The possible consequences of these dietary changes may include alterations in bowel habits and an increased incidence of colon cancer and cardiovascular disease.

An increased incidence of cardiovascular disease is associated with a high intake of dietary cholesterol and saturated fats, but not with the intake of monounsaturated fats. The development of some types of cancer is also associated with diet. A high dietary intake of ω6 polyunsaturated fatty acids may promote tumor growth of some types of cancer. Potential health benefits may be achieved with a diet enriched in ω3 polyunsaturated fatty acids, as suggested by examining the dietary habits of Greenland Eskimos where the incidence of cardiovascular disease, cancer, diabetes, hypertension and chronic diseases associated with abnormalities in immune function and the inflammatory response is virtually nonexistent (Carroll, 1986).

The onset of diabetes mellitus may occur in mature individuals. Increased lipid absorption and hyperlipidemia are features of diabetes that play an important role in the development of cardiovascular disease. Diet may be an important modulator of intestinal function in the presence of chronic conditions such as diabetes. Feeding a polyunsaturated fatty acid diet prevents the increase in nutrient absorption observed with diabetes in animals fed a saturated fatty acid diet (Thomson et al., 1987a, 1987b, 1988a). The mechanisms by which diet and diabetes may influence lipid absorption have not yet been elucidated, nor has it been established whether old diabetics are capable of modifying their nutrient absorption in response to changes in dietary lipids.

Dietary constituents may provide a signal for intestinal adaptation (Thomson and Keelan, 1986). Enterocytes lining the small intestine are continually subjected to changes in the quality and quantity of nutrients in the diet. Accordingly, the intestine must adapt to the variations in dietary load and composition (Diamond, 1991). The response of the mature animal to changes in dietary content and composition is influenced by the type of diets to which the animal is exposed in early life: the ability of the intestine to absorb various nutrients depends on the type of diet fed to the animals at a young age, and has led to the concept of "critical period programming" of the small intestine (Karasov and Diamond, 1983; Karasov et al., 1985; Keelan et al., 1990b; Thomson et al., 1989b). Critical period programming has been defined as "a biological mechanism which is turned irreversibly on or off only once during an individual's lifetime in response to conditions prevailing at some critical stage" (Karasov et al., 1985). The content of the lipids in the diet of the pregnant or nursing rat mother may also influence the intestinal nutrient transport properties in the offspring (Perin et al., 1997; Jarocka-Cyrta et al., 1998).

Changes in the macronutrient content of the diet (protein, carbohydrate, or fat), and specifically changes in the cholesterol content and fatty acid composition result in alterations in BBM lipid composition and nutrient transport (Keelan et al., 1987, 1990a; Thomson et al., 1987c, 1988b). An essential fatty acid-deficient diet results in changes in villus and crypt sizes, as well as epithelial cell ultrastructure, yet does not alter rat BBM cholesterol and phospholipid content. BBM phospholipid fatty acid composition, however, is influenced by feeding an essential fatty acid diet (Christon et al., 1991). The unsaturation of dietary fatty acids influences the lipid composition and function of membranes isolated from many tissues including kidney, brain, heart, liver, and intestine (Clark et al., 1983; Foot et al., 1982; Innis and Clandinin, 1981; Neelands and Clandinin, 1983; Thomson et al., 1986).

Since diets may alter intestinal function, the concept of designing diets as therapeutic nutritional strategies to alter nutrient absorption in the desired direction is an attractive one. An increasing amount of evidence suggests that nutrients play a significant role in the regulation of gene expression (Clarke and Abraham, 1992; Clarke and Jump, 1993, 1994, 1996; McGrane and Hanson, 1992; Jump et al., 1994, 1995; Sanders and Kline, 1995). Very little is known about the nutrient control of gene expression in the intestine, let alone whether this process is altered with aging. Glucose and fructose may play a role in the expression of the genes (SGLT1, GLUT2 and GLUT5) that are responsible for their transport across the BBM and BLM (Shirazi-Beechey et al., 1991; Waeber et al., 1994; Burant and Saxena, 1994; Castello et al., 1995;, Inukai et al., 1993). Long-chain fatty acids may act as signals in the induction of gene expression in adipose cells and liver (Amri et al., 1994; Jump et al., 1994, Kaikaus et al., 1993a, 1993b). Polyunsaturated fatty acids play a role in the hepatic regulation of gene expression of enzymes involved in lipid synthesis either directly or via a response element (Jump et al., 1995; Clarke and Jump 1996). Cholesterol also plays a regulatory role in gene expression of HMG CoA reductase, and enzyme in the cholesterol synthetic pathway (Thumelin et al., 1993). The mechanism(s) by which dietary lipids affect gene expression in the intestine and subsequent lipid absorption have not yet been determined.

VII.   SUMMARY

There is the lack of congruency between human and animal studies, possibly due to different methods and experimental conditions (Holt and Balint, 1993). The data support the possibility that lipid absorption may decrease with aging in healthy individuals, but this decline may not be clinically significant until the individual becomes "stressed," as in feeding a high-fat diet, or concurrently has another disease. The reserve capacity of the intestine compensates for the unpredictable availability of food and food composition, and allows a mechanism by which the intestine can adapt to different conditions, such as cold temperatures and lactation (Ferraris and Diamond, 1997). Adaptation, however, may be energetically expensive and must provide benefit to the individual to be sustained. In the absence of benefit, the adaptation stops resulting in a limit to the reserve capacity. An alteration in the reserve capacity of the intestine may reflect an impaired adaptability of the intestine with aging. The potential of up- or down-regulating intestinal function as needed is an interesting area of research.

More studies need to be done to clarify the effect of aging on lipid absorption. There are several candidates that may cause a reduction in lipid uptake. The gall bladder may have fewer CCK receptors or not bind CCK with the same affinity, and thereby not deliver sufficient bile to solubilize lipids that have been hydrolyzed in the lumen. Pancreatic insufficiency may result in a decrease in pancreatic secretions involved in lipid hydrolysis and thereby reduce lipids available for uptake. Alterations in lipid composition and/or changes in the activity of protein-mediated lipid transport across the BBM may alter the uptake of lipids into the enterocyte. Changes in the activity of re-esterification enzymes and proteins involved in transporting triacylglycerols within the endoplasmic reticulum and the Golgi would alter the packaging of lipids into lipoproteins in preparation for exit from the cell. Accordingly, apoprotein availability would influence the synthesis lipoproteins and alter the rate of exit of lipids from the enterocyte to the lymph. The gene transcription and translation of proteins involved in the many steps of lipid absorption are not well understood. Future studies of the regulation and action of these proteins are needed to provide insight into this complex process of lipid absorption and how it may be affected with aging.

REFERENCES:

1. Aldini, R., Roda, A., Montagnanik M., Roda, E. 1995. Bile acid structure and intestinal absorption in the animal model. *Ital. J. Gastroenterol.* 27:141-144.
2. Amri, E.Z., Aihaud, G., Grimalde, P.A. 1994. Fatty acids as signal transducing molecules: involvement in the differentiation of preadipose to adipose cells. *J. Lipid Res.* 35:930-937.
3. Arora, S., Kassarjian, S., Krasinski, S.D., Croffey, B., Kaplan, M.M., Russell, R.M. 1989. Effect of age on tests of intestinal and hepatic function in healthy humans. *Gastroenterology* 96:1560-1565.
4. Becker, G.H., Meyer, J., Necheles, H. 1950. Fat absorption in young and old age. *Gastroenterology* 14:80-92.
5. Bowman, B.B., Rosenberg, I.H. 1983. Digestive function and aging. *Human Nutr. Clin. Nutr.*. 37C:75-89.
6. Boyden, E.A., Grantham, S.A. 1926. Evacuation of the gall bladder in old age. *Surg. Gynecol. Obstet.* 62: 24-42.
7. Brasitus, T.A., Dudeja, P.K. 1985. Alterations in the physical state and composition of brush border membrane lipids of rat enterocytes during differentiation. *Arch. Biochem. Biophys.* 240:483-488.
8. Brasitus, T.A., Yeh, K.Y., Holt, P.R., Schachter, D. 1984. Lipid fluidity and composition of intestinal microvillus membranes isolated from rats of different ages. *Biochim. Biophys. Acta* 778:341-348.
9. Brasitus, T.A., Dudeja, P.K., Bolt, M.J.G., Sitrin, M.D., Baum, C. 1989. Dietary triacylglycerol modulates sodium-dependent D-glucose transport, fluidity and fatty acid composition of rat intestinal brush border membrane. *Biochim. Biophys. Acta.* 979:177-186.
10. Brown, A.L. 1962. Microvilli of the human jejunal epithelial cell. *J. Cell. Biol.* 12:623-627.
11. Burant, C.F., Saxena, M. 1994. Rapid reversible substrate regulation of fructose transporter expression in rat small intestine and kidney. *Am. J. Physiol.* 237:G71-G79.
12. Carroll, K.K. 1986. Biological effects of fish oils in relation to chronic diseases. *Lipids* 21:731-732.
13. Castello, A., Guma, A., Sevilla, L., Furriols, M., Testar, S., Palacin, M., Zorzano, A. 1995. Regulation of GLUT5 gene expression in rat intestinal mucosa: regional distribution, circadian rhythm, perinatal development and effect of diabetes. *Biochem. J.* 309:271-277.
14. Christon, R., Meslin, J.C., Thevenoux, J., Linard, A., Leger, C., Delpal, S. 1991. Effects of a low dietary linoleic acid level on intestinal morphology and enterocyte brush border membrane lipid composition. *Reprod. Nutr. Devel.* 31:691-701.
15. Cistola, D.P., Sacchettini, J.C., Banaszak, L.J., Walsh, M.T., Gordon, J.I. 1989. Fatty acid interactions with rat intestinal and liver fatty acid-binding proteins expressed in *Escherichia coli. J. Biol. Chem.* 264:2700-2710.
16. Cistola, D.P., Sacchettini, J.C., Gordon, J.I. 1990. 13C-NMR studies fatty acid-protein interactions: comparison of homologous fatty acid binding proteins produced in the intestinal epithelium. *Mol. Cell Biochem.* 98:101-110.

17. Clark, D.L., Hamel, F.G., Queenen, S.F. 1983. Changes in renal phospholipid fatty acids in diabetes mellitus: correlation with changes in adenylate cyclase activity. *Lipids* 18:696-705.
18. Clarke, S.D., Abraham, S. 1992. Gene expression: nutrient control of pre- and posttranscriptional events. *FASEB J* 6:3146-3152.
19. Clarke, S.D., Jump, D.B. 1993. Regulation of gene transcription by polyunsaturated fatty acids. *Prog. Lipid Res.* 32L139-149.
20. Clarke, S.D., Jump, D.B. 1994. Dietary polyunsaturated fatty acid regulation of gene transcription. *Ann. Rev. Nutr.* 14:83-98.
21. Clarke, S.D., Jump, D.B. 1996. Polyunsaturated fatty acid regulation of hepatic gene transcription. *J. Nutr.* 126:1105S-1109S.
22. Corazza, G.R., Frazzoni, M., Gatto, M.R.A., Gasbarrini, G. 1986. Aging and small bowel mucosa: a morphometric study. *Gerontology* 32: 60-65.
23. Davidson, N.O. 1994. Cellular and molecular mechanisms of small intestinal lipid transport. In: *Physiology of the Gastrointestinal Tract*. 3rd ed. Edited by: L.R. Johnson. Raven Press, New York, pp.1909-1934.
24. Diamond, J.M. 1991. Evolutionary design of intestinal nutrient absorption: enough but not too much. *NIPS* 6:92-96.
25. Diamond, J.M., Karasov, W.H. 1987. Adaptive regulation of intestinal nutrient transporters. *Proc. Natl. Acad. Sci. USA* 84:2242-2245.
26. Dietschy, J.M., Sallee, V.L., Wilson, F.R. 1971. Unstirred water layer and absorption across the intestinal mucosa. *Gastroenterology* 61:932-934.
27. Driscoll, D.M., Casanova, E. 1990. Characterization of the apolipoprotein B mRNA editing activity in enterocyte extracts. *J. Biol. Chem.* 265:21401-21403.
28. Einarsson, K., Nilsell, K., Leijd, B., Angelin, B. 1985. Influence of age on secretion of cholesterol and synthesis of bile acids by the liver. *New Engl. J. Med.* 313:377-282.
29. Felgines, C. Mazur, A., Remesy, C., Rayssiguier, Y. 1993. The effect of dietary fiber on apolipoprotein A-1 and A-IV gene expression in rat intestine. *Cell. Mol. Biol.* 39:371-375.
30. Felgines, C., Mazur, A., Rayssiguier, Y. 1994. Effect of the interruption of enterohepatic circulation of bile acids by cholestyramine on apolipoprotein gene expression in the rat. *Life Sci.* 55:1053-1060.
31. Ferraris, R.P., Diamond, J. 1997. Regulation of intestinal sugar transport. *Physiol. Rev.* 77:257-302.
32. Flores, C.A., Hing, S.A.O., Wells, M.A., Koldovsky, O. 1989. Rates of triolein absorption in suckling and adult rats. *Am. J. Physiol.* 257:G823-G829.
33. Foot, M., Cruz, T.F., Clandinin, M.T. 1982. Influence of dietary fat on the lipid composition of rat brain synaptosomal and microsomal membranes. *Biochem. J.* 208:631-640.
34. Funahashi, T. Giannoni, F., DePaoli, A.M., Skarosi, S.F., Davidson, N.O. 1995. Tissue specific, developmental and nutritional regulation of the gene encoding the catalytic subunit of the rat apolipoprotein B mRNA editing enzyme: functional role in the modulation of apolipoprotein B mRNA editing. *J. Lipid Res.* 36:414-428.
35. Gangl, A., Ockner, R.K. 1975. Intestinal metabolism of lipids and lipoproteins. *Gastroenterology* 68:167-186.
36. Gargouri, Y., Moreau, H., Verger, R. 1989. Gastric lipases: biochemical and physiological studies. *Biochim. Biophys. Acta* 1006:255-271.
37. Gordon, J.I., Lowe, J.B. 1985. Analyzing the structures, functions and evolution of two abundant gastrointestinal fatty acid binding proteins with recombinant DNA and computational techniques. *Chem. Phys. Lipids* 38:137-158.
38. Gordon, J.I., Elshourbagy, N., Lowe, J.B., Liao, S., Alpers, Taylor, D.H. 1985. Tissue specific expression and developmental regulation of two genes coding for rat fatty acid binding proteins. *J. Biol. Chem.* 260:1995-1998.
39. Gullo, L., Costa, P.L., Fontana, G., Labo, G. 1976. Investigation of exocrine pancreatic function by continuous infusion of caerulein and secretion in normal subjects and in chronic pancreatitis. *Digestion* 14: 97-107.
40. Gullo, L., Priori, P., Daniele, C., Ventrucci, M., Gasbarrini, G., Labo, G. 1983. Exocrine pancreatic function in the elderly. *Gerontology* 29:407-411.
41. Gullo, L., Ventrucci, M., Naldoni, P., Pezzilli, R. 1986. Aging and exocrine pancreatic function. *J. Am. Geriatr. Soc.* 34:790-792.

42. Haglund, U., Jodal, M. Lundgren, O. 1973. An autoradiographic study of the intestinal absorption of palmitic and oleic acid. *Acta Physiol. Scand.* 89:306-317.

43. Hardin, J.A., Buret, A., Meddings, M.B. Gall, D.G. 1993. Effect of epidermal growth factor on enterocyte brush-border surface area. *Am. J. Physiol.* 264:G312-G318.

44. Hollander, D., Dadufalza V.D. 1983a. Aging: its influence on the intestinal unstirred water layer thickness, surface area and resistance in the unanaesthetized rat. *Can. J. Physiol. Pharmacol.* 61:1501-1508.

45. Hollander, D., Dadufalza, V.D. 1983b. Intestinal exsorption of oleic acid: influence of aging, bile, pH and ethanol. *J. Nutr.* 113:511-518.

46. Hollander, D., Morgan, D. 1979. Increase in cholesterol absorption with aging in the rat. *Exp. Gerontol.* 14:201-204.

47. Hollander, D., Tarnawski, H. 1984. Influence of aging on vitamin D absorption and unstirred water layer dimensions in the rat. *J. Lab. Clin. Med.* 103:462-469.

48. Hollander, D., Dadufalza, V.D., Sletten, E.G. 1984. Does essential fatty acid absorption change with aging? *J. Lipid Res.* 25:129-134.

49. Holt, D., 1981. Intestinal absorption of triglyceride and vitamin D3 in aged and young rats. *Dig. Dis. Sci.* 26:1109-1115.

50. Holt, P.R., Balint, J.A. 1993. Effects of aging on intestinal lipid absorption. *Am. J. Physiol.* 264: G1-G6.

51. Holt, P.R., Yeh, K.Y. 1989. Small intestinal crypt cell proliferation rates are increased in senescent rats. *J. Gerontol.* 44:B9-B14.

52. Holt, P.R., Pascal, R.R., Kotler, D.P. 1984. Effect of aging upon small intestinal structure in the Fischer rat. *J. Gerontol.* 39:642-647.

53. Holt, P.R., Yeh, K.Y., Kotler, D.P. 1988. Altered controls of proliferation in proximal small intestine of the senescent rat. *Proc. Natl. Acad. Sci. USA* 85:2771-2775.

54. Hosoda, S. 1992. The gastrointestinal tract and nutrition in the aging process: an overview. *Nutr. Rev.* 50:372-373.

55. Hosoda, S. Bamba, T., Nishino, H., Nakagawa, M., Nakajo, S. 1976. Mechanisms and malabsorption of fat. *Proceeding of 5th Asian-Pacific Congress of Gastroenterology* 594-597.

56. Hosoda, S., Bamba, T., Nakago, S., Fujiyama, Y., Senda, S., Hirata, M. 1992. Age-related changes in gastrointestinal tract. *Nutr. Rev.* 50:374-377.

57. Imahori, K. 1992. How I undestand aging. *Nutr. Rev.* 50:351-352.

58. Innis, S.M., Clandinin. M.T. 1981. Dynamic modulation of mitochondrial inner-membrane lipids in rat heart by dietary fat. *Biochem. J.* 193:155-167.

59. Inukai, K., Asano, T., Katagiri, H., Ishihara, H., Anai, M., Fukushima, Y., Tsukuda, K., Kikuchi, M., Yazaki, Y., Oka, Y. 1993. Cloning and increased expression with fructose feeding of rat jejunal GLUT5. *Endocrinology* 133:2009-2014.

60. Iseki, S., Kondo, H. 1990a. An immunocytochemical study on the occurrence of liver fatty acid-binding protein in the digestive organs of rats: specific localization in the D cells and brush cells. *Acta Anat.* 138:15-23.

61. Iseki, S., Kondo, H. 1990b. Light microscopic localization of hepatic fatty acid binding protein mRNA in jejunal epithelia of rats using *in situ* hybridization, immunohistochemical and autoradiographic techniques. *J. Histochem. Cytochem.* 38:111-115.

62. Iseki, S., Kondo, H., Hitomi, M., Ono, T. 1990. Localization of liver fatty acid-binding protein and its mRNA in the liver and jejunum of rats: an immunohistochemical and *in situ* hybridization study. *Mol. Cell. Biochem.* 98:27-33.

63. Jarocka-Cyrta, E., Perin, N., Keelan, M., Wierzbicki, E., Wierzbicki, A., Clandinin, M.T., Thomson, A.B.R. 1998. Early dietary experience influences ontogeny of intestine in response to dietary lipid changes in later life. *Am. J. Physiol.* 275:G250-G258.

64. Johnston, L.R., McCormack, S.A. 1994. Regulation of gastrointestinal mucosal growth. In: *Physiology of the Gastrointestinal Tract.* 3rd ed. Edited by: L.R. Johnson, Raven Press, New York, pp. 611-641.

65. Jump, D.B., Clarke, S.D., Thelen, A., Liimatta, M. 1994. Coordinate regulation of glycolytic and lipogenic gene expression by polyunsaturated fatty acids. *J. Lipid Res.* 35:1076-1084.

66. Jump, D.B., Ren, B., Clarke, S., Thelen, A. 1995. Effects of fatty acids on hepatic gene expression. *Prostaglandins Leukotrienes Essential Fatty Acids* 52:107-111.

67. Kaikaus, R.M. Bass, N.M., Ockner R.K. 1990. Functions of fatty acid binding proteins. *Experentia* 46:617-630.
68. Kaikaus, R.M., Chan, W.K., Ortiz de Montellano, P.R., Gass, N.M. 1993a. Mechanisms of regulation of liver fatty acid-binding protein. *Mol. Cell. Biochem.* 123:93-100.
69. Kaikaus, R.M., Sui, Z., Lysendo, N., Wu, N.Y., Oritz de Montellano, P.R., Ockner, R.K., Bass, N.M. 1993b. Regulation of pathways of extramitochondrial fatty acid osication and liver fatty acid-binding protein by long-chain monocarboxylic fatty acids in hepatocytes. *J. Biol. Chem.* 268:26866-26871.
70. Kanda, T., Foucand, L., Nakamura, Y., et al. 1998. Regulation of human intestinal bile acid-binding protein in Caco-2 cells. *Biochem J.* 330:261-265.
71. Kapadia, S., Baker, S.J. 1976. The effects of alterations in villus shape on the intestinal mucosal surface of the albino rat: the relationship between mucosal surface and the crypts. *Digestion* 14:256-268.
72. Karasov, W.H., Diamond, J.M. 1983. Adaptive regulation of sugar and amino acid transport by vertebrate intestine. *Am. J. Physiol.* 245:G443-G462.
73. Karasov, W.H., Solberg, D.H., Chang, S.D., Stein, E.D., Highes, M., Diamond, J.M. 1985. Is intestinal transport of sugars and amino acids subject to critical-period programming? *Am. J. Physiol.* 249:G772-G785.
74. Kardassis, D., Hadzopoulou-Cladaras, M., Ramji, D.P., Cortese, R., Zannis, V.I., Cladaras, C. 1990a. Characterization of the promoter elements required for hepatic and intestinal transcription of the human apoB gene: definition of the DNA-binding site of a tissue specific transcriptional factors. *Mol Cell. Biol.* 10:2653-2659.
75. Kardassis, D., Zannis, V.I., Cladaras, C. 1990b. Purification and characterization of the nuclear factor BA1. A transcriptional activator of the human apoB gene. *J. Biol. Chem.* 265:21733-21740.
76. Kardassis, D., Zannis, V.I., Cladaras, C. 1992. Organization of the regulatory elements and nuclear activities participating in the transcription of the human apolipoprotein B gene. *J. Biol. Chem.* 267:2622-2632.
77. Keelan, M., Walker, K., Thomson, A.B.R. 1985. Intestinal brush border membrane marker enzymes, lipid composition and villus morphology: effect of fasting and diabetes mellitus in rats. *Comp. Biochem. Physiol.* 82A:83-89.
78. Keelan, M., Walker, K., Rajotte, R., Clandinin, M.T., Thomson, A.B.R. 1987. Diets alter jejunal morphology and brush border membrane composition in streptozotocin diabetic rats. *Can. J. Physiol. Pharmacol.* 65:210-218.
79. Keelan, M., Wierzbicki, A.A., Clandinin, M.T., Walker, K., Rajotte, R.V., Thomson, A.B.R. 1990a. Alterations in dietary fatty acid composition alter rat brush border membrane phospholipid fatty acid composition. *Diabetes Res.* 14:165-170.
80. Keelan, M., Thomson, A.B.R., Garg, M.L., Clandinin, M.T. 1990b. Critical period programming of intestinal glucose transport via alterations in dietary fatty acid composition. *Can. J. Physiol. Pharamacol.* 68:642-645.
81. Khalil, T., Fujimura, M., Townsend Jr., C.M., Greeley Jr., G.H., Thompson, J.C. 1984. Different secretagogue responses from pancreatic acini isolated from young and old rats. *Dig. Dis. Sci.* 29:954.
82. Khalil, T., Fujimura, M., Townsend Jr., C.M., Greeley Jr., G.H., Thompson, J.C. 1985. Effect of aging on pancreatic secretion in rats. *Am. J. Surg.* 149:120-125.
83. Kramer, W., Corsiero, D., Friedrich, M., et al. 1998. Intestinal absorption of bile acids: paradoxical behavior of the 14 kDa ileal lipid–binding protein in differential photoaffinity labelling. *Biochem. J.* 333:335-341.
84. Kumar, N.S., Mansback S.M. 1997. Determinants of triacylglycerol transport from the endoplasmic reticulum to the Golgi in intestine. *Am. J. Physiol.* 273:G18-G30.
85. Lenher, R., Kuksis, A. 1995. Triacylglycerol synthesis by purified triacylglycerol synthetase of rat intestinal mucosa. *J. Biol Chem.* 270:13630-13636.
86. Levitt, M.D., Fine, C., Furne, J.K., Levitt, D.G. 1996. Use of maltose hydrolysis measurements to characterize the interaction between the aqueous diffusion barrier and the epithelium in the rat jejunum. *J. Clin. Invest.* 97:2308-2315.
87. Levy, E., Mehran, M., Seidman, E. 1995. CaCo-2 cells as a model for intestinal lipoprotein synthesis and secretion. *FASEB J.* 9:626-635.

88. Lin, M.C., Dramer, W., Wilson, F.A. 1990. Identification of cytosolic and microsomal bile acid-binding proteins in rat ileal enterocytes. *J. Biol. Chem.* 265:14986-14995.

89. Lowe, J.B., Sacchettini, J.C., Laposata, M., McQuillan, J.J., Gordon, J.I. 1987. Purification and comparison of ligand binding characteristics with that of *Escherichia coli*-derived rat liver fatty acid-binding protein. *J. Biol. Chem.* 262:5931-5937.

90. Matsueda, K., Muraaka, A., Umeda, N., Misaki, N., Uchida, M., Kawano, B. 1989. *In vitro* measurement of the pH gradient and thickness of the duodenal mucus gel layer in rats. *Scand. J. Gastroenterol.* 162:31-34.

91. Mayer, R.M., Treadwell, C.R., Gallo, L.L., Vahouny, V.G. 1985. Intestinal mucins and cholesterol uptake in vitro. *Biochim. Biophys. Acta* 833:34-43.

92. Mazur, A. Felgines, C. Nassir, F., Bayle, D., Geux, E., Remesy, C., Rassiguier, Y., Cardot, P. 1991. Apolipoprotein B gene expresssion in rat intestine. The effect of dietary fiber. *FEBS Lett.* 284:63-65.

93. McGrane, M.M., Hanson, R.W. 1992. From diet to DNA: dietary patterning of gene expression. *Nutr. Clin. Prac.* 7:16-21.

94. Meddings, J. 1988. Lipid permeability of rat jejunum and ileum: correlatino with physical properites of the microvillus membrane. *Biochim. Biophys. Acta* 943:305-314.

95. Meddings, J. 1990. Membrane function: its relationship to intestinal absorption and malabsorption. *Can. J. Gastroenterol.* 4:39-46.

96. Meddings, J., Thiessen, S. 1989. Development of rat jejunum: lipid permeability, physical properties, and chemical composition. *Am. J. Physiol.* 256:G931-G940.

97. Meddings, J.B., DeSouza, D., Goel, M., Thiesen, S. 1990. Glucose transport and microvillus membrane physical properties along the crypt-villus axis of the rabbit. *J. Clin. Invest.* 85:1099-1107.

98. Meshkinpour, H., Smith, M., Hollander, D. 1981. Influence of aging on the surface area of the small intestine in the rat. *Exp. Gerontol.* 16:399-404.

99. Minami, H., Kim, J.R., Tada, K., Takahashi, F., Miyamoto, K.K., Nakabour, Y., Sakai, K., Hagihira, H. 1993. *Gastroenterology* 105:692-697.

100. Miyasaka, K., Kitani, K. 1987. Aging and pancreatic exocrine function. Studies in conscious male rats. *Pancreas* 2:523-530.

101. Miyasaka, K., Kitani, K. 1989. Aging and pancreatic exocrine function. Studies in female conscious rats. *Dib. Dis. Sci.* 34:841-848.

102. Miyasaka, K., Nakamura, R., Kitani, K. 1989. Effects of trypsin inhibitor (camostate) on pancreas and CCK release in young and old female rats. *J. Gerontol.* 44:136-140.

103. Montgomery, R.D., Haeney, M.R., Ross, I.N., Sammons, H.G., Barford, A.V., Balakrishnan, S., Mayer, P.P., Culank, L.S., Field, J., Gosling, P. 1978. The aging gut: a study of intestinal absorption in relation to nutrition in the elderly. *Am. J. Med.* 47:197-224.

104. Nakajo, S. 1979. Effect of aging on fat absorption in clinical and experimental studies. *J. Gastroenterol.* 76:1104-1105.

105. Neelands, P., Clandinin, M.T. 1983. Diet fat influence liver plasma membrane lipid composition and glucagon-stimulated adenylate cyclase activity. *Biochem. J.* 212:573-583.

106. Niot, I., Poirier, H., Besnard, P. 1997. Regulation of gene expression by fatty acid: special reference to fatty acid binding protein (FABP). *Biochimie* 79:129-133.

107. Ockner, R.K. 1990. Historic overview of studies on fatty acid-binding proteins. *Mol. Cell Biochem.* 98:3-9.

108. Omodeo-Sale, F., Lindi, C., Marciani, P., Cavatorta, P., Sartor, G., Masotti, L., Esposito, G. 1991. Postnatal maturation of rat intestinal membranes: lipid composition and fluidity. *Comp. Biochem. Physiol.* 100:301-307.

109. Pearse, B.M.R. 1978. On the structural and functional components of coated vesicles. *J. Mol. Biol.* 126:803-812.

110. Peeters, R.A., Veerkamp, J.H. 1989. Does fatty acid-binding protein play a role in fatty acid transport? *Mol. Cell Biochem.* 88:45-49.

111. Pelot, D., LoRusso, J.V., Hollander, D. 1987. The influence of aging on basal and secretin stimulated pancreatic exocrine secretion of the unanaesthetized rat. *Age* 10:1-4.

112. Pelz, K.S., Gottfried, S.P., Soos, E. 1968. Intestinal absorption studies in the aged. *Geriatrics* 23:149-153.

113. Penzes, L., Skala, I. 1977. Changes in the mucosal surface area of the small gut of rats of different ages. *J. Anat.* 124:217-222.

114. Perin, N., Keelan, M., Jarocka-Cyrta, E., Clandinin, M.T., Thomson, A.B.R. 1997. Ontogeny of intestinal adaptation in rats in response to isocaloric changes in dietary lipids. *Am. J. Physiol.* 273:G713-G720.

115. Perkins, W.R., Cafiso, D.S. 1987. Procedure using voltage-sensitive spin-labels to monitor dipole potential changes in phospholipid vesicles: the estimation of phloretin-induced conductance changes in vesicles. *J. Membrane Biol.* 96:165-173.

116. Poirier, H., Degrace, P., Niot, I et al., 1996. Localization and regulation of the putative membrane fatty acid transporter (FAT) in small intestine compared with fatty acid binding protein (FABP). *Eur. J. Biochem.* 238:368-373.

117. Poirier, H., Mathieu, Y., Besnard, P., Bernard, A. 1997. Intestinal lipid esterification and aging in mice and rats. *Comp. Biochem. Physiol.* 116:253-60.

118. Poston, G.J., Singh, P., Draviam, D.J., Upp, J.R., Thompson, J.C. 1988a. Development and age-related changes in pancreatic cholecystokinin receptors and duodenal cholecystokinin, in guinea pigs. *Mech. Aging Dev.* 46:59-66.

119. Poston, G.J., Singh, P., MacLellan, D.G., Yao, C.Z., Uchida, T., Townsend Jr., C.M., Thompson, J.C. 1988b. Age-related changes in gallbladder contractibility and gallbladder cholecystokinin receptor population in the guinea pig. *Mech. Aging Dev.* 46:

120. Proulx, P., Aubry, H.J., Brglez, I., Williamson, D.G. 1984. Studies on the uptake of fatty acids by brush border membranes of the rabbit intestine. *Can. J. Biochem.* 63:249-256.

121. Read, N.W., Barber, D.C., Levin, F.J., Holdsworth, C.D. 1977. Unstirred layer and kinetics of electrogenic glucose absorption in the human jejunum in situ. *Gut* 18:865-876.

122. Sanders, B.G., Kline, K. 1995. Nutrition, immunology, and cancer: an overview. *Adv. Exp. Med. Biol.* 369:185-194.

123. Schachter, D. 1984. Fluidity and function of hepatocyte plasma membranes. *Hepatology* 4:140-151.

124. Schachter, D., Shinitzky, M. 1977. Fluorescence polarization studies of rat intestinal microvillus membranes. *J. Clin. Invest.* 59:536-548.

125. Schneider, B.L., Dawson, P.A., Christie, D.M., Hardikar, W., Wong M.H., Suchy F.J. 1995. Cloning and molecular characterization of the ontogeny of a rat ileal sodium-dependent bile acid transporter. *J. Clin. Invest.* 95:745-754.

126. Schuber, F. 1989. Influence of polyamines on membrane functions. *Biochem. J.* 260:1-10.

127. Scott, J., Wallis, S.C., Davies, M.S., Wynne, J.K., Powell, L.M., Driscoll, D.M. 1989. RNA editing: a novel mechanism for regulating lipid transport from the intestine. *Gut* 30:35-43.

128. Seidel, E.R., Haddox, J.K., Johnson, L.R. 1985. Ileal mucosal growth during intraluminal infusion of ethylamine or putrescine. *Am. J. Physiol.* 249:G434-438.

129. Shepherd, J. 1994. Lipoprotein metabolism: an overview. *Drugs* 47:1-10.

130. Shiau, Y.-F. 1987. Lipid digestion and absorption. In: *Physiology of the Gastrointestinal Tract.* 2nd. ed. Edited by: L.R. Johnson. Raven Press, New York, pp.1527-1556.

131. Shiau, Y.-F. 1990. Mechanism of intestinal fatty acid uptake in the rat: the role of an acidic microclimate. *J. Physiol.* 421:463-474.

132. Shiau, Y.-F., Levine, G.M. 1980. pH dependence of micellar diffusion and dissociation. *Am. J. Physiol.* 239:G177-G182.

133. Shiau, Y.-F., Fernandez, P., Jackson, M.J., McMonagle, S. 1985. Mechanisms maintaining a low pH microclimate in the intestine. *Am. J. Physiol.* 248:G608-G619.

134. Shirazi-Beechey, S.P., Hirayama, B.A., Wang, Y., Scott, D., Smith, M.W., Wright, E.M. 1991. Ontogenic development of lamb intestinal sodium-glucose co-transporter is regulated by diet. *J. Physiol.* 437:669-708.

135. Simko, V., Michael, S. 1989. Absorptive capacity for dietary fat in elderly patients with debilitating disorders. *Arch. Int. Med.* 149:557-560.

136. Small, D.M., Cabral, D.J., Cistola, D.P., Parks, J.S., Hamilton, J.A. 1984. The ionization behavior of fatty acids and bile acids in micelles and membranes. *Hepatology* 4:77s-79s.

137. Sonoyama, K., Nihikawa, H., Kiriyama, S., Niki, R. 1995. Apolipoprotein mRNA in liver and intestine of rats is affected by beef fiber or cholestyramine. *J. Nutr.* 125:13-19.

138. Srivastava, R.A., Tang, J., Krul, E.S., Pfleger, B., Kitchens, R.T., Schofeld, G. 1992. Dietary fat and dietary cholesterol differ in their effect on the *in vivo* regulation of apolipoprotein A-I and A-II gene expression in inbred strains of mice. *Biochim. Biophys. Acta* 1125:251-261.

139. Stremmel, W. 1988. Uptake of fatty acids by jejunal mucosal cells is mediated by a fatty acid binding membrane protein. *J. Clin. Invest.* 82:2001-2010.

140. Stubbs, C.D., Smith, A.D. 1984. The modification of mammalian membrane polyunsaturated fatty acid composition in relation to membrane fluidity and function. *Biochim. Biophys. Acta* 779:89-137.

141. Sweetser, D.A., Lowe, J.B., Gordon, J.L. 1986. The nucleotide sequence of the rat liver fatty acid-binding protein gene. Evidence that exon 1 encodes an oligopeptide domain shared by a family of proteins which bind hydrophobic ligands. *J. Biol. Chem.* 261:5553-5561.

142. Sweetser, D.A., Birkenmeier, E.H., Klisak, I.J., Zollman, S., Sparkes, R.S., Mohandas, T., Lussis, A.J., Gordon, J.I. 1987. The human and rodent intestinal fatty acid binding protein genes. A comparative analysis of their structure expression and linkage relationships. *Biol. Chem.* 262:16060-16071.

143. Sweetser, D.A., Birkenmeier, E.H., Hoppe, P.C., McKeel, D.W., Gordon, J.I. 1988a. Mechanisms underlying generation of gradients in gene expression within the intestine: an analysis using transgenic mice containing fatty acid binding protein-human growth hormone fusion. *Genes. Dev.* 2:1318-1332.

144. Sweetser, D.A., Hauft, S.M., Hoppe, P.C., Birdenmeier, E.H., Gordon, G.I. 1988b. Transgenic mice containing intestinal fatty acid-binding protein-human growth hormone fusion genes exhibit correct regional and cell-specific expression of the reporter gene in their small intestine. *Proc. Natl. Acad. Sci. USA* 85:9611-9615.

145. Swift, L.L., Soule, P.D., Gray, M.E., LeQuire, V.S. 1984. Intestinal lipoprotein synthesis. Comparison of nascent Golgi lipoproteins from chow-fed and hypercholesterolemic rats. *J. Lipid Res.* 25:1-13.

146. Teng, B., Black, D.D., Davidson, N.O. 1990. Apolipoprotein B. Messenger RNA editing is developmentally regulated in pig small intestine: nucleotide comparison of apolipoprotein B editing regions in five species. *Biochem. Biophys. Res. Commun.* 173:74-80.

147. Thomson, A.B.R. 1979a. Limitations of Michaelis-Mentoen kinetics in the presence of intestinal unstirred layers. *Am. J. Physiol.* 236:E701-E709.

148. Thomson, A.B.R. 1979b. Unstirred water layer and age-dependent changes in rabbit jejunal D-glucose transport. *Am. J. Physiol.* 236:E685-E691.

149. Thomson, A.B.R. 1980. Effect of age on uptake of homologous series of saturated fatty acids into rabbit jejunum. *Am. J. Physiol.* 239:G363-G371.

150. Thomson, A.B.R. 1981. Aging and cholesterol uptake in the rabbit jejunum. Role of the bile salt micelle and the unstirred water layer. *Dig. Dis. Sci.* 26:890-896.

151. Thomson, A.B.R., Dietschy, J.M. 1977. Derivation of the equations that describe the effects of unstirred water layers on the kinetic parameters of active transport processes in the intestine. *J. Theor. Biol.* 64:277-294.

152. Thomson, A.B.R., Keelan, M. 1986. Effect of oral nutrition on the form and function of the intestinal tract. *Surv. Dig. Dis.* 3:75-94.

153. Thomson, A.B.R., Keelan, M., Clandinin, M.T., Walker, K. 1986. Dietary fat selectively alters transport properties of rat jejunum. *J. Clin. Invest.* 77:279-288.

154. Thomson, A.B.R., Keelan, M., Clandinin, M.T., Walker, K. 1987a. A high linoleic acid diet diminishes enhances intestinal uptake of sugars in diabetics rats. *Am. J. Physiol.* 252:G262-G271.

155. Thomson, A.B.R., Keelan, M., Clandinin, M.T., Rajotte, R.V., Cheeseman, C.I., Walker, K. 1987b. Treatment of enhanced intestinal uptake of glucose in diabetic rats with a polyunsaturated fatty acid diet. *Biochim. Biophys. Acta* 905:426-434.

156. Thomson, A.B.R., Keelan, M., Garg, M.L. Clandinin, M.T. 1987c. Spectrum of effects of dietary long-chain fatty acids on rat intestinal glucose and lipid uptake. *Can. J. Physiol. Pharmacol.* 65:2459-2465.

157. Thomson, A.B.R., Keelan, M., Clandinin, M.T., Rajotte, R.V., Cheeseman, C.I., Walker, K. 1988a. Use of polyunsaturated fatty acid to treat the enhanced intestinal uptake of lipids in streptozotocin diabetic rats. *Clin. Invest. Med.* 11:57-61.

158. Thomson, A.B.R., Keelan, M., Garg, M.L., Clandinin, M.T. 1988b. Dietary effects of ω3 fatty acids on intestinal transport function. *Can. J. Physiol. Pharmacol.* 66:985-992.

159. Thomson, A.B.R., Keelan, M., Garg, M.L. Clandinin, M.T. 1989a. Intestinal aspects of lipid absorption: in review. *Can. J. Physiol. Pharmacol.* 67:179-191.

160. Thomson, A.B.R., Keelan, M., Garg, M.L. Clandinin, M.T. 1989b. Evidence for critical period programming of intestinal transport function. *Biochim. Biophys. Acta* 1001:302-315.

161. Thomson, A.B.R., Keelan, M., Sigalet, D., Fedorak, R., Garg, M., Clandinin, M.T. 1990. Patterns, mechanisms and signals for intestinal adaptation. *Dig. Dis.* 8:99-111.

162. Thomson, A.B.R., Schoeller, C., Keelan, M., Smith, L., Clandinin, M.T. 1993. Lipid absorption: passing through the unstirred layers, brush border membrane, and beyond. *Can. J. Physiol Pharmacol.* 71:531-555.

163. Thomson, A.B.R., Cheeseman, C.I., Keelan, M., Fedorak, R.N., Clandinin, M.T. 1994. Crypt cell production rate, enterocyte turnover time and appearance of transport along the jejunal villus of the rat. *Biochim. Biophys. Acta* 1191:197-204.

164. Thumelin, S., Forestier, M., Girard, J., Pegorier, J.P. 1993. Developmental changes in mitochondrial 3-hydroxymethyl glutaryl Coenzyme A synthetase gene expression in rat liver, intestine and kidney. *Biochem. J.* 292:493-496.

165. Thurnhofer, H., Hauser, H. 1990a. The uptake of phosphatidylcholine by small intestinal brush border membrane is protein-mediated. *Biochim. Biophys. Acta* 1024:249-262.

166. Thurnhofer, H., Hauser, H. 1990b. Uptake of cholesterol by small intestinal brush border membrane is protein-mediated. *Biochemistry* 29:2142-2148.

167. Tso, P. 1994. Intestinal lipid absorption. In: *Physiology of the Gastrointestinal Tract.* Edited by: L.R. Johnson. Raven Press, New York, pp. 1867-1907.

168. Tso, P., Fujimoto, K. 1991. The absorption and transport of lipids by the small intestine. *Brain Res. Bulletin* 27:477-482.

169. Uchida, K., Nomura, Y., Kadowaki, M., Takase, H., Takano, K., Takeuchi, N. 1978. Age-related changes in cholesterol and bile acid metabolism in rats. *J. Lipid Res.* 19:544-552.

170. Valdivieso, V., Palma, R., Wunkhaus, R., Antezana, C., Severin, C., Contreras, A. 1978. Effect of aging on biliary lipid composition and bile acid metabolism in normal Chilean women. *Gastroenterology* 74:871-874.

171. Vance, J.E., Vance, D.E. 1990. The assembly of lipids into lipoproteins during secretion. *Experientia* 46:560-569.

172. Van der Werf, S.D.J., Huijbregts, A.W.M., Lamers, H.L.M., van Berge Henegowen, G.P., van Tongeren, J.H.M. 1981. Age dependent differences in human bile aid metabolism and 7-alpha-dehydroxylation. *Eur. J. Clin. Invest.* 11:425-431.

173. Vellas, B., Balas, D., Moreau, J., Bouisson, M., Senegas-Balas, F., Guidet, M., Ribet, A. 1988. Exocrine pancreatic secretion in the elderly. *Int. J. Pancreatol.* 3:497-502.

174. Waeber, G., Thompson, N., Haefliger, J.A., Nicod, P. 1994. Characterization of the murine high Km glucose transporter GLUT2 gene and its transcriptional regulation by glucose in a differentiated insulin-secreting cell line. *J. Biol. Chem.* 269:26912-26919.

175. Wang, J.Y., Johnson, L.R. 1992. Luminal polyamines substitute for tissue polyamines in duodenal mucosal repair after stress in rats. *Gastroenterology* 102:1109-1117.

176. Webster, S.G.P., Wilkinson, E.M., Gowland, E. 1977. A comparison of fat absorption in young and old subjects. *Age Ageing* 6:113-117.

177. Weiner, R. Dietze, F., Laue, R. 1984. Age-dependent alterations of intestinal absorption. II. A clinical study using a modified D-xylose absorption test. *Arch. Gerontol. Geriatr.* 3:97-108.

178. Westergaard, H., Dietschy, J.M. 1974. Delineation of the dimensions and permeability characteristics of the two major diffusion barriers to passive mucosal uptake in the rabbit intestine. *J. Clin. Invest.* 54:718-732.

179. Wetterau, J., Aggerbeck, L.P., Bouma, M.-E., Eisenberg, C., Munck, A., Hermier, M., Schmitz, J., Gay, G., Rader, D.J., Gregg, R.E. 1992. Absence of microsomal triglyceride transfer protein in individuals with abetalipoproteinemia. *Science* 258: 999-1001.

180. Wilson, F.A., Dietschy, J.M. 1975. The intestinal unstirred layer: its surface and effect on active transport kinetics. *Biochim. Biophys. Acta* 363:112-126.

181. Wilson, F.A., Sallee, V.L., Dietschy, J.M. 1971. Unstirred water layer in the intestine: rate determinant for fatty acid absorption from micellar solutions. *Science* 174:1031-1033.

182. Winne, D. 1976. Unstirred layer thickness in perfused rat jejunum *in vivo. Experientia* 32:1278-1279.

183. Wong, M.H., Oelkers, P., Craddock, A.L., Dawson, P.A. 1994. Expression cloning and characterization of the hamster ileal sodium-dependent transporter. *J. Biol. Chem.* 269:1340-1347.

184. Wong, M.H., Oelkers, P., Dawson, P.A. 1995. Identification of a mutation in the ileal sodium-dependent bile acid transporter gene that abolishes transport activity. *J. Biol. Chem.* 270:27228-27234.
185. Yuasa, H., Kawanishi, K., Watanabe, J. 1995. Effects of aging on the oral absorption of D-xylose in rats. *J. Pharm Pharmacol.* 47:373-378.
186. Zannis, V.I., Kardassis, D., Cardot, P.I., Hadzopoulou-Cladaras, M., Zanni, E.E., Cladaras, C. 1992. Molecular biology of the human apolipoprotein genes: gene regulation and structure/function relationship. *Curr. Opin. Lipidol.* 3:96-113.

Section IV

Nutritional Therapies and Promotion of Health

19 Nutrition and the Geriatric Surgery Patient

Sheldon Winkler, Meredith C. Bogert, and Charles K. Herman

CONTENTS

I.   INTRODUCTION

The geriatric patient who requires surgical treatment presents a number of problems not encountered in younger patients, the majority of which are the result of the changes that occur with aging or with poor nutrition. Surgical morbidity, postoperative healing, and the patient's return to function may be improved through the application of knowledge of the physical, metabolic, and endocrine changes associated with aging, as well as of the nutritional deficiencies common among this cohort of patients (1).

II.   EFFECTS OF SURGERY ON THE BODY

Any stress, including that from a surgical procedure, causes a dramatic release of ACTH from the anterior pituitary which, in turn, directs the release of cortisol from the adrenal cortex. The circulating cortisol level remains elevated by a factor of 2 to 5 times normal for about 24 hours after the procedure (2), and acts upon skeletal tissue to bring about breakdown of skeletal muscle tissue proteins into amino acids for localized wound healing and for glucose production by the liver.

Concomitantly, epinephrine and norepinephrine are released and remain elevated for up to 48 hours, stimulating breakdown of liver glycogen with the release of glucose for cellular energy needs during the immediate postoperative period (3). The increase in epinephrine suppresses release of insulin (4), glucagon concentrations rise (5), and the liver is stimulated to begin gluconeogenesis to return to preoperative levels and to support the energy requirements of the healing process.

Additional reactions to surgery include alterations in water regulation mediated by release of antidiuretic hormone and aldosterone, which increases water reabsorption in the renal collecting ducts and increases sodium retention in the renal tubules, respectively (6,7). It is believed that the release of these hormones is stimulated by signals from blood-pressure- and osmolarity-sensitive receptors (3). This diminished ability to excrete water in the early postoperative period results in temporary weight gain and a return to normal blood volume (8).

After the above events, the patient enters a metabolic transition period of 1 or 2 days in which the body begins to turn from corticosteroid and epinephrine-initiated breakdown to rebuilding and healing. During this time, shedding of the retained water is effected, while conserving nitrogen and potassium. The slow process of healing and regaining weight can now begin, and is marked by protein synthesis, wound healing, buildup of muscle tissue, and increasing strength (3).

All of these processes occur with a fair degree of predictability in the adequately nourished adult patient. The process is imperiled, as is the prognosis for full recovery, if the adult is elderly and/or malnourished.

III.   GENERAL NUTRITIONAL NEEDS OF THE ELDERLY

A.   PROTEIN

Muscle accounts for 45% of body weight in young adults. This drops to 27% in the very old, who clinically show a marked decrease in the size and strength of all skeletal muscle (9). In the elderly, protein depletion of body stores is seen primarily as a decrease of skeletal muscle mass. Muscle changes are conspicuous in the small muscles of the hands and face and in the muscles of mastication. Chronic dietary protein inadequacy may be involved in depressed immune function, decreasing muscle strength, and poor wound healing in older adults (10). Until recently, it was thought that adults over 50 years of age should ingest 0.8 g of protein per kilogram of weight daily (11), but recent guidelines have suggested from 1 to 1.25 g of high-quality protein per kilogram of weight daily (12).

The best sources of protein for the elderly diet are meat and fish. These foods should be boiled (poached or braised), not fried; boiling prepares meats and fish for the elderly gastrointestinal tract by breaking down the complex proteins into the more easily digested proteoses, whereas frying denatures and coagulates the proteins and makes them difficult to digest (9).

B.   CARBOHYDRATES

It is generally believed that carbohydrate absorption is somewhat impaired in the elderly, although decreased renal function may contribute to carbohydrate loss as well. The increase in lactose intolerance that can occur over time is due to a decrease in lactase activity in the gut lining, but may not be as severe as often believed. Ausman and Russell (13) reported a double-blind study of healthy elderly subjects who were divided into two groups: the first received lactose-containing products, the second received lactose-free products. Approximately 30% of both groups reported bloating and gastrointestinal discomfort, leading to the conclusion that "the true prevalence of lactose intolerance in the elderly is difficult to define."

Current dietary guidelines from the USDA (U.S. Department of Agriculture) (14) suggest that carbohydrates should compose about 60% of daily calories, and the complex carbohydrates (starches) are preferred over simple carbohydrates (sugars).

C. Fat

Generally, the elderly are able to digest and absorb fats in a diet containing 100 g of fat per day; at higher levels (120 g/day), there may be a slightly reduced ability to absorb fats (15). A rare problem with fat absorption can occur with a bacterial overgrowth in the small intestine that interferes with normal bile salt structure and function, but fat malabsorption was not found even in elderly hypochlorhydric individuals (16). The U.S. FDA (Food and Drug Administration) guidelines recommend a diet with less than 30% of its daily caloric intake in the form of fat. In addition, it advises that saturated fat intake be reduced to less than 10% of daily calories, and that cholesterol be limited to less than 300 mg daily (17). These recommendations are for all adults, with no differentiation for the elderly.

D. Water

Water, the most important nutrient in the diet, is essential to all body functions. Water loss must be balanced every day by an adequate intake from drinking water, beverages, soups, and other foods, especially vegetables. If this balance is not maintained, and if water loss exceeds intake, chronic dehydration results. Geriatric patients are particularly susceptible to negative water balance, often caused by excessive water loss through insufficient or damaged kidneys.

Mucosal surfaces become dry and easily irritated in the dehydrated patient. Insufficient fluid consumption in general (and water consumption in particular) can have a deleterious effect on salivary gland function and on overall health in the elderly. The average sedentary adult male must consume at least 2,900 ml of fluid daily, and the average sedentary adult female at least 2,200 ml per day, in the form of noncaffeine, nonalcoholic beverages, soups, and foods. Solid foods contribute approximately 1,000 ml of water, with an additional 250 ml derived from the water of oxidation (18).

E. Fiber

There is no definite requirement for dietary fiber in the daily diet of adults or the elderly. Different kinds of dietary fiber contribute to the motility of the gastrointestinal tract. In studies of different populations, a diet rich in fiber seems to be correlated with decreased rates of cancer and cardiac disease. An increase in dietary fiber is prescribed in the treatment of several diseases common in elderly persons, namely constipation, hemorrhoids, diverticulosis, hiatal hernia, varicose veins, diabetes mellitus, hyperlipidemia, and obesity (13,19). The current recommendation is 20 to 30 g/day, and the U.S. FDA requires that dietary fiber be listed on the nutrition facts panel on food labels (20).

IV. MALNUTRITION IN THE ELDERLY

Malnutrition is a common finding in elderly patients, especially when they are hospitalized. In those patients whose nutritional status is borderline, the stress of illness may bring about deficiencies, and failure to correct malnutrition delays recovery and prolongs the hospital stay (21). The elderly are a more diverse population than any other age group, with individuals having widely varying capabilities and levels of functioning (13); they are at particular risk for marginal deficiencies of vitamins and trace elements. Diagnosis of malnutrition must rely on several methods, for each elderly adult has his or her own energy and intake requirements that must be based upon health status, life situation (whether living independently or institutionalized), activity level, amount of lean muscle mass, and overall frame size. Those individuals who exist in a state of marginal nutritional health may have the balance tipped by illness or other form of stress. The early recognition of malnutrition is a challenge to healthcare providers and caregivers, and prevention of malnutrition can forestall disease development or exacerbation by bolstering immune competence (22).

A. FACTORS CONTRIBUTING TO MALNUTRITION IN THE ELDERLY

Balanced nutrition is a major component of the general well-being of individuals throughout their lives. A vicious cycle exists in that the aging process compromises the body's ability to obtain nutrients from food, and the quality of an individual's nutrition influences how he or she ages (23). Inadequate intake is only one of many causes of nutritional deficiency in the elderly (21).

1. Loss of Appetite and Diminished Taste and Smell

When asked why they don't eat, many elderly patients will say that food doesn't taste good or they are just not hungry. Diminished appetite has many causes (physical, psychological, and social) that can interact to interfere with the ability and/or desire to purchase, prepare, and/or eat food (24).

Depressed taste and smell contribute to loss of appetite. Forty percent of U.S. adults with chronic chemosensory problems (1.5 million persons) are 65 years of age or older (25). In addition to aging, a decline in taste and smell can be caused by medications (26), radiotherapy (27), dental conditions or prostheses, and disease. Those diseases that can affect the senses of taste and smell include nervous system disorders (particularly Alzheimer's and Parkinson's diseases), chronic renal problems, endocrine disorders (diabetes mellitus, hypothyroidism, Cushing's syndrome), local ENT ailments, and viral infections (28,29). Specific nutritional deficiencies (zinc and vitamins B3 and B12) and the nutritional problems relating to cancer can also be involved.

The dimming of taste can result from the degeneration and/or reduction in the total number of taste buds. It is now believed that every taste bud has some degree of sensitivity to all of the primary taste sensations, and that the brain detects the type of taste by the ratio of stimulation of the different taste buds (30). Taste buds normally reproduce themselves approximately every 10 days in a healthy adult; renewal is slowed in the elderly, especially in postmenopausal women suffering from estrogen deficiency. Shortages of protein or zinc also retard taste bud renewal (28).

Olfactory acuity declines with age. The number of olfactory nuclei in the brain decline, and the olfactory receptors in the roof of the nasal cavity regress. Older patients generally have greater difficulty in differentiating among food odors, but are best at discriminating fruits from other stimuli (31). Most studies suggest that the sense of smell is more impaired by aging than the sense of taste (28).

Appetite is also influenced by food palatability. As taste and smell are amalgamated in the determination of palatability and acceptance, the loss of flavor can make foods tasteless with a resultant decline in appetite. Thus, decreased gustatory and/or olfactory ability can have an adverse effect on diet and nutrition.

Psychological and social factors have a significant impact on appetite. Decreased appetite is one of the diagnostic criteria for depression. The prevalence of depression in the community-resident elderly population is estimated to be almost 20% (32). The symptoms of depression in the surgical patient must be differentiated from physical illness, as nearly 20% of older adults with depression present with physical complaints (33). In the elderly, social activities that involve food consumption may also be limited. Absence of these social cues may result in a decrease in appetite.

2. Edentulism

Both partial and complete edentulism, with a reduction in the number and occlusion of teeth, can impact negatively on the patient's ability to masticate food. Decreased masticatory efficiency can contribute to indigestion and a reduction in food intake.

3. Gastrointestinal Malfunction

The gastrointestinal tract of the elderly undergoes changes that contribute to a reduced ability to extract the full nutritional benefits from ingested foods. A reduction in gastric secretion of hydrochloric acid, intrinsic factor, and pepsin occurs in 20% of healthy adults over 60 years of age. The rate of gastric emptying of liquids increases with age, raising the pH in the ileum and negatively affecting the digestion of proteins and fats. If food is improperly digested, the constituent nutrients (proteins, vitamins, minerals, etc.) will not be available to be absorbed and utilized. In addition, a diminution of hepatic size and blood flow results in reduced ability to synthesize albumin and several other plasma proteins, and to metabolize certain medications (34).

4. Loss of Lean Body Mass

A loss of lean body mass accompanies the natural aging process, but the dramatically reduced level of physical activity seen in many of the elderly causes a marked reduction in muscle tissue. The weakness that accompanies this reduction in muscle volume and tone can contribute to difficulties in carrying out daily life activities, including mastication. The vicious cycle of declining energy (anergy), activity, muscle mass, and food intake impacts negatively on quality of life and on overall health and longevity.

B. Malnutrition in the Elderly Surgical Patient

As the geriatric population is projected to increase dramatically over the course of the next 20 years, an increasing number of elderly patients will require both elective and emergency surgery. The risk of malnutrition and subclinical deficiencies (35) of this age group can have a direct impact on postoperative healing ability. The importance of nutrition in the treatment of the elderly hospital patient has frequently been underestimated. The older patient is more likely to be admitted to a hospital with some degree of malnutrition and the metabolic response to surgery is likely to be more severe (36).

The development of in-patient malnutrition often begins long before hospital admission. It may be partially a result of the lengthy time period from onset of symptoms to first presentation at the doctor's office, through presentation at the referred surgeon's office, and finally to the hospital for the surgery. Bowling and Silk (37) conducted a study to assess this time period, and concluded that it could cause many patients to become malnourished prior to admission, which could have implications on the incidence of complications and the length of hospital stay.

V. NUTRITION AND WOUND HEALING

The role of nutrition in wound healing became more clearly defined with the development of intravenous feeding, known as total parenteral nutrition (TPN), in the 1960s. This major advance enabled physicians to provide the patient with a nutritionally complete diet, even if the patient could not eat. In addition, researchers were able to document the adverse effects of nutritional deficiencies on the success of surgical procedures, and how correction of nutritional deficits could alter the surgical/healing outcome for the better (38).

A. THE PROCESS OF WOUND HEALING

Several mechanisms are involved in wound healing, including inflammation, epithelialization, collagen synthesis, angiogenesis, collagen remodeling, and fibronectin-mediated wound contraction. This complex process occurs optimally when there is a sufficient supply of the raw materials — protein, carbohydrate, fat, vitamins, and minerals — that are needed to rebuild the damaged tissues. The lack of any of these important building blocks will adversely affect healing.

B. PROTEIN

Protein deficiency is a major factor in poor wound healing, primarily as a result of depression of fibroblast proliferation and, thus, of the syntheses of connective tissue ground substance (proteoglycans), collagen, new blood vessels, and remodeling of the healing site (39). For surgical patients, the recommended daily intake for protein rises to 2 to 4 g protein per kilogram of body weight per day (40). The essential amino acids are those that cannot be synthesized via transamination; they must be ingested in food. One of these, methionine, has been shown to accelerate the rate of fibroplasia by its conversion to cystine. The mechanism is unclear, but formation of protein-strengthening disulfide bonds in collagen protein synthesis and self-assembly are critical to the stability of this complex molecule, which is essential in scar formation and healing (38). Another essential amino acid, histidine, influences the tensile strength of wounds. Deficiency of histidine in experimental animals reduced the strength of wounds; addition of histidine to the diet restored wound strength to normal levels (41).

In protein deficiency, there is a protraction of the inflammatory phase of wound healing (42), in which proteolytic enzymes are secreted by macrophages and granulocytes, with a resulting 30 to 50% increase in proteolysis of the tissues around the wound site (43). Protein malnutrition is characterized by dry, flaking skin, and by peripheral edema (44), which can mask malnutrition by concealing the amount of muscle wasting that has occurred in the patient (45). In addition, the tissue edema can impair nutrient diffusion to the wound (46). Hair appears dull, lacking normal color, and demonstrates increased pluckability. Muscle cramping and wasting also can be seen (47).

C. CARBOHYDRATES AND FAT

The precise role of carbohydrates and fat in wound healing is less well known than that of proteins. Glucose is utilized as an energy source for cellular metabolism, including metabolism by those cells involved in wound healing. Leukocytes participate in phagocytosis and inflammatory activities, influencing growth factor release that stimulates the proliferation of fibroblasts needed for initial healing activities. Fats are essential components of cell membranes and are needed for synthesis of new cells. However, no known impairment of wound healing has been associated with a deficiency of essential fatty acids (48).

D. IRON AND TRACE MINERALS

Minerals play critical and interrelated roles in wound healing, especially in the processes involved in the synthesis of collagen. The enzymes essential to the synthetic process require cofactors to be present to catalyze the steps in the synthesis. These cofactors include magnesium (48), iron, manganese, copper, and calcium (40). Studies to date have not implicated nutritional deficiencies of manganese or copper in impairment of wound healing in patients with good oral intake, primarily because these elements are present in enough different foods that deficiency usually does not occur. A significant exception has been documented, however, in patients who received long-term TPN without additional supplementation of these minerals (49). Copper is important in erythropoesis and in collagen stability (39).

Severe iron deficiency anemia may reduce the bactericidal competence of leukocytes; this may be offset by a concomitant reduction in rate of bacterial growth (39). Iron is essential for the restoration of normal red blood cell numbers following blood loss from surgery. The serum level of transferrin, a protein used to transport iron, will be higher than normal in the iron-deficient patient, and its level of saturation with iron will be low. Iron is also used as a cofactor in the hydroxylation of proline in the collagen synthetic pathway. A deficiency of iron will decrease the structural integrity of collagen and, hence, decrease wound strength.

F. ZINC

In contrast to the trace minerals, a deficiency of zinc will have markedly adverse effects on wound healing by decreasing the rate of epithelialization, reducing the rate of increase in wound strength, and reducing collagen strength. Zinc has been found to be a cofactor of enzymes responsible for cellular proliferation and protein synthesis (DNA polymerase, RNA polymerase, reverse transcriptase, and ribosomes) (50). A deficiency would interfere with the cellular proliferation required in the wound healing process, including that of inflammatory cells, epithelial cells, and fibroblasts. In addition, zinc acts to stabilize cell membranes by inhibiting lipid peroxidases, and may play a role in the storage of vitamin A in the liver (39). Zinc deficiency also has a negative effect on the immune system by decreasing cellular and humoral immune function; the patient can become more susceptible to infections that may interfere with healing.

Experiments with high levels of zinc supplementation have been tried, in the unsuccessful attempt to accelerate the healing process. It is known that insufficient zinc impairs wound healing, and that a return to normal blood levels will result in a return to the normal rate of healing (51,52). Excessive zinc interferes with copper metabolism and with wound healing by affecting lysyl oxidase, the enzyme crucial to collagen cross-linking (39). The Recommended Daily Allowance for zinc is 15 mg for healthy adults.

Topical zinc oxide as a wound dressing has been found to enhance the re-epithelialization of partial-thickness wounds (53) and to decrease inflammation (54).

F. VITAMINS

Vitamins are essential cofactors in many functions of the body, including wound healing. vitamin C (ascorbic acid) is essential in the synthesis of collagen. vitamin C deficiency will produce a marked alteration in the healing process: without it, the primary sequence of amino acids in the collagen protein is improperly elaborated, the procollagen protein cannot be secreted from the fibroblast, and self-assembly of the collagen polymer cannot occur, as vitamin C is required for the hydroxylation of proline residues.

Consequences of vitamin C deficiency are incomplete wound healing and an increased risk for wound dehiscence (38). Scurvy is the clinical disease resulting from vitamin C deficiency, manifested as decreased integrity of bone, soft tissue, and small blood vessels. Since vitamin C is water-soluble, it is excreted renally and must be replenished frequently. The Recommended Daily Allowance for vitamin C is 60 mg per day. It has been suggested that adequate supplementation of vitamin C be given both pre- and post-operatively, in view of the possibility that surgical patients require more ascorbic acid than healthy persons (55).

Vitamin A can influence the course of patients who receive systemic steroids by reversing the impaired healing effect that steroids have on lysosomal membranes (56–58), and may be a cofactor in collagen synthesis and cross-linking (48). Vitamin A plays a role in cellular differentiation of epithelial cells; deficiency can lead to hyperkeratosis. Like zinc, it has been used as a topical agent to mitigate delayed epithelialization and closure of wounds. Deficiency of vitamin A also plays a role in the increase in the incidence of infections (59). Vitamin A appears to improve host defenses by enhancing cell-mediated immune function (60–64). It increases the number of antibody-producing cells, thus fostering antibody production, and can increase the phagocytic and tumoricidal ability of macrophages (65–68). In a well-nourished patient, vitamin A is stored in the liver in adequate amounts (since it is a fat-soluble vitamin). In a malnourished patient, 25,000 IU of supplemental vitamin A should be taken daily before and after elective surgery. If surgery will interfere with normal eating for a long period, or if the patient develops gastrointestinal complications postoperatively, vitamin A supplementation should be given to the well-nourished patient as well (39).

An excess of vitamin E will delay wound healing and will interfere with the beneficial effects of vitamin A. It is similar to steroids in the inhibition of collagen synthesis and wound healing (69,70). It has been tried as a topical agent for reduction of hypertrophic scar and keloid formation, but has not been found to be particularly effective.

Vitamin K is utilized in the synthesis of prothrombin and clotting factors, and plays a role in bone healing, where it is required for the synthesis of calcium-binding protein (71). Vitamin K deficiency results in excessive bleeding into the wound area during healing, and can predispose the area to the development of infection (39). Other vitamins that contribute on a minor scale by aiding cross-linking of collagen are riboflavin, pyridoxine, and thiamine (72).

VI. CLINICAL STUDIES OF NUTRITION AND WOUND HEALING

Biochemical understanding of the roles of nutrients in wound healing has been gained through the use of animal models. The measurement of wound healing usually requires direct sampling of the wound site by punch biopsy, or manipulation of the wound borders (by tugging at them until they begin to pull apart) to measure the tensile strength of the wound. Since neither of these procedures is possible in the postoperative patient, indirect measurements have been used.

Current nutritional assessment methods (measurements of stored fat, arm muscle circumference, serum albumin, serum prealbumin, transferrin, total plasma protein, and immune status) can only roughly estimate the nutritional status of a patient (38), but should be used conjunctively in an attempt to gauge the patient's preoperative condition. The serum level of albumin is often used as an indicator of an individual's protein intake and of the status of the visceral protein pool (40,42). In one study, it was found to be somewhat useful as a prognostic index for length of hospital stay following major surgery, when corrected for patient age (74). The normal concentration of serum albumin is 4.0 g/dl. A level of 3.5 to 3.9 g/dl indicates mild protein deficiency, 2.5 to 3.5 g/dl is moderately deficient, and less than 2.5 g/dl is considered to be severely protein deficient. However, the serum albumin concentration is not a specific indicator of malnutrition, as patients with hepatic disease and other chronic diseases prevalent in the elderly population commonly demonstrate low levels. Additionally, albumin has a relatively long half-life of 21 days and, therefore, is not reflective of short-term nutritional status. Prealbumin and transferrin have shorter half-lives, but are similarly nonspecific.

A group of 66 patients over 70 years of age who required emergency surgery were followed to determine the incidence of euthyroid sick syndrome (ESS), nutritional abnormalities, and postoperative outcome. The patients were assessed preoperatively for levels of thyroid hormone, catecholamines, cortisol, interleukin-6, interleukin-1, and C-reactive protein. Mortality rates and length of stay in the hospital were related. ESS was diagnosed in 34 patients, and was associated with low serum albumin levels, low triceps skinfold thickness, high cortisol and norepinephrine levels, high death rate, and longer hospital stay. A serum albumin level less than 3.5 g/dl was virtually always associated with ESS (75).

Mullen et al. (76) found that surgical complications doubled in patients with a serum albumin concentration of less than 3.0 g/dl, as compared with levels above 3.0. Patients whose serum transferrin was less than 220 g/dl had a complication rate five times higher than that of patients whose levels were greater than 220 g/dl. Mullen et al. (77) found that preoperative nutritional supplementation in cancer patients reduced surgical complications; Muller et al. (78) showed that preoperative TPN used in malnourished patients with gastrointestinal cancer significantly reduced major complications such as wound dehiscence.

Vaxman et al. (79) studied the effects of high doses of ascorbic acid and pantothenic acid on the wound healing process of human skin. They found that these supplements influenced the levels of trace elements in human skin and scars (Mg, Cu, and Mn levels increased, while Fe levels decreased), and acted to increase the resistance of scars to tensional forces.

The role of nutrition in the development of postoperative orthopedic infections was reviewed by Smith (80), who reported that nutritional deficiencies significantly increased the morbidity and mortality of orthopedic patients (81–83). In addition, poor nutritional status in patients undergoing orthopedic surgery contributed to wound problems (38,84–86), to difficulties with fracture healing (87,88), to development of sepsis (89), and to multiple organ system failure (90,91).

A study of 90 surgical patients receiving intravenous nutrition found that the group who received IV nutrition before and after the procedure had better wound healing than those who received IV nutrition only after the procedure (92). The same investigators also studied a group of 66 surgical patients with three degrees of malnutrition: normal nutritional status, mild protein energy malnutrition, and moderate to severe protein energy malnutrition. Patients with normal nutritional status demonstrated higher amounts of normal collagen (measured by hydroxyproline content) after 7 days, while those with malnutrition had significantly lowered collagen formation. Of interest was the finding that the two protein energy malnourished groups did not differ significantly from each other. This study demonstrated that even mild to moderate protein energy deficiencies will adversely affect healing (93).

A study involving transtibial amputees for occlusive arterial disease found that those patients who received a nutritional supplement had improved wound healing (94). Similarly, a study using nutrition as a prognostic indicator in 47 amputations found that the malnourished patients had a higher frequency of impaired wound healing and an increased risk of postoperative cardiopulmonary and septic complications. All six deaths in the study occurred in the malnourished group (95).

VII.   DISCUSSION

As approximately 50% of hospital patients are malnourished (96), patients admitted to an acute care hospital should undergo a nutritional screening to determine their nutritional intakes. Older patients are more likely to be admitted to the hospital suffering some degree of malnutrition, and the nutritional consequences of their metabolic responses to trauma may be more severe. It is the insidious nature of malnutrition in the elderly that makes the recognition of early warning signs of malnutrition so important. Research is needed to provide more practical age, sex, and culturally specific nutrition parameters. Early detection of malnutrition and appropriate interventions could produce a shift toward prevention (97,98).

Careful planning before surgery can avoid common cognitive, affective, or functional complications in elderly patients. The elimination of medications that cause cognitive dysfunction could help avoid or lessen postoperative confusion. The assessment of preoperative nutritional status could identify patients with significant malnutrition who would be at higher risk for postoperative complications (99), including infection, delay or failure to heal, and/or excessive scarring. Essential to a good surgical outcome are the rapid synthesis of new tissue in the wound area, minimization of contamination, maximization of the patient's immune status, and protection of the wound site. When blood supply, oxygen, and nutrients are available, healing can proceed (100).

A high-carbohydrate, low-fat diet, containing adequate sources of protein, will promote good wound healing by providing sufficient calories to rebuild and heal, while sparing the patient's own muscle mass as an energy source (101). The use of preoperative nutritional supplementation has been more effective for treating protein malnutrition than postoperative supplementation (92). As little as 1 week of preoperative protein supplementation can improve wound healing. Recent protein intake is more important than protein or fat stores (102).

Supplements of amino acids have been found to be beneficial. Methionine and cysteine decrease the length of the inflammatory stage (39) and may protect against oxidative damage (40). Arginine supplementation stimulates development of cytotoxic T-cells, stimulates proliferation of lymphocytes, and increases resistance to infection (103–107).

Nusbaum (108) found that support services such as nutrition, nursing, and physical therapy are very important components in the postoperative care of geriatric patients. In general, advanced age per se is not a contraindication to surgery, but it does require careful preoperative evaluation and vigorous postoperative support. An important parameter of postoperative recovery is the regaining of the patient's preoperative lean body mass. Jensen and Hessov (109) investigated whether a 4-month dietary intervention with dietary advice and home supplementation would impact the speed of regaining muscle in the convalescing patient. They found that patients who received the intervention had a gain of lean body mass after 2 months. After an additional 2 months, both lean body mass and fat were gained. The investigators concluded that, after discharge from the hospital, patients should increase protein intake by taking protein-rich liquid supplements.

A recent weight loss of greater than 10% of lean body mass increases the chances for wound complications (110). Recent preoperative intake of nutrients is most important (92,111); not eating for a week before surgery is worse than eating a limited regular diet for a longer period because nutritional depletion is correlated with wound complications (74,84,93,100).

If the patient has not eaten during the few days before surgery, or if the patient is not expected to eat much postoperatively, nutritional supplementation should be undertaken. Rapid replenishment of depleted nutrients is surprisingly effective, and a few days of parenteral nutrition can return the patient to relatively normal reparative capacity (92).

Surgery should be delayed only if malnutrition is severe (77,92,100,112). If the level of malnutrition is not severe, 2 to 3 days of supplementation should suffice. In all cases, nutritional supplementation begun preoperatively should be carried into the postoperative period (100). Diabetes, if present, must be kept under strict control, for hyperglycemia will decrease vitamin C cellular uptake (113). Increasing the level of vitamin C to 500 to 2000 mg per day can partially overcome this problem.

VIII. SUMMARY

The elderly surgical patient should be evaluated for malnutrition and monitored by the patient's primary physician and surgeon. Preoperative assessment of nutritional status should be the standard of care for the aged. The serum albumin level and the total lymphocyte count can be used to identify patients suffering from malnutrition. Surgery on a malnourished patient should be postponed, if possible, until the nutritional status has been restored to normal levels. A medical evaluation that focuses on the elderly patient's cardiopulmonary and nutritional status should be performed up to 8 weeks before the patient undergoes surgery. Following this evaluation, appropriate dietary, therapeutic, and prophylactic measures to reduce surgical morbidity and mortality can be implemented. The identification and management of nutritional deficiencies in the elderly can be a useful adjunct to successful surgery.

REFERENCES

1. Winkler S. Oral aspects of aging. In: Calkins E, Ford AB, Katz PR, Eds. *Practice of Geriatrics*. 2nd ed. Philadelphia: WB Saunders, 1992:502-512.
2. Birke G, Franksson C, Plantin LO. The excretion pattern of 17-ketosteroids and corticosteroids in surgical stress. *Acta Endocrinol*, 1955;18:201-209.

3. Souba WW, Wilmore D. Diet and nutrition in the care of the patient with surgery, trauma, and sepsis. In: Goodheart RS, Shils ME, Eds. *Modern Nutrition in Health and Disease*. Philadelphia: Lea and Febiger, 1999:1589-1618.

4. Porte D, Graber AL, Kuzuwa T, et al. The effect of epinephrine on immunoreactive insulin levels in man. *J Clin Invest*, 1966;45:228-236.

5. Russell RC, Walker, CJ, Bloom SR. Hyperglucagonaemia in the surgical patient. *Br Med J,* 1975;1(5948):10-12.

6. Traynor C, Hall GM. Endocrine and metabolic changes during surgery: anaesthetic implications. *Br J Anaesth,* 1981; 53(2):153-160.

7. Deutsch S. Effects of anesthetics on the kidney. *Surg Clin North Am,* 1975;55(4):775-786.

8. Philbin DM, Coggins CH. Plasma antidiuretic hormone levels in cardiac surgical patients during morphine and halothane anesthesia. *Anesthesiology,* 1978;49(2):95-98.

9. Massler M. Nutrition and the denture-bearing tissues. In: Winkler, S., Ed. *Essentials of Complete Denture Prosthodontics*. 2nd ed. St. Louis: Ishiyaku EuroAmerica, 1994:15-21.

10. Chernoff R. Effects of age on nutrient requirements. *Clin Geriatr Med*, 1995;11:641-651.

11. Munro HN, Young VR. Protein metabolism is the elderly: observations relating to dietary needs. *Postgrad Med*, 1978;63:143-148.

12. Campbell WW, Crim MC, Dallal GE, et al. Increased protein requirements in elderly people: new data and retrospective assessments. *Am J Clin Nutr*, 1994; 60:501-509.

13. Ausman LM, Russell RM. Nutrition in the elderly. In: *Modern Nutrition in Health and Disease*. Goodheart RS , Shils ME, Eds. Philadelphia: Lea and Febiger, 1999, 869-880.

14. U.S. Department of Agriculture, *Nutrition and Your Health: Dietary Guidelines for Americans*, Home and Garden Bulletin #232, Washington, DC, U.S. Government Printing Office, 1995.

15. Sawaya AL, Saltzman E, Fuss P, et al. Dietary energy requirements of young and older women determined by using the doubly labeled water method*, Am J Clin Nutr*, 1995:62:338-344.

16. Saltzman JR, Kowdley KV, Pedrosa MC, et al. Bacterial overgrowth without clinical malabsorption in elderly hypochlorhydric subjects, *Gastroenterology*, 1994, 106(3): 615-623.

17. Mayfield E. A consumer's guide to fats, in *The FDA Consumer*, U.S. Food and Drug Administration, Washington, DC, U.S. Government Printing Office, 1999.

18. Kleiner SM. Water: an essential but overlooked nutrient, *J Am Diet Assoc*, 1999;99:200-206.

19. Gray DS. The clinical use of dietary fiber. *Am Fam Physician*, 1995; 51(2):419-425.

20. Papazian R. Bulking up fiber's healthful reputation. *FDA Consumer*, U.S. Food and Drug Administration Bulletin FDA 97-2313, Washington, DC, U.S. Government Printing Office, 1997, revised 1998.

21. Zawada ET, Jr. Malnutrition in the elderly. Is it simply a matter of not eating enough? *Postgrad Med*, 1996;100(1):207-208, 211-214, 220-222.

22. Schlienger JL, Pradignac A, Grunenberger F. Nutrition of the elderly: a challenge between facts and needs. *Horm Res*, 1995;43(1-3):46-51.

23. Mirie W. Ageing and nutritional needs. *East Afr Med J*, 1997;74(10):622-624.

24. Russell RM, Sahyoun NR. The elderly. In: *Clinical Nutrition*, 2nd ed. Paige EM, Ed. Washington, DC: C.V. Mosby, 1988;110-116.

25. Hoffman HJ, Ishii EK, Macturk RH. Age-related changes in the prevalence of smell/taste problems among the United States adult population. Results of the 1994 Disability Supplement to the National Health Interview Survey (NHIS). *Ann NY Acad Sci*, 1998;855:716-722.

26. Schiffman SS. Drugs influencing taste and smell perception. In: *Smell and Taste in Health and Disease*. Getchell TV, Doty RL, Bartoshuk LM, Snow JB, Eds. New York: Raven Press, 1991:845-850.

27. Beaven DW, Brooks SE, *Color Atlas of the Tongue in Clinical Diagnosis*, Ipswich, England: Wolfe Medical Publishers, 1988:18.

28. Schiffman SS. Taste and smell losses in normal aging and disease. *JAMA*, 1997;16:1357-1362.

29. Mowe M, Bohmer T. Nutritional problems among home-living elderly people may lead to disease and hospitalization. *Nutr Revs*, 1996;54:S22-S24.

30. Hess MA. Taste: the neglected nutritional factor. *J Am Diet Assoc* 1997; 97(10 suppl 2):S205-207.

31. Schiffman S, Pasternak M. Decreased discrimination of food odors in the elderly. *J Gerontol*, 1979;34:73-79.

32. Murrell SA, Himmelfarb S, Wright K. Prevalence of depression and its correlates in older adults. *Am J Epidemiol*, 1983;117:173.

33. Busse EW, Simpson D. Depression and antidepressants and the elderly. *J Clin Psych*, 1983;44:5(Sec 2):35.

34. Rosenberg IH, Russell RM, Bowman BB. Aging and the digestive system. In: *Nutrition, Aging and the Elderly*. Munro HN, Danford DE, Eds. New York: Plenum Press, 1989:43-60.

35. Blumberg J. Nutritional needs of seniors. *J Am Coll Nutr*, 1997; 16(6):517-523.

36. Williams CM, Driver LT, Lumbers M. Nutrition in the older hospital patient. *J R Soc Health*, 1990;110(2):41-2,44.

37. Bowling TE, Silk BA. How long does it take to operate? The implications for inpatient malnutrition. *Acta Gastroenterol Latinoam*, 1996;26(2): 101-104.

38. Ruberg RL. Role of nutrition in wound healing. *Surg Clin N Am*, 1984;64(4):705-714.

39. Levenson SM, Demetriou AA. Metabolic factors. In: Cohen IK, Diegmann RF, Lindblad WJ, Eds. *Wound Healing: Biochemical and Clinical Aspects*. Philadelphia: W.B. Saunders, 1992:248-273.

40. Mazzotta MY. Nutrition and wound healing. *J Am Podiat Assoc*, 1994;84(9):456-462.

41. Fitzpatrick DW, Fisher H. Carnosine, histidine, and wound healing. *Surgery*, 1982;91:56-60.

42. Keller U, Clerc D, Kranzlin M, et al. Protein sparing therapy in the postoperative period. *World J Surg*, 1986;10(1):12-19.

43. Erlichman RJ, Seckel BR, Bryan DJ, et al. Common complications of wound healing: Prevention and management. *Surg Clin North Am*, 1991;71(6):1323-1351.

44. Gilder H. Parenteral nourishment of patients undergoing surgical or traumatic stress. *J Parenter Enter Nutr*, 1986;10(1):88-91.

45. Wolfe RR. Current thoughts on the assessment of protein metabolism in humans. *J Burn Care Rehabil*, 1991;12(3):211-213.

46. Bobel LM. Nutritional implications in the patient with pressure sores. *Nurs Clin North Am*, 1982;22(2):379-390.

47. Welch PK, Dowson M, Endres JM. The effects of nutrient supplements on high risk long term patients receiving pureed diets. *J Nutr Eld*, 1991;10(3):49-62.

48. Pollack SV. Wound healing: a review. III. Nutritional factors affecting wound healing. *J Dermatol Surg Oncol*, 1979;5(8):615-619.

49. Ruberg RL, Mirtallo J. Vitamin and trace element requirements in parenteral nutrition: An update. *Ohio State Med J*, 1981;77(12):725-729.

50. Solomons NW. Zinc and copper. In: *Modern Nutrition in Health and Disease*. Shils ME, Young VR, Eds. Philadelphia: Lea and Febiger, 1988: 238-262.

51. Chvapil M. Zinc and other factors of the pharmacology of wound healing. In: *Wound Healing and Wound Infection: Theory and Surgical Practice*. Hunt TK, Ed. New York: Appleton-Century Crofts, 1980:135-149.

52. Liszewski RF. The effect of zinc on wound healing: a collective review. *J Am Osteopath Assoc*, 1981;81(2):104-106.

53. Ågren MA, Chvapil M, Franzén L. Enhancement of re-epithelialization with topical zinc oxide in porcine partial-thickness wounds. *J Surg Res*, 1991;50:101-105.

54. Guillard O, Masson P, Piriou A, Brugier J-C, Courtois P. Comparison of the anti-inflammatory activity of sodium acexamate and zinc acexamate in healing skin wounds in rabbits. *Pharmacology*, 1987;34(5):296-300.

55. Schwartz PL. Ascorbic acid in wound healing — a review. *J Am Diet Assoc*, 1970;56(6):497-503.

56. Erlich HP, Hunt TK. Effects of cortisone and vitamin A on wound healing. *Ann Surg*, 1968:167:324-328.

57. Erlich HP, Tarvet H, Hunt TK. Effects of vitamin A and glucocorticoids upon inflammation and collagen synthesis. *Ann Surg*, 1973;177:222-227.

58. Hunt TK. Control of wound healing with cortisone and vitamin A. In: *The Ultrastructure of Collagen*. Longacre JJ, Ed. Springfield, IL: Charles C. Thomas, 1976:497-503.

59. Atukorala TMS, Basu TK, Dickerson JWT. Effect of corticosterone on the plasma and tissue concentrations of vitamin A in rats. *Ann Nutr Metab*, 1981;25:234-238.

60. Barbul A, Thysen B, Rettura G, et al. White cell involvement in the inflammatory wound healing and immune actions of vitamin A. *J Parent Enter Nutr*, 1978;2:129-138.

61. Jurin M, Tannock JF. Influence of vitamin A on immunologic response. *Immunology*, 1972;23:283-287.

62. Medawar PB, Hunt R. Anti-cancer action of retinoids. *Immunology*, 1981;42:349-353.

63. Malkovsky M, Medawar PB, Hunt R, et al. A diet enriched in vitamin A acetate or *in vivo* administration of interleukin-2 can counteract a toleragenic stimulus. *Proc R Soc Lond Biol*, 1984;220:439-445.

64. Seifter E, Rettura G, Levenson SM, et al. A mechanism of action of vitamin A in immunogenic tumor systems. *Curr Chemother Proc*, 10th Int Cong Chemother, vol 2, 1978:1290-1291.

65. Cohen BE, Cohen IK. Vitamin A: adjuvant and steroid antagonist in the immune response. *J Immunol*, 1973;111:1376-1380.

66. Athanassiades TJ. Adjuvant effect of vitamin A palmitate and analogs on cell-mediated immunity. *J Natl Cancer Inst*, 1981;67:1153-1156.

67. Pletsityvi KD, Askerov MA. Effect of vitamin A on immunogenesis. *Vopr Pitan* (English abstract), 1982;11:38-40.

68. Tachibana K, Sone S, Tsubura E, et al. Stimulatory effect of vitamin A on tumoricidal activity of rat alveolar macrophages. *Br J Cancer*, 1984;49:343-348.

69. Greenwald DP, Sharzer LA, Padawer J, et al. Zone II flexor tendon repair: effects of vitamin A,E, beta-carotene. *J Surg Res*. 1990;49:98-102.

70. Erlich HP, Tarver H, Hunt TK. Inhibitory effects of vitamin E on collagen synthesis and wound repair. *Ann Surg*, 1972;175:235-240.

71. Gallop PM, Lian JB, Hawschka PV. Carboxylated and calcium-binding protein and vitamin K. *New Eng J Med*, 1980;302:1460-1466.

72. Alvarez OM, Gilbreath RL. Effect of dietary thiamine on intermolecular collagen cross-linking during wound repair: mechanical and biochemical assessment. *J Trauma*, 1982;22(1):20-24.

73. Stotts NA, Whitney JD. Nutritional intake and status of clients in the home with open surgical wounds. *J Commun Health Nurs*, 1990;7(2): 77-86.

74. Warnold I, Lundholm K. Clinical significance of preoperative nutritional status in 215 noncancer patients. *Ann Surg*, 1984; 3:299-305.

75. Girvent M, Maestro S, Hernandez R, et al. Euthyroid sick syndrome, associated endocrine abnormalities, and outcome in elderly patients undergoing emergency operation. *Surgery*, 1998;123(5):560-567.

76. Mullen JL, Gertner MH, Buzby GP, et al. Implications of malnutrition in the surgical patient. *Arch Surg*, 1979;114(2):121-125.

77. Mullen JL, Buzby GP, Matthews DC, et al. Reduction of operative morbidity and mortality by combined preoperative and postoperative nutrition support. *Ann Surg*, 1980;192(5):604-613.

78. Muller JM, Brenner U, Denst C, et al. Preoperative parenteral feeding in patients with gastrointestinal carcinoma. *Lancet*, 1982;1(8263):68-71.

79. Vaxman F, Olender S, Lambert A, et al. Can the wound healing process be improved by vitamin supplementation? *Eur Surg Res*, 1996;28:306-314.

80. Smith TK. Nutrition: its relationship to orthopedic infections. *Orthoped Clin N Am*, 1991;22(3):373-377.

81. Foster MR, Heppenstall RB, Friedenberg ZB, et al. A prospective assessment of nutritional status and complications in patients with fractures of the hip. *J Orthop Trauma*, 1990;4(1):49-57.

82. Jensen JE, Jensen TG, Smith TK, et al. Nutrition in orthopaedic surgery. *J Bone Joint Surg Am*, 1982;64(9):1263-1272.

83. Mandelbaum BR, Tolo VT, McAfee PC, et al. Nutritional deficiencies after staged anterior and posterior spinal reconstructive surgery. *Clin Orthop*, 1988;234:5.

84. Dickhaut SC, DeLee JC, Page CP. Nutritional status: importance in predicting wound healing in amputations. *J Bone Joint Surg Am*, 1984;66(1):71-75.

85. Kay SP, Moreland JR. The effect of malnutrition on below-knee amputations. *Scientific Program, American Academy of Orthopedic Surgeons Meeting*, New Orleans, LA, 1986.

86. Young ME. Malnutrition and wound healing. *Heart Lung*, 1988;17(1):60-67.

87. Cuthbertson DP. Post-traumatic metabolism: a multidisciplinary challenge. *Surg Clin N Am*, 1978;58(5):1045-1054.

88. Einhorn TA, Levine B, Michel P. Nutrition and bone. *Orthop Clin North Am*, 1990;21(1):43-50.

89. Keusch GT, Farthing MJG. Nutrition and infection. *Annu Rev Nutr*, 1986;6:131-154.

90. Smith TK. Prevention of complications in orthopedic surgery secondary to nutritional depletion. *Clin Orthop*, 1987;222:91-97.

91. Smith TK. Recognition and treatment of nutritional deficits in the multiply-injured patient. In: *The Multiply-Injured Patient with Complex Fractures.* Meyers MH, Ed. Philadelphia: Lea and Febiger, 1984.

92. Haydock DA, Hill GL. Improved wound healing response in surgical patients receiving intravenous nutrition. *Brit J Surg*, 1987;74(4):320-323.

93. Haydock DA, Hill GL. Impaired wound healing in surgical patients with varying degrees of malnutrition. *J Parent Enter Nutr*, 1986;10(6):550-554.

94. Eneroth M, Apelqvist J, Larsson J, Persson BM. Improved wound healing in transtibial amputees receiving supplementary nutrition. *Int Orthop*, 1997;21(2):104-108.

95. Pedersen NW, Pedersen D. Nutrition as a prognostic indicator in amputations. A prospective study of forty-seven cases. *Acta Orthop Scand*, 1992;63(6):675-678.

96. Lipkin EW, Bell S. Assessment of nutritional status. The clinician's perspective. *Clin Lab Med, 1993;13(2):329-352.*

97. Barrocas A, Belcher D, Champagne C, Jastram C. Nutrition assessment — practical approaches. *Clin Geriatr Med*, 1995;11(4):675-713.

98. McWhirter JP, Pennington CR. Incidence and recognition of malnutrition in hospital. *Br Med J*, 1994;308(6934):945-948.

99. Hirsch CH. When your patient needs surgery: how planning can avoid complications. *Geriatrics*, 1995;50(2):39-44.

100. Hunt TK, Hopf HW. Wound healing and wound infection — what surgeons and anesthesiologists can do. *Surg Clin N Am*, 1997;77(3):587-606.

101. Nirgiotis JG, Hennesey PJ, Black CT, et al. Low fat, high carbohydrate diets improve wound healing and increase protein levels in surgically stressed rats. *J Pediatr Surg*, 1991;26(8):925-928.

103. Windsor J, Knight G, Hill G. Wound healing response in surgical patients: recent food intake is more important than nutritional status. *Br J Surg*, 1988;75(2):135-137.

103. Reynolds JV, Daly JM, Zhang S, et al. Immunomodulatory mechanisms of arginine. *Surgery*, 1988;104(2):142-151.

104. Reynolds JV, Daly JM, Shou J, et al. Immunologic effects of arginine supplementation in tumor-bearing and non-tumor-bearing hosts. *Ann Surg*, 1990;211(2):202-210.

105. Efron DT, Kirk SJ, Regan MC, et al. Nitric oxide generation from L-arginine is required for optimal human peripheral blood lymphocyte DNA synthesis. *Surgery*, 1991;110(2):327-334.

106. Daly JM, Reynolds J, Thom A, et al. Immune and metabolic effects of arginine in the surgical patient. *Ann Surg*, 1988, 208(4):512-523.

107. Daly JM, Reynolds J, Sigal RK, et al. Effect of dietary protein and amino acids on immune function. *Crit Care Med*, 1990;18(2 suppl):S86-93.

108. Nusbaum NJ. How do geriatric patients recover from surgery? *South Med J*, 1996;89(10):950-957.

109. Jensen MB, Hessov I. Dietary supplementation at home improves the regain of lean body mass after surgery. *Nutrition*, 1997;13(5):475-476.

110. Orgill D, Demling RH. Current concepts and approaches to wound healing. *Crit Care Med*, 1988;16(9):899-908.

111. Goodson WH, Lopez SA, Jensen JA, et al. The influence of a brief preoperative illness on post-operative healing. *Ann Surg*,1987;205:250-255.

112. Delany HM, Demetriou AA, Teh E, et al. Effect of early postoperative nutritional support on skin wound and colon anastomosis healing. *J Parent Enter Nutr*, 1990;14(4):357-361.

113. Marhoffer W, Stein M, Maeser D, et al. Impairment of polymorphonuclear leukocyte function and metabolic control of diabetes. *Diabetes Care*, 1992;15:256-260.

20 Tube Feeding in the Nursing Home

Carlene Russell

CONTENTS

I.   INTRODUCTION

Adequate nutrition is basic to life. Food and fluids are necessary to maintain health and to support normal body functions. When oral intake of nutrients is not adequate, it is medically appropriate to provide for nutritional needs by other methods. Enteral nutrition is the delivery of nutrients via tube into the gastrointestinal tract for the purpose of meeting nutritional needs consistent with the plan of care for maintenance, rehabilitation, or palliation. If there is a fully or partially functioning gastrointestinal system present, then delivery of nutrients via an enteral feeding tube is a means of maintaining adequate nutrition.

In the nursing home setting, a tube feeding may be required due to functional disabilities associated with neurologic deficits, dementia, stroke, Parkinson's disease, Alzheimer's disease and related disorders; increased requirements resulting from fractures, pressure ulcer, or surgery. Where residents have difficulty eating and nursing home staff have limited time to assist them, insertion of feeding tubes for the convenience of staff is an unacceptable rationale for use.

The major rationale for tube feeding is a demonstrated medical need to prevent or reverse malnutrition or dehydration. Prior to initiating tube feeding, all possible alternatives should be explored. Restoration to oral feeding is a goal throughout the treatment program when consistent with diagnosis. When a tube feeding is implemented, the potential for the resident to return to oral feedings needs to be reviewed at least quarterly by the interdisciplinary care plan team.

0-8493-2228-6/01/$0.00+$.50
© 2001 by CRC Press LLC

II.   ADVANCED DIRECTIVES

The wishes or advance directives of the residents and their families need to be reflected in the plan to proceed with a tube feeding. This becomes very important in an environment where the nursing home regulations emphasize maintaining or improving level of health. With this emphasis, nursing homes are feeling pressure to do whatever is needed to prevent the decline of the residents' health. Many elderly residents have chronic debilitating conditions that in the natural progression of the disease or aging process result in a poor oral intake. An oral intake that is consistently below estimated needs results in a gradual decline in health status eventually leading to death. When the prognosis does not warrant aggressive nutrition support, tube feeding is contraindicated.

When residents are unable to communicate their wishes in regard to tube feeding, the issue of whether a resident has expressed wishes in writing through an advance directive or other medical guideline is a key point. When someone is no longer capable of discussing his or her wishes, it is imperative to communicate the consequences of discontinuing or not initiating enteral feedings to the guardian or individual with power of attorney so that an educated decision about tube feeding is made (1,2).

The Patient Self Determination Act (1991) as a part of Omnibus Budget Reconciliation Act of 1990 (OBRA) specifies that all Medicare and Medicaid nursing facilities have written policies and procedures to implement the resident's right to make decisions concerning their medical care, including their right to accept or refuse medical treatment and the right to execute advance medical directives; document presence of advance directive in the resident's medical record; and provide education about advance directives.

III   ENTERAL FEEDING ACCESS

Determining the optimal access route for enteral nutrition depends on the anticipated duration of therapy, the adequacy of gastric function, lower esophageal sphincter competence, and the risk of aspiration.

Feeding tubes are named for the site of entry into the body and the location of the tip of the tube. Common access sites for enteral tube feedings are as follow:

Nasoenteric, which includes the following:
 Nasogastric — through the nose into the stomach
 Nasoduodenal — through the nose into the duodenum
 Nasojejunal — through the nose into the jejunum
Gastrostomy — through the abdominal wall directly into the stomach
Jejunostomy — through the abdominal wall into the jejunum

A. NASOGASTRIC FEEDING

Residents who require enteral nutrition support for a short period of time (i.e., less than 4 weeks) may benefit from a nasogastric feeding tube placed in the stomach, duodenum, or proximal jejunum. Patients with gastroparesis, diseases involving the stomach, or those at risk of pulmonary aspiration should have a tube placed beyond the pylorus into the small bowel. Nasoduodenal and nasojejunal feeding tubes may be placed by a variety of methods, including spontaneous passage, in which the tube migrates to the small bowel by peristalsis or with the help of prokinetic agents (e.g., metclo-pramid, erythromycin), active bedside placement, or fluoroscopic and endoscopic methods. The method used depends on the training of the clinician and availability of equipment.

B. ENTEROSTOMY FEEDING

Residents who require tube feedings longer than 4 weeks may have a gastrostomy or jejunostomy tube surgically or endoscopically placed. Gastrostomy tubes are indicated when gastric emptying is normal, a gag reflex is present, and there is no esophageal reflux.

Jejunostomy feeding tubes are generally placed at the time of a surgical procedure, or they may be placed endoscopically. Candidates for jejunal feeding tubes include those at risk of aspiration, severe esophageal reflux, obstruction, stricture, fistulae, or ileus of the upper gastrointestinal tract.

Complications of enteral feedings include introduction of feedings through tubes that are inadvertently positioned in the respiratory tract and pulmonary aspiration secondary to gastroesophageal reflux. To minimize these occurrences, nasoenteral feeding-tube placement should be checked on initial insertion, before each intermittent feeding, and at least once per shift during continuous feedings. In nursing homes, radiographic confirmation of tube placement is often not an option. Visual inspection of aspirates from feeding tubes along with auscultation of air insufflated through a feeding tube are recommended methods for checking tube placement. Accuracy of these two methods is improved when combined with use of pH testing of aspirates (3). Gastrostomy tube placement is checked by measuring the length of the tube extending from the abdomen.

IV. ENTERAL FEEDING TUBES

Feeding tubes are made of soft, biocompatible materials such as polyurethane or silicone. Enteral tubes are generally described in terms of their external diameter, composition, length, and the presence or absence of a weighted tip. The outer diameter of the feeding tube is described in French units; each French unit equals 0.33 mm. Most adults tolerate a tube diameter of 8 to 10 French with a length of 110 cm for nasogastric or transpyloric placement. Larger tubes, nasally placed, may cause esophagitis, pharyngitis, otitis, and pressure necrosis in the nasolabial area. They also may compromise lower esophageal sphincter competency, increasing the potential for gastric reflux and pulmonary aspiration of gastric contents. Larger tubes may interfere with swallowing and are uncomfortable for the resident. Gastrostomy tubes are usually greater than 12 French and conventional jejunostomy tubes are greater than 6 French.

Foley catheters have been used for gastrostomy tubes. There are several disadvantages associated with this practice: the foley catheter is not biocompatible; the balloon deteriorates in the presence of gastric acid; the balloon may migrate across the pylorus and obstruct the small bowel; there is not a skin disc and no way to close the end of the tube; and foley catheters are often made of latex, which is a problem for latex-sensitive individuals.

V. NUTRIENT NEEDS

Nutrient needs are affected by physical characteristics, activity level, nutritional status, medical condition, and degree of metabolic stress. Established equations can be used to estimate calorie needs. The Harris–Benedict equation uses sex, height, weight, and age to estimate resting energy needs. Factors for activity and injury are included in the equation. Protein needs will generally range from 0.8 to 2.0 gm/kg of body weight, with the higher end of this range required for surgery or wound healing. Estimated fluid needs will average 30 ml/kg, with lesser amounts of 25 ml/kg in congestive heart failure or higher amounts of 40 ml/kg to address urinary tract infections or fluid losses. The tube feeding formula that best matches estimated nutrient needs should be selected (4).

VI. FORMULA SELECTION

Formulas can be grouped into three main categories: polymeric, predigested, and modular. Selection of formula is based on several factors, including digestive and absorptive capacity, volume status, and overall disease state.

Polymeric formulas are nutritionally complete, predominately lactose-free, and are casein or soy protein isolate based. Normal digestion and absorption are required. Polymeric formulas are available in the following varieties: standard, high-nitrogen, fiber supplemented, concentrated, and disease specific.

Predigested formulas require minimal or no digestion for absorption. These formulas are usually low in fat and/or provide a portion of the fat in the form of medium-chain triglycerides.

Modular formulas are single macronutrients such as carbohydrate, protein, and fat that may be used to alter the calorie or protein content of a base formula or create a new tube feeding formula.

Indications for use of specialty products (5):

1. Residents diagnosed with HIV or AIDs with one of the following symptoms: CD4 < 400; Serum albumin < 3.0; >5% weight loss; intractable diarrhea.
2. Significantly delayed gastric emptying: (a) repeated vomiting or high gastric residuals on standard products, or (b) jejunal feeding with intolerance to other products.
3. Maldigestion/malabsorption:(a) intolerance to intact nutrients evidenced by diarrhea; or (b) anticipate malabsorption of intact nutrients due to history of diarrhea or extensive GI pathology; or (c) clinical or biochemical evidence of impaired gut function (positive xylose, mannitol, or lactulose tests).
4. Insulin-dependent diabetes mellitus with unstable glucose labels documented on standard formula is then controlled on specialty formula.
5. Pancreatic diseases: elevated serum lipase and/or amylase or abdominal pain with intact nutrients; requires bowel rest to reduce pancreatic stimulation.
6. Renal disease: tolerates less than 50 g protein per day. Increased BUN (>40) and creatinine (>2.0). Serum electrolytes are elevated (Na, K, PO4, Mg).
7. Pulmonary impairment diseases: residents exhibit retention of CO_2 in the serum due to pulmonary insufficiency or weaning from chronic mechanical ventilation.
8. Sepsis/infection (non-HIV immunocompromised): metabolic stress with or at risk of infection including sepsis, infected pressure ulcers and infected ventilator-dependent residents. Albumin <3.0.

VII. ENTERAL FEEDING ADMINISTRATION

The method of administration to provide enteral nutrition support depends on the location of the feeding tube, tolerance to the feeding regimen, ease of administration, and overall nutritional goals. The three methods of tube feeding administration are bolus, intermittent, and continuous.

1. Bolus feeding is characterized as the rapid delivery (10 minutes of less) of 200 to 400 ml of formula several times a day. A large syringe connected to the feeding tube is generally used to administer the feeding. Bolus feedings may result in nausea, abdominal bloating, cramps, diarrhea, or aspiration, more so than with other administration methods.
2. Intermittent feedings may be delivered by slow gravity drip or by a feeding pump. Usually 250 to 400 ml formula is given over a 30- to 60-minute period five to eight times per day. This schedule of administration simulates the meal pattern. Intermittent administration is generally indicated for gastric feedings, since the small bowel does not tolerate large volumes of formula at one time. Gastric residuals should be checked prior to

administration of formula to assess tolerance. This type of administration is contraindicated when the risk of aspiration is high.

3. Continuous feedings are preferred when the tube feeding is initiated; the resident has not been fed for 3 or more days; the resident is unstable or critically ill, including residents at risk for aspiration; and when the duodenal or jejunal feeding sites are used. Continuous may be given by gravity drip or by feeding pump. Gastric residuals should be checked every 4 to 8 hours to assess patient tolerance.

VIII.   TUBE FEEDING MONITORING

A continual monitoring system is needed to evaluate weight, hydration status, bowel movements and other signs to indicate response to the tube feeding. *The Resident Assessment Protocol: Feeding Tubes* is a required assessment form in nursing facilities participating in Medicare and Medicaid. Medicare daily charting guidelines for tube-fed patients include the following information:

- Vital signs
- Presence or absence of nausea/vomiting, aspiration, abdominal distention, drainage/odor or signs of infection around stoma, irritation around nares
- Type of tube, tube placement check, and results
- Name of formula, calories received
- Checking for residual
- How resident is tolerating the feeding
- Results of check for gastric residual and amount of residual
- Head of bed elevated
- Percentage, type of food taken orally, if applicable
- If used, mittens removed every 2 hours
- If receiving speech therapy, response to therapy to improve swallowing ability

IX.   MEDICATIONS

The administration of medications through enteral feeding tubes increases risk of tube occlusion and incompatibility of medications with tube feeding formula. Enteral formulas may interfere with the absorptive or therapeutic effect of some medications (6). Medications should never be added directly to the formula. The following guidelines are established to minimize problems:

1. Flush feeding tube with 15 to 60 ml of water before and after medication is infused.
2. Do not crush enteric-coated or timed-released tablets or capsules.
3. Administer each medication separately.
4. Dilute hypertonic medications with water.
5. Avoid potential drug–medication interactions by using alternative administration routes, alternative formulas or medication, altering feeding or medication schedules as indicated, and multidisciplinary team input.
6. If feeding tube is placed into jejunum, check with pharmacist before administering medication.

X.   MEDICARE REIMBURSEMENT

In general, enteral nutrition may be reimbursed under Medicare Part B coverage. To be reimbursed by Medicare, enteral nutrition must be ordered by a physician and must be considered reasonable and necessary for a patient with a functioning GI tract who, due to pathology or permanent nonfunction of the structures that normally permit food to reach the digestive tract, cannot swallow or take sufficient nutrients orally to maintain weight or strength commensurate with the patient's general condition. The test of permanence is considered to be met if the medical record indicates that the impairment is anticipated to continue for a period of more than 3 months. Enteral nutrition is not covered for patients with a normally functioning GI tract whose need for enteral nutrition is due to lack of appetite, unwillingness or refusal to eat, inability to cooperate with a feeding program, or convenience (7).

To ensure reimbursement, documentation identifying the physiologic need for enteral therapy must exist in the medical record. Coverage of enteral nutrition requires documentation of medical necessity in the following areas:

1. Diagnosis
2. Functional impairment
3. Pump justification
4. Calorie justification
5. Product justification

XI. NURSING HOME REGULATIONS

Nursing home regulations support the use of tube feeding after adequate assessment of the resident's condition determines its need. Several federal requirements address tube feedings in the nursing home.

1. *Resident Assessment.* The facility must conduct initially and periodically a comprehensive, accurate, standardized, reproducible assessment of each resident's functional capacity. The intent is for each resident's nutritional needs and capabilities to be properly assessed and identified, and care planned for by the facility.
2. *Quality of Care.* Each resident must receive and the facility must provide the necessary care and services to attain or maintain the highest practicable physical, mental, and psychosocial well-being, in accordance with the comprehensive assessment and plan of care. The intent is for each resident to have appropriate high-quality nutritional care and services to avoid decline in health status and to reach and maintain levels of physical and mental health that are attainable.
3. *Nasogastric Tubes.* Based on the comprehensive assessment of a resident, the facility must ensure that a resident who has been able to eat enough alone or with assistance is not fed by nasogastric tube unless the resident's clinical condition demonstrates that use of a nasal was unavoidable, and a resident who is fed by a nasogastric or gastrostomy tube receives the appropriate treatment and services to prevent aspiration pneumonia, diarrhea, vomiting, dehydration, metabolic abnormalities, and nasal-pharyngeal ulcers and to restore, if possible, normal eating habits. The intent is for the nasogastric tube feeding to be utilized only after adequate assessment, and the resident's clinical condition makes this treatment necessary.
4. *Quality of Life.* A facility must care for its residents in a manner and in an environment that promotes maintenance of each resident's quality of life. The intent is that each resident has a right to nutritional care/services that promote self-esteem, poise, self-respect, and individuality.

The nursing home survey process focuses on specific quality indicators. Quality indicators that will trigger a more in-depth survey include fecal impaction, urinary tract infection, weight loss, tube feeding, decline in activities of daily living, and pressure ulcers. Additionally, residents with the following dehydration risk factors of vomiting/diarrhea resulting in fluid loss; elevated temperatures and/or infectious processes; use of medications including diuretics, laxatives, and cardiovascular agents; or renal disease will receive chart review to determine adequate assessment and interventions are being used to ensure adequate hydration. Residents receiving enteral nutrition support must have orders for sufficient amount of free water and the water and feeding must be administered in accordance with the physician order.

Residents identified to be at risk for developing pressure ulcers must have an adequate assessment with preventive interventions implemented. Risk factors include diabetes, peripheral vascular disease, chronic obstructive pulmonary disease, a terminal condition, hip fractures or other surgical interventions that limit mobility, cerebral vascular accident, immobility, hemiplegia/hemiparesis, physical restraints, decreased sensory perception, history of pressure ulcers, incontinence, edema, compromised nutritional status such as unintended weight loss, or malnutrition. Residents who have an existing pressure ulcer need care plan interventions to provide an aggressive program of treatment.

The interdisciplinary care plan directs consistent quality care in the nursing home. The care plan must include the resident's clinical conditions and risk factors for developing problems. The interventions identified on the care plan must be accurately reflected in the care that is provided to the resident.

XII. BEST PRACTICE GUIDELINES FOR TUBE FEEDINGS IN NURSING HOMES (8)

Standard 1 Selection and administration of tube feeding is consistent with the overall care plan and goals for therapy and is delivered in an ethical manner.

Criterion 1.1 The wishes/advance directives of the resident /family are reflected in the tube feeding plan.

Criterion 1.2 Goals for the tube feeding (maintenance, repletion, palliation) are stated and consistent with the tube feeding plan.

Criterion 1.3 The client's rights to privacy and dignity are reflected in the tube feeding plan.

Criterion 1.4 Tube feeding is discontinued when the resident is able to eat an adequate oral diet or when the tube feeding is no longer consistent with the overall care plan and goals for therapy.

Standard 2 Selection of tube feeding formula and volume meets nutritional needs based on a comprehensive resident assessment.

Criterion 2.1 Tube feeding formula selection is based on the resident's nutritional and metabolic needs and medical condition.

On average, most people need 30 ml water per kilogram body weight per day or 1 ml of water for every kilocalorie fed. Most 1 cal/ml formulas are about 80% water, 1.2 to 1.5 cal/ml formulas are about 75% water, and 1.5 to 2.0 cal/ml formulas are 50% water, so additional water must be given.

Fever, elevated environmental temperature, low environmental humidity, dry oxygen, and air-fluidized bed therapy cause evaporative water loss. Additional water must be given in these cases.

Vomiting, diarrhea, excessive ostomy drainage, and other GI fluid losses cause loss of water and electrolytes. These losses must be replaced with an oral or IV hydration solution that contains water and electrolytes in appropriate amounts.

Standard 3 The type and location of the feeding tube is appropriate based on the medical conditions and goals for care.

Criterion 3.1 A nasogastric tube is considered when tube feeding is expected to be of short (generally less than 3 weeks) duration. An ostomy tube (such as a gastric or jejunal tube) is considered when tube feeding is expected to be needed for longer than 3 weeks.

Criterion 3.2 Tube feeding infusion can be via an open or closed delivery system. An open system utilizes a syringe, or formula is decanted in an administration container. The volume prescribed must be delivered within 4 to 12 hours to maintain microbial quality. A closed system is prefilled with a commercially sterile formula that usually contains a least a liter of product, and hangtime can extend to 24 hours.

Criterion 3.3 Use of feeding pumps reduces risk of tube feeding intolerance due to unintentional bolus infusion of formula. A closed delivery system and jejunostomy feeding generally require delivery of formula via pumps.

Standard 4 The initial tube feeding plan, including routine monitoring to prevent problems and monitoring progress toward nutritional and medical goals, is documented in the medical record.

Criterion 4.1 A routine monitoring schedule is established and followed.

Standard 5 Potential problems associated with tube feeding are identified and preventive actions taken.

Criterion 5.1 Body weight, biochemistries, and vital signs are routinely evaluated to identify the potential for and to prevent metabolic problems.

Metabolic problems that have been associated with tube feeding include fluid/electrolyte and blood glucose abnormalities.

Criterion 5.2 Stool changes, abdominal pain/distention, nausea and vomiting — symptoms of gastrointestinal problems — are evaluated to determine their cause and provide appropriate preventive or therapeutic actions.

Gastrointestinal symptoms may be due to non-tube feeding causes — medical condition, malnutrition, medications, constipation or impaction. Tube feeding-related gastrointestinal symptoms may be due to formula type, administration rate or delivery method, unsanitary handling methods during formula preparation and/or administration, and prolonged hangtime of formula at the bedside.

Criterion 5.3 Potential mechanical problems associated with the feeding tube — displacement or migration, pulmonary aspiration of gastric contents, tube degradation, balloon rupture or inability to deflate it, tube clogging, and infection or irritation at the tube site — are identified and steps taken to prevent or treat them.

Use of appropriate feeding tubes and feeding sites, routine irrigation with clear water, routine verification of tube placement, use of clean technique during tube and site care, and securing tubes properly are preventive steps.

Standard 6 Principles of food safety are applied to preparation, storage, delivery, and administration of tube feeding.

The Hazard Analysis Critical Point system (HAACP), a system for maintaining food safety, can be used to help maintain the safety of tube feeding.

Criterion 6.1 Food safety hazards associated with the formula are identified and preventive measures taken.

Hazards associated with tube feeding formula include touch contamination during preparation and administration, adding substances (e.g., water, medications) to formula, prolonged hangtime at the bedside, and unsafe storage and transport conditions.

Criterion 6.2 Food safety hazards associated with the tube feeding administration system are identified and preventive measures taken.

Hazards associated with tube feeding administration system include touch contamination during set up and use, and use of feeding sets or containers for more than 24 hours, or reuse of system components marked for single-use only.

Criterion 6.3 Food safety hazards associated with the tube-fed resident are identified and preventive measures taken.

Hazards associated with the resident include retrograde contamination and increased susceptibility to illness due to microbial contamination.

REFERENCES

1. Position of the American Dietetic Association: Issues in feeding the terminally ill adult. *J. Am. Diet. Assoc.*, 92, 996, 1992.
2. Position of the American Dietetic Association: Legal and ethical issues in feeding permanently unconscious patients. *J. Am. Diet. Assoc.*, 95, 231, 1995.
3. Metheny, N., Verification of feeding tube placement. *Curr. Issues Enteral Nutr. Support*, (Sept), 34,1995.
4. Niedert, K., *Nutrition Care of the Older Adult*. Chicago, IL: The American Dietetic Association, 1998, chap.11 and 14.
5. Hall, J., Campbell, S., Gallaher-Allred, C., *Best Practice Guidelines for Tube Feeding: A Nurse's Pocket Manual*. Columbus, OH: Ross Products Division, Abbott Laboratories: 1997.
6. ASCP. *Enteral Therapy Policy and Procedure Manual for Assisted Living, Home Care, and Nursing Facilities*. Alexandria, VA: American Society of Consultant Pharmacists, 1999.
7. Smith, D., *Medicare Nursing Home Enteral Nutrition Reimbursement Manual*, 4th ed. Columbus, OH: Ross Products Division, Abbott Laboratories, 1997.
8. Health Care Financing Administration. *Enteral Feeding: Current Practices and Outcome Measures*. March 24, 1997.

21 Effective Nutrition Education Strategies to Reach Older Adults

U. Beate Krinke

CONTENTS

I. INTRODUCTION

Older adults at all socioeconomic levels are willing to adopt new dietary behaviors that they believe will help them to live independently;[1-4] they rank nutrition and exercise among key health habits that can contribute to independence. Older adults want to avoid being a burden to others; furthermore, no individual person can live to old age without making numerous dietary changes. First, people's tastes and habits shift as their social cohort changes. Second, technology and the food supply do not remain constant. Today's supermarket looks nothing like the grocery stores of the early 1900s. The old grocery or dry-goods store was too small to hold the thousands of food items available to consumers in today's "supermarket." In the early 1900s, when today's older adults learned their food habits, there was no access to extensive deli sections, fresh produce from all over the world, and aisle after aisle of frozen food. As the food supply has grown during the last century, so have consumers' choices and range of decisions regarding what to eat, how to procure, and how to prepare foods. Older adults have learned how to use or deal with "new" kitchen appliances and equipment (microwaves, toaster ovens, refrigerators, stick blenders), cookbooks (recipes for the new, leaner, red meats), and social practices related to food (fast-food restaurants, frozen meals, take-out food, car-food, grazing). Overall, older adults have had to learn many new dietary practices in order to keep pace with the changing marketplace.

Individuals who developed their eating habits in the early 1900s have heard, and likely adapted to, several iterations of dietary guidance. Models used to design a health-promoting diet have been based on the Seven Food Groups, the Basic Four food groups, and now the Food Guide Pyramid, which educators and counselors are adapting for the special needs of an older audience.[5] Also, older adults have had to interpret changing dietary advice such as "maintain ideal weight," "avoid too much sodium,"[6] "maintain appropriate body weight," "achieve an ideal weight," and "limit total daily intake of salt to 6 or less."[7] Especially in the areas of dietary fat and cholesterol, new scientific findings have led to speculation, disagreement, and conflicting changing dietary recommendations. Older adults are no strangers to changes in diet or to changes in food and nutrition advice.

Just as in any other age group, some older individuals will be resistant to adopting desirable health-promoting behaviors. But compared with younger people, older adults are especially motivated to stay independent and maintain their abilities, and thus wish to learn behaviors and practices that will contribute to maximum health.[1,2,8] Older adults can, and do, change the way they eat. For instance, while developing a nutrition education program for older adults, Goldberg et al.[3] surveyed older adults to conclude that "many older people have modified their diets in an effort to reduce their risk of chronic disease."

II.   EFFECTIVE NUTRITION EDUCATION RESULTS IN BEHAVIOR CHANGE

Nutrition educators have defined nutrition education as "any set of learning experiences designed to facilitate the voluntary adoption of eating and other nutrition-related behaviors conducive to health and well-being."[2] The U.S. Department of Health and Human Services defined nutrition education for Title III C programs of the Older Americans Act (Elderly Nutrition Programs) as the provision of "knowledge, skills and/or assistance to older adults to enable them to eat nutritiously, thus contributing to the maintenance of optimum health."[9] It follows from these definitions that nutrition education is more than dispensing information; it is an intervention process designed to change behaviors and lead an individual to achieve better health and subsequently a better quality of life. For example, older adults can learn nutrition information and new nutrition behaviors to cope with conditions associated with aging, such as arthritis, osteoporosis, heart disease, and diabetes. They may also benefit from nutrition education to help them deal with bereavement and changes in functional, social, and economic status. Nutrition education goes beyond providing nutrition information because the desired outcome of nutrition education is achievement of health-promoting food and nutrition behaviors.

To achieve behavior change in their target audiences, nutrition educators use instructional strategies that facilitate: (1) gains in food and nutrition knowledge, (2) development of skills needed to practice beneficial nutritional habits, and (3) acquisition or reinforcement of the confidence and commitment needed to achieve and maintain health-promoting nutrition behaviors.

Nutrition education "works" when learners know how to select foods that will nourish them; when they understand basic relationships between food, nutrients, and their own body; and when they use that knowledge to improve their own health. Evidence of effective nutrition education in an older adult audience has been reported in a variety of settings. For instance, it was seen in improved food intake (greater consumption of targeted foods including low-fat dairy products, water, and of fiber from fruits and vegetables) after individuals participated in an educational community gardening project[10] as well as in a health promotion program that yielded improved health risk scores and decreased insurance claims.[11,12]

III. LITERATURE REVIEWS OF NUTRITION EDUCATION

Several major reviews reported that effective nutrition education programs are behaviorally based and theory-driven.[2,13-15] The review authors found that a good educational plan begins by identifying the needs and motivations of a target audience, selecting behaviors to target for change, designing and implementing learning experiences that facilitate adoption of selected behaviors, and helping learners identify support systems to maintain desired behaviors. In 1973, Whitehead reported on studies done since 1900, concluding that, too often, educators had focused on disseminating nutrition information and expecting, but not achieving, behavior change. Johnson and Johnson[13] conducted a meta-analysis of the nutrition education literature for youth and adult programs, suggesting that goals be identified as short- or long-term in generating a synthesis of effective nutrition education. The more a participant became engaged in the learning process, the more likely that desired short- or long-term nutrition goals would result. The two instructional strategies involving or engaging participants to the greatest extent were cooperative learning situations (achieve mutual learning goals) and structured academic controversies (take opposing sides, discuss, reach consensus). Johnson and Johnson[13] reported that factors found to influence nutrition practices are conforming to group norms, making a public commitment, emulating social models, receiving personalized information, cognitive processing, teaching others, having continuing motivation, and responding to gain or loss appeals, i.e., trying to achieve perceived benefits or avoid losses.

A U.S. Department of Agriculture-contracted, comprehensive review of nutrition education programming for older adults by Maloney and White[14] identified elements of successful programs, namely that they are audience centered, use personalized approaches and known motivating factors, engage learners to be active participants, continue to reinforce new behaviors, and are sensitive to the functional status of their audiences (limitations in vision or hearing). These elements support Johnson and Johnson's 1985 meta-analysis and synthesis. Maloney and White searched seven computerized databases and contacted health and aging organizations, a university, and trade associations in order to find examples of nutrition education interventions that have been evaluated, but "only a few studies met the methodological criteria specified for their review."[14]

In reviewing all past nutrition education literature and intervention studies geared to older adults, Contento et al.[2] found only 14 studies that met their criteria for sound design, which included measurement of behavioral outcomes. Contento et al. reiterated the elements of successful nutrition interventions that Maloney and White[14] presented. Reviewers agree that programs based on disseminating information did not result in behavior change, which is integral to the process of nutrition education. Increased knowledge alone does not automatically lead to attitudinal shifts or to more desirable nutrition behaviors.

IV. THE FRAMEWORK OF EFFECTIVE NUTRITION EDUCATION

The purpose of nutrition education is to facilitate development of improved dietary practices in a target audience. Learning and maintaining new dietary practices requires that the individual learner integrate new knowledge skills and attitudes. Four essential elements must come together for the individual learner: (1) cognition or knowledge of issues being addressed, (2) capability or skill to carry out new behaviors, (3) commitment to change, and (4) confidence that one is able to change. These four elements are important, because facilitating improved dietary practices through educational programs is a complex process, not only because each learner approaches dietary behavior change from their unique situation, but also because educators vary in their approaches to curriculum development and program implementation. Dissemination of nutrition information is only one component of nutrition education; by itself, it typically does not result in behavior change.

A. COGNITION: GAINING KNOWLEDGE OF NUTRITION FACTS AND PRINCIPLES

Cognition, or knowledge, is one of the cornerstones of nutrition education, as pictured in Figure 21.1. Understanding enough about food, nutrition, and one's health or lifestyle results from cognitive processing; the learner engages in mental processes to integrate new information into an existing knowledge network. Knowing what to do or why to perform a specific dietary practice is a prerequisite for acquiring desired dietary behaviors.

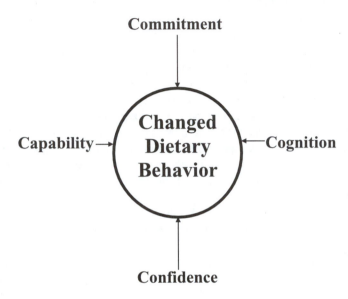

FIGURE 21.1 Essential elements for achieving and maintaining individual behavior change.

Knowledge about "what should be done" is one aspect of nutrition education that can be learned in many ways. What "should be done" is also taught in many different ways, depending on the educator. Educators tend to favor one of several educational perspectives; each educator's unique perspective affects his or her teaching.

A developmental view of education suggests that teachers focus on the learner's personal stage of cognitive, emotional, or moral development. The curriculum will then be designed to match the particular developmental stages of the learner, which may range from dependency (wanting to be told what to do) to self-actualization (integrating facts and concepts to enhance life-style). Self-directed learning modules accommodate varied developmental stages, because the learner can control the scope and progress of the lesson.

Another educational view, the social learning perspective, assumes that individuals concentrate on learning things that are culturally and socially reinforced. In that case, a curriculum would feature social interactions and support; strategies might include mentoring, peer-teaching, and group discussions. An example of using a social learning perspective approach is the senior peer educator program developed by Ness et al.[16] where a network of peer educators grew from 18 to 35 active peer educators in roughly 6 years. In all, 95 peer educators trained during those years branched out their services to develop community programs, initiate fund drives, and eventually generate community ownership of the program.

Yet another educational view focuses on learners as they construct knowledge by relating new information to existing information. In this constructionist perspective, educators facilitate cognitive processes such as insight, perception, and memory by structuring the curriculum so that learners can link new information to existing knowledge structures. This process is sometimes called "scaffolding." The constructionist educator approaches teaching with the belief that brains do not merely absorb knowledge as a sponge absorbs water but that each learner builds knowledge domains by actively selecting and integrating new information found to be interesting.

A constructionist approach can be used in adult education because it is based on the principle that learners come to new situations with a large repertoire of beliefs, attitudes, and knowledge. Instructional theory in this constructionist approach[17] has been classified into three categories of teaching. Each will result in a different approach to nutrition education. First, the "transport of knowledge" type of teaching treats content as a commodity. Giving lectures, pamphlets, and newsletters, is an example of the transport of knowledge approach to teaching that Paul[18] calls the didactic approach. The teacher chooses content and presents it to the learner. The teacher might report that "I gave them the lesson," or "they got the diet instructions." Second, the "application of algorithms" type of teaching assumes that following a specific formula or routine will lead to learning new facts and skills. Following the steps of a curriculum (like a recipe), will result in the desired information or skill. The third type of teaching uses a "transfer of responsibility" model.[17] The teacher acts as facilitator, arranging experiences and structuring discovery or inquiry learning situations while the learner acts as an apprentice, developing new knowledge and skills under the guidance of a more experienced person. The transfer of responsibility is complete when the learner or apprentice can perform the desired skills without guidance.

B. CAPABILITY: HAVING RELEVANT SKILLS

Capability is different from cognition because it involves an action or a skill. Being capable of a new dietary behavior means that an individual not only knows what is expected but also has the ability to carry out an appropriate action. Capabilities targeted in nutrition education programs might be skills such as label reading in order to choose cereal that fits a whole-grain, high-fiber diet, cooking skills to substitute canola or olive oils for butter or margarine in food preparation, and choosing nutrient-dense food items when eating away from home. While eating at a restaurant, it is not enough to know that premixed salads tend to be high in fat; one must be able to ask the wait-staff to bring salad dressing "on the side" or to suggest substitutions. Knowing "how to do something," as opposed to knowing "about something," is sometimes referred to as *instrumental knowledge* as opposed to *procedural knowledge*. Both types of knowledge should be acquired; one does not substitute for another. A nutrition education program that includes skill development opportunities such as food shopping trips can enhance the learners' capability to make health-promoting food choices.

C. COMMITMENT AND CONFIDENCE: BELIEVING IN THE OUTCOMES

Most often, nutrition education revolves around the relationships of nutrition to health, such as eating five servings of fruits and vegetables a day to decrease risk of developing cancer. In the health field, there is accumulating evidence for the theory that "a personal sense of confidence and control not only enhances health but also produces a positive effect in terms of recovery from illness and the day-to-day management of personal health habits."[19] In both health behavior research and learning theory research, this sense of feeling self-confident and capable is linked to self-efficacy and locus of control issues, and has been shown to be related to an individual's actual health-promoting behavior.[20-22] Developing individual confidence together with competence or capability can contribute to desired behavior changes. "Nothing breeds success like success" should be the curriculum designer's motto to ensure that lessons are structured to teach simple skills and constructs before the more difficult ones. For example, plans for a fiber-rich menu might use small steps to build an understanding of the required dietary adjustments together with the confidence to be able to make those adjustments. A learner who knows that dietary fiber increases should be achieved slowly and that adequate fluid intake should accompany a fiber increase, and who understands what a reasonable amount of daily fiber intake is, can slowly gain confidence about making appropriate personal menu planning decisions in various situations.

Being knowledgeable, capable, and confident about following a modified eating pattern will yield only desired behaviors if the individual also makes the commitment to change. Nutrition educators strive to help learners develop the attitudes as well as the knowledge and the skills to make wise food-related choices day-in and day-out. Effective nutrition educators enable learners to develop self confidence to modify their diets. The terms "empowered" and "activated" are sometimes used to describe commitment and committed individuals who use their knowledge to solve problems and make decisions, whether diet-related or not.

Practicing positive nutritional health habits as an activated consumer requires nutrition knowledge (cognition and capability), commitment to act on this knowledge, and the confidence that one is capable of achieving the desired goals. These four C's of nutrition education: Cognition, Capability, Commitment, and Confidence, interact to support changed dietary behaviors. Together, these elements contribute to nutrition education that works.

V. THEORETICAL BASES FOR NUTRITION EDUCATION

Because food and nutrition behavior change is a complex subject, models for nutrition education can come from a variety of fields including communications, psychology, community organization, and motivational theory. The following brief synopsis highlights some of the more commonly used theories and examples of how they fit into nutrition education. The Contento et al.[2] review and the Glanz et al.[21] text are excellent resources for exploring these potential theoretical frameworks; they are useful development tools for nutrition educators. Theories underlying effective nutrition education programs help planners clarify their goals and typically include Social Cognitive Theory (pre-1986; the related framework was called Bandura's Social Learning Theory), the Health Belief Model, and Prochaska's Theory of the Stages of Change, also called the Transtheoretical Model.[20-23]

Bandura's Social Cognitive Theory explains human functioning in terms of three major interdependent components (examples in parentheses):

1. Behavior
   - The induction of psychological change (adopting a new attitude toward health-promoting snacks)
   - Generalization of change across situations (selecting whole grain instead of refined cereal, and also switching to whole grain bread and whole grain pasta)
   - Maintenance of change over time (drinking 1% milk instead of whole milk, in restaurants as well as at home)
2. Cognitive and other personal factors
   - Ability to use symbols (using label information to make food purchase decisions)
   - Using forethought or ability to visualize the future (limiting fatty foods during the week in order to "save up" for a weekend party)
   - Modeling or observational learning (mimicking exercise behavior of a respected role model, or "Jane uses mustard instead of mayo for bread so I do too")
   - self-regulatory ability, seeing discrepancies between one's own standards and potential actions (not eating the onion ring appetizer, even though friends are eating it, because of the decision to lose 10 pounds in the next half-year)
   - self-reflective capabilities and confidence in self (understanding that fitness requires consistent activity, and therefore sticking to one's walking plan, rain or shine)
3. Environmental supports
   - Change takes place within a social network; group members agree on group norms, including attitudes toward food and health (forming a walking group that brings water bottles on hikes rather than soda or "sport drinks")

- Community events and activities can support or sabotage personal change efforts (the cookie sale fund raiser makes dieting more difficult, while a fun-run or walk can promote health and fitness)

Bandura found that self-efficacy and mastery experiences were powerful predictors of behavior change; in other words, confidence in one's capabilities to make behavior changes successfully is followed by successful behavior change. Educators help learners achieve their goals when learners develop an "optimistic and resilient sense of personal efficacy."[20] In nutrition education, mastering nutrition knowledge and health-promoting eating patterns builds learners' well-being. Bandura said "self-doubters are easily wiped out." In other words, nothing breeds success like success.

The Health Belief Model explains the relationship between one's beliefs about a problem and one's subsequent behaviors. For instance, if one believes that the risks of a heart attack can be decreased by eating more vegetables and fruits as well as less saturated fat, then one is more likely to change dietary patterns in that direction. According to the Health Belief Model, whether one changes a behavior depends on the three following factors as well as the relationship among these factors (examples in parentheses):

1. Threat
   - Perception of susceptibility to the condition ("How likely is it that I will have a heart attack?")
   - Perception of seriousness of the condition ("Will a heart attack leave me permanently disabled?")
2. Outcome expectations
   - Perception of benefits of the action ("Will I live better if I skip my evening bowl of ice cream?)
   - Perception of barriers or costs of that action ("Will I miss my evening bowl of ice cream?")
3. Efficacy expectations
   - Perception of one's ability to carry out an action ("Will I be able to follow through on my good intentions to eat five servings of fruit and vegetables every day?")

The health belief model has been successfully used in smoking cessation programs.

The Transtheoretical Model (sometimes referred to as the Stages of Change Theory) integrates constructs from other psychological and behavioral theories and is currently being tested in nutrition education.[24] The Transtheoretical Model[21,25] suggests that nutrition interventions be tailored to the different psychological processes individuals undergo as they progress through change:

- Pre-contemplation (satisfied with the status quo)
- Contemplation (acknowledge a problem)
- Preparation (intention to make a change soon/within 6 months)
- Action (change in behavior)
- Maintenance (continuing the new behavior)

In some cases, such as substance addiction, there is an additional stage called termination (no further temptation, confidence to remain smoke-free).

To progress from one stage to the next, the individual makes a decision based on the benefits and costs of change. The decisional balance during the contemplation stage might be "less saturated fat in my diet improves my cardiac risk profile, which is important to my health because my father has heart disease," versus "I like the taste of cream in my coffee and don't want to give that up." Processes of change in this transtheoretical model include such factors as (examples in parentheses):

- Consciousness-raising (learning again that eggs are a nutrient-dense food and can easily be part of a healthy diet)
- Self-reevaluation (eating to become a more fit and healthier person is part of who I am)
- Helping relationships (a walking buddy makes fitness routines easier)
- Contingency management (planning ahead for ordering at a restaurant, acting in the belief that choosing the fruit dessert is more rewarding than eating the chocolate mousse)
- Stimulus control (not buying ice cream to keep at home)

There are other theoretical models for nutrition education; the Glanz et al.[21] text and the *Journal of Nutrition Education* are prime resources for readers seeking a deeper understanding of available options.

VI.   ENGAGING THE LEARNER TO CHANGE DIETARY PRACTICES

Opportunities to engage learners in nutrition education are everywhere. Figure 21.2 shows some common areas through which to reach adults, especially older adults. It shows some situations or areas that affect the dietary practices of adults, especially older adults. All of these arenas have potential as venues for nutrition education program development because they are channels through which people procure food and drink or information about eating and drinking. These are places to catch people's attention about their diets.

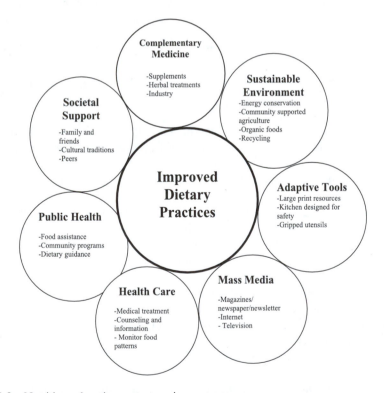

FIGURE 21.2   Nutrition education can occur in many arenas.

We do not know yet which instructional strategy will be effective for each specific audience under specified circumstances, but we do know that certain strategies result in increased knowledge, enhanced skills, and changed attitudes.[2,13] Effective instructional strategies include cooperative learning, inquiry learning, nutrition experiments, and working through academic controversies. The key is to engage the learner.

The following are examples of instructional strategies that engage older learners.

A. COOPERATIVE LEARNING

For cooperative learning, small groups or teams work together, exchanging information, teaching each other, *holding each other accountable* to achieve common goals, and providing support and assistance to each other. Key features of cooperative learning are goal achievement that stems from interdependent action, everyone sharing in responsibilities, a structured set of parameters, and group members participating as active learners. Cooperative learning is not simply working side-by-side as individuals in small groups.

Advantages	Disadvantages
Diverse groups share strengths, perspectives	Takes time to build group/team empathy
Makes use of knowledge from other content areas	Group may take longer to accomplish an outcome than
Once group is set, learners generate new information	an individual
More solutions are generated by the group than by one	Need commitment of learners and teacher to make it
Flexible method, it allows work with varied group sizes	work
(from 2 on up)	

Potential nutrition activities using cooperative learning:

- Develop a cable program on coping with special diets for diabetics.
- Participate in a community garden project.
- Compare food patterns of several cultures to develop a file of multicultural, health-promoting recipes.

B. INQUIRY LEARNING

Inquiry learning begins with a given problematic situation. Learners select data sources, gather and analyze information, describe the problem, and examine potential alternative solutions to the problem based on the collected data. Key features of inquiry learning are to identify data sources and investigate information to define the problem, to compare and contrast information, to determine what is not known but must be found out, and to seek missing information in order to reach conclusions. The discovery process of working to define and solve problems enhances analysis skills. Inquiry learning does not consist of looking up answers to specific questions such as "What is the fiber content of an apple?" or simply asking for the answer to a question.

Advantages	Disadvantages
Flexibility; learners can pursue a topic at their own speed and choose a specific direction	Learners who want direction may feel lost
Learners work out their own conclusion; it's not told to them	Need to allow enough time for learners to develop inquiry strategies (what is available and accessible to them: reference texts? interviews? Internet?)
Teacher doesn't need to think of all possible alternatives for potential answers; in fact, groups of learners can brainstorm many strategies and often generate more diverse answers	Learner needs to be able to distinguish types of information sources, such as distinguishing between accurate, objective information and biased information; learner must decide whether the bias affects the needed information, e.g., an advertising message for a food will be unlikely to present reasons it may not be a good food choice

Potential activities for inquiry learning:

- Play out scenarios related to food safety: What to bring to a social potluck and how to handle food items during and after the meal to keep food safe.
- Explore the organic food issue — local sources, reasons for use, differences in taste, price, nutrition, and storage requirements.
- Develop a plan to feed themselves nutritiously for a week on the current food stamp allowance (information needed includes food stamp eligibility requirements and food stamp allowances, grocery costs, what makes a meal nutritious, what is required to eat well for a week).

C. Nutrition Experiments

The experimental approach to nutrition education means trying out various approaches to a "problem" and comparing and evaluating the results. Key features of the experimental approach are that it uses trial and error to test ideas; uses experiments when there is a "what if" question; develops a "let's try it and see" attitude, because learning comes from the process of trying (what works, why; what didn't work, why not?). Nutrition experiments are not cooking vegetables by a single method without comparing alternatives such as cooking times, temperatures, ingredients, or taste. Learning from experiments relies on the comparison of alternative outcomes.

Advantages	Disadvantages
Attempting to forecast outcome stimulates curiosity	Only certain lessons can be learned through experiments
Maintains motivation through planning and in analyzing results	Can be costly; need facilities, materials, space
Reinforces analytical thinking about food, nutrition	Need time to plan and carry out experiments
Learners participate at their own level, arrive at their own conclusions	
Learners construct their own meanings to build structures for subsequent learning	

Potential nutrition experiment activities:

- Preserving garden produce by drying, freezing, refrigeration.
- Preparing foods by a variety of methods and comparing results (e.g., baked, pan-fried, broiled, or steamed hamburger patties).
- Making baked potatoes by various methods, in microwave and in oven, baking red and white, in foil or paper or unwrapped, then comparing results (time, energy used, resulting product texture, taste).

D. Structured Academic Controversies

Structured academic controversies in nutrition involve "having participants take opposing sides of an issue, explore their differences in opinion and information, and come to a consensus that incorporates the best ideas from both sides."[13] An academic controversy is similar to debate, in that parties examine and defend opposing views, but adds a step, namely that the group must arrive at consensus. Key features of the structured academic controversy method are that the educator chooses an issue that can be approached from two or more sides such as, "Should the government regulate the sale of vitamins and minerals?" Learners examine two or more sides of an issue through discussion, debate; the learner needs to pick a position on a topic and defend it; after positions are presented and discussed, the group continues discussion to arrive at consensus about the issue; it integrates both cooperative learning and inquiry learning into its process.

Advantages	Disadvantages
Having a position to defend engages and stimulates the learner to think through the topic	To properly develop academic controversies takes time and careful consideration of the learners' abilities, interests
Learners examine the issue in their own way, and in presenting their position, use information that is meaningful or relevant to them	Emotions may run high (good because the learner is engaged); requires a skilled, sensitive facilitator to diffuse when it goes too far
Topics chosen can mirror current dilemmas faced by learners and therefore help them develop useful coping strategies	Each learner's opinion must be treated with respect as group tries to reach consensus, need atmosphere of listening to each other
Practicing intellectual defense of a stance and anticipating opponents' arguments promotes critical (dialogical) thinking	

Potential activities using structured academic controversies:

- Examine the dietary guideline about limiting fat in the diet and apply it to proposed modifications of a senior nutrition program menu. Teams for and against the change would each present their cases, then both teams together would discuss the merits of the cases and decide on how they would proceed as a group. For teams of two, each individual would present either the pro or the con position, then each team would try to decide which recommendation to make.
- Explore and answer, "If vitamin D is a problematic nutrient for most older adults, should foods other than milk be fortified with vitamin D for the general public?" "Should vitamin/mineral supplements be regulated as drugs?"

The strategies named (cooperative learning, inquiry learning, nutrition experiments, and structured academic controversies) are effective because they use techniques that promote reflective thinking and support learner involvement. Based on reviews of nutrition education, behavior change theories, and the constructionist view of teaching, learner involvement or engagement is crucial to effective nutrition education.[2,17]

Curricular strategies to engage older learners must take into consideration some of the potential limitations associated with old age, such as declines in visual acuity and hearing loss. Figure 21.3 presents a summary of suggestions to enhance written materials.

- **12–16-point font**
- **Serif lettering**
- **Bold type**
- **High contrast (black on white)**
- **Avoid glossy paper to decrease glare**
- **Avoid blue, green, and violet (paper and print color) due to decreased ability to discriminate between these colors**
- **Use personal pronous such as I, you, we**
- **Short 10–12-word sentences**
- **5th- to 8th-grade reading level**

Figure 21.3   Tips for written nutrition education materials[26,27,28]

VII.　CONCLUSIONS

"You can't teach an old dog new tricks" is a cliche that does not apply to older adults. When material is perceived as relevant and useful to enhance personal health and well-being, older adults are likely to learn new dietary patterns. In fact, to achieve old age, an individual adjusts and adapts constantly. In *Living to 100*,[29] Perls and Silver found that the single thread connecting centenarians is their adaptive capability — they are resilient, dealing with the stresses of life efficiently and effectively. Adjusting eating patterns to support health can be one such mechanism for successful aging.

ACKNOWLEDGMENTS

The author wishes to thank Jennifer Bertrand, R.D., M.P.H. candidate at the University of Minnesota School of Public Health Nutrition Program, for selecting literature, preparing the figures, and providing constructive feedback for this chapter. Jennifer's work on this chapter was supported by the Marguerite J. Queneau Scholarship Fund.

REFERENCES

1. Maloney SK, Fallon B, Wittenberg CK. Executive summary. Aging and health promotion: Market research for public education. Washington, DC: Office of Disease Prevention and Health Promotion, U.S. Department of Health and Human Services, PHS, 1984.
2. Contento I, Balch GI, Bronner YL, et al. The effectiveness of nutrition education and implications for nutrition education policy, programs, and research: A review of research. *J Nutr Ed* 1995;27:339-46.
3. Goldberg JP, Gershoff SN, McGandy RB. Appropriate topics for nutrition education for the elderly. *J Nutr Ed* 1990;22:303-10.
4. Krinke UB. Nutrition information topic and format preferences of older adults. *J Nutr Ed* 1990;22:292-7.
5. Russell RM, Rasmussen H, Lichtenstein AH. Modified Food Guide Pyramid for people over seventy years of age. *J Nutr* 1999;129:751-3.
6. U.S. Department of Agriculture, U.S. Department of Health and Human Services. *Nutrition and Your Health: Dietary Guidelines for Americans*. Washington, DC: U.S. Government Printing Office, 1980.
7. Committee on Diet and Health (Food and Nutrition Board; National Research Council). *Diet and Health. Implications for Reducing Chronic Disease Risk*. Washington, DC: National Academy Press, 1989.
8. Pocinki KM. Writing for an older audience: Ways to maximize understanding and acceptance. *J Nutr Elderly* 1991;11:69.
9. Hutchings LL, Tinsley AM. Nutrition education for older adults: How Title III-C Program participants perceive their needs. *J Nutr Ed* 1990;22:53-8.
10. Hackman RM, Wagner EL. The Senior Gardening and Nutrition Project: Development and transport of a dietary behavior change and health promotion program. *J Nutr Ed* 1990;22:262-70.
11. Fries JF, Bloch DA, Harrington H, Richardson N, Beck R. Two-year results of a randomized controlled trial of a health promotion program in a retiree population: The Bank of America Study. *Am J Med* 1993;94:455-62.
12. Leigh JP, Richardson N, Beck R, et al. Randomized controlled study of a retiree health promotion program. The Bank of American Study. *Arch Intern Med* 1992;152:1201-6.
13. Johnson DW, Johnson RT. *Nutrition education: A model for effectiveness, a synthesis of research. J Nutr Ed* 1985;17:S44.
14. Maloney SK, White SL. *Nutrition Education for Older Adults: A Review of Research*. Alexandria, VA: U.S. Department of Agriculture Food and Nutrition Service, Office of Analysis and Evaluation, 1994.
15. Sims LS. Nutrition education research: Reaching toward the leading edge. *J Am Diet Assoc* 1987;87:S10-8.
16. Ness K, Elliott P, Wilbur V. A peer educator nutrition program for seniors in a community development context. *J Nutr Ed* 1992;24:91-4.

17. Thomas R, Johnson S, Anderson L. *Alternative Perspectives of Instruction and Cognitive Theory: Implications and Proposals*. Berkeley, CA: National Center for Research in Vocational Education, University of California at Berkeley, 1992.
18. Paul RW. *Critical Thinking: What Every Person Needs to Survive in a Rapidly Changing World*. Rohnert Park, CA: Center for Critical Thinking and Moral Critique, Sonoma State University, 1990.
19. Igoe J. Empowerment of children and youth for consumer self-care. *Am J Health Promotion* 1991;6:55-64.
20. Bandura A. *Social Learning Theory*. Englewood Cliffs, NJ: Prentice-Hall, 1977.
21. Glanz K, Lewis FM, Rimer BK. *Health Behavior and Health Education. Theory, Research, and Practice*. San Francisco, CA: Jossey-Bass, 1997.
22. Houts SS, Warland RH. Rotter's social learning theory of personality and dietary behavior. *J Nutr Ed* 1989;21:172-9.
23. Greene GW, Rossi SR. Stages of change for reducing dietary fat intake over 18 months. *J Am Diet Assoc* 1998;98:529-34.
24. Horwath C. Applying the transtheoretical model to eating behavior change. Seminar presented at the Division of Epidemiology, University of Minnesota. Minneapolis, MN, 1998.
25. Greene GW, Rossi SR, Reed GR, Willey C, Prochaska JO. Stages of change for reducing dietary fat to 30% of energy or less. *J Am Diet Assoc* 1994;94:1105-10.
26. Arditi A. *Making Text Legible: Designing for People with Partial Sight*. New York, NY: Lighthouse International, 1999.
27. Arditi A. *Effective Color Contrast: Designing for People with Partial Sight and Color Deficiencies*. New York: Lighthouse International, 1999.
28. Weinrich SP, Boyd M. Education in the elderly. Adapting and evaluating teaching tools. *J Gerontol Nurs* 1992;18:15-20.
29. Perls TT, Silver MH. *Living to 100. Lessons in Living to Your Maximum Potential at Any Age*. New York: Basic Books, 1999.

22 Nutritional Modulation of Neurodegenerative Disorders

Hunter Yost and Evan W. Kligman

CONTENTS

As healthcare providers move from a disease-focused model to health promotion and disease management based on patient uniqueness and evidence based medicine, their tools will include improved understanding of the genetic uniqueness of the patient, the factors that modify genetic expression and the intercellular modulators of function that give rise to increased risk of age-related disease.

Jeffrey Bland, Ph.D.
Improving Intercellular Communication in Managing Chronic Illness:
1999 Seminar Series Syllabus, Institute of Functional Medicine

I. INTRODUCTION

The emerging paradigm of the functional and nutritional medicine approach to chronic illnesses including neurodegenerative disorders offers clinicians and scientists a broader perspective for understanding and managing problems becoming increasingly prevalent in an aging society. In keeping with the theme of this book, the role of cruciferous vegetables, other nutrients, and herbs will be discussed. We will explore a variety of key biological processes and interactions that can lead to neurodegenerative disease and where effective evidence-based nutritional treatment programs can be devised: methylation defects (involving vitamins B-12, B-6, and folate) which lead to widespread neurologic damage from elevated levels of homocysteine; impairments in liver detoxification processes and their relationship to Parkinson's disease; disruption of intracellular communication through messenger molecules like nitric oxide and the relationship to dementia; and the increased levels of oxidative stress due to free radical damage contributing to most neurodegenerative diseases. Examples of functional and nutritional treatments for the following conditions will be provided: multiple sclerosis; epilepsy; Alzheimer's disease; and Parkinson's disease. Scientific documentation to support these nutritional approaches for impacting causative metabolic processes is provided as alternatives or complementary treatments to the new pharmaceutical "smart drugs." A wise physician once said, "If you are sitting on a nail, it's going to take a whole lot of aspirin to feel better." Indeed, by removing impediments to health, beneficial substances are much more likely to be effective.

This chapter is intended to be a brief overview of the role of nutrition in neurodegenerative conditions and is not intended as a treatment manual for these disorders. The reader is encouraged to consult with a physician knowledgeable in the area of functional medicine.

II. NUTRITIONAL MODULATION OF NEURODEGENERATIVE DISORDERS

A wealth of research over the past 10 to 15 years has confirmed that there are significant nutritional influences on genetic expression and mitochondrial functioning in the nervous system. In addition, mechanisms of nutritional regulation of detoxification processes in the liver and other organs that directly affect neuronal functioning have been studied. Steventon et al. point out that individuals who have a genetic propensity toward poor detoxification of specific compounds may run a higher risk for neurodegenerative diseases unless they can avoid exposure to these substances or improve the expression of genes involved with their detoxification (1). Researchers at Johns Hopkins School of Medicine recently suggested that the sulforaphane present in members of the cruciform family (broccoli, cabbage, cauliflower, Brussels sprouts) can increase the liver's ability to engage in phase II conjugation reactions, thus helping the body convert chemicals that might be cancer-producing into nontoxic substances. Animals given a concentrated extract of this substance derived from cruciferous vegetables are able to resist potentially cancer-causing chemicals (2). A possible role for sulforaphane in neurodegenerative disease has also been postulated.

Protection against both endo- and exotoxins appears to require proper gene expression of the xenobiotic detoxification pathways. A variety of nutrients are known to influence the activity of these pathways, including dietary sulfate, glutathione, N-acetylcysteine, glycine, pantothenic acid, vitamin C, and molybdenum (3). A simple noninvasive test exists to evaluate the body's detoxification processes, with critical implications for the nervous system. The acetaminophen challenge test involves an oral dose of acetaminophen followed by a urine collection of its metabolites to assess phase II glucuronidation, sulfation, or amine acid conjugation. Variations in phase II detoxification can be determined through the levels of acetaminophen conjugates, glucuronide, sulfate, or mercapturate. Difficulties in the body's ability to properly detoxify acetaminophen in this challenge test can be used as a metabolic marker of risk for a number of neurodegenerative diseases, including Parkinson's, where inadequate phase II sulfation and glutathione conjugation have been documented. (4, 5).

Research on the relationship between diet and various nutrients and nervous system function indicates that many neurotransmitters are synthesized from essential dietary nutrients. For example, serotonin is derived from tryptophan, the dopamine group of neurotransmitters from phenylalanine and tyrosine, and acetylcholine from choline, a B-complex nutrient. Choline, the precursor to acetylcholine, is not synthesized in the neurons and is primarily dependent on dietary intake. If there is not enough choline in the diet, CNS levels of acetylcholine decrease. Many studies have shown that cholinergic neurons decline with aging. Cholinergic neurons may be a "weak link" in age-related cognitive decline and Alzheimer's disease.

Innovative research by Wurtman at MIT suggests that where there is an unmet CNS need for choline-containing phospholipids necessary for the synthesis of acetylcholine, a process of auto-cannibalization of cholinergic neuronal membranes may result during times of stress, drug treatment, and disease. These conditions may increase the risk for neurodegenerative diseases such as Alzheimer's (6). At these times, increasing dietary choline-containing phospholipids, such as phosphatidylcholine or choline itself, may have a beneficial effect in maintaining cholinergic neuronal membrane integrity and CNS neuronal choline reserves. Wurtman's research indicates further that dietary composition may play an important role in increasing or reducing the risk of various age related neurodegenerative diseases.

Evidence accumulated over the past 20 years suggests that the pathogenesis of many neurological disorders may involve injury to the neurons resulting from overstimulation of receptors by excitatory amino acids. These disorders include stroke, hypoglycemia, epilepsy, chronic conditions such as Huntington's chorea, the neurodegeneration from AIDS, and possibly Alzheimer's and Parkinson's diseases. According to Perlmutter, "the cornerstone of this emerging model seems to focus on the critically important role of mitochondrial energy metabolism and its relationship to the toxic effects of excitatory neuro-transmitters. In this model, excitatory neuro-transmitters (predominately glutamate) stimulate specific neuronal receptors, which, when altered by deficient mitochondria ATP production, leads to a self perpetuating cascade of events ultimately culminating in neuronal death" (7). Understanding the importance of the NMDA receptor on the mitochondrial membrane, which is specific for the excitatory neurotransmitter glutamate, and its nutritional regulation can be of immense value in understanding functional neuronal processes in Parkinson's, Huntington's, and Alzheimer's diseases. The NMDA receptor, under normal conditions of mitochondrial ATP production, is blocked by the magnesium ion. When mitochondrial oxidative phosphorylation activity is decreased, changes in the transmembrane potential alleviate the magnesium block of the NMDA receptor. Then, under conditions of stimulation by glutamate during cerebral ischemia, neurotoxin exposure, or other sources of oxidative stress, there is an influx of calcium into the mitochondria. This calcium influx initiates a cascade of events leading to neuronal destruction including activation of nitric oxide synthase, increased free radical production, and activation of proteases and lipases.

Traditionally, amantadine, a NMDA antagonist, has been used to treat Parkinson's. Newer NMDA antagonists, such as gabapentin and riuzole, are also now available for treatment. Other pharmacological agents such as neurontin, lamotrigene, diphenylhydantion, and carbamazepine, are NMDA antagonists.. A Chinese herbal medicine, Huperzine A (Qian Ceng Tan), was recently reported in the *Journal of the American Medical Association* as a new treatment possibility for Alzheimer's disease. Huperzine A specifically inhibits glutamate stimulation of the NMDA receptor and has acetylcholinesterase inhibitory activity (8).

From a nutritional medicine perspective, upregulating neuronal mitochondrial activity through biochemical cofactors and dietary antioxidants is critical. Coenzyme Q10 has documented activity in transporting electrons in the mitochondria as well as functioning as an antioxidant in free radical scavenging activities. It has been shown to be effective in specific mitochondrial myopathies such as Kearn-Sayre syndrome and chronic progressive external opthalmoplegia (9). Idebenone, a coenzyme Q10 derivative with increased blood–brain barrier penetration, produced enhanced cerebral metabolism in a 36-year-old man with MELAS (mitochondrial myopathy, encephalopathy, lactic acidosis, and stroke-like episodes) during a 5-month treatment period with idenbenone up to 270 mg per day (10).

Acetyl-l-carnitine has been shown to increase ATP production, reduce production of mitochondrial free radicals, maintain transmembrane mitochondrial potential, and enhance NAD/NADH electron transfer (11). Thal and colleagues at the University of California San Diego evaluated the efficacy of acetyl-l-carnitine, 1 g t.i.d. for 12 months in a multicenter, placebo controlled study of 431 patients with Alzheimer's disease, 83% of whom completed the 1 year study. Their results showed "a trend for early onset patients on acetyl-l-carnitine to decline more slowly than early onset Alzheimer's patients on placebo" (11).

Phosphatidylserine (PS) is a naturally occurring phospholipid that is found in all cells of the body, with particularly high concentrations in the brain. PS is an essential cell membrane building block for nerve cells. As a unique phospholipid constituent of all known cell membranes, PS helps to ensure membrane integrity in conjunction with other phospholipids. PS enhances both neuronal and mitochondrial stability and activity, reduces mitochondrial free-radical production, and reduces cortisol production. Excessive cortisol levels have been associated with memory impairment and altered neuronal glucose metabolism. Researchers at Stanford treated a group of 149 patients meeting criteria for "age associated memory impairment" over a period of 12 weeks with either PS 100 mg t.i.d or placebo. Actual improvement on psychometric testing related to learning and memory was seen in a majority of patients in the treatment group, specifically those who had scored above the expected range of cognitive performance associated with dementing disorders such as Alzheimer's disease, but who were performing in the low normal range for persons' of the same age. The authors report "results of this study suggest that phosphatidylserine may be a promising compound for the treatment of memory deficits that frequently develop in the later decades of adulthood." Effects were present on a number of outcome variables related to important activities of daily living such as learning and recalling names, faces, and numbers (12–14).

Alpha lipoic acid, "the universal antioxidant" with its dual solubility in both water and lipid, is gaining support as a promising nutrient for neuronal protection in neurodegenerative disorders. It easily crosses the blood–brain barrier, acts as a chelator for ferrous iron, copper, and cadmium, and participates in the regeneration of endogenous antioxidants including vitamins E, C, and glutathione. An excellent review provides a solid framework for its clinical usage (15).

Glutathione, in the form of glutathione peroxidase, protects neurons from excessive ROS. Reduced levels of glutathione have been associated with neuronal damage from peroxynitrate and sulfite, two toxins commonly found in the food supply. Sulfite occurs in pollution and food preservatives. Peroxynitrate, an oxidant, results from nitric oxide combining from superoxide ions produced in immune reactions. These two toxins damage DNA protein, and lipids and may accelerate neuronal damage associated with Parkinson's disease. Consistent with these findings is the observation that the substantia nigra, where dopamine is produced in the brain, is often depleted of glutathione in patients with Parkinson's. Thus, adequate antioxidants, effective detoxification processes, and reduction or elimination of sulfites in the diet might protect against or attenuate the progression of Parkinson's and possibly other neurodegenerative disorders (16).

III. NITRIC OXIDE, NEURONAL TOXICITY, AND DIETARY MODULATION

Nitric oxide (NO) is a small, unstable molecule with one unpaired electron and is classified as a free radical. Its role in neurodegenerative diseases is now receiving considerable attention. NO is synthesized from l-arginine in the urea cycle through the action of nitric oxide synthase (NOS). Two forms of NOS have been identified, a constitutive and an inducible form. The inducible form is quantitatively increased in response to the stimulus/need for additional NO production. The constitutive form is relatively constant.

NOS-activated macrophages and various enzymes participate in the production of reactive oxygen species (ROS), which interfere with neuronal mitochondrial functioning. Simultaneous production of NO and ROS within the nervous system can result in the production of peroxynitrite, a powerful free-radical oxidant that can damage neurons and other cells.

Elevated levels of NOS have been found in the brains of patients with multiple sclerosis. NO may be involved in the pathogenesis of Alzheimer's disease (17). NO also plays a role in the cascade of events leading to neuronal death following glutamate stimulation of the NMDA receptor.

Research shows that nutritional insufficiencies and/or nutrient manipulations significantly influence the activity of NOS. Nutrients such as riboflavin, niacin, folate, B-12, l-arginine, omega-3 fatty acids, and antioxidants play important roles in modulating the function and activity of NOS. In fact, in the CNS, high levels of NO can react with the cobalt atoms in B-12 molecules . This can result in a functional deficiency of intracellular B-12 that would not be identified by measuring serum levels (18).

Maintaining a functional balance between NO and NOS production is desirable. In conditions where there is an insufficiency of NO, administration of l-arginine, B-12, folate and other B vitamins can be helpful. In conditions involving excess NO production, use of sulfur-containing antioxidants (glutathione, *N*-acetyl-cysteine, and lipoic acid) and coenzyme Q-10 may be helpful along with citrulline-rich foods, such as watermelon (100 mg of citrulline per 100 g of watermelon). Additionally, the administration of oral l-citrulline and l-lysine may help to reduce NO production (19).

IV. ENVIRONMENTALLY ACQUIRED NEUROTOXINS AND NEUROTOXIC METABOLITES

A report in the *Wall Street Journal* October 14, 1991 illustrated the clinical manifestations of an environmentally acquired neurotoxin. A man in his 40s experienced severe headache, nausea, dizziness, and eventually seizures after cutting his grass. He had fertilized his lawn earlier that day with diazinon, a common pesticide. After a thorough evaluation, he was diagnosed with pesticide poisoning. While many other homeowners had used diazinon without incident, health history revealed that this individual was taking cimetidine at the time of the incident. Cimetidine (Tagamet) is a known inhibitor of hepatic phase I P450 detoxification enzymes. Mr. Latimer suffered from an iatrogenically induced neurotoxicity because his detoxification processes were inactivated by cimetidine, causing neurologic damage.

Many other environmental chemicals have been identified as neurotoxic agents, such as the herbicide paraquat. Individuals exposed to paraquat have neurologic damage due to the release of superoxide (OH) in the brain (20).

Stress-induced catecholamines (i.e., norepinephrine and epinephrine) can adversely affect brain function and memory. Detoxification of catecholamines releases reactive oxygen species (ROS) and neurotoxic metabolites (i.e., adrenochrome). Since neuronal function is primarily generated within the mitochondria, situations of increased ROS will adversely affect this functioning. Stress can be considered to be a neurotoxic factor that can increase the risk for neurodegenerative diseases.

V. COMPREHENSIVE FUNCTIONAL AND NUTRITIONAL APPROACH FOR NEURODEGENERATIVE DISORDERS

The following approach may be useful to clinicians in treating various neurodegenerative diseases with nutritional interventions (21):

1. Recognize genetic susceptibilities through history and functional testing.
2. Nutritional support for detoxification of both endo- and exotoxins.
3. Nutritional support of neuronal mitochondrial oxidative-phosphorylation.
4. Nutritional support for the reestablishment of appropriate (balanced) redox.
5. Reduce excess dysfunctional activation of the immune and adrenal systems by lowering antigenic load and stress factors.

VI. EXAMPLES OF NUTRITIONAL FACTORS IN SPECIFIC NEURODEGENERATIVE CONDITIONS

A. MULTIPLE SCLEROSIS

In multiple sclerosis (MS), there is increased risk of macrocytosis, low serum/CSF vitamin B12, and raised homocysteine; MS and pernicious anemia have very similar epidemiology and B12 is critical for myelin synthesis (22).

Elevated levels of nitric oxide synthase (NOS) have been found in the brains of patients with MS (23). Nutritional approaches that increase dietary citrulline help to reduce nitric oxide formation. (watermelon, *citrullus vulgaris*, contains 100 mg/100 g of citrulline) (24).

Supplementation with magnesium, vitamin D, and cod liver oil decreased the number of exacerbations over a 1- to 2-year period by 50% in a group of MS patients with unambiguous exacerbations during the 12 to 24 months prior to the study (25). Studies show a high prevalence of vitamin D deficiency in patients with multiple sclerosis (%).

Swank and Dugan found that increasing cod liver oil intake is normally accompanied by a decrease in saturated fat intake by as much as 2 g for every 1 g increase, suggesting that decreased saturated fat intake might be a factor contributing to improvement(25).

Other beneficial dietary changes that might slow the progression of MS include minimizing protein intake, avoiding polyunsaturated oils, using black currant oil, and eating sardines or flaxseed as a source of omega-3 essential fatty acids.

B. EPILEPSY

Thiamine deficiency may be associated with risk of seizures. In one study, patients with a diagnosed thiamine deficiency had epileptiform manifestations on EEG that were attributable to the deficiency state. Thiamine deficiency may provoke epileptic manifestations in patients who have a subclinical predisposition to seizures (26).

Based on their urinary glycoprotein-peptide complex patterns, four epileptic children with autistic syndrome who were receiving anticonvulsants were treated with either a gluten-free and milk-reduced, or a milk-free and gluten-reduced diet. Three out of the four children had a reduction in seizure frequency. In addition, urinary peptide secretion was reduced and some behaviors improved (27).

Carnitine is an amino acid that is excreted in large amounts when antiseizure medications such as valproic-acid or carbamazepine are taken, leading to hepatotoxicity. Carnitine supplementation is effective in reducing valproic acid-associated hyperammonemia (28).

C. ALZHEIMER'S DISEASE

A study in 1997 showed that 2000 IU of vitamin E daily delayed admission to a nursing home by an average of 230 days over placebo for patients with Alzheimer's disease (AD). Dr. Graff-Radford, a neurologist at the Mayo Clinic, Jacksonville, Florida, recommends giving vitamin E in the early stages of AD. Patients on warfarin and high-dose vitamin E are at risk of hemorrhage (30).

Estrogen replacement and anti-inflammatory medications may also be protective. The relative risk of developing AD may be reduced to as low as 0.40 in patients taking NSAIDS (31). In a trial using indomethacin, modest improvement in cognitive functioning was noted among the treatment group vs. an eight-fold decline in the placebo group (32). With estrogen replacement therapy, a relative risk was 0.46 as compared with nonusers (33). The mechanism of action appears to be estrogen's role as an antioxidant and in stimulating neuronal development in the limbic system, cerebral cortex, and basal forebrain. Estrogen also appears to improve the growth of cholinergic neurons. Further, NMDA receptors in the hippocampus are regulated by estratrienes, which develop with estrogen interaction with glutathione (34).

One hundred patients aged 55 or older, with a clinical diagnosis of AD, including 76 patients with histologically confirmed AD, were compared with 108 controls. Results showed that total homocysteine levels were significantly higher, and serum folate and B-12 levels were lower in patients with AD than controls. In a 3-year follow-up with the AD patients, radiological evidence of disease progression was greater among those with higher homocysteine levels at entry to the study. The stability of these findings over time and the lack of relationship with the duration of symptoms argue against these findings being a consequence of the disease (35).

Nutrients such as B-1, ginkgo biloba, NADH, and zinc are noted to have a positive effect in AD. However, single evaluation of any nutrient against a chronic disease will probably yield minimal results. Every patient with a neurological disorder, according to Hamilton, should have

B-1, folate, B-12, total homocysteine, and methylmalonic acid levels, as well as amino acid and essential fatty acid profiles (36).

Electron transport defects have also been noted in AD. This defect may render neuronal cells more sensitive to environmental toxins and lead to mitochondrial encephalopathies (37). Similar defects have been found in Parkinson's disease (PD).

D. PARKINSON'S DISEASE

In evaluating 5342 independently living individuals without dementia between 55 and 95 years of age, including 31 individuals with PD, the odds ratio for PD was 0.5 per 10 mg daily vitamin E intake, 0.06 per 1 mg beta carotene intake, 0.09 per 100 mg vitamin C intake, and > 0.09 per 10 mg flavanoid intake. The association for vitamin E intake was dose-dependent. A high dose of vitamin E may be protective against the occurrence of Parkinson's disease (38).

In an open trial of 885 patients with PD, half of these patients received NADH by intravenous infusion over 30 minutes, and another group of patients obtained 5 mg NADH orally by capsules. Both the infused and the oral treatments were given every other day for 14 days. In about 80% of patients, a beneficial clinical effect was observed (39).

Intake of specific foods and food groups have also been associated with risk of developing PD. Those subjects with higher potato consumption had an odds ratio of 0.43, and those with a history of consuming red meat had an odds ratio of 1.78 in a study by Hellenbrand et al. (40). Increased intake of animal products may increase the risk of PD by as much as 5.3 times (41).

Metabolic differences have also been noted in patients with PD. For instance, those with an inherited CYP2D6 cytochrome P450 enzyme had an increased risk of 2.4 times for developing the condition (42).

VII. CONCLUSIONS

Research over the past 15 years has suggested that functional and nutritional medicine approaches to the neurodegenerative diseases may help reduce the risk as well as the progression of certain chronic conditions. Mechanisms of action include dietary supplementation with vitamins and/or herbs to attenuate key biological processes such as impaired methylation, environmental neurotoxins and neurotoxicity, impaired detoxification, oxidative stress, and impaired mitochrondrial function. Essential to the investigation of possible causative or promoting agents of neurodegenerative disorders is recognition of the individual's unique biochemical and genetic susceptibilities, identification of various toxic (including pharmaceutical) exposures, oxidative stress load, and existing nutrient deficiency states. Important in the therapeutic aspects of intervention is nutritional support for optimal mitochondrial function, reestablishment of appropriate redox, and reduction of excess dysfunctional activation of immune and adrenal systems.

REFERENCES

1. Steventon GB, Heafield MT, Waring RH, Williams AC. Xenobiotic metabolism in Parkinson's disease. *Neurology* 39:883-887, 1989.
2. Zhang Y, Tallalay P, Cho CG, Posner GH. A major inducer of anticarcinogenic protective enzymes from broccoli: Isolation and elucidation of structure, *Proc. Nat. Acad. Sci.* 89; 2399-2403, 1992.
3. McFadden, SA. Phenotypic variation in xenobiotic metabolism and adverse environmental response: Focus on sulfur-dependent detoxification pathways. *Toxicology* July 17:111(1-3):43065, 1996.
4. Tanner CM, Liver enzyme abnormalities in Parkinson's disease. *Geriatrics*, August 46:60-63, 1991.
5. Standard liver detoxification profile performed by Great Smokies Diagnostic Laboratory, Ashville, North Carolina, U.S. (1-800-522-4762).

6. Wurtman RJ, Zeisel SH. Brain choline: Its sources and effects on the synthesis release of acetylcholine. *Aging;* 19:303-313, 1982.

7. Perlmutter D. Functional therapeutics in nerodegenerative disease. *Sixth International Symposium on Functional Medicine syllabus,* 1999.

8. Skolnick A. Old Chinese herbal medicine used for fever yields possible new Alzheimer's disease therapy. *JAMA* March, 1997.

9. Bresolin N, et al. Clinical and biochemical correlations in mitochondrial myopathies treated with coenzyme Q-10,. *Neuro* June 38(6): 892-9, 1988.

10. Ikejiri Y. et al. Idebennone improves cerebral mitochondrial oxidative metabolism in a patient with MELAS. *Neuro* 47:583-585, 1996.

11. Thal LJ. A one year multi-center placebo controlled study of Alzeheimer's disease. *Neuro* 47: 705-711, 1996.

12. Crool TH et al. Effects of phosphotidylserine in aged-associated memory impairment. *Neuro* 41:644-649, 1991.

13. Lombardi GF et al. Pharmacological treatment with phostidylserine of 40 ambulatory patients with senile dementia syndrome, *Minerve Med* 80: 599-602, 1989.

14. Delwaide PJ et al. A double blind randomized controlled study of phosphatidyl serine in senile demented patients. *Acta Neurol Scand* 73:136-1986.

15. Packer L et al. Neuroprotection by the metabolic antioxident alpha lipoic acid. *Free Radical Biology Med;* 22:359-378, 1997

16. Marshall K-A et al. The neuronal toxicity of sulfite plus peroxynitrate is enhanced by glutathione depletion: Implications for Parkinson's disease. *Free Radical Medicine;* 27(5):515-520, 1999.

17. Bagasra O. Activation of the inducible form of nitric oxide synthase in the brains of patients with multiple sclerosis. *Proc Natl Acad Sci USA* Dec 19: 92 (26); 12041-5, 1995.

18. Flippo TS, Holder WD. Neurologic degeneration associated with nitrous oxide anesthesia in patients with vitamin B12 deficiency. *Arch Surg.* 128;1391-1395, 1993.

19. Larrick JW. Metabolism of arginine to nitric oxide: An area for nutritional manipulation of human disease? *J Optimal Nutr.* 3(1):22-31, 1994.

20. Liu D, Yang J, McAdoo D. Paraquat, a superoxide generator kills neurons in the rat spinal cord. *Free Rad Biol Med.* 18(5):861-867, 1995.

21. Bland J. New perspectives in nutritional therapies: Improving patient outcomes. *Functional Neuro.* 1996.

22. Reynolds, EH. Multiple sclerosis and vitamin B-12 metabolism. *J Neuroimmunology,* 1992; 40.

23. Larick JW. Metabolism of arginine to nitric oxide: An area for nutritional manipulation of human disease? *J Optimal Nutr.* 3 (1):22-31, 1994.

24. Goldberg P et al. Multiple sclerosis: Decreased relapse rate through dietary supplementation with calcium, magnesium and vitamin D. *Med Hypothesis* 21 (2):193-200, 1986.

25. Swank RL, Dugan BB. Effects of low saturated fat diet in early and late cases of multiple sclerosis. *Lancet* 336:37-39, 1990.

26. Nieves, J et al. High prevalence of vitamin D deficiency and reduced bone mass in multiple sclerosis. *Neurology* September 1994.

27. Keyser A. Epileptic manifestations and vitamin B-1 deficiency. *Euro Neurol.* 31:121-5, 1991.

28. Reichelt KL et al. Gluten, milk proteins and autism: Dietary intervention effects on behavior and peptide secretion. *J Appl Nutr.* 42 (1):1-11, 1990.

29. Kelly RI, The role of carnitine supplementation in valproic acid therapy. *Ped* June, 93 (6): 891-892, 1994.

30. Zwillich T, Vitamin E high on list of Alzeheimer's therapies. *Family Practice News* 27, August 15,1999.

31. Stewart WF et al. Risk of Alzheimer's disease and duration of NSAID use. *Neurology,* March 1997.

32. Rogers, J et al. Clinical trial of indomethacin in Alzheimer's disease. *Neurology,* August 1993.

33. Kawas MD et al. A prospective study of estrogen replacement therapy and the risk of developing Alzheimer's disease. *Neurology,* June 1997.

34. Green PS et al. Nuclear estrogen receptor-independent neuroprotection by estratrienes: a novel interaction with glutathione. *Neuroscience* May 1998.

35. Clarke et al. Folate B-12, and serum homocysteine levels in confirmed Alzheimer's disease. *Arch Neurology* Nov. 1998: 55: 1449-1455.

36. Hamilton K. Comment on Alzeheimer's conditions. *Clinical Pearls News* 9(3), March 1999.

37. Parker WD et al. Electron transport defects in Alzheimer's diseased brains. *Neurology* (44), 1994.

38. de Rijk, MC, "Dietary Antioxidents and Parkinson's disease: The Rotterdam Study", *Arch Neurol.* 54: June 1997762-765.

39. Birkmeyer, JG et al. Nicotinamide adenine dinucleotide (NADH) - A new therapeutic approach to Parkinson's disease: Comparisons of oral and parenteral applications, *Acta Neurol Scand*, 87: suppl. 146:32-35, 1993.

40. Hellenbrand, W et al. Diet and Parkinson's disease: A possible role for the intake of specific foods and food groups. *Neurology* September 1996.

41. Logroscino, C et al. Dietary lipids and antioxidants in Parkinson's disease: a population-based, case-controlled study. *Ann Neurol*, January 1996.

42. Chan P. Genetically determined differences in xenobiotic metabolism as a risk factor in Parkinson's disease. *Fundam Appl Toxicol.* (30), 1996.

23 Antioxidants as Therapies of Diseases of Old Age

Teresa Bermejo Vicedo and
Francisco Jose Hidalgo Correas

CONTENTS

I. INTRODUCTION

The production and action of free radicals (FRs) have been linked to the general aging process, as it is known that these substances generated constantly in living cells lead to a series of changes in the body that contribute to this phenomenon. The FRs are oxidizing substances to which the various organs and systems of the body react in different ways as well as being able to change their different mechanisms according to the damage produced by Frs. As a result, FRs may form part of the etiology leading to aging and the degenerative processes associated with age in the various organic systems of humans. It is also necessary to consider that other substances in the body, known as antioxidants (AO), compensate for the harmful effects of FRs and represent an important defense mechanism against oxidative stress. These substances also have antiaging properties and specific protective functions for some diseases.

In an experimental model with animals, Ambrosio et al.[1] showed that old cells cannot produce antioxidant enzymes, thus leading to the accumulation of high levels of FR reacting with other molecules in the cell to cause damage. For these researchers, the lengthening of lifetimes is connected with a diminished production of FRs and, as a result, a reduction in the damage they cause, in the same way as a reduction in longevity would be related to an increase in FR levels. Kyriazis[2] argued that the biological study of aging is especially important for the study of illness, suggesting the existence of three factors involved in the aging process: genetic predisposition, physical injury, and the inability of the human body to repair such injury.

On many occasions, great age is associated with chronic illnesses responsible for a large number of disabilities. Many of these disabilities are associated with the action of FRs, including arteriosclerosis, cancer, diabetes-related complications, cataracts, Alzheimer's and Parkinson's diseases, amyotrophic lateral sclerosis, reperfusion ischemia, senile macular degeneration, rheumatoid arthritis, respiratory distress syndrome, sepsis, ulcerative colitis, and Crohn's disease. In such situations, the primary prevention of these conditions through the administration of antioxidants should be a specific and important aim.[3]

The present chapter will review the formation of FRs in the cell and the mechanisms compensating their harmful effects through the so-called antioxidants, which might be described as endogenous or exogenous, depending on their origin. We will describe their mechanism of action, the recommended doses and administration methods, and the last part will include a review of the various diseases currently related with the action of FRs in elderly patients.

II. SOURCES FOR THE PRODUCTION OF FREE RADICALS OR OXIDIZING MOLECULES AND THEIR EFFECTS ON THE BODY

In living organisms, there are many chemical compounds with two or more elements linked by bound electrons in covalent pairs allowing them to remain stable. Several factors may cause this binding to be broken, giving rise to a loss of stability in the molecule and the generation of free radicals. The causes leading to this molecular break-up include the presence of preexisting FRs, energy, and various enzymes.[4-7]

FRs are chemical compounds with or without a charge and with an unpaired electron in their outermost orbit. As a result, they are extremely reactive and cause chemical chain reactions leading to cell damage.[1-3] For this reason, it is necessary to establish defense mechanisms to cut short these reactions, either through an antioxidant or by means of the interconnection of two FRs.[7]

The FRs produced in the body as cell metabolism products include active oxygen compounds (AO), lipidic radicals, and hemo-group related radicals.[7]

In aerobic organisms, 98% of O_2 is required for cell feasibility and is used as the final sum of the electrons coming from the oxidation of the immediate substances by converting them to water. It is involved in many basic reactions generating intermediate compounds such as super-oxide and hydroxyl radicals (AO), unstable molecules[5-7] requiring the action of antioxidants to prevent potential cell damage. These AO are generated by many different routes in living beings. Other compounds such as oxygen singlets and hydrogen peroxide are also generated and, in the presence of free transition metals (particularly iron and copper), these generate the hydroxyl radical, which is extremely reactive. It has lately been assumed that this molecule is initially responsible for the oxidative destruction of biomolecules.[8]

There are various endogenous sources in living organisms for the production of FRs, the most important being the mitochondrial electron transport chain, the metabolism of fatty acids into peroxisomes, the reactions of cytochrome P450 and phagocytic cells,[7,8] formed by the action of various intracellular enzymes (oxidases, cyclooxygenases, lipoxygenases, dehydrogenases, peroxidases) of the different small organs (mitochondria, lysosomes, peroxisomes, nucleus, endoplasmic reticulum, plasma membrane and cytosol). Similarly, the phagocytic cells attack pathogenic particles with a mixture of oxidants and FRs including the oxygen singlet, hydrogen peroxide, nitrite, and hypochlorite.[9-11] In infections, neutrophils are stimulated by the capture of oxygen to form AO and also, if they are stimulated by the action of myeloperoxidase, which produce halogenated compounds that kill off bacteria through phagocytosis in vacuoles.[7]

There are other mechanisms for the production of FRs in various organs, and many investigator groups are researching their potential relationship with the origin of illnesses such as Alzheimer's disease, Parkinson's disease, and other degenerative conditions considered below.

Free radicals mainly act on biological macromolecules (lipids, nucleic acids, and proteins), damaging them through oxidation. Their main effect **on lipids** is lipidic peroxidation of the unsaturated lipids in the cell membrane, producing a loss of fluidity and alterations in the membrane protein bonds and finally cell destruction. In the peroxidation process, the hydroperoxyl radical is formed, and this maintains the oxidating process until it is stopped by the antioxidant molecules. If this lipid peroxidation process is not interrupted, it will give rise to the creation of reactive cyclical endoperoxides and unsaturated aldehydes, which might act as mutagenic agents, disable enzymes, or react with proteins and nucleic acids.[12-14] **On nucleic acids,** the FRs damage the DNA and may produce mutagenesis and carcinogenesis. **With enzymes,** also through thiol groups (-SH) and other proteins, the FRs bring about their deactivation and denaturalization, producing the oxidation of sulfhydryl groups, peptide fragmentation, breaking of bonds between proteins, etc., and finally, they act on **carbohydrates** by altering the cell functions such as those associated with the activity of interleukins and the formation of prostaglandins, hormones, and neurotransmitters.

III. ANTIOXIDANT SUBSTANCES

The **antioxidant defenses** are to be found in the body's cell compartments in the form of **enzymatic and nonenzymatic antioxidants.** The **nonenzymatic** ones are found naturally in the diet and include vitamins (A, C, E, -carotenes), taurine, cysteine, and glutathione (GSH). These absorb the FRs from the intracellular and intravascular spaces. The **enzymatic antioxidants** include metallo-enzymes containing selenium as glutathione peroxidase, superoxide dismutases, and catalases.[4]

Apart from these two types of defense mechanisms, there are transition metal sequestration systems. Transition metals like iron and copper are involved as catalysts in redox reactions, and it is therefore very important for these metal ions to be stored safely in proteins such as ceruloplasmin and transferrin, rather than ferritin and lactoferrin.[4,15] On the other hand, several substances exist such as calcium channel blockers, nonsteroid antinflammatory drugs, manitol, albumin, and glutamine, which work as exogenous antioxidants.

There now follows a description of the basic characteristics of the natural antioxidants: vitamins E, A, C, selenium, and GSH, their mechanism of action, pharmacokinetics, side effects, and toxicity profile. Although there are other micronutrients forming part of the antioxidants enzymes (Zn, Cu, Mn, Fe), there is currently insufficient literature on the subject for the role of these substances to be clearly defined alongside the free radicals in the development of certain pathologies.

A. Vitamin E

This is the name given to a group of natural liposoluble antioxidants (tocopherols and tocotrienols) found in the oils of certain plants (soybean, safflower, and corn), vegetable oil products (margarine), nuts and seeds, whole grains, wheat germ, and green, leafy vegetables. Their biological activity is due to alpha-tocopherol. vitamin E is a liposoluble vitamin.

Vitamin E (tocopherol) is the most prevalent antioxidant in the cell membrane and prevents the onset and propagation of lipidic peroxidation due to FRs, thus preserving the membrane's integrity.[16] It can also be found in organic fluids and inside the cell in connection with LDL and other lipidic molecules.[4] Its effect is carried out through the capture of FRs in the biological membranes and its transformation into the neutral stable radical, tocopheril, which gives rise to vitamin E through the participation of GSH and vitamin C[4,6]; this system means that the reduced form of vitamin E[16] remains at stable concentrations. Tocopherol can also react with the oxygen singlet.[7]

When vitamin E is not available in the body at a suitable concentration, there is an increase in the degree of lipidic and protein oxidation, thus leading to the destruction of the cell functions and the inactivation of cell enzymes.[16] It also has an important role to play in immunocompetence through an increase in the production of humoral antibodies, resistance to bacterial infections, cell immunity, the response of T lymphocytes, the production of tumor necrosis factor (TNF), and the activity of the natural killer cells. It inhibits the formation of mutagens and nitrosamines, avoiding damage to the DNA.

Vitamin E is absorbed in the intestine, for which it requires the presence of bile. If there is no bile or pancreatic juices, absorption is very limited, and this may lead to a deficit of this vitamin in patients with biliary obstruction, choleostatic disease, pancreatitis, and cystic fibrosis. It is distributed together with lipoproteins, mostly VLDL and LDL, and is released into tissues for storage (adipose tissue, liver, muscle). The plasma levels are related to the total amount of plasma lipids, but this does not indicate an appropriate status of vitamin E reserves. Thus, in hypolipidemias, even though the lipid levels are low, the vitamin E reserves might not be. In hyperlipidemias, the opposite situation might occur.[17-19]

The liver is responsible for controlling alpha-tocopherol in plasma and for releasing it into the peripheral tissues. As a result, patients with alcohol-related hepatic disease or hemochromatosis may have diminished concentrations of plasma alpha-tocopherol. Blood concentration level is 0.7 to 2 mg/dl and it is excreted through the kidneys.[17-19]

A deficiency in this vitamin may lead to hemolytic anemia, neuronal degeneration, edema, hemorrhage, reticulocytosis, and thrombocytosis.[17,19] On the other hand, the symptoms of the toxic effects of hypervitaminosis are fatigue, weakness, nausea, headache, blurred vision, flatulence, and diarrhea. These are generally mild and transitory conditions, and it has been shown that, in patients receiving dosages of between 200 and 1,000 IU/day over periods of more than 11 years, only 0.6% of them presented any gastrointestinal side effects, dermatitis, or fatigue.[20]

In a clinical trial carried out by Meydani et al.,[21] it was concluded that the supplementary administration of alpha-tocopherol at doses less than or equal to 60 to 800 IU/day had no adverse effects on elderly patients and improved their immune function.

Vitamin E cannot be administered together with oral anticoagulants, as it may increase the risk of excessive bleeding; its supplementary administration at high doses in patients with malabsorption of vitamin K may even exacerbate clotting disorders.[20]

B. Vitamin A

Nature provides carotenoids (pro-vitamin A) as well as the compounds retinol, retinoic acid, and retinal and its esters. The beta-carotenes (pro-vitamin A) are converted to retinol in the intestinal mucosa; the ester forms of retinol are changed into retinol by the action of pancreatic esterases. It is a liposoluble vitamin found in yellow vegetables (cantaloupe, carrots) and green leafy vegetables, and yellow-orange fruits.

Beta-Carotene is the main precursor of vitamin A, an antioxidant found together with vitamin E in the cell membranes of lisosomes and microsomes. These may prevent the peroxidation induced by the oxygen singlet and by other FRs among the liposomal membranes.[22]

It is absorbed in the small intestine, requiring for the purpose the presence of biliary salts, pancreatic lipase, and dietary fat. It is stored in the liver (80–90%), the retina, lungs, and kidneys. It is distributed through the retinol-bound protein complex (RBP). The plasma concentration of

RBP is 40 to 50 µg/ml (without the presence of malnutrition). Normal serum concentrations of vitamin A are 30 to 80 mcg/dl. It is excreted in the bile.[17,19]

Vitamin A deficiency produces xerophthalmia, night blindness, keratinization, and an increased incidence of infections.

When β-carotenes are taken orally to the point where they produce a concentration in blood of 0.4 mg/dl, they may lead to carotenodermia (a reversible and benign yellowish coloring of the skin). Rarely, there have also been cases reported of arthralgias, echimosis, and diarrhea.[20]

The safety of vitamin A has been established at doses between 15 and 50 mg/day. It must be administered with caution in patients with liver and kidney conditions.[20]

C. Vitamin C

Vitamin C is found in nature in citrus fruits and vegetables, including tomatoes, potatoes, green and red peppers, and green leafy varieties (spinach, collard greens). It is a hydrosoluble vitamin. It is a scavenger of superoxide, hydroxyl, and nitrosyl radicals, producing the breakdown of the FR chain reactions. It inhibits the conversion of nitrites into nitrosamines and nitrosamides, which are carcinogenic.[23,24] It increases the immune response.[17]

Vitamin C is involved in the body's redox cycles by transferring hydrogen ions. vitamin C is a redox agent that behaves like an antioxidant when taken with the diet. If it is taken as a dietary supplement, it may act as an antioxidant or as an oxidant, depending on the circumstances: it acts as an oxidant when it is administered together with iron or when there are high iron reserves in the body.[25] Its administration is, therefore, contraindicated in patients with hemochromatosis and in those cases requiring an extra dose of iron.[20]

Vitamin C is absorbed in the small intestine by a saturable transporter, thus implying that very high doses do not lead necessarily to increased absorption. The maximum capacity of absorption is achieved at doses of 3 g/day. Its storage within the body is limited (20 mg/kg), so that this will be the maximum level attained even with excess consumption.

The concentration in serum must be 0.2 mg/dl. It is excreted through the kidneys, by means of tubular resorption in an active and saturable process that may compete with the excretion of uric acid. Its main metabolite is in the form of an oxalate of which the amount produced daily varies between 30 and 40 mg, with 30 to 40% of it being excreted per day.[17,19]

Vitamin C deficiency produces delays in the healing of wounds, petechiae, echimosis, perifollicular hemorrhage, bleeding spongy gums, irritability and, in the most extreme cases, with the onset of scurvy.

Administration of vitamin C may lead to the formation of oxalate and urate kidney stones, either because it is taken per os at high doses or following intravenous administration, as well as in patients with prior chronic kidney failure.[26,27]

The administration of 100 mg three times a day over 8 weeks produced an increase of 12% in the number of leukocytes, whereas a daily dose of 2 g over 15 days diminished antibacterial activity.[28]

Side effects have been observed at the gastrointestinal level when it is taken at high doses. These include local esophagitis caused by prolonged contact with the mucosa, stomach cramps, nausea, and diarrhea, mainly osmotic.[17]

D. Glutathione

Glutathione is a tripeptide of great importance as a catalyst. It acts as an antioxidant and takes part in the redox cycle, where the reduced GSH is also capable of capturing FRs and peroxides directly through oxidation to GSSG, preventing the lipidic oxidation of the cell membrane and its subsequent harmful effect on cell functions.[29] But it also forms part of the antioxidant enzymes capturing FRs. It has been shown to be more effective than catalase in the detoxification of hydrogen peroxide.

GSH has an important role to play in organs exposed to exogenous toxins, such as the liver, kidneys, lung, and intestine and in other organs with lower concentrations of other antioxidant enzymes (SOD and catalase).

The greatest concentration of GSH is found in the fluids of the respiratory tract, where it acts as the captor of inhaled toxins and FRs produced by the activated phagocytes in the lungs.[29] It may be depleted when there is oxidative stress, such as in the presence of atmospheric pollutants, tobacco smoke and during antitumor therapy.[29]

The role of GSH in various pathologies such as acute respiratory distress syndrome, acquired immunodeficiency syndrome, aging, and kidney diseases is currently under investigation.[29] It also has an important role as an antidote in cases of poisoning.

GSH is known to exist at low concentrations in the elderly, associated with the increased risk of chronic diseases such as kidney failure, malignant illnesses, diabetes, alcoholism, Parkinson's disease, and the formation of cataracts. Julius et al.[30] measured the GSH concentrations in 33 patients between 60 and 79 years of age and related the health index, number of illnesses, and other chronic illness risk factors, proving the existence of a direct relationship between the highest concentrations of GSH and increased age with good health in all the age groups. They also found that people with chronic diseases had lower concentrations of GSH than those who were free of disease.

Nutall et al.[31] also determined the plasma concentrations of GSH and lipidic hydroperoxides in healthy young people, adults, and elderly volunteers as well as in elderly nonhospitalized patients with chronic diseases and elderly patients admitted to hospital with acute illnesses. The markers of oxidative damage were low in healthy youths, high among healthy adults, and even higher among the sick elderly than among the healthy ones. For this reason, they concluded that aging is associated with a reduction of AO in plasma and an increase in oxidation damage even among elderly volunteers in good health. Acute severe ill health requiring admission to hospital is associated with a change in the levels of AO and greater oxidative damage.

E. SELENIUM

Selenium forms part of the antioxidant enzymes. It is a key component of glutathione peroxidase, which has been shown to prevent the growth of some types of cancer. The levels of selenium in cereals and plants depend on the soil content. Some foods such as garlic, fungi, and asparagus also have a high percentage of this micronutrient.

It may be an essential component for the protection of the coronary endothelium against oxidative damage. It is currently known that there is an inversely proportional relationship between the concentrations of selenium and the severity of coronary arteriosclerosis.[20]

IV. FUNCTIONS OF THE ANTIOXIDANTS ON IMMUNITY

The evidence that micronutrients have a positive influence on the immune function in the elderly has been shown in clinical trials with micronutrients on their own and in combination. It is a known fact that aging reduces the production of antibodies, the mass of thymic tissue, hypersensitivity, the production of monoclonal immunoglobulins, production of autoantibodies, etc.

Several trials have concluded that certain immune function markers in the elderly are positively influenced when they are administered a dietary supplement with high doses of vitamin E (alpha-tocopherol, 800 mg/day), pyridoxin (50 mg/day), and beta-carotenes (15–60 mg/day); on the other hand, other micronutrients such as Zn (100–150 mg/day) had a negative effect on immunity.[32]

The enhancement in immunity brought about by vitamin E on the T lymphocytes may be based on an indirect effect on macrophages and not merely through its antioxidant properties. Activated macrophages secrete suppression factors such as hydrogen peroxide and E2 prostaglandins, which depress the proliferation of lymphocytes.[33]

Few clinical trials, however, have been carried out with beta-carotenes on the immune function in the elderly. In these studies, the authors have found a significant increase in the percentage of CD4 lymphocytes, natural killer cells, cells expressing interleukin-2 receptors, and transferrin receptors in subjects taking from 30 to 60 mg of beta-carotene daily when compared with placebo. No changes were observed in the total T lymphocytes or in CD8 lymphocytes. The beta-carotenes may act through an increase in the effects of cytochines and prostaglandins on natural immunity.[33]

V. DIETARY INTAKE OF ANTIOXIDANTS AND RECOMMENDATIONS FOR DAILY CONSUMPTION

The plasma levels of antioxidant vitamins are influenced by a series of factors such as diet (how food is prepared, content, and type of fat), homeostatic regulatory mechanisms, and other variables such as lifestyle or smoking. A well-balanced diet provides a suitable daily consumption of vitamins, which leads to optimal levels in plasma among healthy adults not subjected to oxidative stress.

The regular consumption of fresh fruit, particularly citrus fruits, ensures an adequate intake of vitamin C. At the same time, the consumption of carotenes through eating vegetables provides the necessary amount of beta-carotene. As for vitamin E, this is taken together with vegetable oils (olive oil, sunflower oil), cereals, and walnuts, and in margarines and mayonnaise sauce, and these should be preferred over oils from cartamo, rapeseed, soy, and grape as these have a lower vitamin E content.

Looking specifically at the elderly, it is necessary to take into account the physiological changes occurring at this age and possibly leading to an increase or reduction in the absorption of vitamins, as well as the frequent fact that they often have an unsuitable or insufficient food intake, all contributing to vitamin deficiency. As a result, the elderly should be encouraged to increase their consumption of fruit and vegetables in the diet due to the high levels of these foods in carotenoids, phenolic antioxidants, trace elements, vitamin B, and fibre.[34]

There is currently no official recommendation on the daily dose of antioxidants to be administered, perhaps because it is difficult to quantify the amount of FRs produced and, therefore, the amount of antioxidants required to neutralize them. The Recommended Dietary Allowances (RDAs) are available for vitamins in the elderly, but these recommendations have been changed in countries such as Germany, Canada, or France, which propose their own daily recommendations (Table 23.1).

Other authors such as Lachance have put forward recommendations for an appropriate intake of antioxidant vitamins in the diet: 145 mg vitamin C, 23 mg vitamin E, and 32 mg carotenes.[35] As you can see, these recommendations are equivalent to three times the RDAs established in 1989 (10th edition).

TABLE 23.1
Recommended Dietary Allowances in Different Countries

Vitamin	RDA	1991 UK	1991 Germany ENZ	1990 Canada RNI/ANR	1992 France ANC
Vitamin A (μg retinol)	800–1000	700	800–1000	800–1000	800
Vitamin E (mg)	8–10		12	6/7–5/7	12
Vitamin C (mg)	60	40	75	30/40	80

On the other hand, various clinical trials have been carried out to discover the effects of a suitable dietary intake of vitamins on the elderly. Johnson and Porter designed a randomized, double-blind, placebo-controlled clinical trial to determine the effects of low doses (<2 times the RDAs) of micronutrient supplements (zinc and selenium) and/or vitamins (vitamin C, alpha-tocopherol, and beta-carotenes) on the incidence of respiratory and urogenital infections in the elderly residents of nursing homes.[32] After a 2-year study, there was a considerable reduction in the number of infections in the elderly when supplementary trace elements are given but not when the supplements were low doses of vitamins.

Another descriptive study of 24 elderly hospitalized patients, carried out to assess the status of antioxidant vitamins through daily intake by determination of the associated biochemical indicators (levels of beta-carotenes, alpha-tocopherol, and vitamin C), concluded that the average intake of vitamin C (21 mg/day) and vitamin E (3.1 mg of alpha tocopherol) were below RDA levels.[36] More than 85% of the elderly patients studied had an intake that was two thirds lower than the RDAs for these vitamins and 50% of them had insufficient intake of vitamin A (800 µg of retinol equivalent per day).

Other studies with elderly patients have shown that a daily supplement of antioxidant vitamins has a beneficial effect on this age group. Thus, Wartanowicz et al.[37] indicated that vitamin C and E supplements produce a reduction in the concentrations of lipidic peroxides. Other authors have concluded that supplements of vitamin E and selenium improve general condition. For example, Tolonen et al.[38] indicated that the plasma concentrations of lipidic peroxides were initially higher in the elderly, but the values diminished down to control group levels (young volunteers) 3 months after beginning administration of dietary supplements with vitamins E, C, B$_6$, beta-carotenes, zinc, and selenium.

VI. BENEFITS OF ANTIOXIDANTS IN CERTAIN DISEASES

It is currently believed that FRs are involved in the development of a large number of degenerative processes and illnesses. In these cases, the administration of antioxidants (AO) is proposed to prevent or improve the progress of the disease. In this sense, some of the most recent and significant publications concerning these illnesses are reviewed below.

A. CARDIOVASCULAR DISEASE

Low-density lipoproteins (LDL) are clearly involved in arteriosclerotic processes. Polyunsaturated fatty acids, which are susceptible to lipidic peroxidation, may form FRs harming the endothelium and heart muscle cells, provoking the proliferation of smooth muscle, and reducing the mobility of tissue macrophages. When this occurs, the LDL (together with cholesterol and oxidized fatty acids) are phagocyted by the macrophages and phagocytes, thus initiating the process of formation of arteriosclerotic plaques. According to current scientific data, vitamin E reduces the susceptibility of LDL to oxidation.[39]

It has also been seen that, during myocardial ischemia and reperfusion, the GSH and the GSH/GSSG ratio are reduced in ischemic tissues, and the area of the myocardium damaged is inversely proportional to the GSH content of the heart muscle.[40] In patients with coronary artery disease undergoing cardiopulmonary bypass surgery, the levels of hydrogen peroxide did not increase significantly during or after this surgery in those patients receiving vitamin E before surgery.[41,42]

The clinical trials carried out (control case studies and cohort surveys) and the observational studies are based on the hypothesis that the dietary or supplementary antioxidants provide protection against conditions such as arteriosclerosis and coronary disease, but the conclusions of these studies do not allow the assumption of a causal link between the intake or serum levels of antioxidants and the onset of cardiovascular disease.

Since atherosclerotic disease develops throughout the life of the individual affected, it is important to review the papers published on the role of natural antioxidants in this disease, although the results are contradictory, particularly with regard to the benefits of vitamin C. The studies published in this field follow.

The World Health Organization's "Monica" Group carried out an epidemiological study[43] in 20 European populations regarding the risk factors involved in death through ischemic coronary disease. It was found that there was a direct correlation between the low serum levels of vitamins E and C and increased mortality. The mortality was inversely related to an increased intake of vegetables, and a low mortality risk was also significantly inversely related to high levels of vitamins C and E in plasma, but the same was not found with beta-carotenes.

Furthermore, with a population of 6000 inhabitants in Scotland, a case control study[44] was carried out to determine whether the plasma concentrations of antioxidant vitamins might be related to the risk of suffering angina. An inversely proportional relationship was found between the incidence of angina and the plasma concentrations of beta-carotenes and vitamins C and E. Nonetheless, the incidence is only significant for vitamin E. Hence, populations with a high incidence of coronary disease may be able to benefit from diets rich in vitamin E.

In 1993 and over 8 years [sic], the "Nurses Health Study" was carried out with a cohort of over 80,000 healthy American women, and a significant reduction of 13% was found in the risk of suffering coronary diseases among those women who regularly took preparations containing vitamin E[45] over 2 years. Although several doses were analyzed, only levels of 100 IU/day reduced the risk of suffering heart disease.

In that same year, a 4-year prospective study[46] was carried out with a group of 39,000 healthy volunteers from the nursing profession, aged between 40 and 75 years. The conclusion was that the intake of 100 IU/day of vitamin E during at least 2 years (regardless of the consumption of vitamins C and A) reduces the risk of cardiovascular disease by 17%.

With regard to vitamin C in this group of disorders, there are also several studies published. The results of Enstrom et al.[47] in a population of 11,000 men indicate that mortality due to cardiovascular disease or any other cause is inversely related to the intake of vitamin C. Knetk et al.[48] found that the consumption of vitamin C produces a significant reduction in the risk of death due to cardiovascular disease among women, but not among men. The reduction in the risk for women was 51% with doses above 90 mg/day and less with 60 mg/day. But the results of these surveys must be analyzed with caution, because they did not consider the intake of vitamin E.

The isolated influence of carotenes has been studied in a survey of a cohort of 1899 participants with type II hyperlipidemia included in the placebo group[49] of the Lipid Research Clinics Coronary Primary Prevention Trial, which explored the relationship between carotenoids in plasma and the risk of suffering cardiovascular disease. After adjusting the factors, an inverse relationship was identified between the serum concentrations of carotenoids and cardiovascular disease events. A greater carotenoid content in plasma was linked to a reduction of 36% in cardiovascular accidents.

Greenberg et al.[50] documented 285 cases of mortality in a cohort of 1700 men and women aged 60 years during a period of approximately 8 years. The people with initially higher plasma levels of beta-carotenes showed a drop of 48% in the risk of death from cardiovascular disease, as opposed to those presenting lower concentrations.

In 1986, working with a group of 34,486 post-menopausal women without cardiovascular disease, Kushi et al.[51] performed a survey to identify their eating habits (sources of vitamins A, E, and C). These subjects were followed up over 7 years, during which time 242 women died from cardiovascular disease. After adjusting the results for age, calorie intake, and other potential masking variables, the authors found an inverse relationship between the consumption of vitamin E and the risk of death by cardiovascular disease. Those women with a higher intake of this vitamin reduced their risk by 60%. This association was not found with the consumption of vitamins A and C .

The "Cambridge Heart Antioxidant Study," a controlled trial with 2002 patients with coronary disease (coronary arteriosclerosis),[52] was carried out to assess the impact of vitamin E on cardio-vascular disease. In this study, the patients were randomized to receive vitamin E (at doses of 800 IU/day or 400 IU/day) or placebo. The treatment with both doses of vitamin E significantly reduced the risk of myocardial infarction and cardiovascular incidents by 77% and 47%, respectively, depending on the dose. There was no reduction, however, in the number of deaths due to cardio-vascular disease. In the ATCB study of individuals with a prior history of myocardial infarction, this risk was reduced by 38% among those patients receiving alpha-tocopherol. Nonetheless, the risk of death from this pathology was not reduced.[53]

Other studies have related diminished concentrations of selenium in serum with an increased risk of cardiovascular disease. In several of these studies,[54,55] an association has been found between the plasma levels of selenium and the incidence of cardiovascular disorders and myocardial inf-arction. There is, however, some controversy about the role of selenium in this context, as other studies[43,56] have not established any clear connection between the levels of selenium in serum and the risk of suffering cardiovascular disease.

Finally, it must be pointed out that with regard to cardiovascular disease, the American Health Association recommends that the general population eat a balanced diet with special emphasis on fruit and whole green vegetables that are rich in antioxidants instead of a dietary supplement.[57]

B. PLATELET AGGREGATION

Platelet hyperaggregability is a significant factor in the progress of arteriosclerosis and other cardiovascular diseases.[58] There is evidence that vitamin E inhibits platelet aggregation and the production of prostaglandins *in vitro,* as it prevents the peroxidation of arachidonic acid, and may thus have a significant role at this level.[59] In this sense, the results of a study carried out into a group of healthy adults who were administered a daily supplement of 400 IU of vitamin E over 4 weeks finally conclude that there is a significant reduction in platelet adhesion.[60]

C. CANCER

Antioxidants are implicated in the development of certain types of cancer. In this way, vitamin E and other AO may act as anticancer agents by FR chelation.

Although numerous epidemiological studies have shown the protective effect of fruit and vegetables in different types of cancer such as cancer of the lung, esophagus, pancreas, and stomach as well as colorectal and bladder cancer, or cancer of the uterus, ovary, and endometrium, and breast cancer,[61] other studies carried out in different populations to whom antioxidant supplements were administered failed to find a lower incidence of this kind of pathology.[62-65]

Although there are only limited controlled trials in humans, the results of the epidemiological studies into the administration of vitamin E (on its own or in combination with other AO) indicate a lower incidence of certain types of cancer. vitamin E protects cellular DNA and prevents the development of cancer in the colon, breast, liver, and skin, whereas a deficiency in this vitamin causes alterations in the cell membrane, basically in reproductive cells and red globules.[5,58]

Greenberg et al.[66] administered β-carotenes (25 mg/d), ascorbic acid (1 g/d), α-tocopherol (400 mg/d), alone and in association, to patients with colorectal adenoma for 4 years and found that this treatment did not protect against recurrent colorectal adenoma among those patients in whom a tumor had been excised before admission to the study.

The concomitant administration of 50 μg of Se, 15 mg/d of beta-carotene and 30 mg/d of alpha-tocopherol reduced cancer mortality by 9% in a study of a Chinese population with a high risk of suffering from cancer of the stomach and esophagus.[67]

With regard to skin cancer, the population exposed to high levels of UV radiation is known to show an increase in the incidence of all kinds of melanoma. This incidence may be reduced through the administration of vitamin E.

Finally, it should be pointed out that the use of AO also seems appropriate as an adjuvant therapy in patients undergoing chemotherapy treatment. In this sense, in a randomized, double-blind placebo-controlled study, Wadleigh et al.[68] assessed the efficacy of the topical application of 1 ml of an oil-based vitamin E solution at a concentration of 400 mg/ml twice daily over 5 days vs. a placebo in the treatment of mucositis in cancer patients who were being given chemotherapy, and this group of researchers found that a statistically significant number of ulcers were cured in the group with vitamin E.

D. Degenerative Diseases

1. Arthritis

Fairburn et al.,[69] found that the levels of tocopherol were normal in patients with rheumatoid arthritis, but the concentration in synovial fluid was severely depleted. In connection with this finding, some authors have found that vitamin E therapy is effective in the alleviation of the pain and in improving the mobility of patients with osteoarthritis.[70,71] Blankenhorn carried out a double-blind study of patients with this condition and showed that vitamin E not only improves their pain and mobility but also reduces the need to administer analgesic and the morbidity rate.[71] For Smidt and Bayer,[72] vitamin E is as effective as diclofenac in the treatment of ankylosing spondylitis.

2. Cataracts

The photooxidative mechanisms and the formation of FRs are important factors to consider in the development of this pathology, leading to sight problems and eventually blindness in elderly patients.[73] In this respect, it has been put forward that it might produce oxidation of the proteins in the lens and that vitamins C and E and the carotenoids may play a significant role in the protection against cataracts and macular degeneration.

Robertson et al.[74] carried out an epidemiological study to ascertain the effect of an antioxidant vitamin supplement on the risk of cataracts among adults over the age of 55 years and concluded that it is reduced with a daily supplement of vitamin E, C, or a combination of both. In addition, other authors found that vitamin C supplements over 10 years or longer reduce the opacity of lenses by 80%.[75]

Seddon et al.[76] examined 350 people aged between 55 and 80 years and suffering from a disease diagnosed during the first year of inclusion in the study. The control group comprised 520 individuals with another ocular affection. An association was found between the high consumption of carotenoids and the low risk of macular degeneration.

3. Tardive Dyskinesia

This degenerative neurological illness has a higher incidence among persons over the age of 65 years. In various studies, the administration of vitamin E has been put forward for this condition. Lohr and Calguiuri[77] collated results founded in the literature, and of the 12 studies carried out before 1996, nine of them showed that the administration of vitamin E produced some improvement in the condition (mainly in those cases, slight to moderate), with no benefit being apparent in the others.

4. Alzheimer's Disease

Alzheimer's is a progressive neurological disease characterized by a degeneration of the neurones and cognitive deterioration. Various studies have suggested that lipidic peroxidation is one of the main causes of the membrane dysfunction and subsequent cell death in Alzheimer's cases. A post mortem analysis of Alzheimer's patients showed they had significantly lower levels of phospholipids and cholesterol in the cell membrane of the white matter and other brain tissues and an even greater proportion in the frontal cortex. It is also known that the brain is particularly vulnerable to the formation of FRs due to its high oxygen demands even though it has a low concentration of antioxidant enzymes.[78]

Several hypotheses have been proposed regarding which FRs have an effect on this condition. In this sense, it seems that iron, ferritin, mercury, and copper would lead to lipidic peroxidation. It is also believed that the catabolism of dopamine is a source generating FRs, and for this reason those areas with high concentrations of catecholamines are very susceptible to oxidative destruction. Catecholamines can auto-oxidize to free radical forms or increase the formation of hydrogen peroxide through the action of monoamine-oxidases.[78]

It has also been proposed that glutamate may be toxic for nerve cells, as the stimulation of its receptors leads to neuronal death through the increased production of hydrogen peroxide.[78] Other mechanisms may also be responsible for the pathogenesis of Alzheimer's disease but, in any case, the generation of free radicals may increase the advance of this condition.

On the other hand, the prevention of the disease through antioxidants has not been widely studied in the elderly population, so it is necessary to clarify many aspects of the safety and efficacy of these products in this disease

For all these reasons, clinical trials have been carried out with AO in this pathology. Sano et al.[79] carried out a multi-center, randomized, double-blind, placebo-controlled study including 341 patients with moderate Alzheimer's disease. For 2 years, vitamin E (2000 IU/day) on its own, selegiline (10 mg/day) on its own, both together, or placebo were administered to these subjects. It is an accepted fact that selegeline may act as an antioxidant by reducing the oxidative deamination and the resulting neuronal toxicity. The authors concluded that the drugs studied, either on their own or in combination, delayed the functional deterioration of the neurones. With the combination of both substances, they achieved lower benefits (either through interaction between molecules or through action of different mechanisms). They propose the preferential use of vitamin E over selegiline due to the interactions associated with the latter.

5. Parkinson's Disease

The generation of FRs has been hypothesized as an important factor in the development of this pathology, with consideration of vitamins C and E in its treatment.

The "Deprenyl and Tocopherol Antioxidative Therapy of Parkinsonism Study"[80] assessed the administration of vitamin E and selegiline in these patients, concluding that there was no delay in the progress of the condition through the administration of tocopherol.

Other authors[81] considered the combination of high doses of vitamin E (3200 IU/day) and vitamin C (3000 mg/day) in patients with Parkinsonism, concluding that the antioxidant treatment reduced the need for treatment with levodopa more than 2.5 years.

REFERENCES

1. Ambrosio G, Abete P, Rengo F, Chiariello M. Oxigen free radicals and cardiac aging. *Cardio Elderly* 1993;1(6):531-535.
2. Kiriazys M. Free radicals and aging. *Care Elderly* 1994; 6 (7):260-262.
3. Stähelin HB. The impact of antioxidants on chronic disease in aging and in old age. *Int J Vitam Nutr Res* 1999;69 (3):146-149.
4. Grimble RF. The maintenance of antioxidant defenses during inflammation. In DW Wilmore and Carpentier YA, Eds., *Metabolic support of the Critically Ill Patient*. Springer-Verlag, Berlin, 1993.
5. Cortés Saavedra MP, Fernandez Bernardo E, Cárdenas Díaz AM. Antioxidantes y especies activas del oxígeno: importancia biológica y clínica. *Farmacoterapia* 1990;7;246-253.
6. Deby C, Hartstein G, Deby-Dupont G, Lamy M. Antioxidant therapy. Bion J, Bouchardi H, Dellinger RP, Dobb GJ, Eds. *Currents Topics in Intensive Care*, Vol. 2, W.B. Saunders, London, 1995, pp. 175-205.
7. Bendich A. Antioxidant nutrients and inmune functions — introduction. *Advances Exper Med Biol* 1990;262:1-12.

8. Beckman KB, Ames BN. The free radical theory of aging matures. *Physiol Rev* 1998;78 (2):547-581.

9. Chanock SJ, BJ, Smith R, Babior BM. The respiratory burst oxidase. *J Biol Chem* 1994;269:24519-24522.

10. Moslen MT. Reactive oxygen species in normal physiology, cell injury and phagocytosis. *Adv Exp Med Biol* 1994;336:17-27.

11. Robinson JM, Badwey JA. Production of active oxygen species by phagocytic leukocytes. *Immunol Ser* 1994;60:159-178.

12. Marnett LJ, Hurd HK, Hollstein MC, Kevin DE, Esterbauer H, Ames BN. Naturally ocurring carbonyl compounds are mutagens in Salmonella tester strain TA104. *Mutat Res* 1985;148:25-34

13. Cao G and Cutler RG. Protein oxidation and aging. II. Difficulties in measuring alkaline protease activity in tissues using the fluorescamine procedures. *Arch Biochem Biophys* 1995;320:195-201.

14. Szweda LI, Uchida K, Tsai L, Stadtman ER. Inactivation of glucose-6-phosphate dehydrogenase by 4-hydroxy-2-nonenal. Selective modification of an active-site lysine. *J Biol Chem* 1993;268:3342-3347.

15. Eddleston JM, Braganza JM. Antioxidants. The pivotal key to the management of protease-linked acute pancreatitis. In: Mutz NJ, Koller W, Benzer H, Eds. *7th European Congress on Intensive Care Medicine.* Bologna (Italy). Monduzzi Eds.1994:41-46

16. Packer L. Interactions among antioxidants in health and disease: vitamin E and redox cycle. P.S.E.B.M. 1992;200:271-276.

17 Meuers DG, Maloley PA, Weeks D. Safety of antioxidant vitamins. *Arch Intern Med* 1996;156:925-935.

18. Traber MG. Vitamin E in humans: demand and delivery. *Annu Rev Nutr* 1996;16:321-347.

19. De Juana P, Bermejo T. Vitaminas y oligoelementos en nutrición parenteral. In: S Celaya Perez, Ed. *Tratado de Nutricion Artificial.* Tomo I. Ed Aula Médica. Pag 261-279.

20. Odeh RM, Cornish LA. Natural antioxidants for the prevention of atherosclerosis. *Pharmacotherapy* 1995;15 (5):648-659.

21. Meydani SN, Meydani, Blumer J, Leka L, Pedrosa M, Diamond R. Assessment of the safety of supplementation with different amounts of vitamin E in healthy older adults. *Am J Clin Nutr* 1998;68:311-318.

22. Paloza P, Moualla S and Krinsky N. Effects off b-carotene and a-tocopherol on radical initiated peroxidaion of microsomes. Free Radical Biol Med 1992;13:127-136.

23. Borek C. Antioxidants and cancer. *Sci Med* 1997:52-61.

24. Hercberg S, Galan P, Preziosi P, Alfarez MJ, and Vazquez C. The potential role of antioxidant vitamins in preventing cardiovascular diseases and cancers. *Nutrition* 1998;14:513-520.

25. Herbert V. Viewpoint does mega-c do more good than harm, or more harm than good? *Nutr Today* 1993:28-32.

26. McMichael AJ. Kidney stone hospitalization in relation to changes in vitamin C consumption in Australia 1966-1976. *Commun Health Stud* 1978;2: 9-13.

27. Roth DA. Vitamin C and oxalate stones. *JAMA* 1977;237:2080.

28. Bendich A, Cohen M. Ascorbic acid safety analysis of factors affecting iron absorption. *Toxicol Lett* 1990;51:189-201.

29. Lomaestro BM, Malone M. Glutathione in health and disease pharmacotherapeutic issues. *Ann Pharmacother* 1995;29:1263-1273.

30. Julius M, Lang CA, Gleiberman L, Harburg E, Difranceso W, Schork A. Glutathione and morbidity in a community-based sample of elderly. *J Clin Epidemiol* 1994-;47:1021-1026.

31. SL Nuttall, U Martin, AJ Sinclair, MJ Kendall. Glutathione: in sickness and in health. *Lancet* 1998;352:645-646 (letters).

32. Johnson MA, Porter KH. Micronutrient supplementation and infection in institutionalized elders. *Nutr Rev* 55:400-404.

33. Meydani SN, Wu D, Santos MS, Hayek M. Antioxidants and inmune response in aged persons: overview of present evidence. *Am J Clin Nutr* 1995;62 (suppl):1462S-1476S.

34. Biesalki HK, Böhles H, Esterbauer H, Fürst P, Gey F Hundsdörfer G, Kasper H, Sies H, Weisburger J. Antioxidant vitamins in prevention. *Clin Nutr* 1997;16:151-155.

35. Lachance PA. Future vitamin and oxidant RDAs for health promotion. *Preventive Med* 1996;25:46-47.

36. Schmuck A, Ravel A, Coudray C, Alary J, Franco A, Roussel AM. Antioxidant vitamins in hospitalized elderly patients: analysed dietary intakes and biochemical status. *Eur J Clin Nutr* 1996;50:473-478.

37. Wartanowicz M, Panczenko-Kresowska B, Ziemlanski S, et al. The effect of alpha tocopherol and ascorbic acid on the serum lipid peroxide level in elderly people. *Ann Nutr Metab* 1984;28:186-191.

38. Tolonen M, Sarna S, Halme M, et al. Antioxidant supplementation decreases TBA reactants in serum of elderly. *Biol Trace Element Res* 1988;17:221-228.

39. (Diaz MN, Balz F, Vita JA, Keaney JF. Antioxidants and atherosclerotic heart disease. *New Eng J Med* 1997;337:408-414.

40. Singh A. Lee KJ, Lee CY, Goldfarb RD, Tsan MF. Relation between myocardial glutathione content and extent of ischemia-reperfusion injury. *Circulation* 1989;80:1975-1804.

41. Cavarocchi NC, England MD, O'Brien JF, et al. Superoxide generation during cardiopulmonary bypass: is there a role for vitamin E? *J Surg Res* 1986;40:519-527.

42. Hodis HN, Mack WJ, LaBree L, et al. Serial coronary angiographic evidence that antioxidant vitamin intake reduces progression of coronary artery atherosclerosis. *JAMA* 1995;273 (23):1849-1854.

43. Gey KF, Puska P, Jordan P, Moser UK. Inverse correlation between plasma vitamin E and mortality from ischemic heart disease in cross-cultural epidemiology. *Am J Clin Nutr* 1991;53:1-9.

44. Riemersma RA, Wood DA, Macintyre CCA, Elton RA, Gey KF, Liver MF. Risk of angina pectoris and plasma concentration of vitamins A, C, and E and carotene. *Lancet* 1991;337:1-5.

45. Stampfer MJ, Hennekens CH, Manson JE, et al. Vitamin E consumption and the risk of coronary disease in women. *New Engl J Med* 1993;328:1444-1449

46. Rimm EB, Stampfer MJ, Ascherio A, et al. Vitamin E consumption and the risk of coronary heart disease in men. *New Engl J Med* 1993;328:1450-1456.

47. Enstrom JE, Kanim LE, Klein MA. Vitamin C intake and mortality among a sample of the United States population study. *Epidemiology* 1994;3:194-202.

48. Knetk P, Reunanen A, Jarvinen R, Seppanen R, Heliovaara M, Aromaa A. Antioxidant vitamin intake and coronary mortality in a longitudinal population study. *Am J Epidemiol* 1994;139:1180-1190.

49. Morris DL, Kritchevsky SB, Dave CE. Serum carotenoids and coronary heart disease: The Lipid Research Clinics Coronary Primary Preventions trial and follow-up study. *JAMA* 1994; 272:1439-1441.

50. Greenberg ER, Baron JA, Karagas MR, Stukel TA, Nierenberg DW, Stevens NM, et al. Mortality associated with low plasma concentrations of beta carotene and the effect of oral supplementation. *JAMA* 1996;275:699-703

51. Kushi LH, Folsom AR, Prineas RJ, Mink PJ, Wu Y, Bostick RM. Dietary antioxidant vitamins and death from coronary heart disease in postmenopausal women. *New Engl J Med* 1996;334:1156-1162.

52. Stephens NG, Parsons A. Schofield PM et al. Randomized controlled trial of vitamin E in patients with coronary disease: Cambridge Heart Antioxidant Study (CHAOS). *Lancet* 1996;347:781

53. The Alpha-Tocopherol Beta Carotene Cancer Prevention Study Group. The effect of vitamin E and beta-carotene on the incidence of lung cancer and other cancers in male smokers, *New Engl J Med* 1994;330:1029-1035.

54. Wang YX, Bocker K, Reuter H et al. Selenium and myocardial infarction: glutathione peroxidase in platelets. *Klin Wochenschr* 1981;59:817-818.

55. Salonen JT, Salonem R, Lappetelainen R, Maenpaa PH, Alftham G, Pusica P. Risk of cancer in relation to serum concentration of selenium and vitamins A and E: matched case-control analysis of prospective data. *BMJ* 1985;290:417-420.

56. Salonen JT, Salonen R, Penttilae R et al. Serum fatty acids, apolipoproteins, selenium and vitamin antioxidants and the risk of death from coronary artery disease. *Am J Cardiol* 1985;56:226-231.

57. Krauss RM, Deckelbaum RJ, Ernst N, Fisher E, Howard BV, Knopp RH, et al. Dietary guidelines for healthy American adults: a statement for health professionals from the Nutrition Committee, American Heart Association. *Circulation* 1996;94:1795-1800.

58. Packer L. Protective role of vitamin E in biological systems. *Am J Clin Nutr* 1991;53:1050 S-1055 S.

59. Szczekllik A, Gryglewski RJ, Domagala B, et al. Dietary supplementation with vitamin E in hyper-lipoproteinemias: effects on plasma lipid peroxides, antioxidants activity, prostacyclin generation and platelet aggregability. *Thromb Haemost* 1985;54:425-430.

60. Jandak J, Steiner M, Richardson PD, et al. Reduction of plateled adhesiveness by vitamin E supplementation in humans. *Thromb Haemost* 1988;49:393-404.

61. Block G, Patterson B, Subar A. Fruit, vegetables, and cancer prevention: a review of the epidemiological evidence. *Nutr Cancer* 1992;18:1.

62. Omenn GS, Goodman GE, Thornquist MD, Blames J, Cullen MR, Glass A, et al. Effects of a combination of beta carotene and vitamin A on lung cancer and cardiovasuclar disease. *New Engl J Med* 1996;334:1150-155.

63. Hennekens CH, Buring JE, Manson J, Stampfer M, Rosner B, Cook NR, et al. Lack of effect of long term supplementation with beta carotene on the incidence of malignant neoplasms and cardiovascular disease. *New Engl J Med* 1996;334:1145-1149.

64. Willett WC, Polk BF, Underwood BA, et al. Relation of serum vitamins A and E and carotenoids to the risk of cancer. *New Engl J Med* 1984;310:430-434.

65. Nomura AMY, Stemmermann GN, Heilbrun LK, et al. Serum vitamin levels and the risk of cancer specific sites in men of Japanese ancestry in Hawaii. *Cancer Res* 1985;45:2369-2372.

66. Greenberg ER, Baron JA, Tosteson TD, et al. A clinical trial of antioxidant vitamins to prevent colorectal adenoma. *New Engl J Med* 1994;331(3):141-147.

67. Blot WJ, Li J-Y, Taylor PR, Guo W, Dawsey S, Qang G-Q, et al. Nutrition intervention trials in linxian, china:supplementation with specific vitamin/mineral combinations, cancer incidence, and disease-specific mortality in the general population. *JNCI* 1993;85:1483-1492.

68. Wadleigh RG, Redman RS, Graham ML, Krasnow SH, Anderson A, Cohen MHs. Vitamin E in the treatment of chemotherapy-induced mucositis. *Am J Med* 1992;92:481-484.

69. Fairburn K, Grootveld M, Ward RS, et al. A-tocopherol, lipids and lipoproteins in knee joint synovial fluid and serum from patients with inflammatory joint disease. *Clin Sci* 1992;83:657-664.

70. Machtey I, Ouaknine L. Tocopherol in osteoarthritis: a controlled pilot study. *J Am Geriatr Soc* 1978;26:328-330.

71. Blankenhorn G. Clinical efficacy of spondyvit (vitamin E) in activated arthroses. A multicenter, placebo-controlled, double-blind study. *Z Orthop* 1986;124:340-343.

72. Smidt KH, Bayer W. Efficacy of vitamin E as a drug in inflammatory joint disease. *Adv Exp Med Biol* 1990;264:147-150.

73. Jacques PF, Chylack LT, McGandy RB, Hartz SC. Antioxidant status in persons with and without cataracts. *Arch Opththalmol* 1988;106:337-340.

74. Robertson J, Donner AP, Trevithick JR. Vitamin E intake and risk of cataracts in humans.*Ann NY Acad Sci* 1989;570:372-382.

75. Jacques PF, Taylor A, Hankinson SE, et al. Long-term vitamin C supplement use and prevalence of early age-related lens opacities. *Am J Clin Nutr* 1997;66:911-916.

76. Seddon JM, Ajani U, Sperduto RD, Hiller R, Blair N, Burton TC, et al. Dietary carotenoids, vitamins A, C, and E, and advance age-related macular degeneration. *JAMA* 1994;272:1413-1420.

77. Lohr JN, Caligiuri MP. A double-blind placebo controlled study of vitamin E treatment of tardive dyskinesia. *J Clin Psychiatry* 1996;57:167-173

78. Pitchumoni S, Murali P. Current status of antioxidant therapy for Alzheimer's disease. *J Am Geriatric* 1998;46:1566-1572.

79. Sano M, Ernesto C, Thomas RG, Klauber MR, Schafer K, Grundman M, et al. Controlled trial of selegiline, alpha tocopherol, or both as treatment for Alzheimer's disease. *New Engl J Med* 1997;336:1216-1222.

80. Parkinson Study Group. Effects of tocopherol and deprenyl on the progression of disability in early Parkinson's disease. *New Engl J Med* 1993;328:176-183.

81. Fahn S. A pilot trial of high-dose alpha-tocopherol and ascorbate in early Parkinson's disease. *Ann Neurol* 1992;32 (suppl):S128-132.

82. Recommended dietary allowances for elderly in USA, UK, Germany, Canada and France. Appendix I. Facts and Research in Gerontology 1994 (Supplement: Nutrition).

Index